Byung-Ho Choi, Seung-Mi Jeong, Jihun Kim, Wilfried Engelke

Flapless Implantology

Flapless Implantology

Byung-Ho Choi, DDS, MS, PhD
Seung-Mi Jeong, DDS, PhD
Jihun Kim, DDS, MS
Wilfried Engelke, DDS, MD, PhD

QUINTESSENCE PUBLISHING

London, Berlin, Chicago, Tokyo, Barcelona, Beijing, Istanbul, Milan,
Moscow, New Delhi, Paris, Prague, São Paulo, Seoul and Warsaw

Translation of Flapless Implantology, 1st edition:
by Byung-Ho Choi

British Library Cataloguing in Publication Data
Flapless implantology.
1. Dental implants. 2. Flaps (Surgery)
I. Choi, Byung-Ho.
612.6'93-dc22

ISBN: 9781850971955

Quintessence Publishing Co. Ltd,
Grafton Road, New Malden, Surrey KT3 3AB,
Great Britain
www.quintpub.co.uk

Editing: Quintessence Publishing Co. Ltd, London
Layout and Production: Jens Girke and Ina Steinbrück, Quintessenz Verlags-GmbH, Berlin

Printed and bound in Germany by Hofmann Druck, Nuremberg, Germany

Preface

Flapless implant surgery is thought by many to be a procedure with many limitations, including the inability to save the keratinized mucosa because a tissue punch removes some of this tissue; a lack of proper drilling depth assessment as it is difficult to see lines on the drill at the bone crest; an inability to assess the location of the implant because there is no direct visualization of the bone; and an inability to correct peri-implant defects as they are not exposed during surgery. As a result, guidelines on the flapless procedure were that it should be used only when the bone has abundant width and when the soft tissue has sufficient amounts of keratinized mucosa. Based on these guidelines, there are few cases in which the flapless procedure can be applied.

There are two ways to view flapless implant surgery, either as having possibilities or as possessing limitations. This book shows how to overcome the limitations and how to take advantage of its extraordinary benefits. Flapless implant surgery has numerous advantages, including the preservation of circulation, soft tissue architecture, and hard tissue volume at the site, decreased surgical time, improved patient comfort, and accelerated recuperation. This book shows definitive outcomes and scientific proof of the efficacy of flapless implant surgery as well as the best techniques necessary to obtain its greatest benefits. It also addresses the application of flapless implant surgery to a variety of clinical situations and includes specific techniques for the management of challenging cases. A final chapter focuses on flapless implant surgery for specific implant systems.

Practical information is provided for the reader who wishes to learn flapless implant surgery. We sincerely hope it will serve as a useful fund of knowledge as well as a guide for those who are interested in flapless implant surgery. Finally, I would like to thank Quintessence Publishing for recognizing the value of flapless implant surgery and the need for a book on its clinical applications.

Authors

Byung-Ho Choi, DDS, MS, PhD
Professor
Department of Oral and Maxillofacial Surgery
College of Dentistry, Wonju College of Medicine
Yonsei University, Korea

Jihun Kim, DDS, MS
Lecturer
Department of Dentistry
Wonju College of Medicine
Yonsei University, Korea

Seung-Mi Jeong, DDS, PhD
Professor
Department of Prosthodontics
Wonju College of Medicine
Yonsei University, Korea

Wilfried Engelke, DDS, MD, PhD
Professor
Department of Oral Surgery
School of Dentistry
Georg-August-University, Göttingen, Germany

Contents

CHAPTER

1

Comparison of Flap and Flapless Implant Surgeries

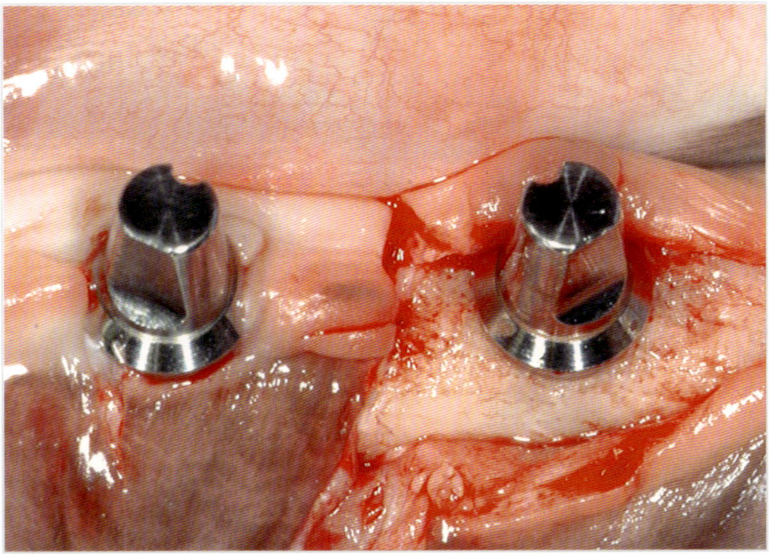

Key point

Flap elevation on the alveolar crest can have a butterfly effect in implant treatment.

Overview

A minor incident that produces a drastic result is called the "butterfly effect." It describes the possibility that "something as small as the flutter of a butterfly's wing can ultimately cause a typhoon halfway around the world." In implant treatment, the gingival incision can have a subsequent large-scale effect that is similar to the butterfly effect. The flap implant procedure is a method of implant placement in which the mucoperiosteum is elevated to expose the underlying bone after making an incision in the gingiva of the alveolar crest; implant placement is performed, and then the flap is sutured back in place (Fig 1-1). In contrast, the flapless implant procedure does not reflect the crestal soft tissue. Instead, a core of gingival tissue (the size of the implant diameter) over the crestal bone is removed, or a crestal mini-incision and local undermining (the range of the implant diameter) are performed at the implant site. Implant osteotomy is then performed at the center of the core of the exposed bone (Fig 1-2). This chapter addresses the effect of such a small difference between flap and flapless implant surgery on the healing of peri-implant tissues.

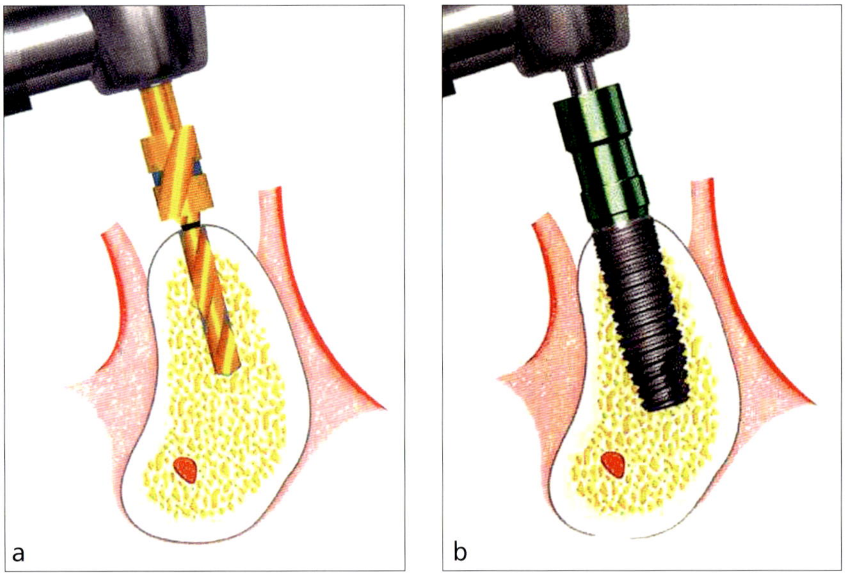

Fig 1-1 (a and b) The flap implant procedure is a method of implant placement in which the mucoperiosteum is elevated to expose the underlying bone after an incision in the gingiva of the alveolar crest.

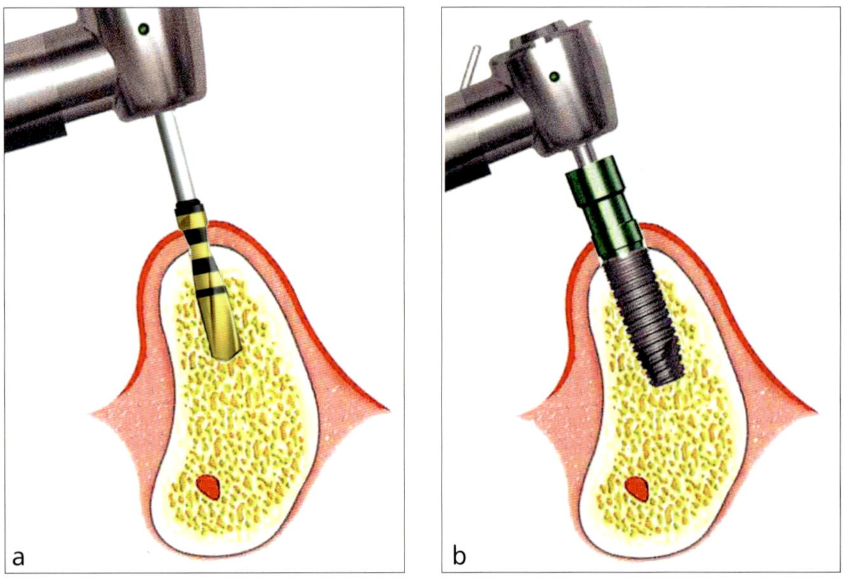

Fig 1-2 (a and b) The flapless implant procedure is a method that does not reflect the crestal soft tissue. Instead, a core of gingival tissue (the size of the implant diameter) is removed over the crestal bone.

Effect on healing of peri-implant mucosa

Incision line opening is the most common postoperative complication of flap implant surgery.[1] In other words, after surgery, the sutured area opens where the reflected soft tissues are approximated and sutured (Fig 1-3). The opening of the sutured area aggravates and lengthens the inflammatory phase of repair, leaving an extensive scar (Fig 1-4). Opening of the incision line does not occur in flapless implant surgery as it does not require sutures. Moreover, the peri-implant mucosa has small, clean, closed wounds after a flapless procedure. This may improve the ability of the peri-implant mucosa to heal quickly with little scar formation (Fig 1-5). Scar tissue is vulnerable in terms of defense (Fig 1-6). The level of tissue injury influences the speed and quality of the healing process.[2-4]

Effect on thickness of peri-implant mucosa

When implants are placed with flap elevation, the mucosa around the implants thickens after surgery (Fig 1-7). According to Cardaropoli et al.,[5] the thickening of the adjacent mucosa eases over time. However, after one year, the adjacent mucosa had thickened by approximately 1 mm and maintained this thickness. When implants were placed without flap elevation, the adjacent mucosa thickened by approximately 0.7 mm as a result of postoperative edema formed immediately after the surgery. Three months later, the adjacent mucosa resolved to the original level and then maintained its level (Figs 1-8 and 1-9). After flap implant surgery, the increase in mucosal thickness spreads towards the bone, resulting in bone loss (Figs 1-10 and 1-11). The flapless procedure is quite advantageous in terms of maintaining the original form and thickness of the mucosa surrounding the implants.

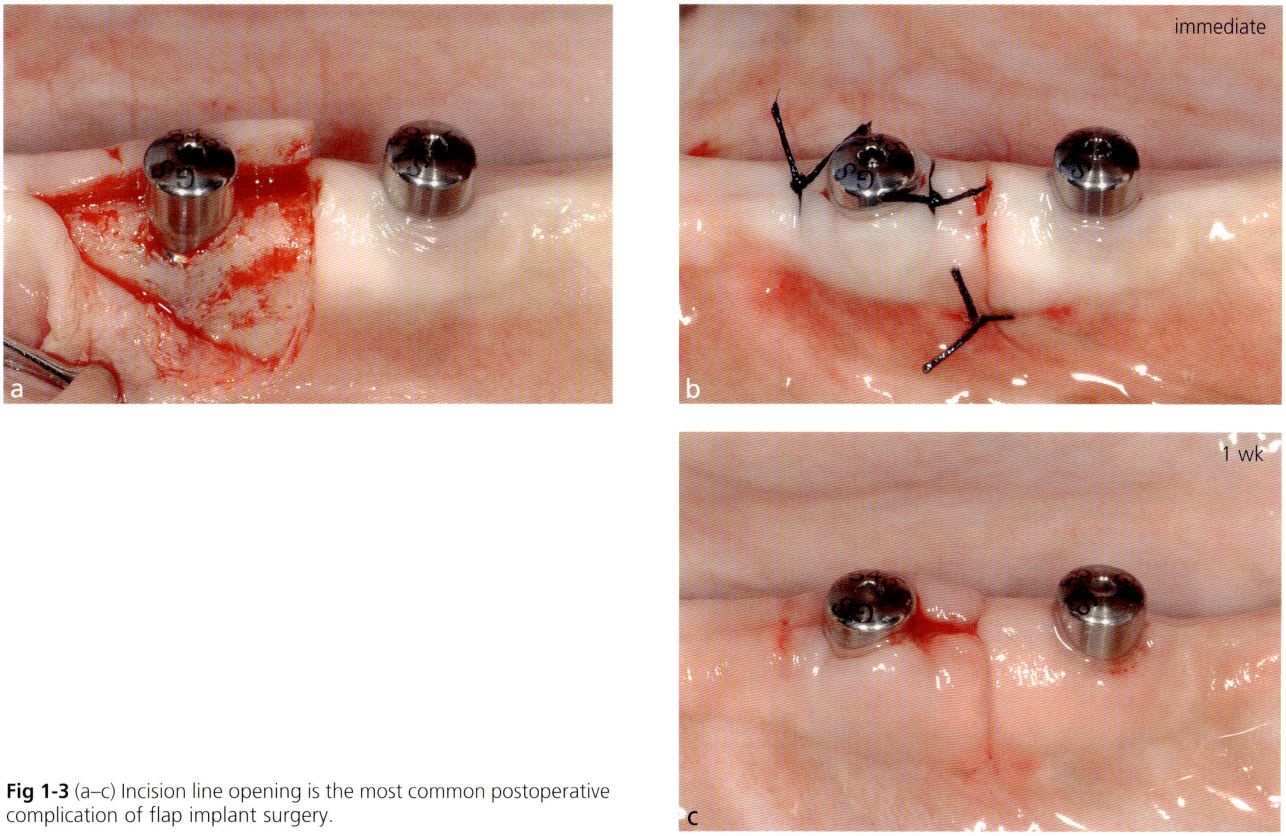

Fig 1-3 (a–c) Incision line opening is the most common postoperative complication of flap implant surgery.

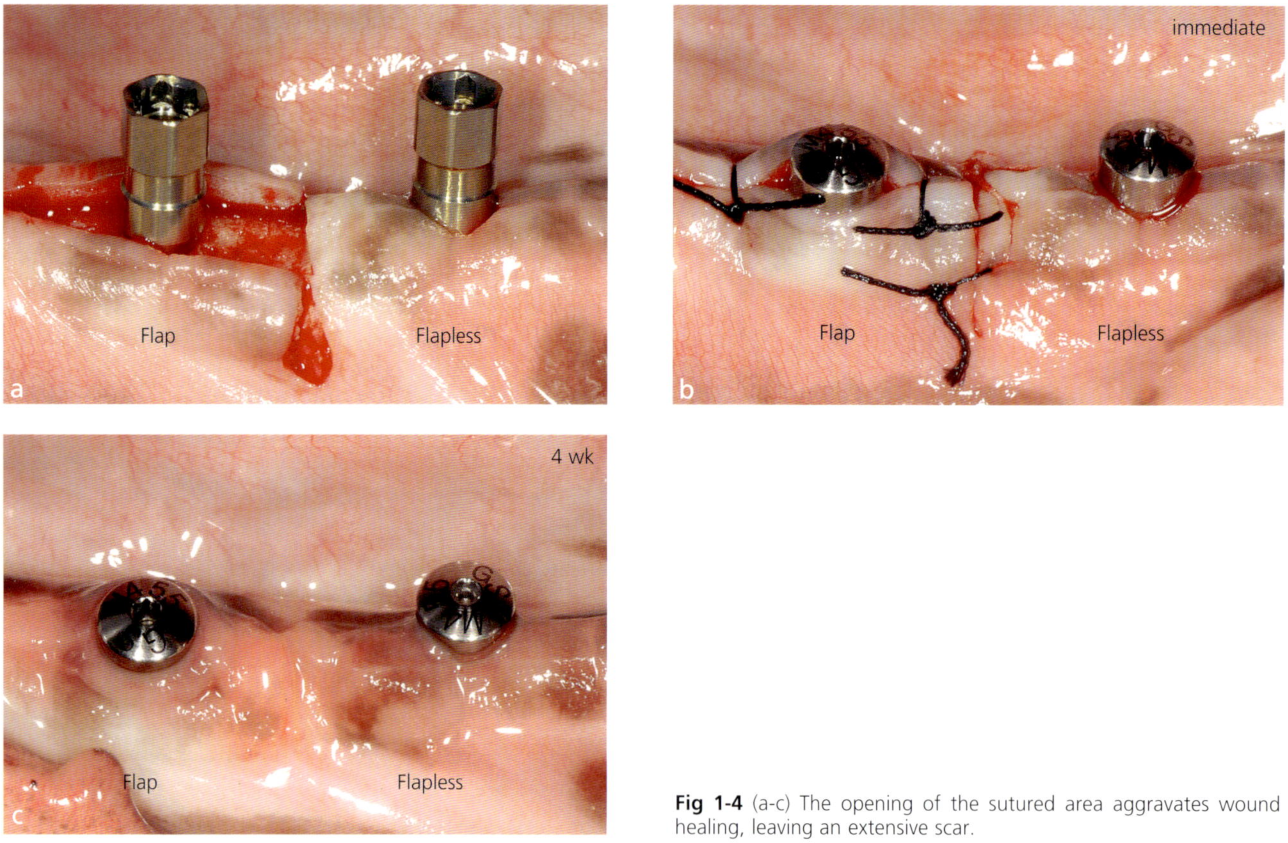

Fig 1-4 (a-c) The opening of the sutured area aggravates wound healing, leaving an extensive scar.

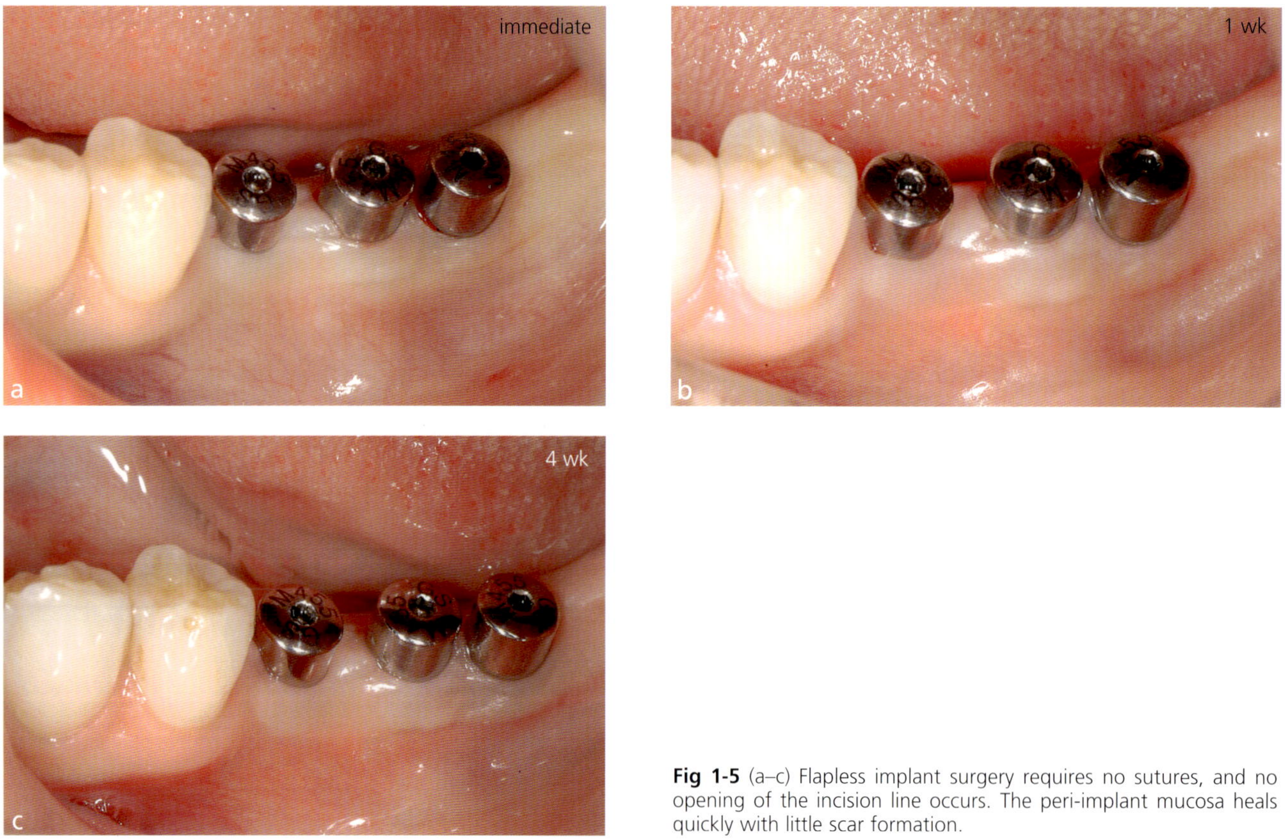

Fig 1-5 (a–c) Flapless implant surgery requires no sutures, and no opening of the incision line occurs. The peri-implant mucosa heals quickly with little scar formation.

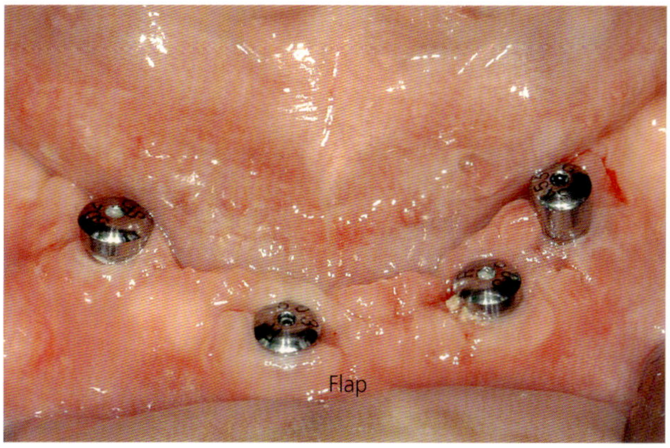

Fig 1-6 Intraoral view after the flap implant procedure. The peri-implant mucosa heals with extensive scar formation.

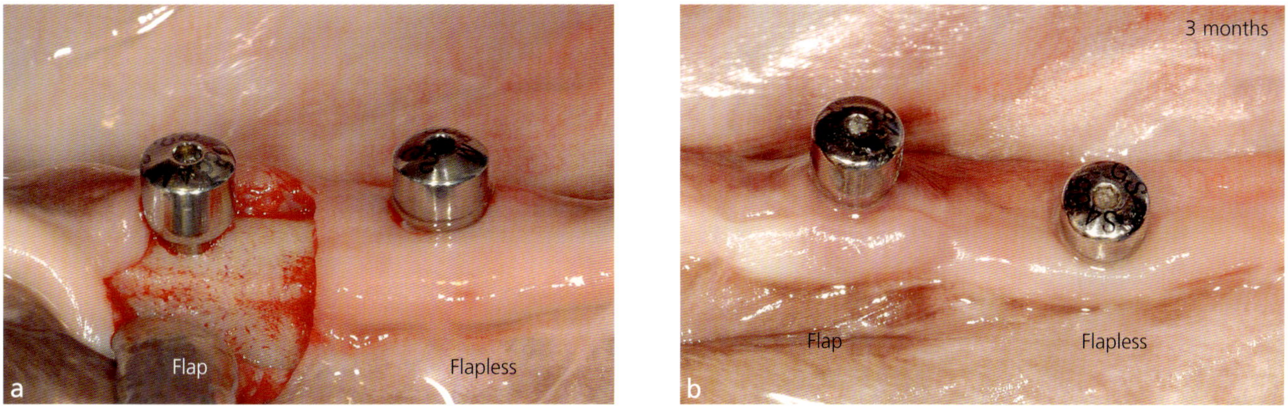

Fig 1-7 (a and b) When implants are placed with flap elevation, the mucosa around the implants thickens after surgery.

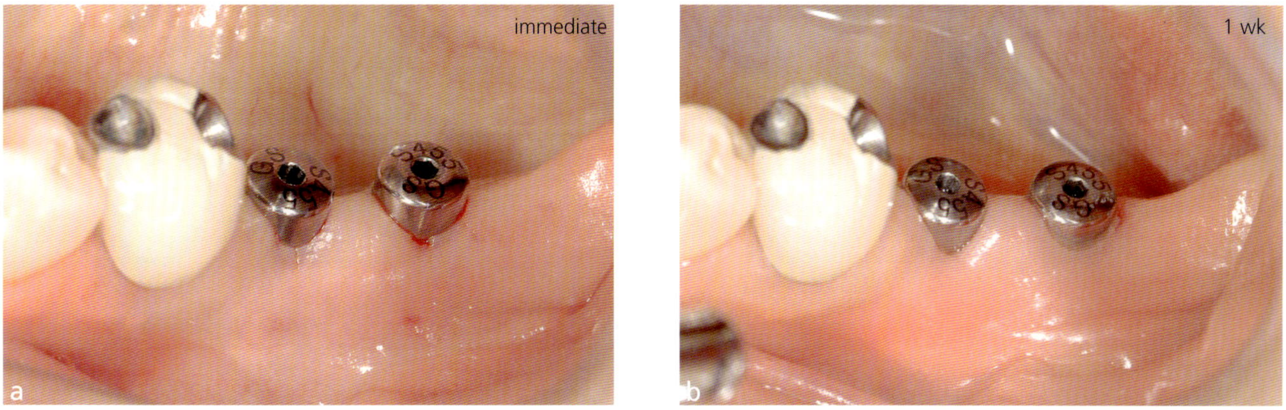

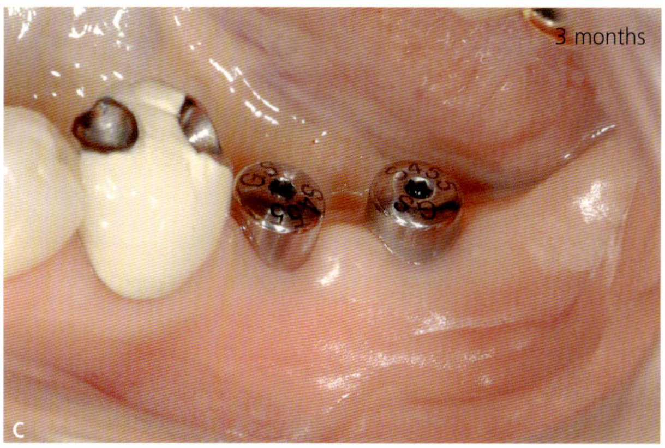

Fig 1-8 (a–c) When implants are placed without flap elevation, the adjacent mucosa thickens as a result of postoperative edema immediately after surgery. The adjacent mucosa thickness reduces to almost the original thickness 3 months later.

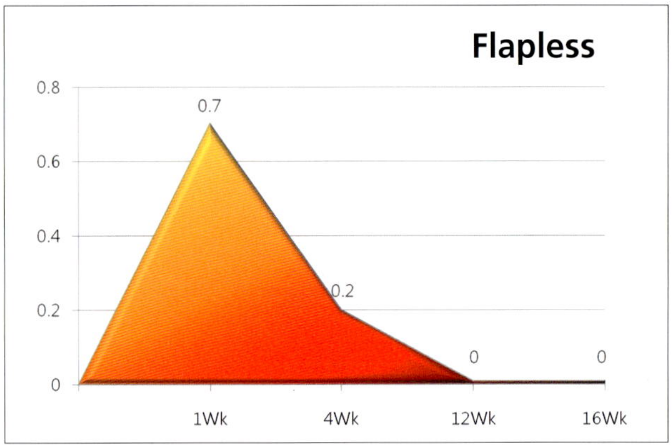

Fig 1-9 When implants are placed without flap elevation, the adjacent mucosa thickens by approximately 0.7 mm owing to postoperative edema immediately after the surgery. Three months later, the adjacent mucosa resolves to the original level and then maintains its level.

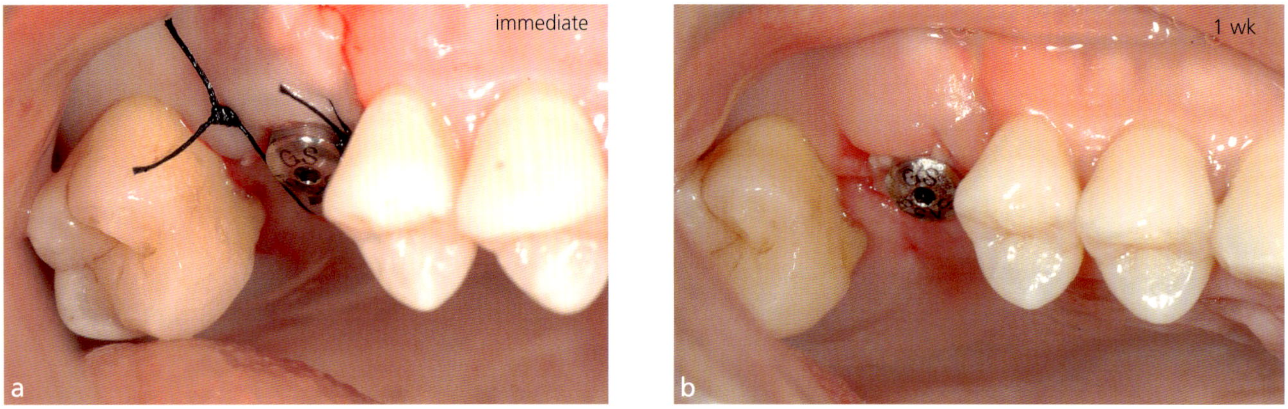

Fig 1-10 (a and b) Intraoral view of the peri-implant mucosa after the flap implant procedure.

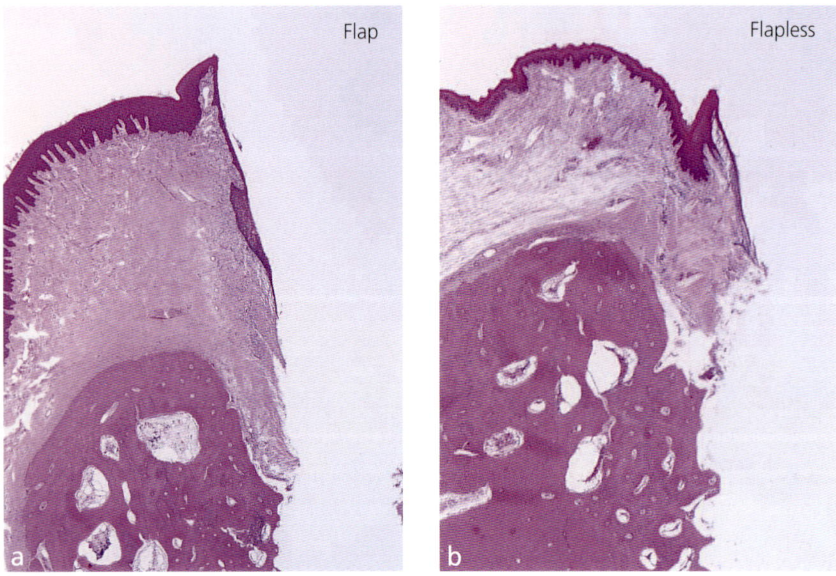

Fig 1-11 (a and b) After flap implant surgery, an increase in mucosal thickness results in bone loss.

Effect on sulcus depth around the implant

A comparison of the flap and flapless procedures showed that the sulcus depth was significantly deeper in the implants placed using the flap procedure than in those placed using the flapless procedure. Approximately three months after implant placement, the average pocket probing depths for the flap and flapless procedures were 1.7 mm and 1.0 mm, respectively (Fig 1-12). Flapless implant surgery is quite advantageous in terms of reducing the sulcus depth around the implants.

The effectiveness of hygiene decreases with increasing sulcus depth.[6] Therefore, the sulcus depth should be reduced in order to enable the patients to perform effective daily hygiene. Maintaining a good environment for the health of the tissue adjacent to the implant will ensure the success of the implant.

Effect on morphogenesis of peri-implant mucosa

For flap implants, the implant–mucosa barrier comprises the junctional epithelium that is approximately 2 mm in length, and a connective tissue compartment that is approximately 1–1.5 mm high.[7,8] When implants were placed without flap elevation, the lengths of the junctional epithelium and the zone of connective tissue integration were approximately 1.2 mm and 1.0 mm, respectively,[9] indicating that the junctional epithelium extends more apically in flap implants than in flapless implants (Figs 1-13 and 1-14). The more apically positioned junctional epithelium is related directly to an increased sulcus depth around the implant, which provides an environment that is more conducive to peri-implantitis.

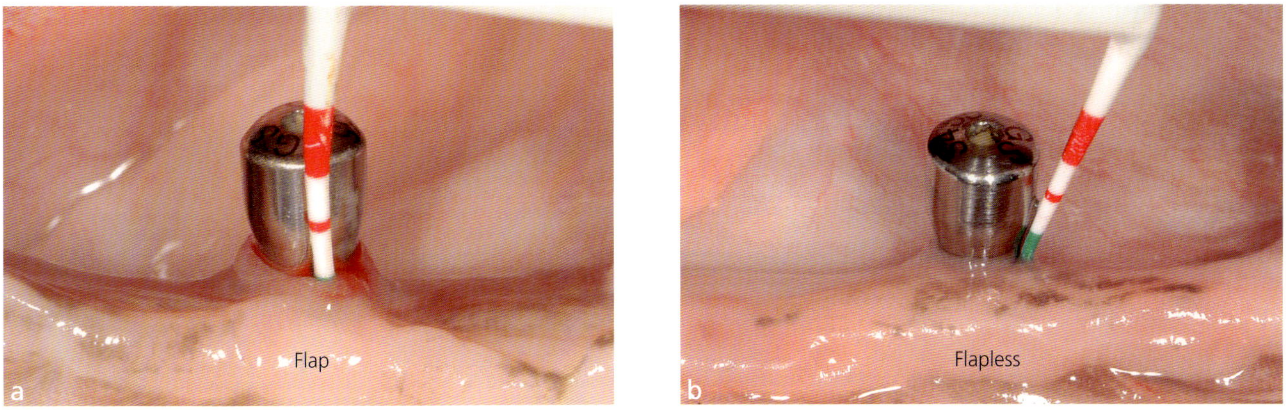

Fig 1-12 (a and b) The sulcus depth is deeper in implants placed with the flap procedure than in implants placed with the flapless procedure.

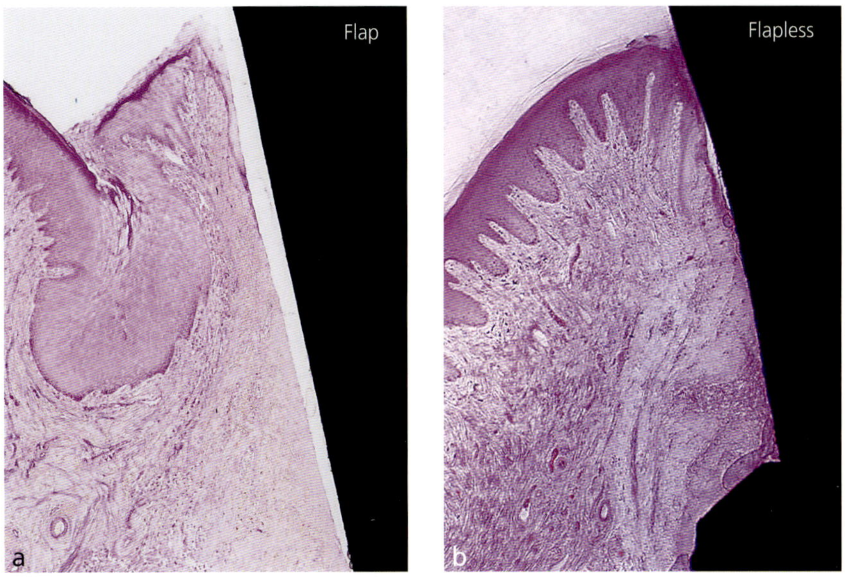

Fig 1-13 (a and b) The junctional epithelium extends more apically in flap implants than in flapless implants. The more apically positioned junctional epithelium is related directly to an increased sulcus depth around the implant.

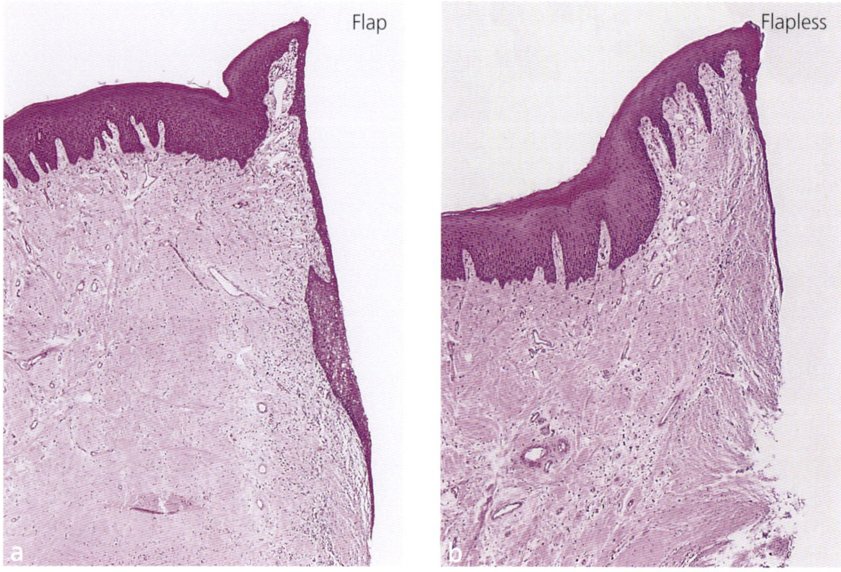

Fig 1-14 (a and b) The junctional epithelium extends more apically in flap implants than in flapless implants.

Effect on blood vessels of peri-implant mucosa

For flap implants, the connective tissue surrounding the implants heals with extensive scar formation and a scarcity of blood vessels.[10,11] However, for flapless implants, such tissue heals with little scar formation and an increase in the distribution of blood vessels (Fig 1-15),[12] which will improve the healing and defensive ability.

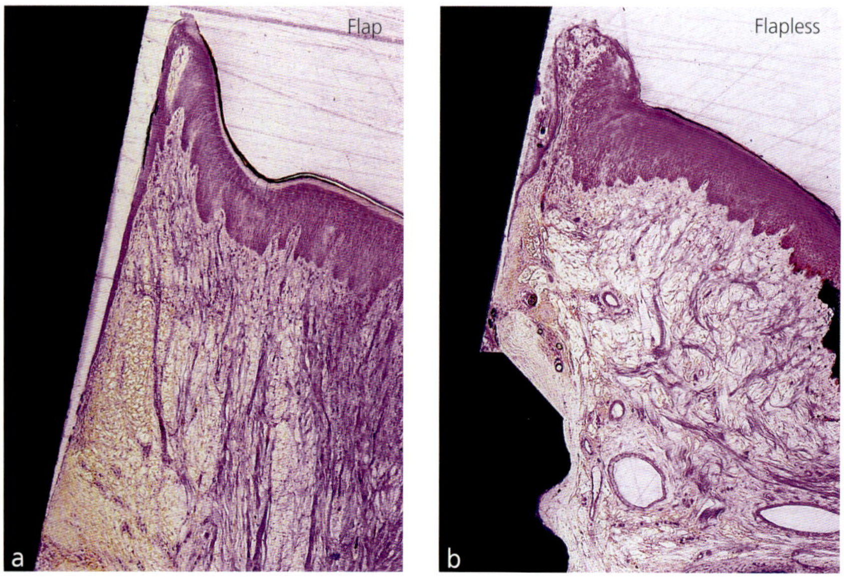

Fig 1-15 (a and b) With flap implants, the connective tissue surrounding the implants heals with extensive scar formation with few of blood vessels. With flapless implants, the tissue heals with little scar formation with an increase in distributed blood vessels.

Effect on inflammation resistance of peri-implant mucosa

An animal experiment was carried out to determine the effect of flapless implant surgery on the inflammation resistance of the peri-implant mucosa using a canine mandible model. The gingival index, probing pocket depth, and bleeding on probing were evaluated 3 months after the flap and flapless implant procedures. The flapless implant placement had lower values of all of these measurements compared with the flap implant placement (Fig 1-16).[9] This suggests that the flapless implant method is more effective in developing inflammation resistance in the soft tissue surrounding the implants. The soft tissue adjacent to the implant contained more blood vessels after flapless surgery, which might have strengthened its resistance to inflammation.

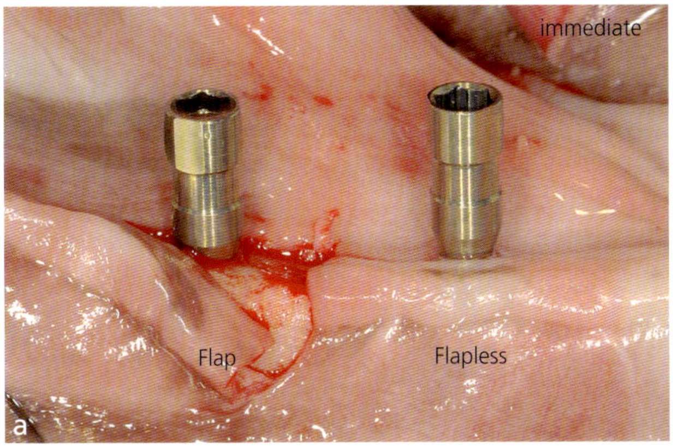

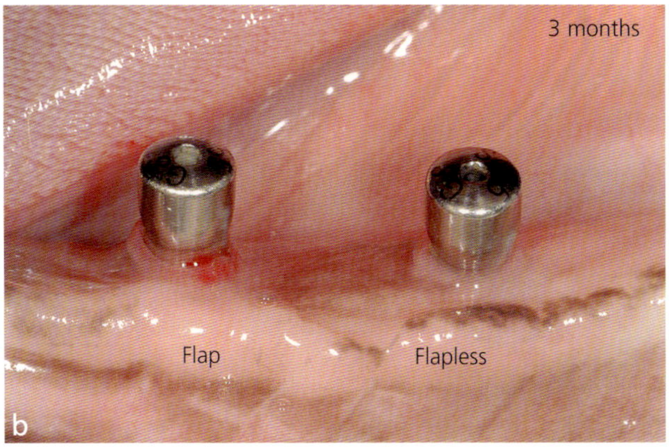

Fig 1-16 (a and b) Flapless implant placement has lower gingival indices and less bleeding on probing compared with flap implant placement.

Effect on peri-implant bone loss

It was reported that most crestal bone loss occurs in the early phase (3–4 months) after implant placement.[13,14] Significantly higher rates of crestal bone resorption occur during this period than in any other post-loading periods. A comparison of the flap and flapless procedures revealed higher crestal bone loss in the implants placed with the flap procedure during the early postsurgical period (Figs 1-17 to 1-20).[15] The mean crestal bone loss was approximately 1 mm more in the implants placed with the flap procedure than in the implants placed with the flapless procedure (Table 1-1). The authors obtained a similar result in both the animal experiments and clinical study (Figs 1-21 to 1-23).[16]

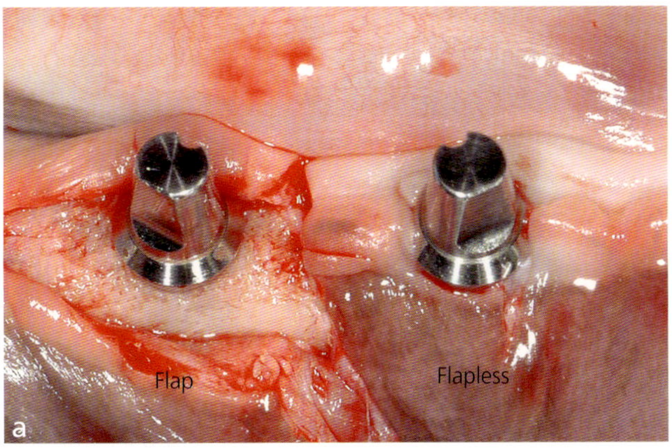

Fig 1-17 The effect of flap and flapless surgery on the peri-implant bone loss was compared using a canine mandible model.

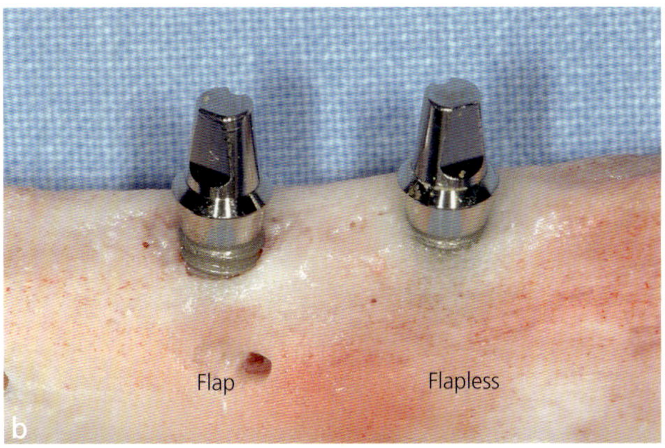

Fig 1-18 There was more crestal bone loss during the 3-month postsurgical period in implants placed with the flap procedure.

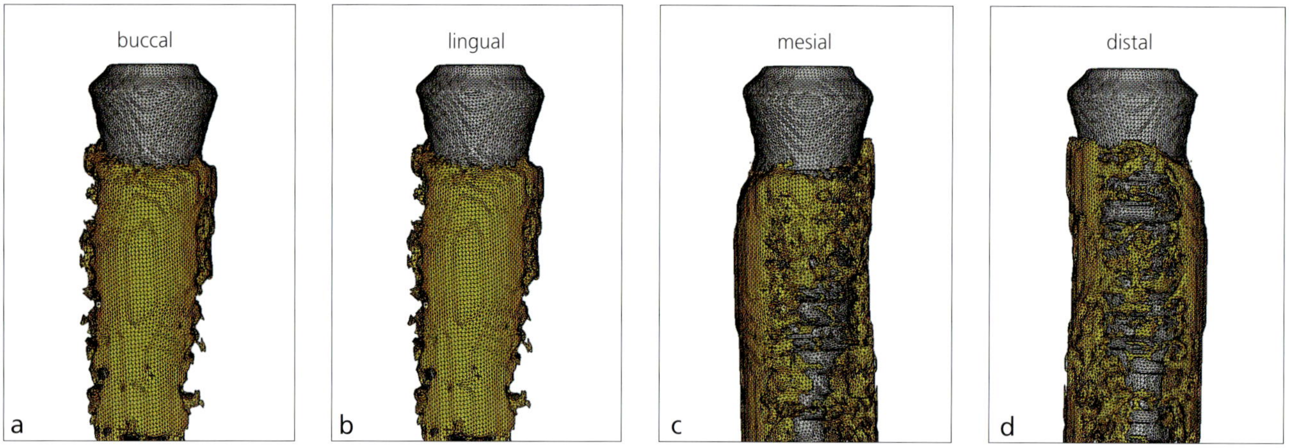

Fig 1-19 (a–d) Three-dimensional micro-CT showing the bone (yellow) around implants (gray) placed without a flap. Buccal = buccal side of the alveolus; lingual = lingual side of the alveolus.

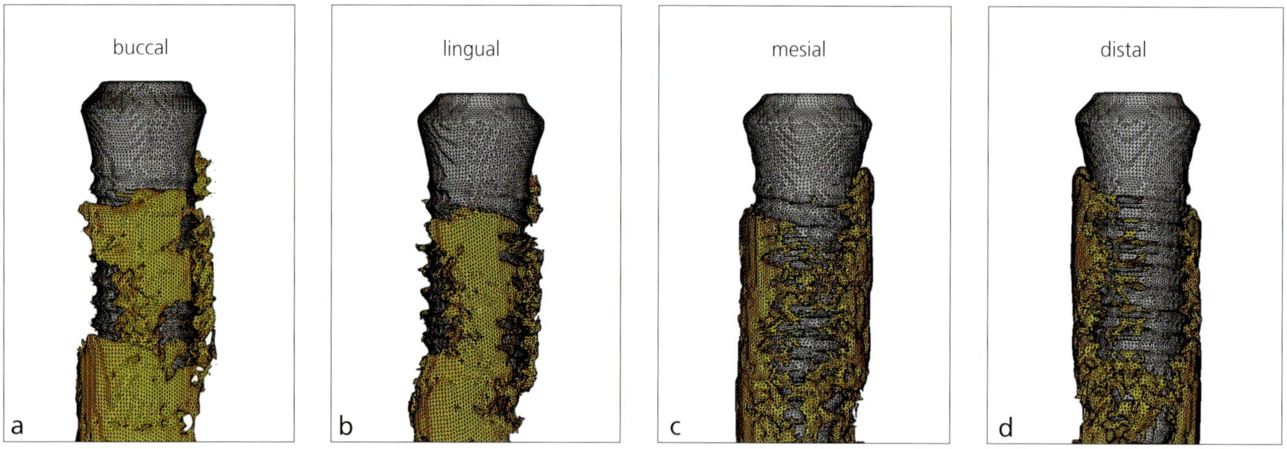

Fig 1-20 (a–d) Three-dimensional micro-CT showing the bone (yellow) around implants (gray) placed with a flap. Buccal = buccal side of the alveolus; lingual = lingual side of the alveolus.

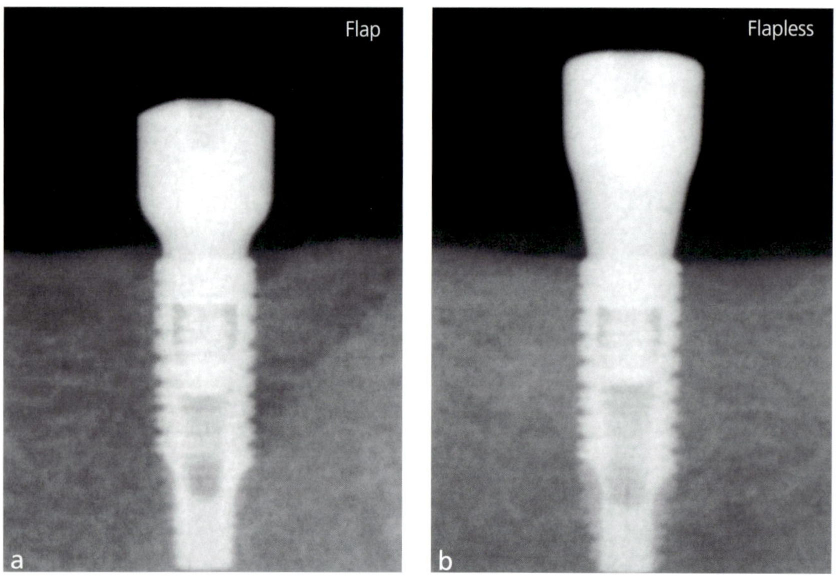

Fig 1-21 (a and b) Radiographs taken 3 months after implant placement. Note the marginal bone resorption at the flap implant site and no bone resorption at the flapless implant site.

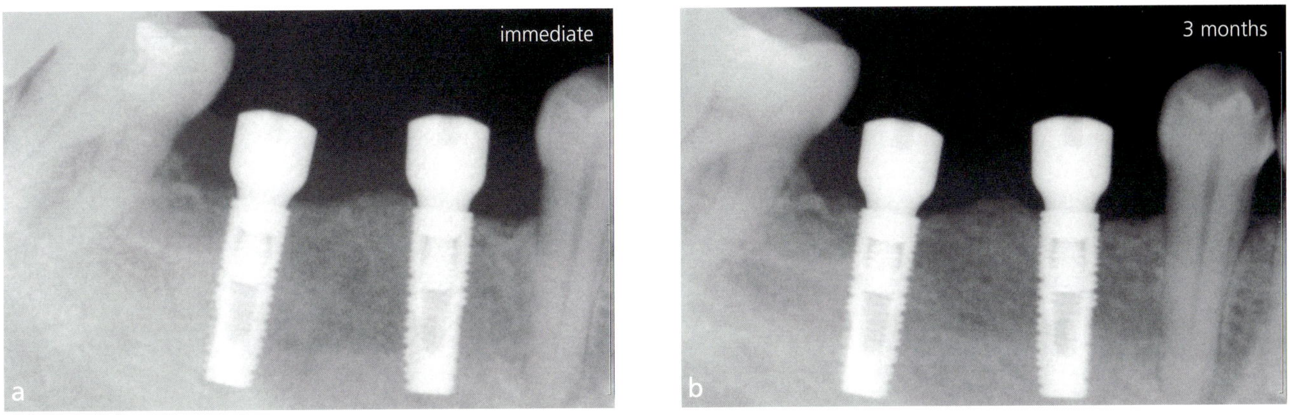

Fig 1-22 (a and b) Radiographs taken immediately and 3 months after the flapless procedure.

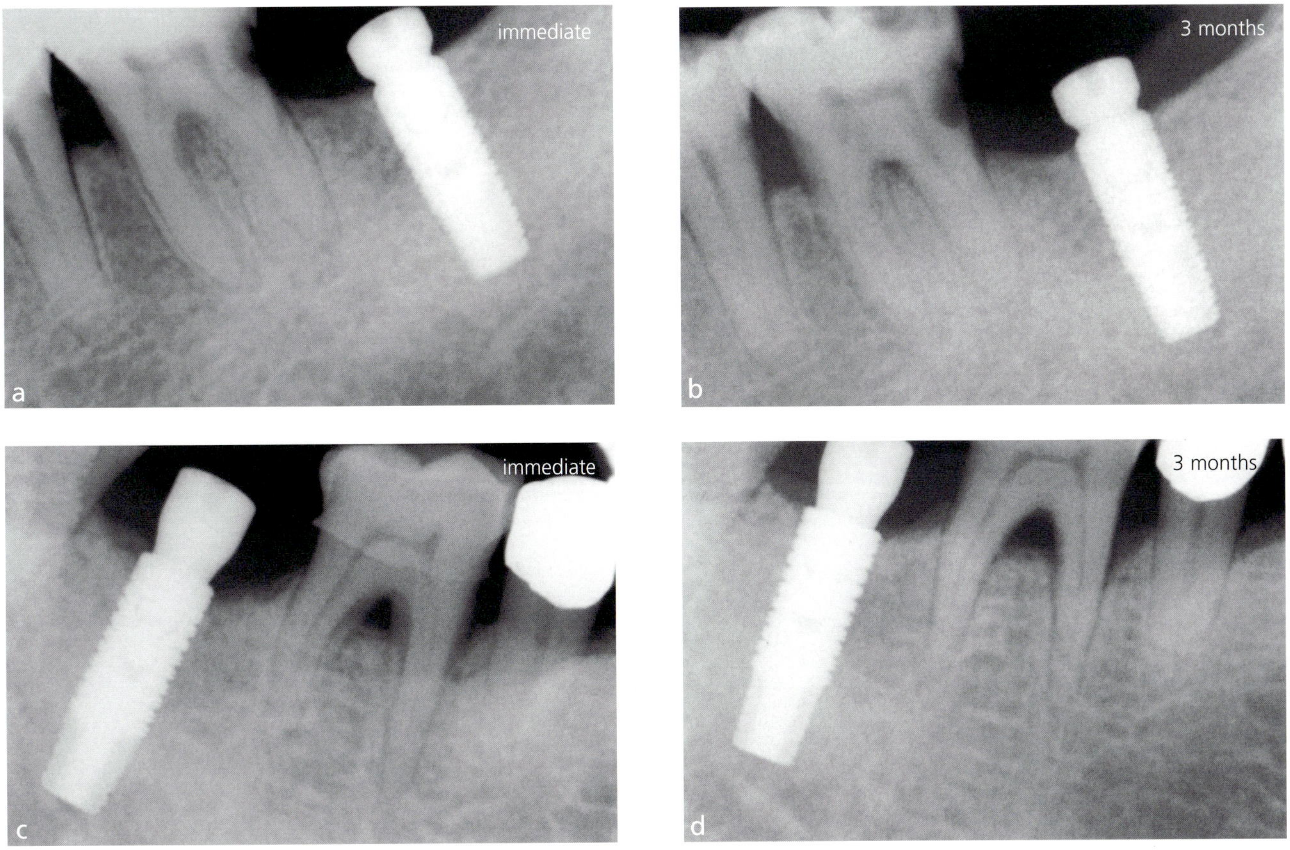

Fig 1-23 (a–d) Radiographs taken immediately and 3 months after the flapless procedure.

Effect on osseointegration of implants

Implant stability is closely related to the bone–implant contact area. This means that the stability of implant anchorage increases with increasing osseointegration rate. A comparison of the flap and flapless procedures showed more osseointegration at the flapless sites than at the flap sites. Therefore, flapless implant surgery improves the osseointegration of dental implants after surgery (Figs 1-24 and 1-25; see Table 1-1).[15,16] The enhanced osseointegration of dental implants resulting from flapless implant surgery improves the implant stability.

Effect on bone density adjacent to the implant

The effect of flap and flapless surgery on bone density in the region adjacent to the implant was compared using a canine mandible model. The bone density was approximately 10% higher around the implants placed using the flapless procedure than those placed using the flap procedure. In particular, the largest difference in bone density between the two procedures occurred in the area where the buccal periosteum was elevated. This suggests that flapless implant surgery plays a key role in enhancing bone density adjacent to the implant (Figs 1-26 and 1-27; see Table 1-1).

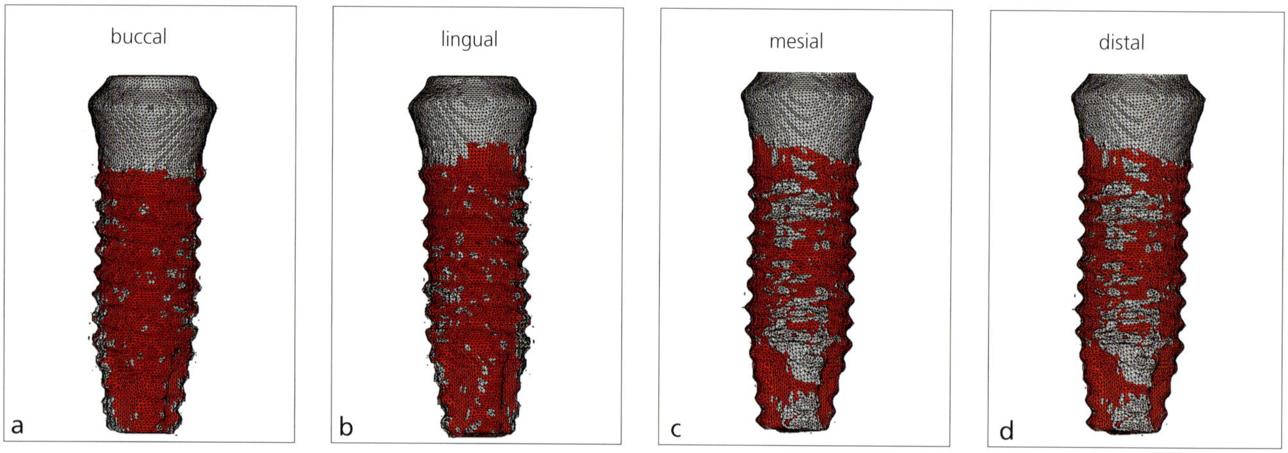

Fig 1-24 (a–d) Three-dimensional micro-CT overview of the bone-to-implant contact area (red) around the implant (gray) placed without a flap.

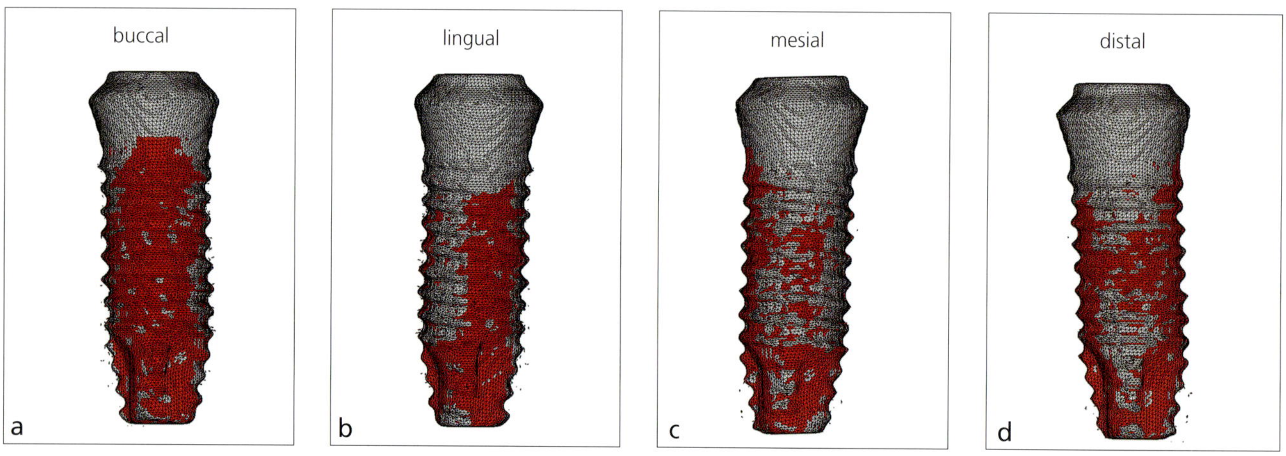

Fig 1-25 (a–d) Three-dimensional micro-CT overview of the bone-to-implant contact area (red) around the implant (gray) placed with a flap.

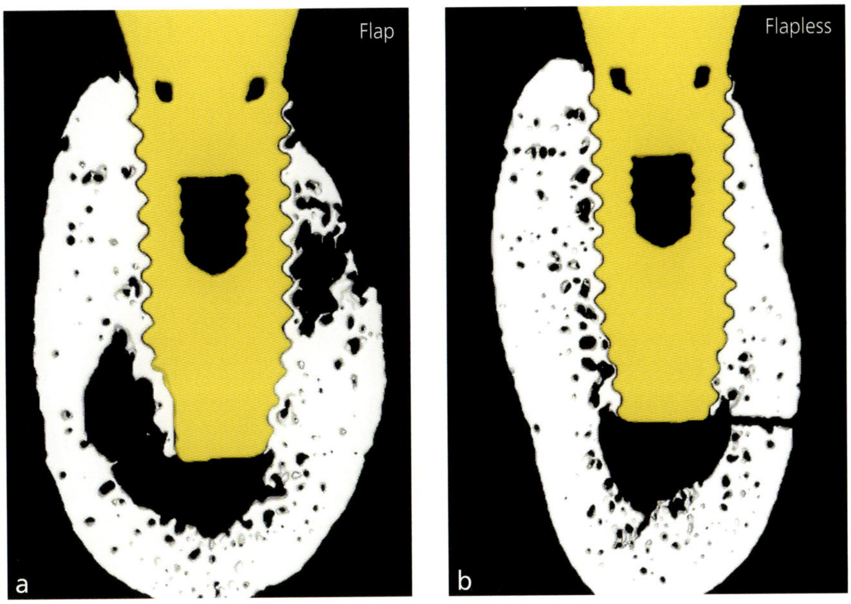

Fig 1-26 (a and b) The bone density is higher around the implants placed using the flapless procedure than those placed using the flap procedure.

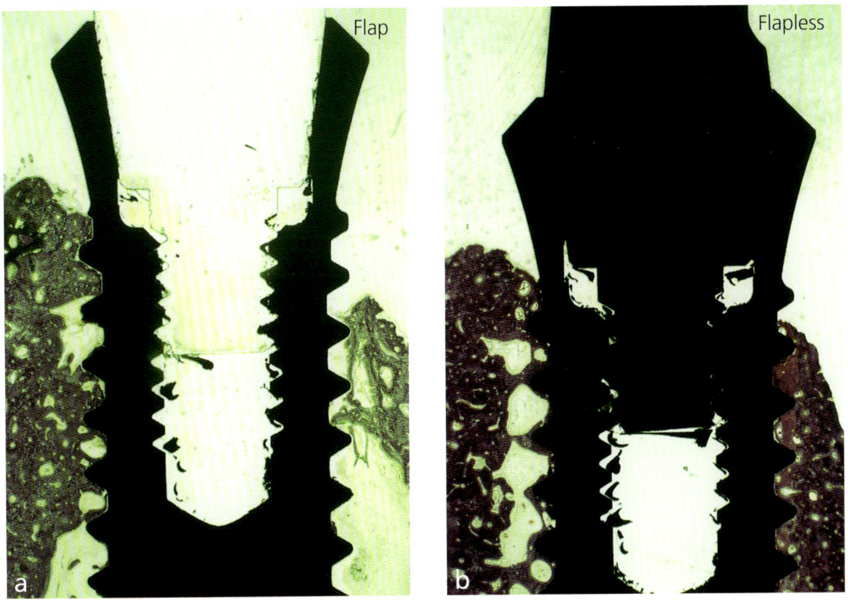

Fig 1-27 (a and b) View of the specimens showing the bone density around the implants placed using either the flap or the flapless procedures.

Table 1-1 Parameters (mean values and standard deviation) of bone height, bone-to-implant contact, and bone density around dental implants when placed either without or with a flap.

	Flapless group	Flap group	*P* value
Bone height (mm)	10.1 ± 0.5	9.0 ± 0.7	< .05
Bone-to-implant contact (%)	70.4 ± 6.3	59.5 ± 6.3	< .05
Bone density (%)	65.1 ± 7.5	55.0 ± 6.7	< .05

Effect on implant stability

The effects of flap and flapless surgery on implant stability were compared using a canine mandible model. Implants stabilized more quickly without flap elevation than with flap elevation. For flapless implants, the increase of stability occurred after two weeks, without a period of decreasing stability. However, for flap implants, a shift in implant stability from decreasing stability to increasing stability occurred after two weeks (Fig 1-28). This suggests that flapless implant surgery plays a crucial role in enhancing implant stability.

Effect on early plaque control

Early plaque control plays an important role in healing the tissue surrounding the implant. Cleaning the implants immediately after flap implant surgery may be quite difficult because a long sutured wound in the incision area is vulnerable to mechanical irritation. For these reasons, the patients are instructed to use a 0.12% chlorhexidine rinse for a 2-week period (Fig 1-29). However, the chlorhexidine rinse is ineffective in removing plaque. Plaque accumulation on the marginal portion of the implant abutments has previously been reported to cause an inflammatory reaction in the peri-implant mucosa. After flapless implant surgery, the implant surface is in close contact with the surrounding mucosa without sutures, which is why flapless implants can be cleaned effectively on a daily basis using a plaque control procedure immediately after implant placement (Fig 1-30).

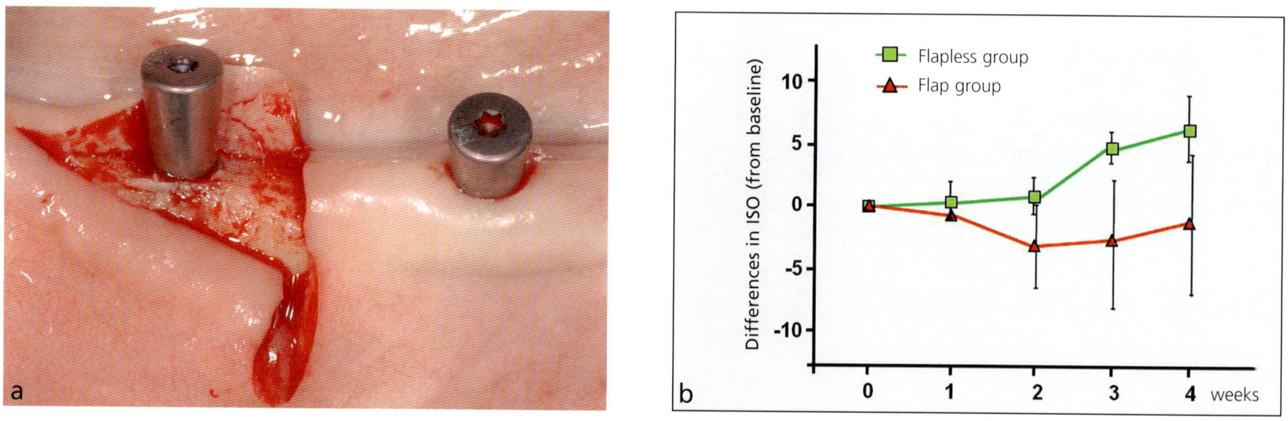

Fig 1-28 (a and b) Effect of flap and flapless surgery on the implant stability was compared using a canine mandible model. Implants stabilized more quickly without flap elevation than with flap elevation. When implants (Straumann® SLActive) were placed without flap elevation, the increase of stability occurred after 2 weeks without a period of decreasing stability. ISQ – implant stability quotient.

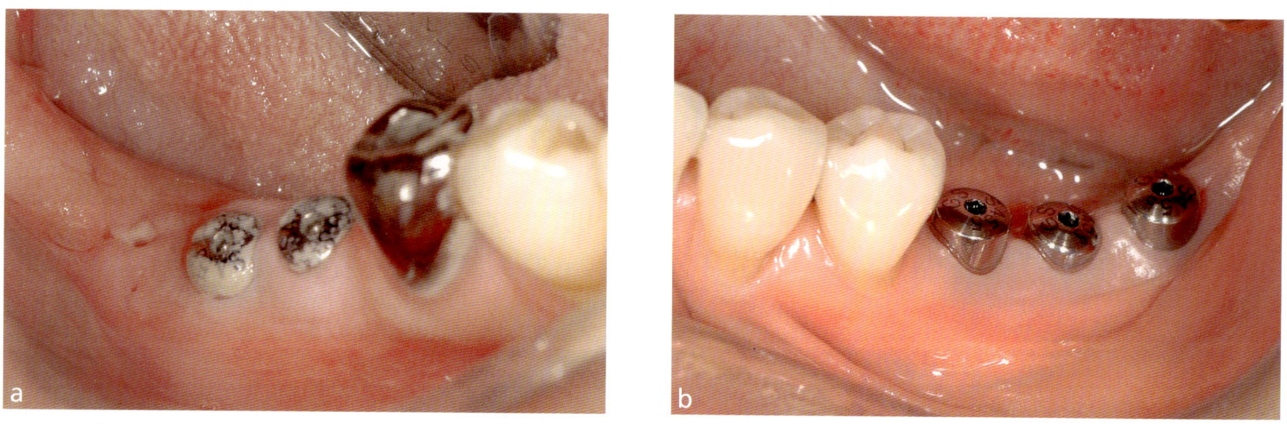

Fig 1-29 (a) Intraoral view showing that a chlorhexidine rinse is not effective at removing plaque. (b) Intraoral view showing that flapless implants can be cleaned effectively with a plaque control procedure immediately after implant placement.

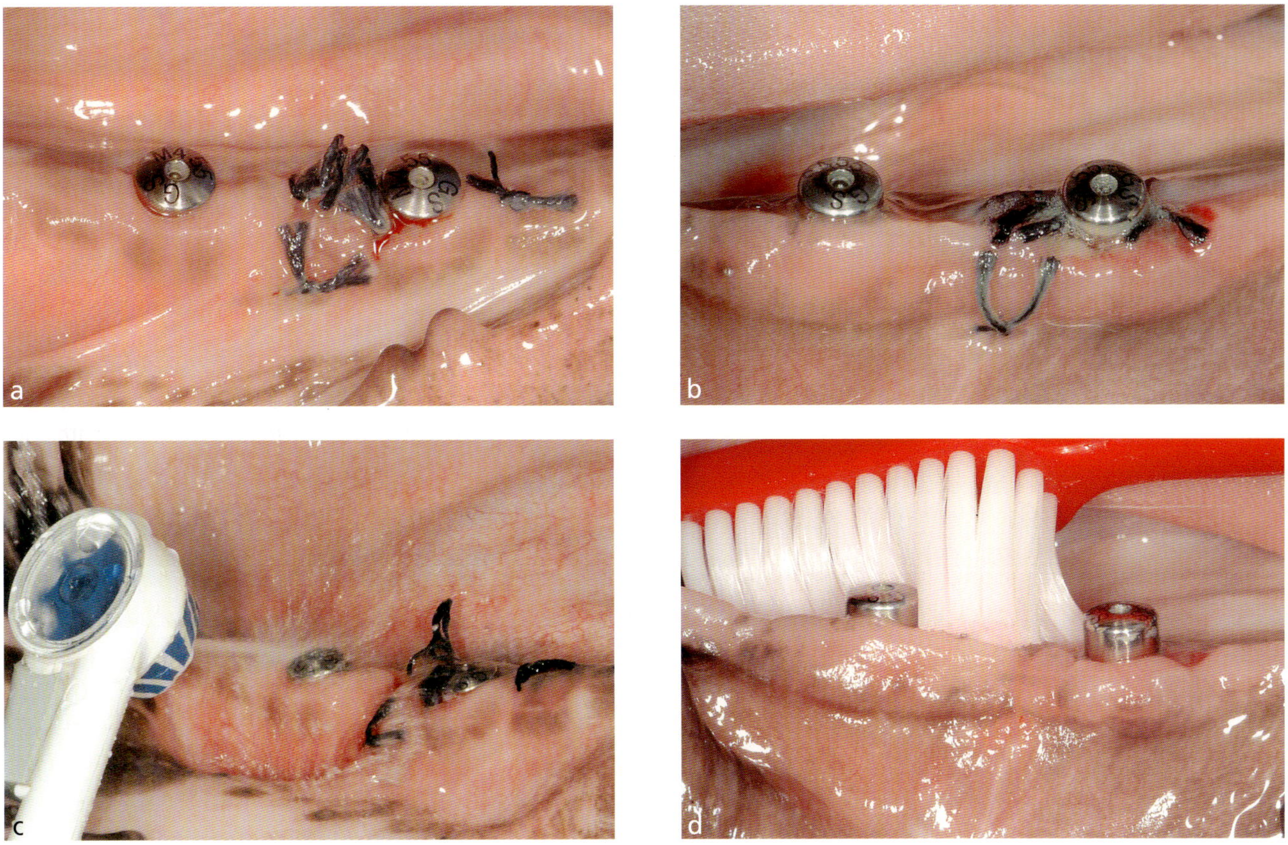

Fig 1-30 (a–d) Cleaning the implants immediately after flap implant surgery may be quite difficult because a long sutured wound in the incision area is vulnerable to mechanical irritation. However, the flapless implants can be cleaned effectively using a plaque control procedure immediately after implant placement.

Precision of flapless implant placement

There is some concern that implants cannot be placed precisely by the flapless approach, because both the drilling and implant placement procedures are controlled above the mucosa without looking at the alveolar bone. In the author's experience, provided the mucosal thickness is measured precisely and the shape of the alveolar bone is properly evaluated, implant placement can be performed precisely even without exposing the bone surface (Fig 1-31).

Summary

When implants are placed using the flapless procedure, there is little scar formation in the soft tissue adjacent to the implants, an increase in the blood vessels of the peri-implant mucosa, and a decrease in peri-implant bone loss. This procedure also boosts the osseointegration of the implants, enhances the bone density adjacent to the implants, and enables the use of an effective method of early plaque control. If these advantages of flapless implants accumulate over time after surgery, this procedure can produce a subsequent large-scale effect, akin to the butterfly effect.

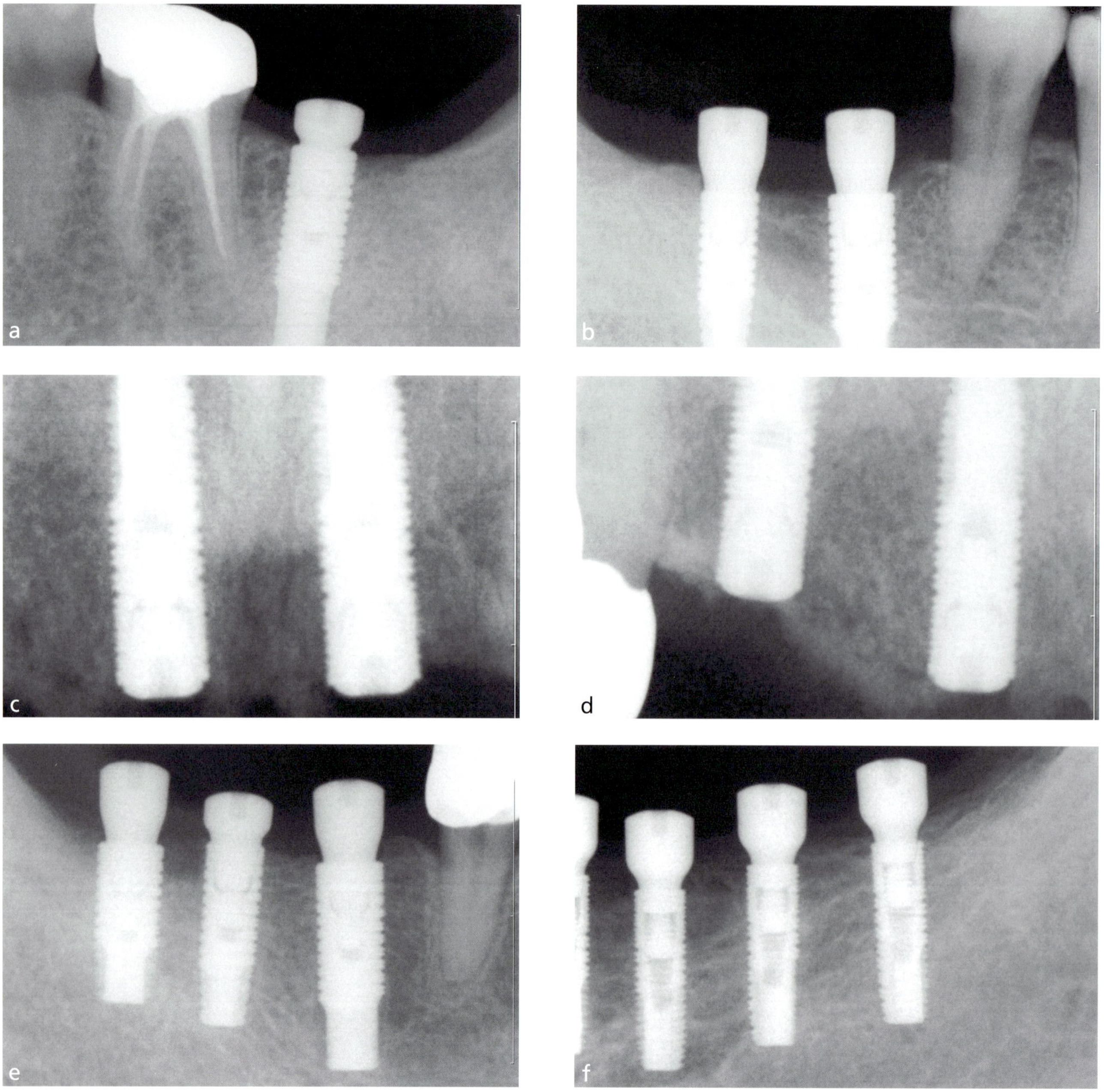

Fig 1-31 (a–f) Radiographs showing that implant placement can be performed precisely even without exposing the bone surface.

References

1. Misch CE. Contemporary Implant Dentistry, ed 3. St Louis, MO: Mosby, 2008:68–91.
2. Homans J. A Textbook of Surgery. Springfield, IL: Charles C Thomas, 1945:1–30.
3. Sabiston DC, Lyerly HK. Textbook of Surgery: The Biological Basis of Modern Surgical Practice. Philadelphia, PA: WB Saunders, 1997: 207–220.
4. Mathes SJ. Plastic Surgery. Philadelphia, PA: Saunders Elsevier, 2006: 209–234.
5. Cardaropoli G, Lekholm U, Wennstrom JL. Tissue alterations at implant supported single tooth replacement: a 1-year prospective clinical study. Clin Oral Implants Res 2006;17:165–171.
6. Becker W, Becker BE, Newman MG. Clinical and microbiologic findings that may contribute to dental implant failure. Int J Oral Maxillofac Implants 1990;5:31–38.
7. Berglundh T, Lindhe J. Dimension of the peri-implant mucosa: biological width revisited. J Clin Periodontol 1996;23:971–973.
8. Berglundh T, Lindhe J, Ericsson I, Marinella CP, Liljenberg B, Thomsen P. The soft tissue barrier at implants and teeth. Clin Oral Implants Res 1991;2:81–90.
9. You TM, Choi BH, Li J, Xuan F, Jeong SM, Jang SO. Morphogenesis of the peri-implant mucosa: a comparison between flap and flapless procedures in the canine mandible. Oral Surg Oral Med Oral Pathol Oral Radiol Endod 2009;107:66–70.
10. Berglund T, Lindhe J, Jonsson K, Ericsson I. The topography of the vascular systems in the periodontal and peri-implant tissues in the dog. J Clin Periodontol 1994;21:189–193.
11. Moon IS, Berglundh T, Abrahamsson I, Linder E, Lindhe J. The barrier between the keratinized mucosa and the dental implant: an experimental study in the dog. J Clin Periodontol 1999;26:658–663.
12. Kim JI, Choi BH, Li J, Xuan F, Jeong SM. Blood vessels of the peri-implant mucosa: a comparison between the flap and flapless procedures. Oral Surg Oral Med Oral Pathol Oral Radiol Endod 2009; 107:508–512.
13. Pham AN, Fiorellini JP, Paquette DP, Williams RC, Weber HP. Longitudinal radiographic study of crestal bone levels adjacent to non-submerged dental implants. J Oral Implants 1994;10:26–34.
14. Hermann JS, Cochran DL, Nummikoski PV, Buser D. Crestal bone changes around titanium implants: a radiographic evaluation of unloaded nonsubmerged and submerged implants in the canine mandible. J Periodontol 1997;68:1117–1130.
15. Jeong SM, Choi BH, Li J et al. Flapless implant surgery: an experimental study. Oral Surg Oral Med Oral Pathol Oral Radiol Endod 2007;104:24–28.
16. Jeong SM, Choi BH, Li J, Ahn KM, Lee SH, Xuan F. Bone healing around implants following flap and mini-flap surgeries: a radiographic evaluation between stage I and stage II surgery. Oral Surg Oral Med Oral Pathol Oral Radiol Endod 2008;105:293–296.

CHAPTER

2

Possibilities and Limitations of Flapless Implantology

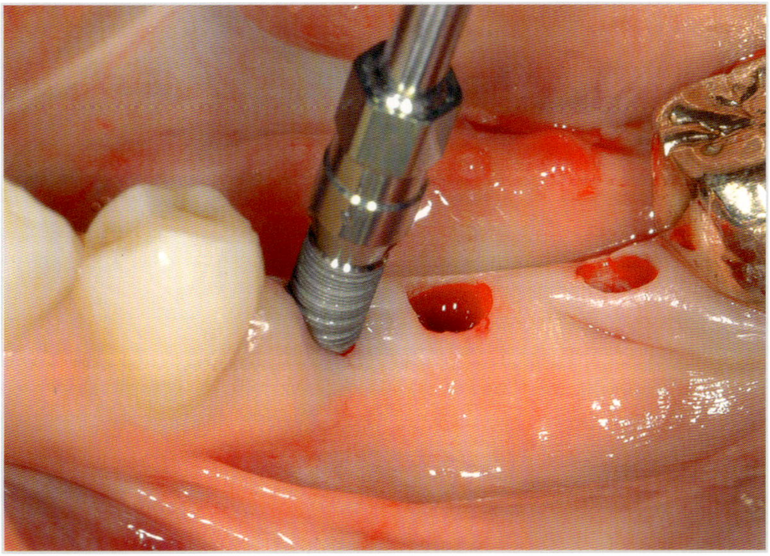

Key point
Visualization difficulties can be overcome.

Overview

Advances in implant surface processing technology have given modern implants considerably enhanced osseointegration ability, and developments in radiographic technology have greatly improved the precision of site preparation. Now is the time to shift to minimally invasive implant surgery in order to provide more predictable results, as well as better function, esthetics, and comfort. When implants are placed without flap elevation, there is little scar formation in the soft tissue adjacent to the implants, an increase in blood vessels of the peri-implant mucosa, a decrease in the sulcus depth around the implants, and a reduction in peri-implant bone loss. This procedure also improves the esthetic results by maintaining the original form and thickness of the mucosa surrounding the implant. However, one major limitation with this surgery is the lack of visibility of the hard tissue contours during the procedure. This chapter describes the possibilities and limitations of flapless implant surgery as well as how to compensate for these restrictions.

Advantages of flapless implant surgery

The ability to protect soft tissue

The amount of tissue injury can influence the speed and quality of the healing process.[1-3] Surgical trauma can damage the soft tissues when implants are placed with flap elevation (Fig 2-1). Furthermore, the conditions for wound healing around implants are poor when the soft tissues are approximated around the permucosal healing abutment with a suture (Fig 2-2). This is because the wound edges around the implants are not completely closed and hematomas can form beneath the flap. However, there is less soft tissue trauma in flapless implant surgery because the tissues are not reflected.

The most common postoperative complication of flap implant surgery is opening of the incision line (Fig 2-3).[4] The opening of the sutured area aggravates and lengthens the inflammatory phase of repair, leaving more scar tissue (Fig 2-4). With flapless implant surgery, no opening of the incision line can occur because the procedure does not require sutures. Moreover, the peri-implant mucosa has small, clean, closed wounds after the flapless procedure. This may improve the ability of the peri-implant mucosa to heal quickly, with little scar formation. Scar tissue is an area deficient of blood vessels, which impairs the defense system. If the defense mechanisms are impaired, smaller bacterial concentrations will be needed to initiate an infectious process. This can partly explain why extensive progression of inflammation often occurs in the peri-implant mucosa.[5]

The ability to protect blood vessels of the peri-implant mucosa

Several authors[6-8] have reported that, when using a flap procedure, an approximately 300–500 µm wide zone of supracrestal connective tissue apical to the junctional epithelium surrounding the implant is almost devoid of vessels. The results of an animal study showed that there were almost twice as many vessels in the flapless implant group as in the flap implant group.[9] This suggests that the peri-implant mucosa is more richly vascularized in a flapless implant than in a flap implant. The more richly vascularized peri-implant mucosa is directly related to an increased blood supply around the implant, which may improve the healing and defensive abilities.

The circulation of blood within the mandible is centrifugal under normal conditions; that is, the blood circulates from the inside of the bone to the outside and ends up in the vessels located in the periosteum and soft tissues associated with the bone. However, the direction of blood flow may reverse with aging and tooth extraction. The changes in the patterns of blood flow to the edentulous ridge are of particular importance in implant dentistry. Mucoperiosteal flap reflection can easily reduce blood supply to the bone surface in situations where the blood supply to the bone is reversed so that the direction of flow is from the outside to the inside of the bone. Understanding the changes in blood flow is of great significance in implant dentistry. Therefore, we now address the changes in blood supply to the jaw with aging and tooth extraction.

Vascular changes in the alveolar bone after tooth extraction and with aging

The inferior alveolar artery is the major artery supplying blood to the mandible. This artery runs within the mandibular body and supplies blood from the marrow (medullary) region outward through the cortical bone to the end in vessels located in the periosteum and soft tissues associated with the bone. As a result, the circulation of blood within the mandible is centrifugal. Within the marrow spaces, the artery forms a network of vessels known as the endosteal or medullary plexus. Vessels from this plexus enter the cortical bone and eventually reach the bone surface. Once the vessels reach the outer surface of the bone, they anastomose with the vessels within the fibrous layer of the periosteum or with the arteries supplying the soft tissues. The network of vessels associated with the periosteum is called the periosteal plexus. In addition to these vascular networks, the periodontal plexus is associated with the teeth.[10,11] When teeth are present, the inferior alveolar artery sends branches into the alveolar process and to the teeth. The periodontal plexus, in turn, connects to the vessels of the periosteal plexus.

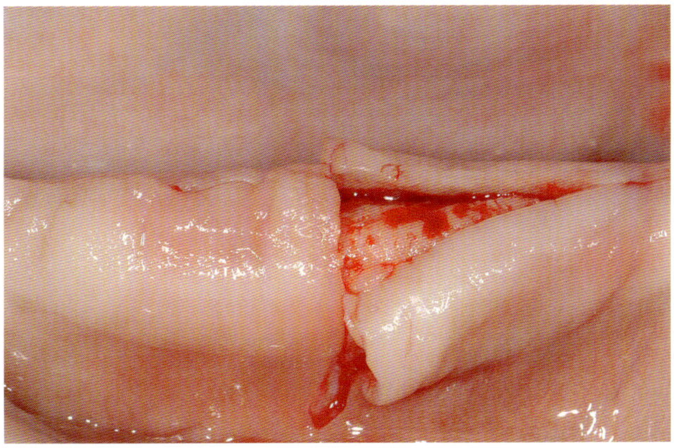

Fig 2-1 When tissue is cut or damaged by surgery, wound repair processes begin to restore tissue integrity, leaving a scar.

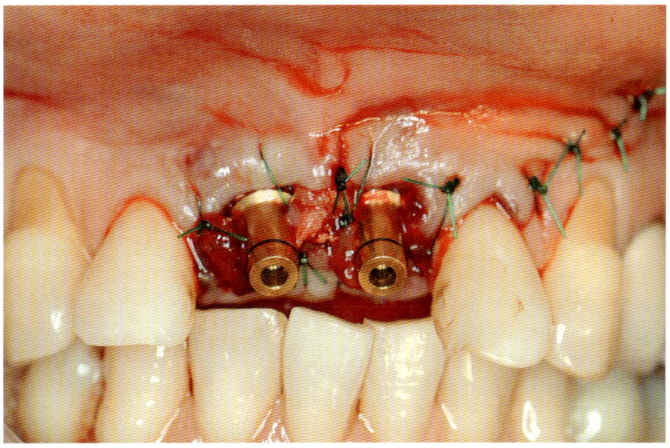

Fig 2-2 When the flap implant procedure is used, the soft tissues are approximated around the permucosal healing abutments with a suture. The conditions for wound healing around implants are poor.

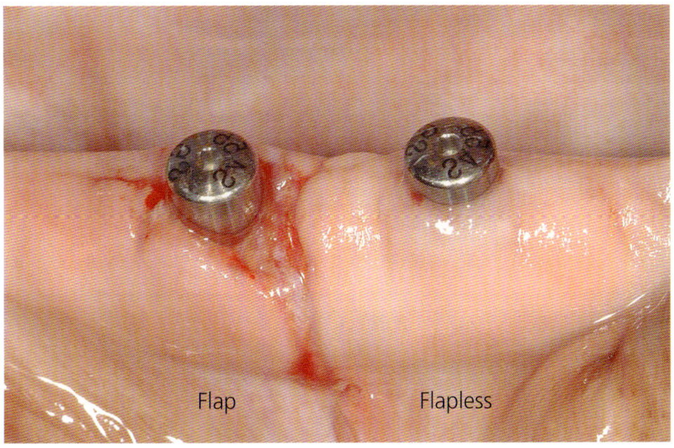

Fig 2-3 The most common postoperative complication of flap implant surgery is incision line opening. The opening of the sutured area aggravates wound healing, leaving an extensive scar.

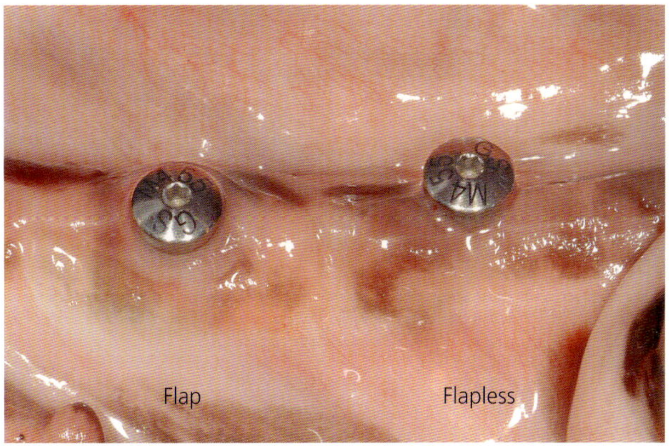

Fig 2-4 The mucosa around the implants thickens after surgery when implants are placed with flap elevation.

Once a tooth is removed, its periodontal plexus is lost. Tooth extraction may lead to a decrease in flow within the inferior alveolar artery (Fig 2-5).

Furthermore, a blockage of the inferior alveolar artery can occur with aging. It has been reported that the inferior alveolar artery is susceptible to arteriosclerotic changes and tends to become tortuous and narrow with age.[12,13] A blockage of the inferior alveolar artery occurs years before there is any clinical evidence of a blockage in the carotid vessels. Angiographic studies of living human subjects of all ages demonstrated a blockage of the inferior alveolar artery in 79% of all individuals studied, and no arterial flow in 33% of patients. The incidence of an absence of flow in the inferior alveolar artery increases with age.

When abnormal circulatory conditions exist within the mandible with aging, such as an occlusion of the nutrient artery, the blood supply to the bone is reversed and the direction of the flow is from the outside to the inside of the bone. In these cases, the blood supply to the mandible is dependent on the external blood supply located within the periosteum and soft tissues. As a result, when the periosteum is reflected off the crestal bone of an aged edentulous mandible, the cortical bone blood supply is affected dramatically, causing osteoblast death on the surface through lack of nutrition. The reduced blood supply in an aged edentulous mandible is also associated with occasional postoperative incision line opening. Overall, successful implant placement in an aged edentulous mandible requires careful protection of the blood vessels.

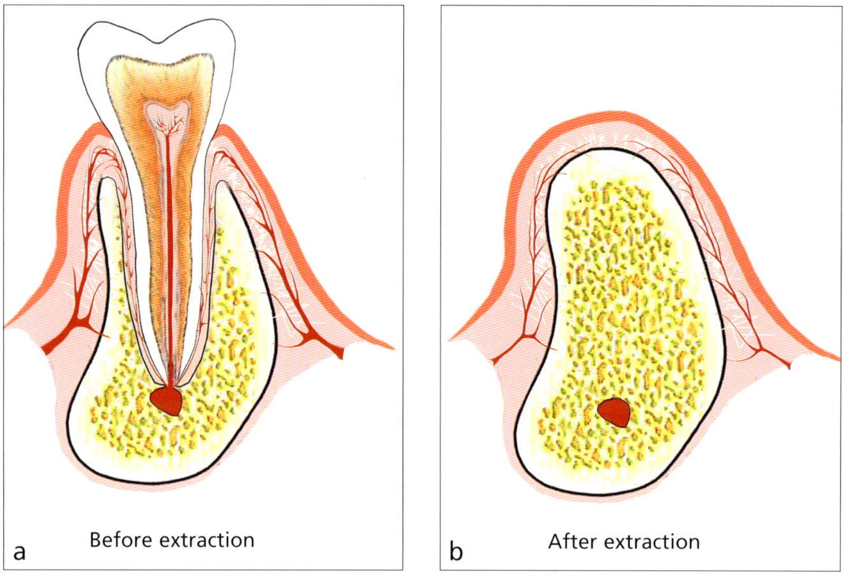

Fig 2-5 (a and b) Once a tooth is removed, its periodontal plexus is lost. Tooth extraction may lead to a decrease in flow within the inferior alveolar artery.

Vascular changes in the alveolar mucosa after tooth extraction

Once a tooth is extracted, the site may heal by repair or regeneration of the bone. The tooth socket regenerates bone by secondary intention, and the tissue in the socket area heals as scar tissue with few blood vessels. In addition, once a tooth is removed, its periodontal plexus is lost, leading to a decrease in blood flow within the inferior alveolar artery. Eventually, a 1–2 mm wide avascular zone is created in the crestal area of the edentulous alveolar ridge (Fig 2-6).[14] Therefore, the alveolar mucosa in the crestal area of the edentulous alveolar ridge is likely to become a problematic area for wound healing.

The ability to protect peri-implant mucosa health

For flap implants, the implant–mucosa barrier consists of junctional epithelium approximately 2 mm in length, and a connective tissue compartment approximately 1–1.5 mm high.[8,15] When implants are placed without flap elevation, the length of the junctional epithelium is approximately 1.2 mm, and the zone of connective tissue integration is 1.0 mm in length, which suggests that the junctional epithelium extends more apically in flap implants than in flapless implants.[16] The more apically positioned junctional epithelium is related directly to an increased sulcus depth around the implant, which provides an environment more conducive to peri-implantitis.

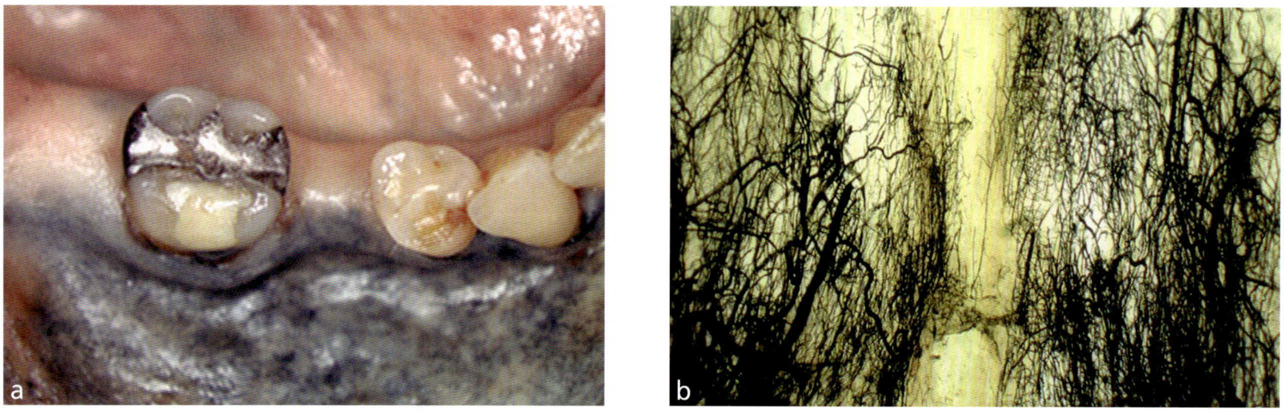

Fig 2-6 (a and b) Once a tooth is extracted, a 1–2 mm wide avascular zone is created in the crestal area of the edentulous alveolar ridge. Reproduced from Kleinheinz et al.[14] with permission.

Flapless implant surgery is advantageous in terms of reducing the sulcus depth around the implants because the effectiveness of hygiene decreases with increasing sulcus depth.[17] Maintaining a good environment for the health of the tissue adjacent to an implant will ensure the success of the implant.

The ability to protect the periosteum

It has been reported that bone regeneration is almost entirely dependent on the periosteum, with a minor contribution from the bone edges.[18,19] The bone regeneration capability of the periosteum can be damaged by surgical trauma. Since the mucoperiosteum is not elevated by surgery, flapless implant surgery causes less surgical damage to the periosteum. As a result, the bone regeneration ability of the periosteum is maintained after the flapless implant procedure. Furthermore, most of the blood supply is associated with the periosteum in the mandible. The cortical bone blood supply is affected significantly when the periosteum is reflected off the crestal bone.

Effect of the periosteum on bone regeneration

It has been reported that bone regeneration in discontinuity defects in the mandible is dependent almost entirely on the periosteum, with minor contributions from the bone edges.[18] The author's animal study[19] strongly supports this contention (Figs 2-7 to 2-9). When the periosteum was removed, mandibular defects >10 mm failed to heal across the entire defect (Fig 2-8). However, when the periosteum was preserved, bone formation occurred both from the periosteum and from the bone edges. There was sufficient bone formation to allow bone bridging across the 30 mm and 40 mm defects (Fig 2-9). These findings suggest that the periosteum plays a major role in bone regeneration.

The ability to protect peri-implant bone

When comparing flap and flapless procedures, the crestal bone loss occurring during the early postsurgical period was significantly greater in the implants placed with the flap procedure.[20] The mean crestal bone loss was approximately 1 mm more in the implants placed with the flap procedure than in the implants placed with the flapless procedure.[21]

The ability to maintain the original form of the mucosa

When implants are placed without flap elevation, the adjacent mucosa thickens by approximately 0.7 mm due to postoperative edema, which occurs immediately after surgery, resolves to the original level 3 months later, and then maintains its level. The flapless procedure is advantageous in terms of maintaining the original form and thickness of the mucosa surrounding the implants.[16] As a result, flapless implant surgery has been applied in the anterior esthetic zone to optimize the esthetic results (Fig 2-10).[22]

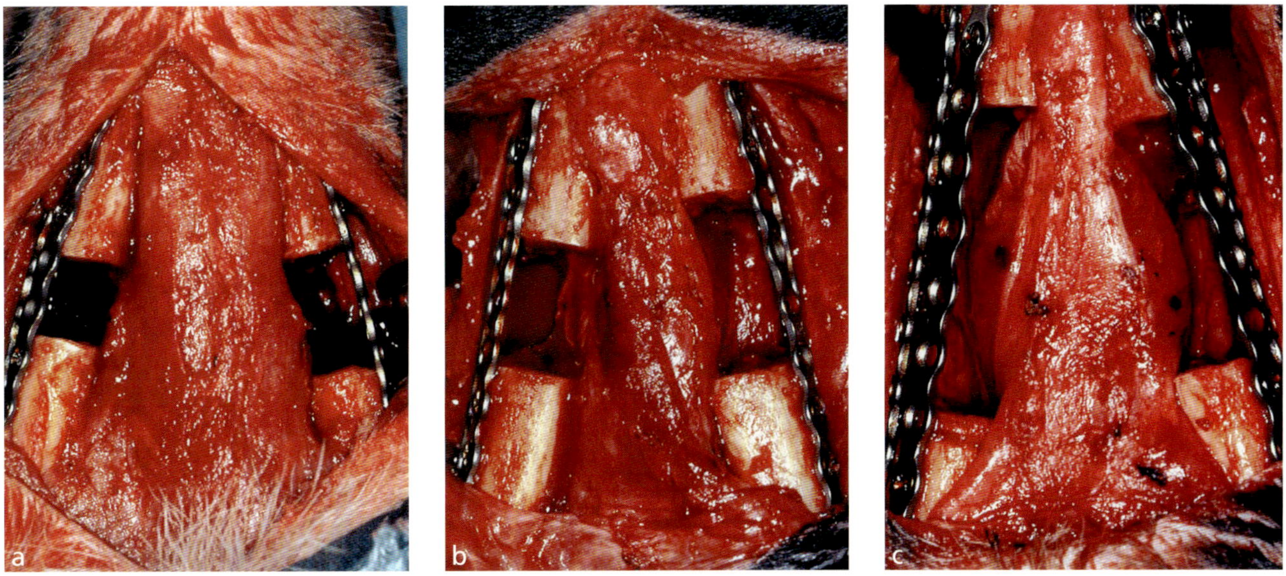

Fig 2-7 (a–c) Animal study on bone regeneration in discontinuity defects in the canine mandible. In eight animals, segments measuring 5, 10, 15, and 20 mm were excised with the surrounding periosteum. In the remaining eight dogs, segments measuring 30, 40, 50, and 60 mm were excised preserving the periosteum.

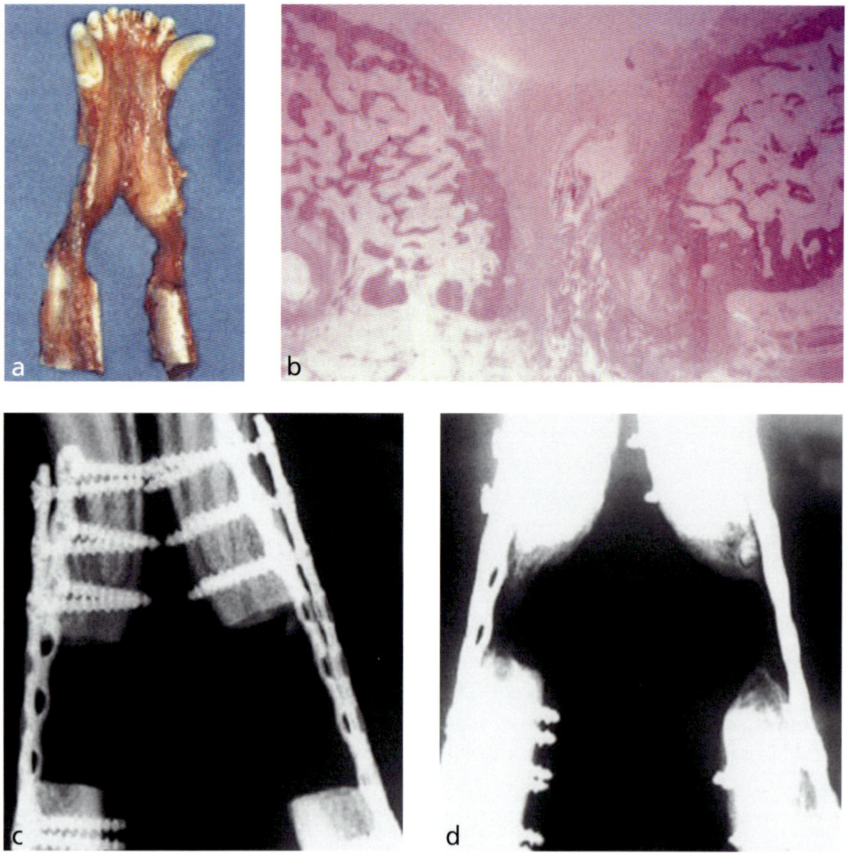

Fig 2-8 Mandible in which 15 mm and 20 mm defects with periosteal resection were created. (a) Photograph of a specimen. (b) Histological appearance showing nonunion. (c) Radiograph taken 2 weeks postoperatively. (d) Radiograph taken 12 weeks postoperatively. In defects longer than 15 mm, bone bridging was incomplete and a fibrous band was noted.

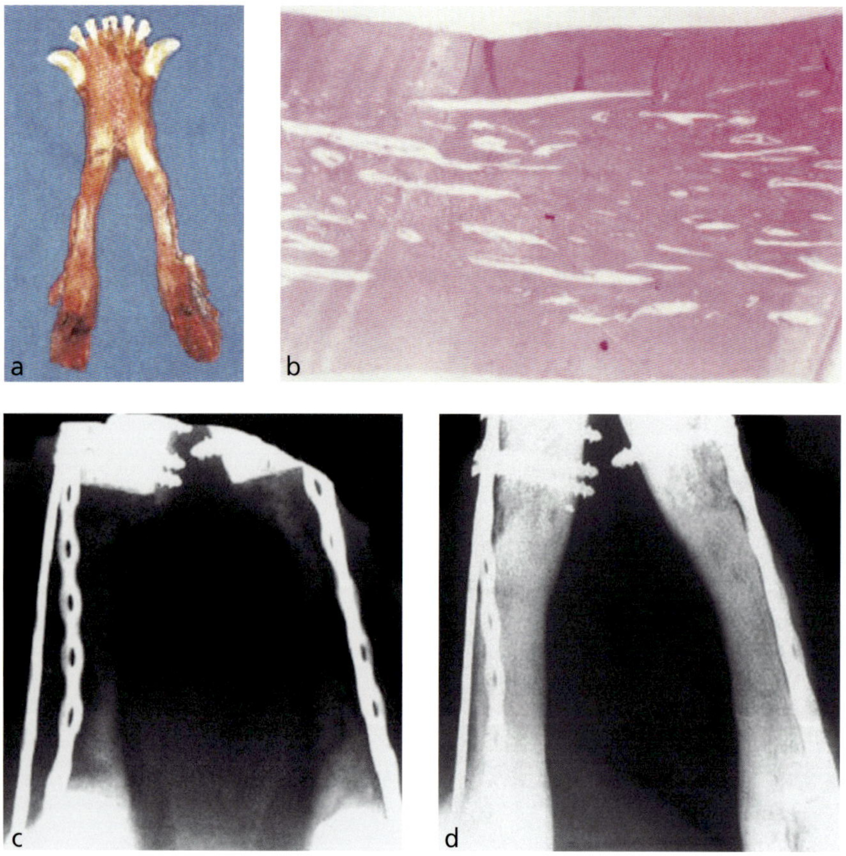

Fig 2-9 Mandible in which 30 mm and 40 mm defects were created preserving the periosteum. (a) Photograph of a specimen. (b) Histological appearance showing bone bridging. (c) Radiograph taken 2 weeks postoperatively. (d) Radiograph taken 12 weeks postoperatively. In the mandibles where the periosteum had been preserved, the 30 mm and 40 mm defects showed complete bony union.

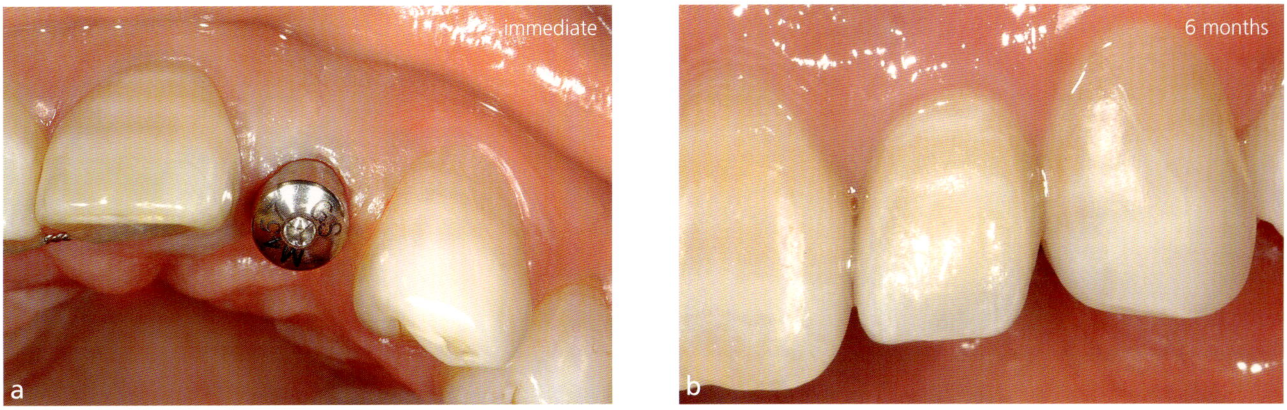

Fig 2-10 (a) Clinical photograph immediately after flapless implant placement and (b) 6 months after placement.

The ability to increase resistance to postoperative infection

When the mucoperiosteum is cut and elevated by surgery, blood vessels are damaged, leading to a subperiosteal hemorrhage. Edema and swelling can develop beneath the flap, which is accompanied by hematoma formation. The severity of the swelling and edema increases with increasing elevation of the flap. A hematoma can be a source of infection. In addition, incision line opening occurs as a result of tension created by the hematoma. Wound dehiscence can trigger an infection. Infections adjacent to the implants are closely related to peri-implant bone loss. In particular, an infection occurring during the first two weeks of healing after implant placement plays a crucial role in early bone loss around the implants (Fig 2-11). Therefore, preventing both hematomas and wound dehiscence is crucial for preventing infections and reducing early bone loss around the implants.

Another disadvantage of flap implant surgery on wound healing is the need for sutures, which serve as an infection locus in the mucosa. Sutures generate an immune response because they are foreign bodies that are susceptible to infection. Moreover, when sutures are present, it is quite difficult to clean the implants, which increases plaque accumulation and the risk of infection.

The flapless implant procedure is performed in the attached mucosa without reflecting the crestal soft tissue. Postoperative infections are less likely to occur because the attached mucosa around the implants is in close contact with the underlying bone. In addition, there is little dead space between the implants and surrounding mucosa immediately after placing the implant as a result of the tight contact. After flapless implant surgery, the flapless implants can be cleaned effectively on a daily basis using a plaque control procedure immediately after implant placement. These factors also increase the resistance to postoperative infection (Figs 2-12 and 2-13). Moreover, the preserved vessels help to maintain the resistance to infection.

Convenience of treatment

The flapless implant procedure is performed in the attached mucosa area without extensive flaps, making implant placement simple and easy. The procedure allows clinicians to place implants in less time with less bleeding. In addition, there is usually minimal discomfort, pain, and swelling after implant placement.

Limitations of flapless implant surgery and solutions

Assessment of bone volume

The primary disadvantage of flapless implant surgery is the inability to assess the bone volume during an implant osteotomy or insertion. Therefore, flapless implant surgery requires preoperative images of the shape of the jaw bone to evaluate the available bone height and width. The images consist mainly of panoramic and cross-sectional views of the jaw bone. In complex cases, computerized tomography or computer imaging software may help to assess the bone volume before flapless implant surgery.

Figure 2-14 shows the planned placement of an implant at the site of the mandibular first molar. The data were transferred to a surgical template. It should be noted that only a part of the bone can be seen even when the bone is exposed by flap elevation. The bone structure can be evaluated using support immersion endoscopy during flapless implant surgery.[23,24] A direct view of the walls of the implant cavities using the endoscopy enables the surgeon to select the appropriate mode of bone preparation and implant. Figure 2-15 shows various types of bone structure.

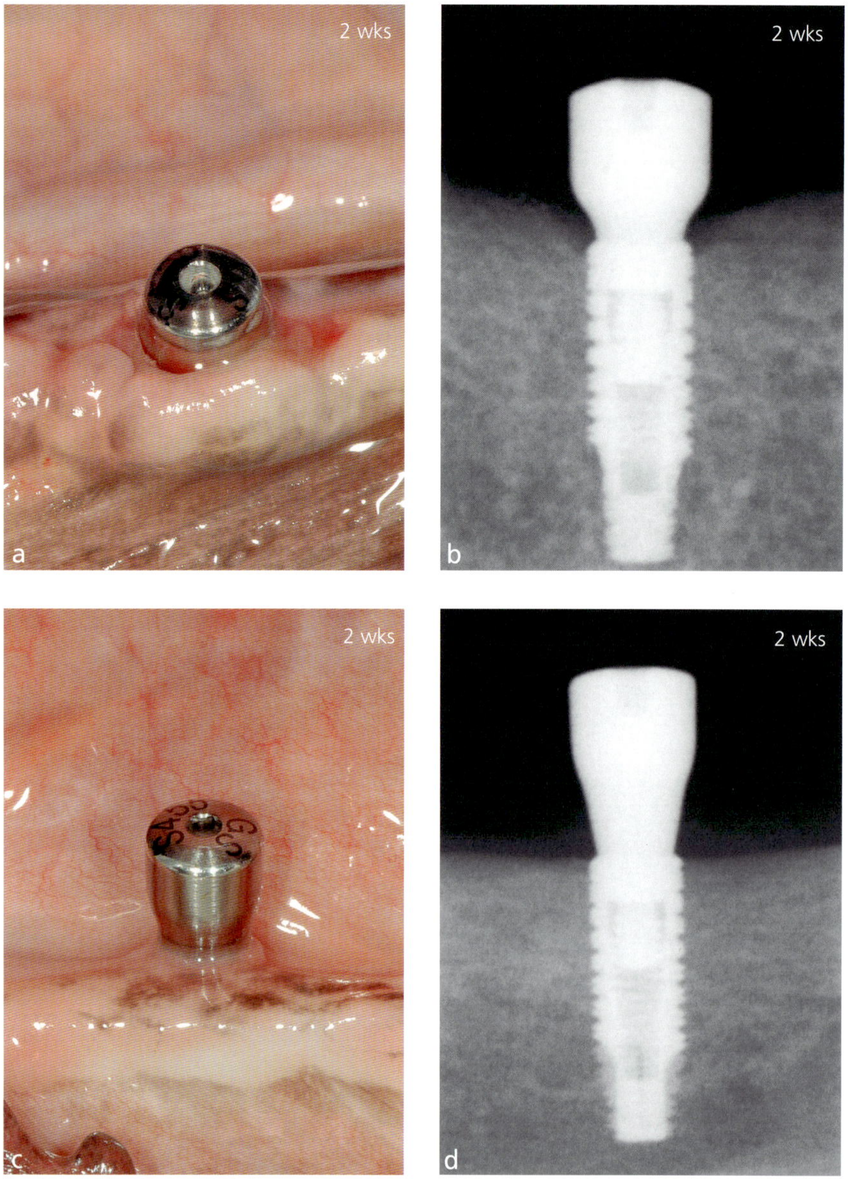

Fig 2-11 (a–d) Views of the peri-implant mucosa and bone 2 weeks after implant placement. An infection occurring during the first 2 weeks of healing plays a crucial role in early bone loss around the implants.

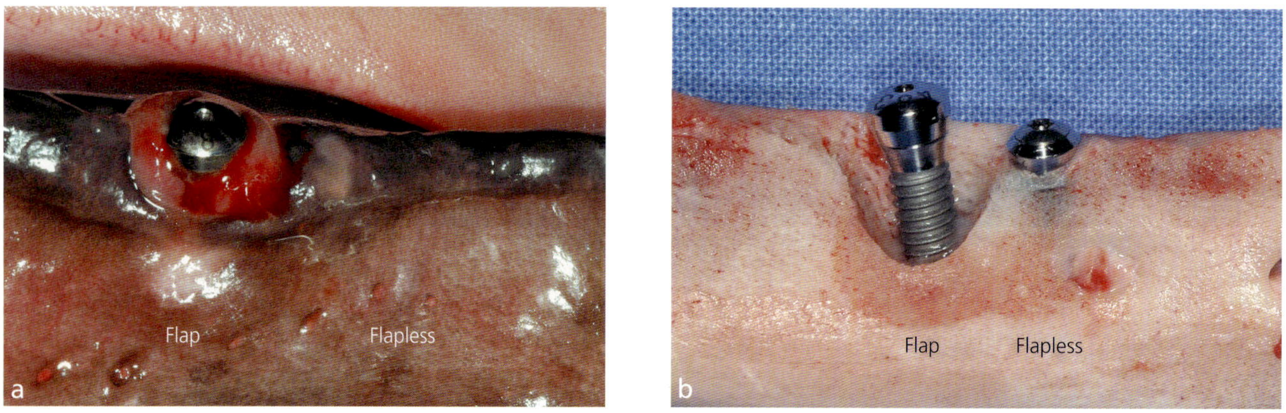

Fig 2-12 (a and b) An experiment was carried out to examine the effect of flap and flapless implant surgery on the inflammation resistance of the peri-implant mucosa using a canine mandible model. The flapless implant method was more effective in developing inflammation resistance of the tissue surrounding the implants.

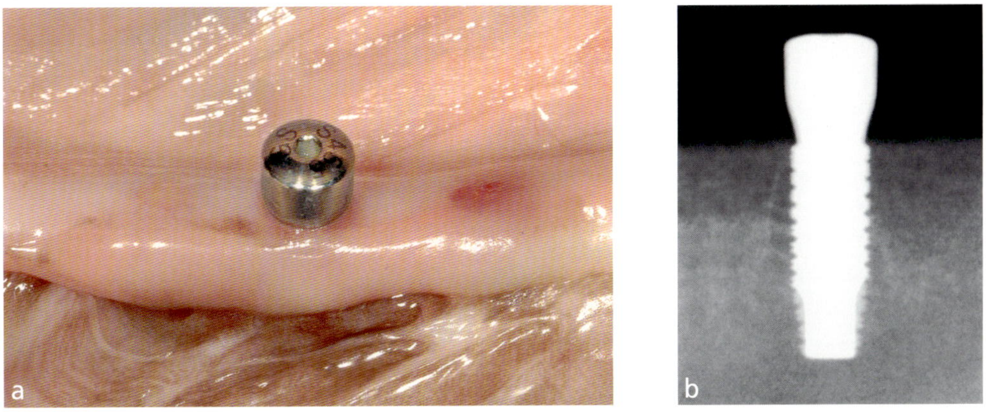

Fig 2-13 (a and b) Views of the peri-implant mucosa and bone 3 months after a flapless implant procedure. Note the healthy peri-implant mucosa and bone.

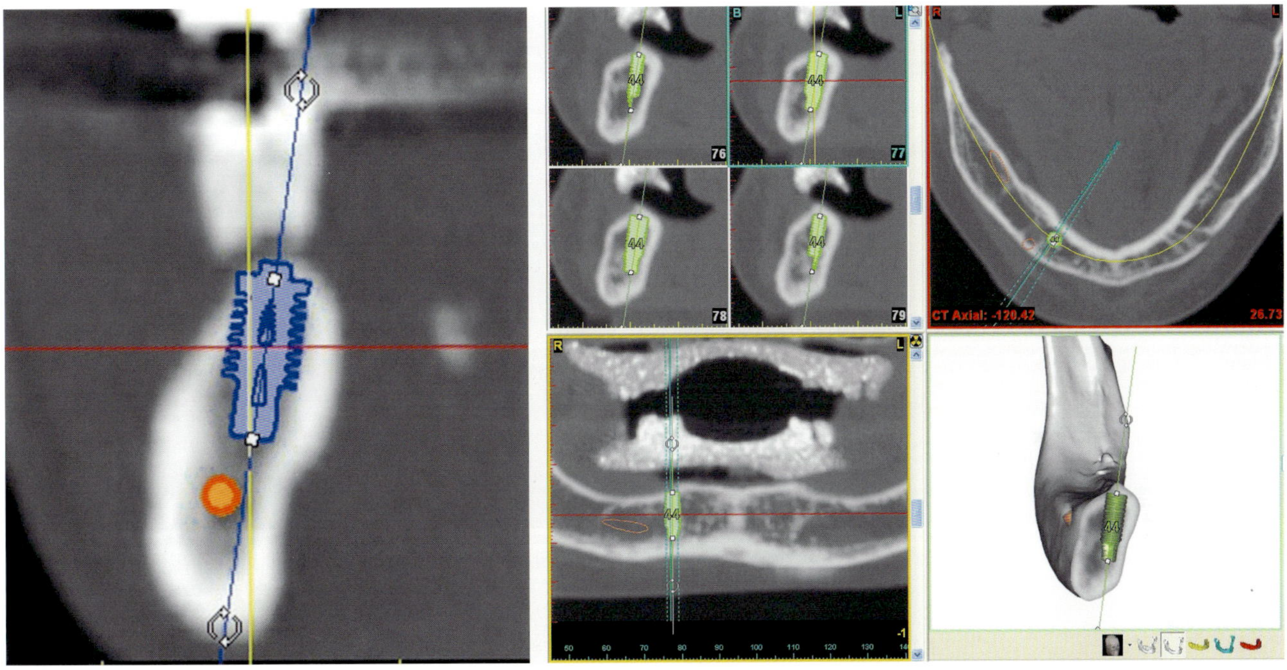

Fig 2-14 The planned placement of an implant at the site of the mandibular first molar using computer imaging software.

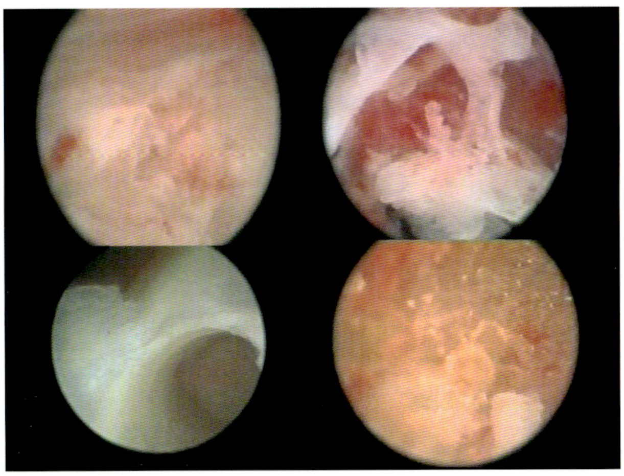

Fig 2-15 Endoscopic images of cortical (left) and trabecular (right) bone structures. The bone marrow on the right side below shows fatty degeneration that is unsuitable for implant placement.

Assessment of the direction of implant drilling

Drilling in flapless implant surgery is performed without visualization of the bone. This blind procedure increases the risk of cortical bone perforation owing to a lack of visibility of hard tissue contours. The use of carefully planned surgical guides helps the surgeon to drill in the precise planned position (Fig 2-16).[25,26]

Computerized tomography or computer imaging software may help increase the precision of surgical templates in guiding the direction of implant drilling. Precision of implant site preparation has been improved significantly using three-dimensional planning based on computerized tomography (CT).[27–29] Flapless implant surgery offers ease of use of a surgical guide because the guide can be stabilized on the mucosa. Even with the surgical guide, precautions should be taken during the drilling procedure. Throughout, the surgeon must palpate the cortical plate to detect any perforation of the plate. Incorrect angulation of the implant drills can perforate the plate, usually on the buccal aspect. Perforation of the buccal plate is generally detected by palpation. An unintended deviation of the bone cavity can also be detected by an endoscopic examination.

Figure 2-17 shows the exposure of an adjacent tooth during cavity preparation of an implant. The periodontal ligament at the edges of the exposed root can be visualized clearly.

Assessment of the depth of drilling

Since the crest of the ridge is below the soft tissue, it is difficult to observe the lines on the drill to access the drilling depth. Therefore, flapless implant surgery requires measurements of the mucosal thickness at the implant site to control the depth of drilling above the mucosa.

The simplest method of measuring the mucosal thickness is by use of a needle. The needle is inserted into the bone surface going through the mucosa, and the depth is marked with a rubber stop. The thickness of the mucosa covering the alveolar crest can be determined in a panoramic view. A cross-sectional view of a CT scan can also be used to determine the mucosal thickness. Prior to drilling, the mucosal thickness is measured using a periodontal probe or a depth gauge to verify the height of the mucosa at the implant site (Fig 2-18). The sum of the length of the implant and the thickness of the mucosa is marked on the drills. Stops on the drill can be used for the mark.

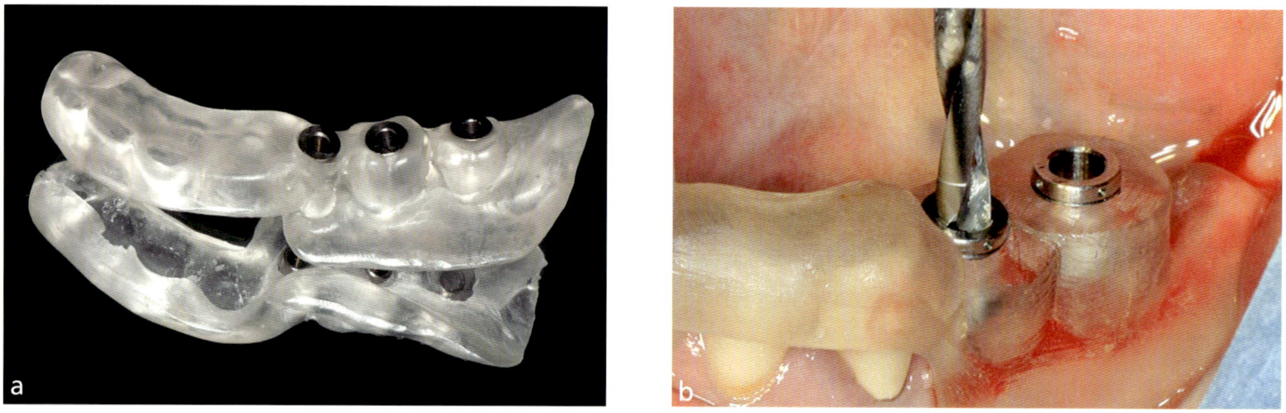

Fig 2-16 (a) Surgical guide and (b) osteotomy using a surgical guide.

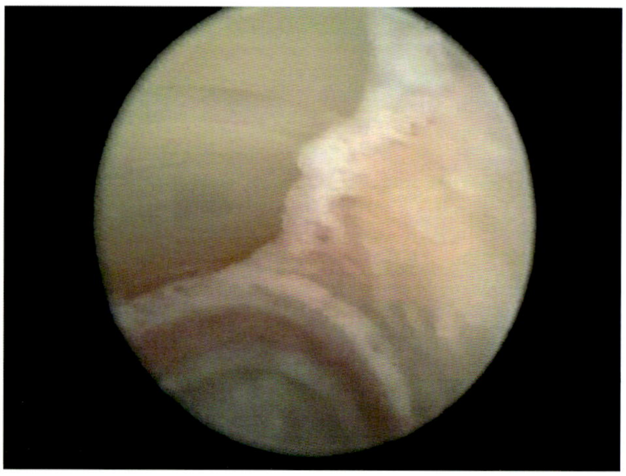

Fig 2-17 Exposure of an adjacent tooth root.

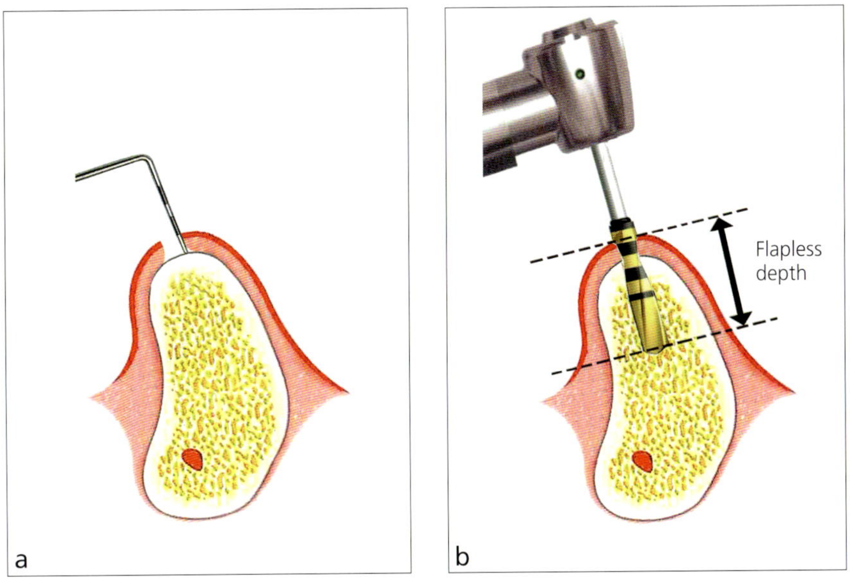

Fig 2-18 (a and b) Prior to drilling, the mucosal thickness is measured and the sum of the length of the implant and the thickness of the mucosa is marked on the drills.

An endoscopic assessment of the mucosal thickness above the alveolar bone surface can help to determine the drilling depth. A final check of the implant cavities prior to insertion as well as the alignment of the implant can be made using support immersion endoscopy (Fig 2-19). Visualization of the implant interface with support immersion endoscopy can help to overcome the lack of a direct view during flapless implant placement.

Assessment of location of the implant crest module in the alveolar crest

The surgeon will also have trouble assessing the location of the implant crest module in relation to the crest of the bone, because flapless implant surgery does not provide direct visualization of the bone. Therefore, there is some concern that flapless implants cannot be placed precisely. In the author's experience, implant placement can be performed precisely provided the mucosal thickness is measured exactly and the shape of the alveolar bone is evaluated properly, even without exposing the bone surface. The most effective way of assessing the location of the implant crest module is peri-implant probing around the implant using a probe or an explorer and carried out immediately after implant placement to verify that the implant crest module is located at the level of the bone crest (Fig 2-20).

Inability to maintain keratinized mucosa

A soft tissue punch may inadvertently remove all the keratinized mucosa on the facial aspect of the implant. For this reason, many clinicians consider flapless implant surgery only in areas with sufficient amounts of keratinized tissue.[4] Based on animal experiments, the optimal tissue punch size is 3.0–3.5 mm when a 4.5 mm permucosal healing abutment is used (Fig 2-21). The peri-implant mucosa heals quickly with little scar formation when the peri-implant mucosa is in tight contact with the implants after implant placement. These results suggest that the amount of keratinized tissue sacrificed by the soft tissue punch at the flapless implant site does not exceed 3.0–3.5 mm in width.

Flapless implant placement can also be performed using a mini-incision technique (Fig 2-22). Mini-incision implant placement requires a crestal mini-incision, approximately 5 mm in length, horizontal to the alveolar crest at the center of the implant site. The mini-incision technique is beneficial in saving the keratinized mucosa.

It should be noted that drills can damage the adjacent soft tissue. Therefore, the use of drills with cutting surfaces on the tips and rounded surfaces on the other parts is advisable (Fig 2-23).

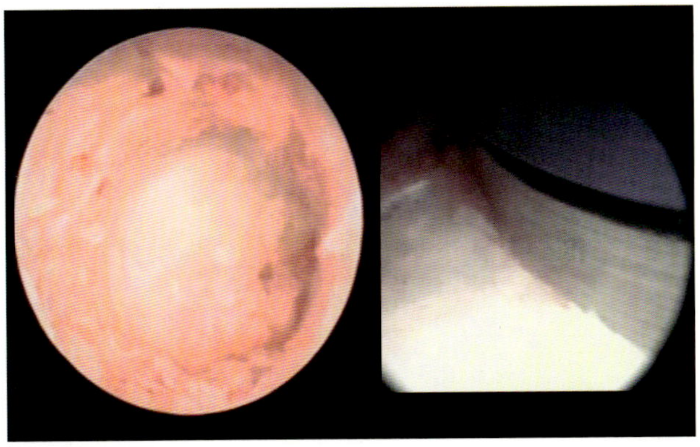

Fig 2-19 An implant cavity in the right posterior mandible (left). An implant with a cover screw after insertion at the crestal level (right).

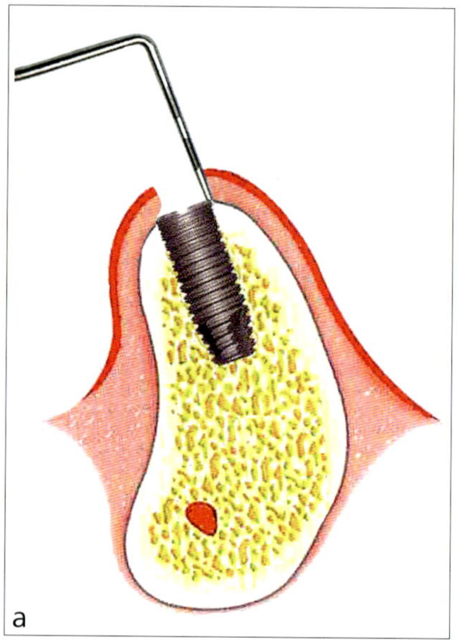

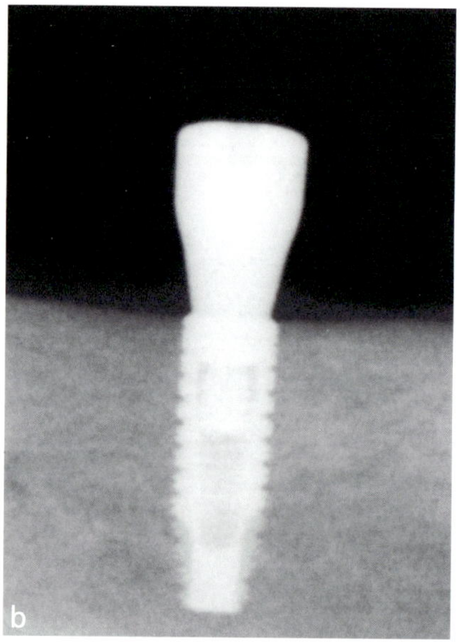

Fig 2-20 (a) Assessment of the location of the implant crest module using a probe. (b) Radiographic results after flapless implant surgery.

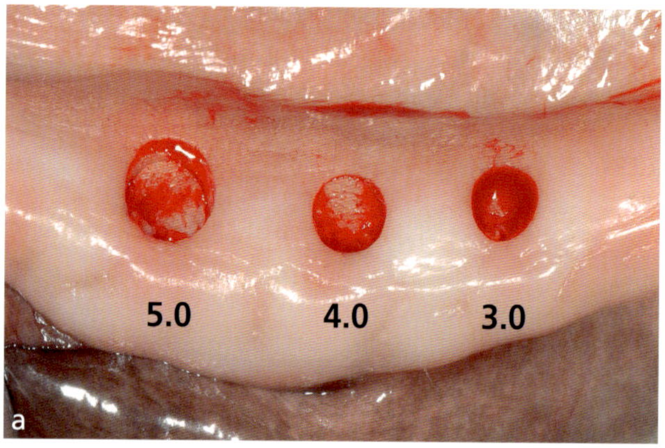

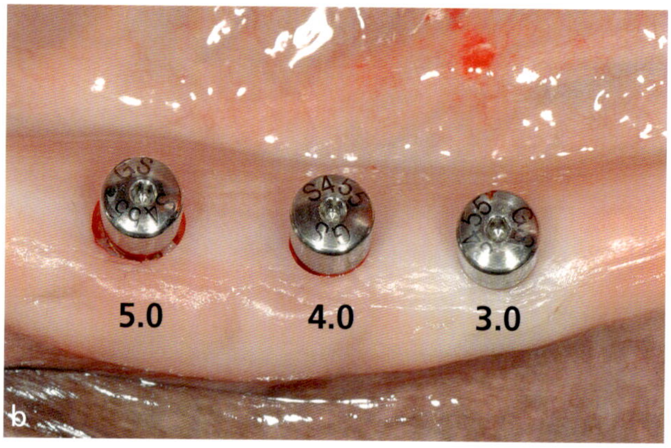

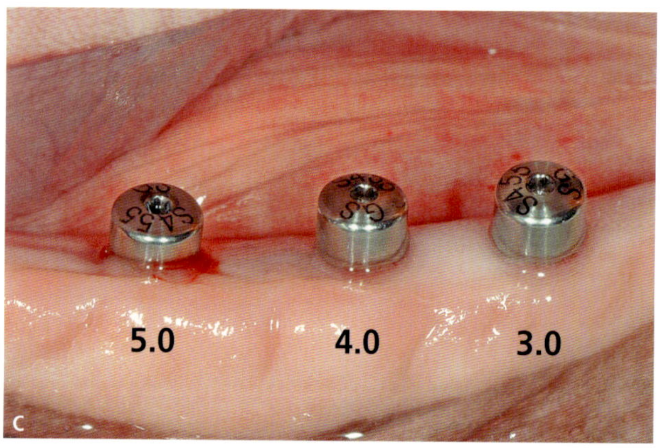

Fig 2-21 (a–c) Effect of the size of a tissue punch on the healing of peri-implant tissue. The optimal tissue punch size for peri-implant tissue healing is 3.0–3.5 mm.

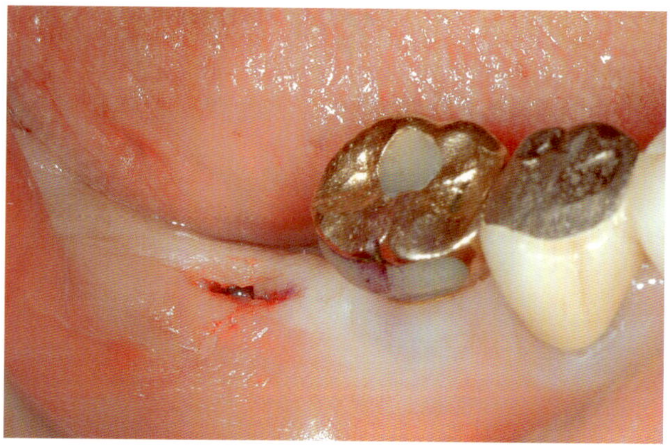

Fig 2-22 Flapless implant placement can also be performed using a mini-incision technique.

Correction of peri-implant defects

Because flapless implant surgery does not provide direct visualization of the bone, there is some concern that no bone defects can be corrected during implant insertion. However, the bone defects can be covered at the time of implant placement with a graft material using a subperiosteal tunneling procedure(Fig 2-24).[30]

The subperiosteal tunneling procedure permits flapless implant placement in the crestal area of the edentulous alveolar ridge where the mucosa is likely to become a problematic area for wound healing. For making subperiosteal tunnels, a vertical incision is made approximately 8 mm away from the implant. The graft material is introduced to the peri-implant defects through the subperiosteal tunnel. The biggest advantage is that lateral ridge augmentation can be performed simultaneously with flapless implant placement. However, in the case of vertical bone resorption, implants are inserted using a flapless procedure after augmenting the ridge using the subperiosteal tunneling

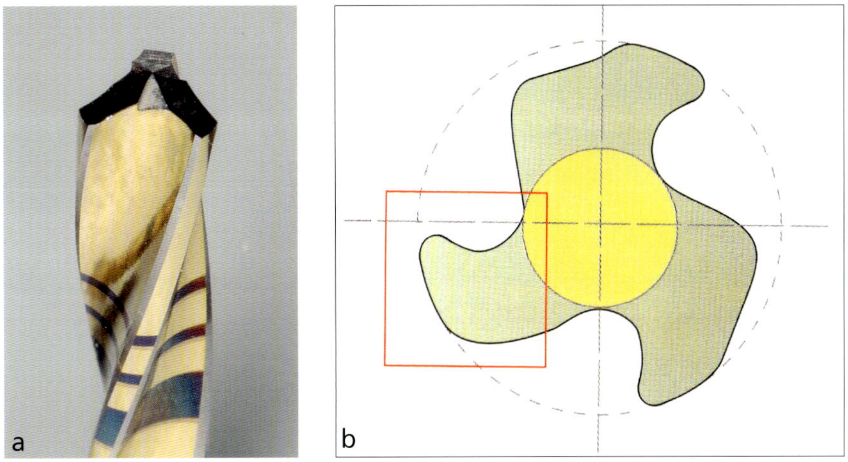

Fig 2-23 (a and b) A drill with a cutting surface on the tip and rounded surface on the other parts.

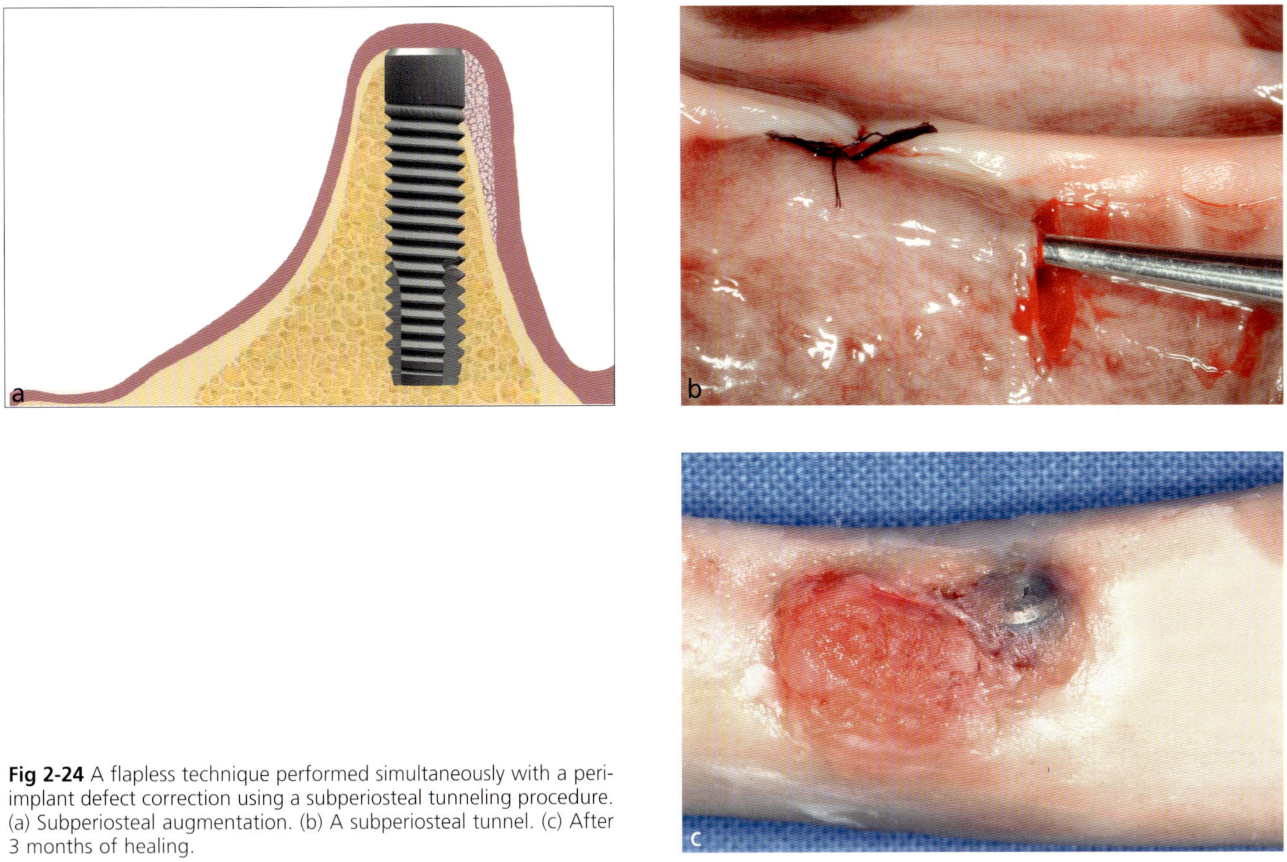

Fig 2-24 A flapless technique performed simultaneously with a peri-implant defect correction using a subperiosteal tunneling procedure. (a) Subperiosteal augmentation. (b) A subperiosteal tunnel. (c) After 3 months of healing.

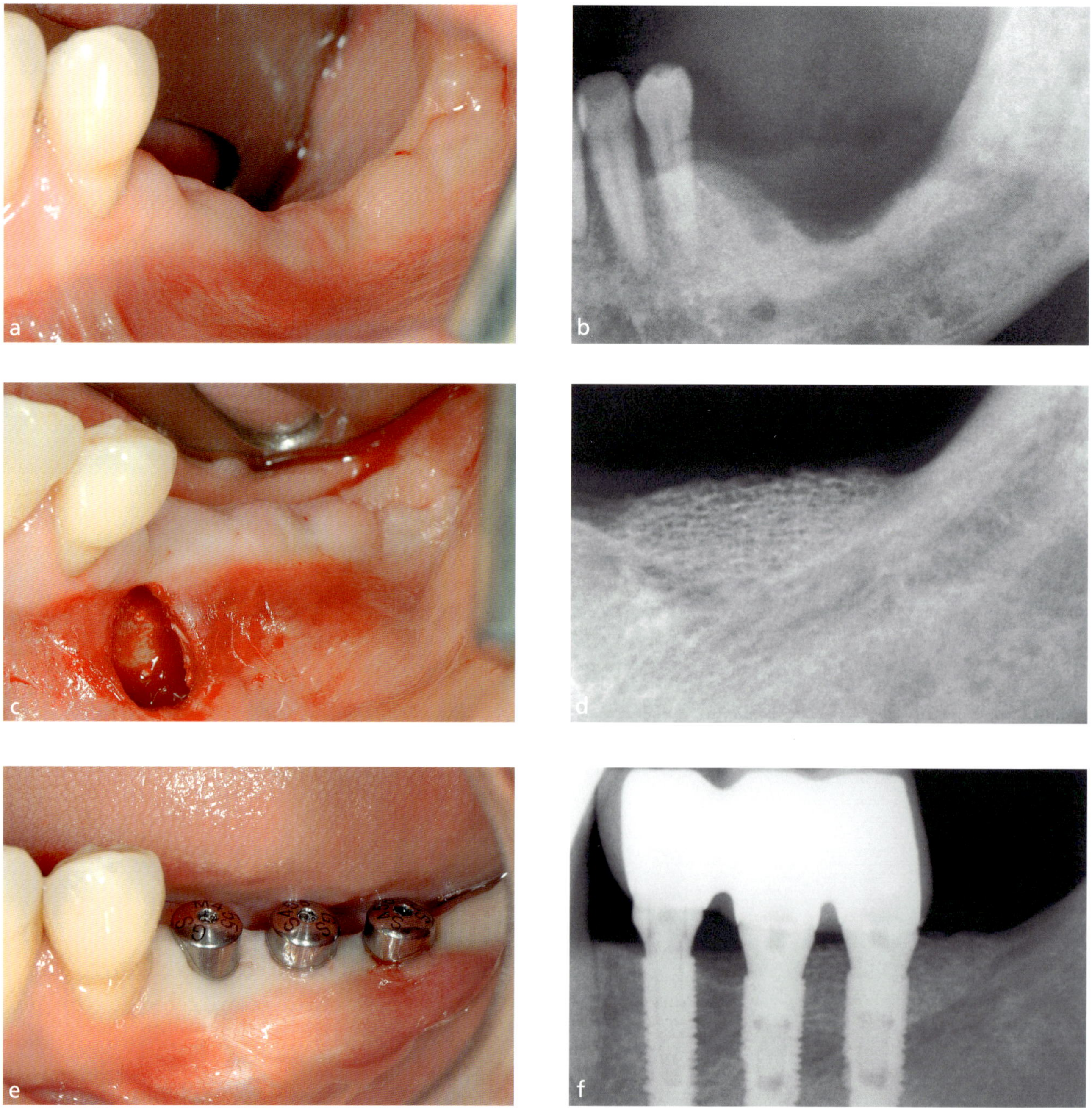

Fig 2-25 In the case of vertical bone resorption, the flapless implant placement is delayed as a secondary procedure after vertical ridge augmentation using the subperiosteal tunneling procedure. (a) Intraoral view of the missing teeth in the left posterior mandible. (b) Radiograph of the patient. (c) Intraoperative view of vertical augmentation using a Bio-Oss® block. (d) Radiograph after 6 months. (e) Immediately after flapless implant placement. (f) One year later.

procedure (Fig 2-25). Placement of a bone graft material on the implant surface using the subperiosteal tunnel technique can be controlled endoscopically. Figure 2-26 shows an exposed implant surface and augmentation with bone particles via a subperiosteal tunnel.

Contamination of the implant by soft tissue contact

The implant surface may be contaminated by soft tissue contact during the flapless implant procedure (Fig 2-27). Some authors have argued that it is important to avoid contamination of the implant surface with bacteria and biological molecules: that is, to avoid saliva and foreign

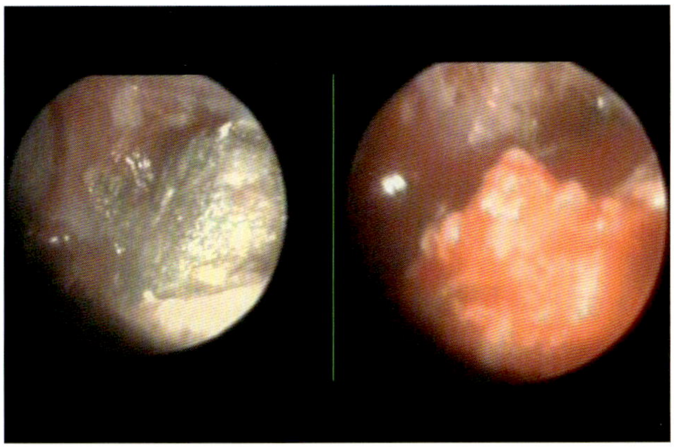

Fig 2-26 Augmentation of an exposed implant surface (left) with graft material (right).

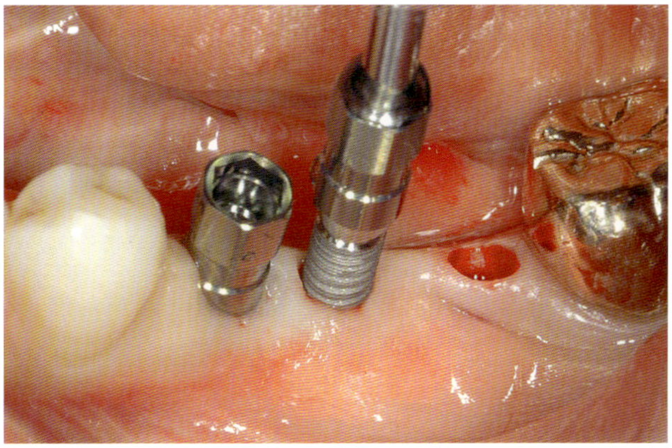

Fig 2-27 The implant surface can be contaminated by soft tissue contact during the flapless implant procedure. However, the soft tissue does not prevent osseointegration.

body contamination during the surgical insertion of implants in the jaws.[31] To prevent contamination of the implant surface, the mucoperiosteum is elevated to expose the underlying bone and keep the mucosa away from the implants during surgical insertion in the jaw.

In contrast, Ivanoff et al.[32] reported that preoperative soft tissue contamination of titanium implants does not prevent osseointegration. They examined the differences in bony contact between biologically contaminated implants and standard controls. There were no major morphological differences between the control and test sites with regard to their bone or marrow structures and bone–implant contacts. Esposito et al.[33] reported that clinical observations and experimental evidence failed to indicate any soft tissue contact-related causes for implant failures.

Our study of the effect of soft tissue contamination on osseointegration produced results similar to those of Ivanoff et al. and Esposito et al. (Fig 2-28). Nevertheless, the following form of management is recommended for flapless implant surgery: meticulous preoperative disinfection should be performed, particularly in the area of the mucosa through which the implants pass (Fig 2-29). It is also recommended that soft tissue should not be inserted into the bone holes during implant placement (Fig 2-30).

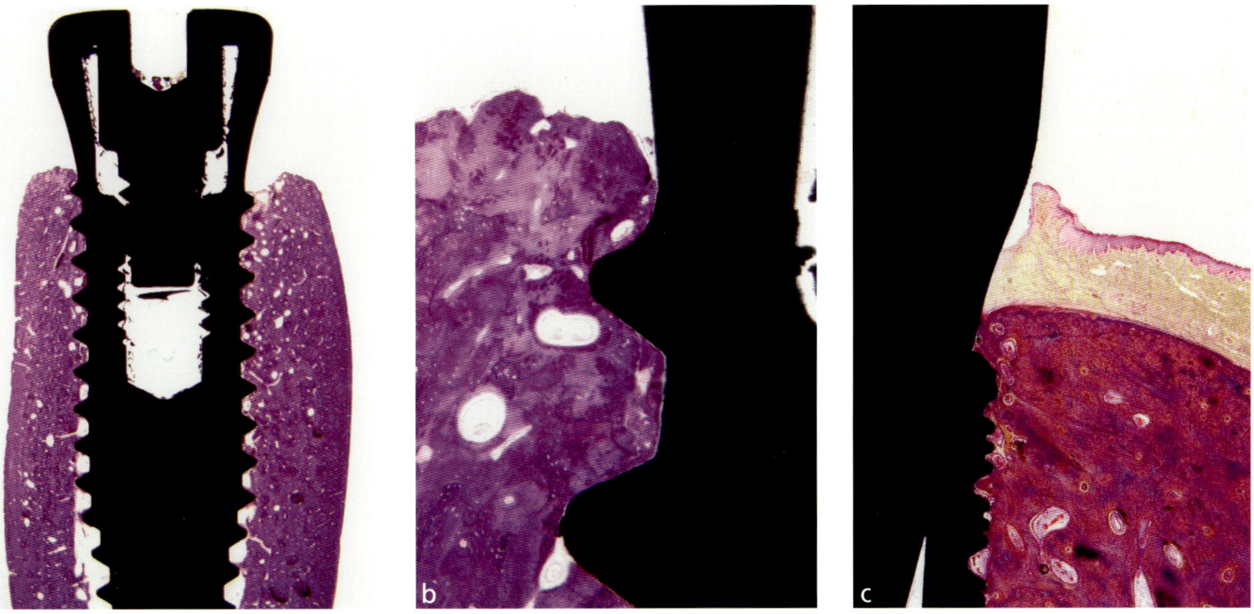

Fig 2-28 (a–c) Experimental evidence failed to indicate any soft tissue contact-related causes for implant failures. Note the osseointegration and soft tissue attachment around the implant 3 months after flapless implant placement.

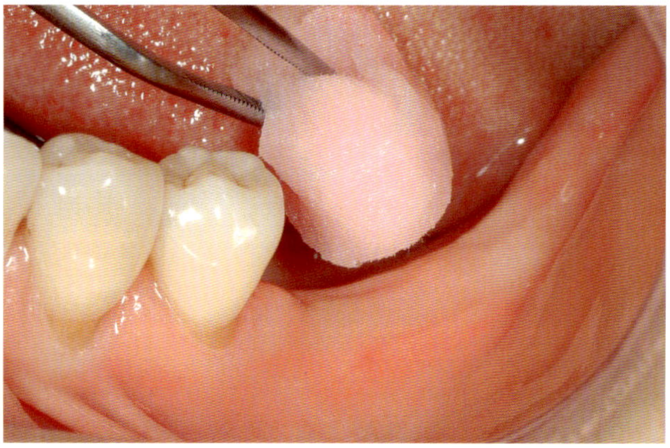

Fig 2-29 It is advisable to avoid contamination of the implant surface with bacteria and biological molecules – i.e. to avoid saliva and foreign-body contamination during surgical insertion of implants. Meticulous preoperative disinfection should be performed, particularly in the area of the mucosa through which the implants pass.

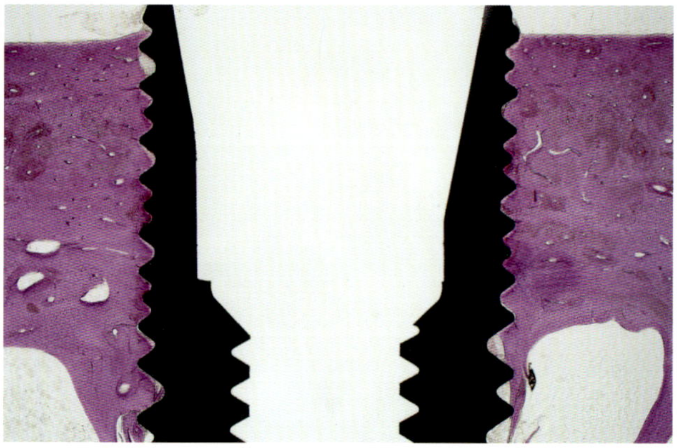

Fig 2-30 View of a specimen immediately after implant placement showing that soft tissue has not been inserted into the bone holes during the flapless procedure.

Summary

The flapless implant procedure is performed in the attached mucosa without reflecting the crestal soft tissue. The rationale for flapless implant surgery is to protect the soft tissue and ensure favorable conditions for the healing of soft tissue adjacent to the implant. The advantages of flapless procedures include a shorter procedure time, as well as a decrease in intraoperative bleeding and postoperative patient discomfort. Wounds around the implants heal quickly with little scar formation. It also increases resistance to postoperative infections by preserving the vessels around the implants. Flapless implant surgery is recommended for its advantages, even though there is some difficulty in evaluating the alveolar bone shape and angulation during the procedure. Furthermore, it is important to find a new technique to extend the use of flapless procedures in implant surgery.

References

1. Homans J. A Textbook of Surgery. Springfield, IL: Charles C Thomas, 1945:1–30.
2. Sabiston DC, Lyerly HK. Textbook of Surgery: The Biological Basis of Modern Surgical Practice. Philadelphia, PA: WB Saunders, 1997:207–220.
3. Mathes SJ. Plastic Surgery. Philadelphia, PA: Saunders Elsevier, 2006; 209–234.
4. Misch CE. Contemporary Implant Dentistry, ed 3. St Louis: Mosby, 2008:68–91.
5. Berglundh T, Lindhe J, Jonsson K, Ericsson I. The topography of vascular systems in the periodontal and peri-implant tissues in the dog. J Clin Periodontol 1994;21:189–193.
6. Abrahamsson I, Berglundh T, Wennström J, Lindhe J. The peri-implant hard and soft tissues at different implant systems: a comparative study in the dog. Clin Oral Implants Res 1996;7:212–219.
7. Berglundh T, Lindhe J, Ericsson I, Marinello C, Liljenberg B, Thomsen P. The soft tissue barrier at implants and teeth. Clin Oral Implants Res 1991;2:81–90.
8. Buser D, Weber HP, Donath K, Fiorellini JP, Paquette DW, Williams RC. Soft tissue reactions to non-submerged unloaded titanium implants in beagle dogs. J Periodontol 1992;63:226–236.
9. Kim JI, Choi BH, Li J, Xuan F, Jeong SM. Blood vessels of the peri-implant mucosa: a comparison between the flap and flapless procedures. Oral Surg Oral Med Oral Pathol Oral Radiol Endod 2009;107:508–512.
10. Bell WH. Biologic basis for maxillary osteotomies. Am J Phys Anthropol 1973;38:279–290.
11. Bell WH. Revascularization and bone healing after anterior maxillary osteotomy: a study using adult rhesus monkeys. J Oral Surg 1969;27:249–255.
12. Bradley JC. Age changes in the vascular supply of the mandible. Br Dent J 1972;132:142–144.
13. Bradley JC. A radiological investigation on the age changes of the inferior dental artery. Br J Oral Surg 1975;13:82–90.
14. Kleinheinz J, Büchter A, Kruse-Lösler B, Weingart D, Joos U. Incision design in implant dentistry based on the vascularization of the mucosa. Clin Oral Implants Res 2005;16:518–523.
15. Berglundh T, Lindhe J. Dimension of the peri-implant mucosa: biological width revisited. J Clin Periodontol 1996;23:971–973.
16. You TM, Choi BH, Li J, Xuan F, Jeong SM, Jang SO. Morphogenesis of the peri-implant mucosa: a comparison between flap and flapless procedures in the canine mandible. Oral Surg Oral Med Oral Pathol Oral Radiol Endod 2009;107:66–70.
17. Becker W, Becker BE, Newman MG. Clinical and microbiologic findings that may contribute to dental implant failure. Int J Oral Maxillofac Implants 1990;5:31–38.
18. Lemperle SM, Calhoun CJ, Curran RW, Holmes RE. Bony healing of the large cranial and mandibular defect protection from soft tissue interposition: a comparative study of spontaneous bone regeneration, osteoconduction, and cancellous autografting in dogs. Plast Reconst Surg 1998;101:660–672.

19. Huh JY, Choi BH, Kim BY, Lee SrH, Zhu SJ, Jung JH. Critical size defect in the canine mandible. Oral Surg Oral Med Oral Pathol Oral Radiol Endod 2005;100:296–301.
20. Jeong SM, Choi BH, Li J et al. Flapless implant surgery: an experimental study. Oral Surg Oral Med Oral Pathol Oral Radiol Endod 2007:104;24–28.
21. Jeong SM, Choi BH, Li J, Ahn KM, Lee SH, Xuan F. Bone healing around implants following flap and mini-flap surgeries: a radiographic evaluation between stage I and stage II surgery. Oral Surg Oral Med Oral Pathol Oral Radiol Endod 2008:105;293–296.
22. Kan JY, Rungcharassaeng K, Ojano M, Goodacre CJ. Flapless anterior implant surgery: a surgical and prosthodontic rationale. Pract Periodont Aesthet Dent 2000;12:467–474.
23. Engelke W. In-situ examination of implant sites with support immersion endoscopy. Int J Oral Maxillofac Implants 2002;17:703–706.
24. Engelke W. Die Untersuchung von Implantatkavitäten mit der Stützimmersionsendoskopie. Z Zahnärztl Implantol 2002;18:36–40.
25. Rocci A, Martignoni M, Gottlow J. Immediate loading in the maxilla using flapless surgery, implants placed in predetermined positions, and prefabricated provisional restorations: a retrospective 3-year clinical study. J Clin Implant Dent Relat Res 2003;5(suppl 1):29–36.
26. Campelo LD, Camara JR. Flapless implant surgery: a 10-year clinical retrospective analysis. Int J Oral Maxillofac Implants 2002;17: 271–276.
27. Meyer U, Wiesmann HP, Runte C. Evaluation of accuracy of insertion of dental implants and prosthetic treatment by computer-aided navigation in minipigs. Br J Oral Maxillofac Surg 2003;41:102–108.
28. Fortin T, Champleboux G, Bianchi S, Buatois H, Coudert JL. Precision of transfer of preoperative planning for oral implants based on cone-beam CT-scan images through a robotic drilling machine. Clin Oral Implants Res 2002;13:651–656.
29. Jacobs R, Adriansens A, Naert I, Quirynen M, Hermans R, Van Steenberghe D. Predictability of reformatted computed tomography for pre-operative planning of endosseous implants. Dentomaxillofac Radiol 1999;28:37–41.
30. Jeong SM, Choi BH, Li J, Xuan F. Simultaneous flapless implant placement and peri-implant defect correction: an experimental pilot study in dogs. J Periodontol 2008;79:876–880.
31. Adell R, Lekholm U, Brånemark PI. Surgical procedures. In: Brånemark PI, Zarb GA, Albrektsson T (eds) Tissue-integrated Prostheses: Osseointegration in Clinical Dentistry. Chicago,IL: Quintessence, 2000.
32. Ivanoff CJ, Sennerby L, Lekholm U. Influence of soft tissue contamination on the integration of titanium implants. Clin Oral Implants Res 1996;7:128–132.
33. Esposito M, Hirsch JM, Lekholm U, Thomsen P. Biological factors contributing to failures of osseointegrated oral implants. I: Success criteria and epidemiology. Eur J Oral Sci 1998;106:527–551.

CHAPTER

3

Comparison of Soft Tissue Punch and Mini-incision Techniques

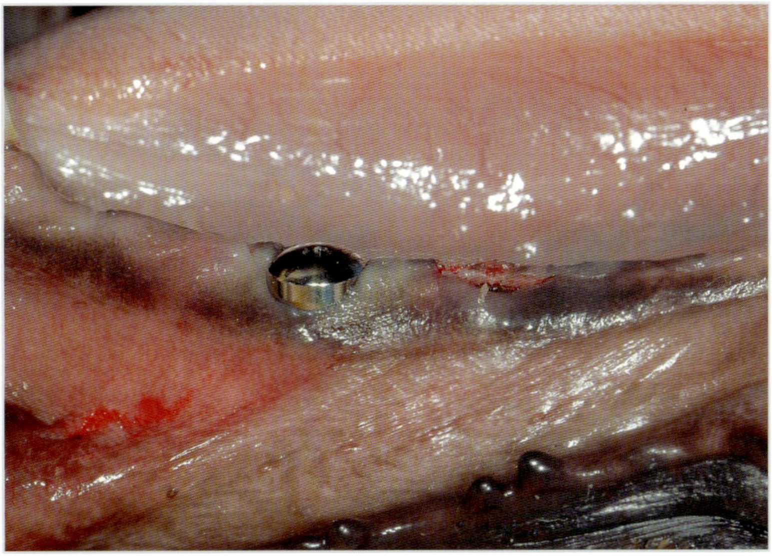

Key point

A mini-incision is a second flapless technique.

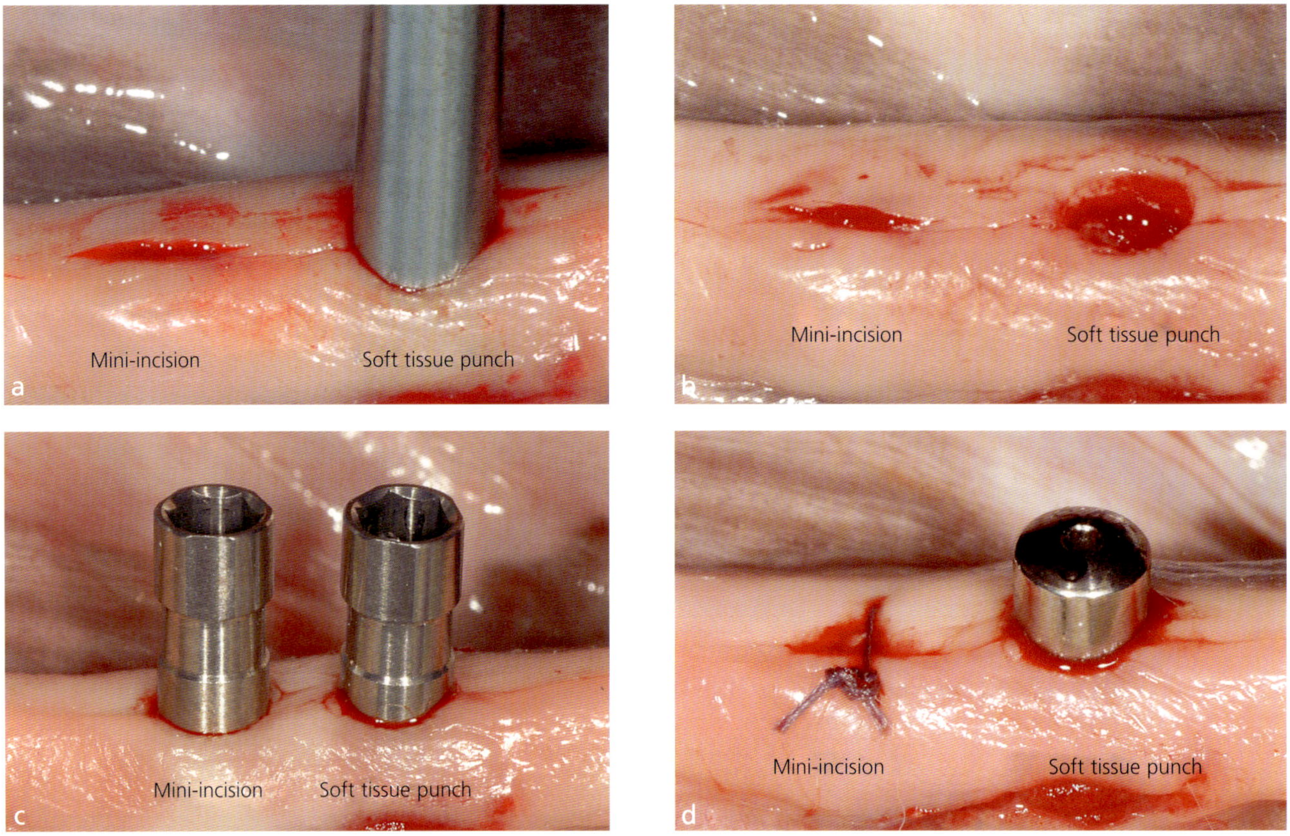

Fig 3-1 Clinical features of implant placement using a soft tissue punch or mini-incision. (a) The soft tissue is incised or is pierced with a punch. (b) Immediately after the incision and punch. (c) Immediately after implant placement. (d) The incised gingiva is sutured to submerge the fixture at the mini-incision site, and an abutment is connected to the fixture at the punch site.

Overview

Flapless implant surgery can be classified into two types, the soft tissue punch technique and the mini-incision technique (Fig 3-1). The first requires a circumferential incision in the gingiva at the center of the implant site with the removal of some attached gingiva (the size of the implant diameter). After implant placement, abutments are connected immediately to the fixtures such that the coronal portion of the abutments remains exposed to the oral cavity. In contrast, mini-incision implant placement requires a crestal mini-incision and local undermining (the range of the implant diameter) at the implant site. After implant placement, the crestal incision is closed, submerging the implant. The soft tissue punch technique is used for a one-stage surgical approach, whereas the mini-incision technique is used for either a one-stage or a two-stage surgical approach. The two-stage surgical process places the implant body below the soft tissue until bone healing has occurred. The choice is dependent on the bone quality and primary implant stability. In general, either a soft tissue punch nonsubmerged or a mini-incision nonsubmerged procedure is used for the mandible with thick cortical bone and a highly stable primary implant, while the mini-incision submerged procedure is used for the posterior maxillae with either poor bone quality or a relatively unstable primary implant. This chapter addresses the healing process for the bone and soft tissue around the implants installed using these procedures. Flapless implant surgery using these two techniques is described in more detail in Chapter 5.

Comparison of peri-implant bone loss

It is unclear whether nonsubmerged or submerged healing provides a better prognosis for dental implants. Levy et al.[1] examined healing around both submerged and nonsubmerged implants in beagles and reported that the "bone-to-implant contact" was greater in the submerged implants than in the nonsubmerged implants. However, some studies reported that the osseointegration achieved by these two implant methodologies is almost identical.[2–6] It is generally believed that there are no differences in

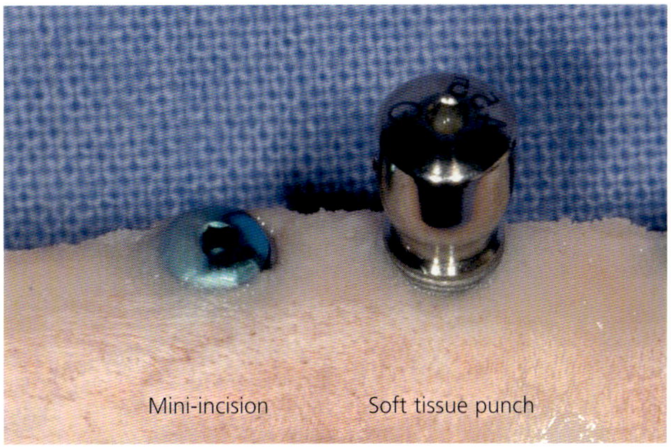

Fig 3-2 Mandible showing the peri-implant bone 3 months after implant placement using mini-incision submerged and soft tissue punch nonsubmerged techniques. Note that new bone is formed above the rough/smooth border on mini-incision submerged implants.

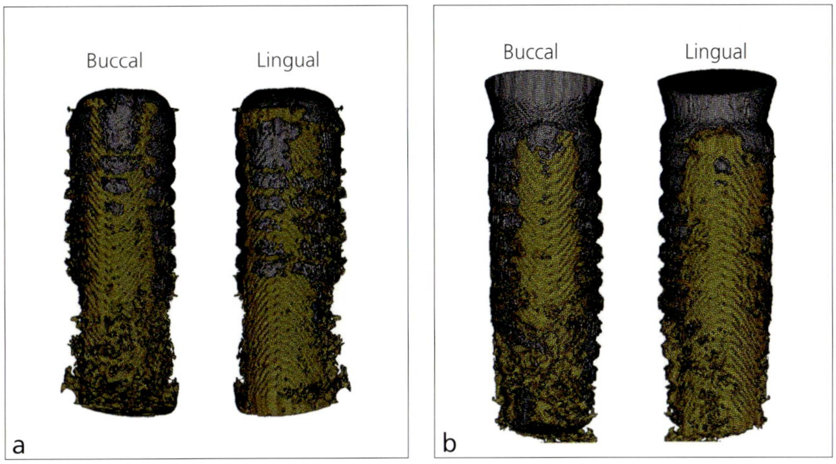

Fig 3-3 Three-dimensional micro-CT showing that the mini-incision submerged implants (a) have higher peri-implant bone levels compared with the soft tissue punch nonsubmerged implants (b).

Table 3-1 Peri-implant bone levels 3 months and 5 months after implant placement using mini-incision submerged and soft tissue punch nonsubmerged techniques.

Months	Bone height (mm)		*P* value
	Soft tissue punch nonsubmerged group (n = 12)	Mini-incision submerged group (n = 12)	
3	9.8 ± 0.4	10.3 ± 0.5	< .05
5	9.6 ± 0.4	9.8 ± 0.3	> .05

peri-implant bone loss between the submerged and nonsubmerged implants based on studies that evaluated the implants placed with flap elevation.[7–11] Based on a review of the current literature, there are no reports on the influence of flapless submerged or nonsubmerged implant surgery on bone loss around the implants. We have examined the effects of flapless nonsubmerged and submerged surgery on changes in the crestal bone in a canine mandible model.[12] In particular, one group of implants was nonsubmerged using the soft tissue punch technique, while the other group of implants was submerged using the mini-incision technique. At 3 months (from stage I to stage II surgeries), the submerged implants had significantly higher peri-implant bone levels than the nonsubmerged implants (Figs 3-1 to 3-3; Table 3-1). These results suggest that when implants are submerged with mini-incision surgery, the bone height around the implants in the early phase after implant placement is significantly greater than when the implants are not submerged. One interesting finding was the formation of new bone above the rough/smooth border on the submerged implants (see Fig 3-2), suggesting that bone loss is related to the exposure of implants through the mucosa after implant placement.

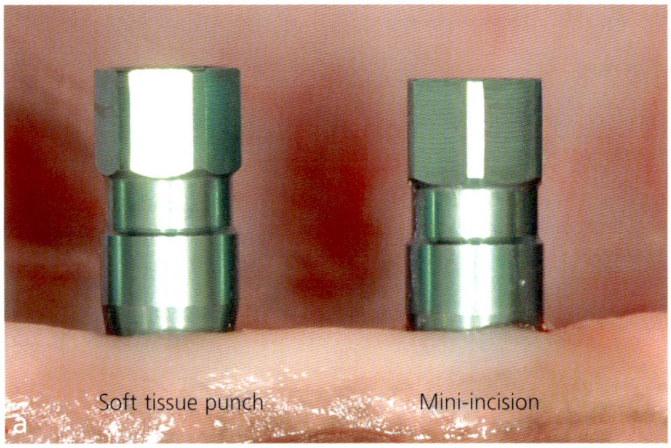

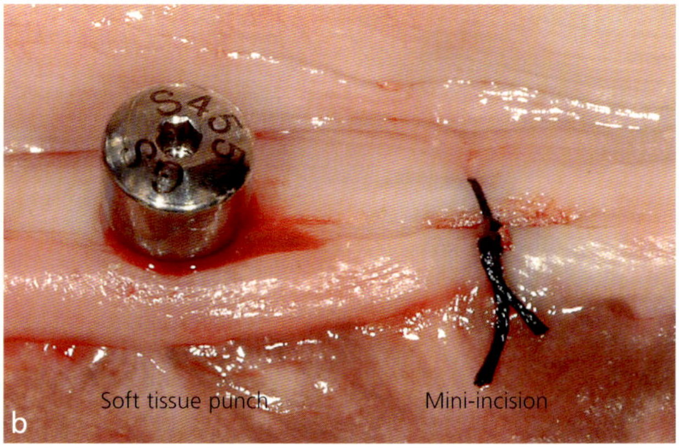

Fig 3-4 Clinical features of implant placement using soft tissue punch or mini-incision techniques. (a) Soft tissue immediately after implant placement. (b) An abutment is connected to the fixture at the punch site, and the incised gingiva is sutured to submerge the fixture at the mini-incision site.

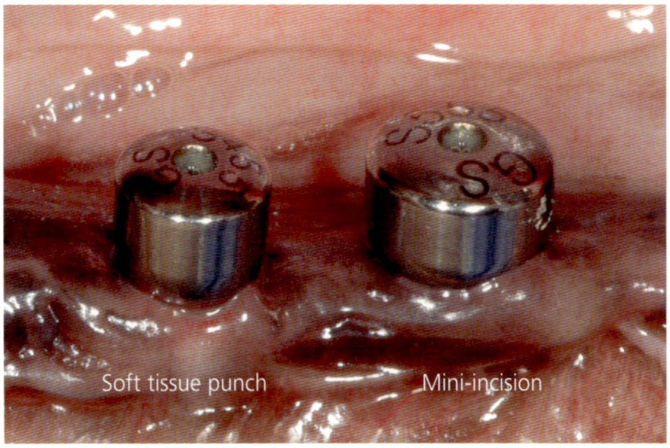

Fig 3-5 Three months after implant placement, second-stage surgery and transmucosal abutment connection is performed for the mini-incision submerged implants.

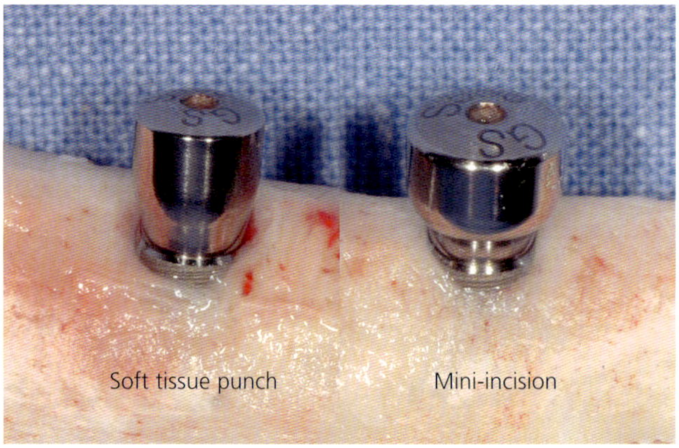

Fig 3-6 Mandible showing the peri-implant bone 5 months after implant placement (2 months after stage II surgery) using soft tissue punch (left) and mini-incision (right).

The peri-implant bone levels for the soft tissue punch and mini-incision approaches were also compared from stage I surgery to 5 months. After 3 months, second-stage surgery and transmucosal abutment attachment was performed for the implants that had been submerged using the mini-incision technique. The changes in the crestal bone were evaluated after a 2-month healing period (5 months after stage I surgery). With respect to differences between the soft tissue punch and mini-incision procedures, there were no significant changes in the peri-implant bone levels during the healing period (stage I to 5 months after surgery). With the mini-incision submerged implants, there was no bone loss around the implants within the osseointegration period between the stage I and II surgeries. However, a small amount of bone resorption was observed after reentry surgery and attachment of the transmucosal abutment. With the soft tissue punch nonsubmerged implants, a small amount of bone loss occurred immediately after implant placement, which then stabilized (Figs 3-4 to 3-7; see Table 3-1).

Although there were no differences in the overall degree of peri-implant bone loss between soft tissue punch nonsubmerged and mini-incision submerged approaches, the mini-incision approach was more effective in improving the implant anchorage in the early phase after implant placement. In addition, the small amount of bone loss that occurred after both the soft tissue punch and mini-incision methods was related to the exposure of the implants through the mucosa after implant placement.

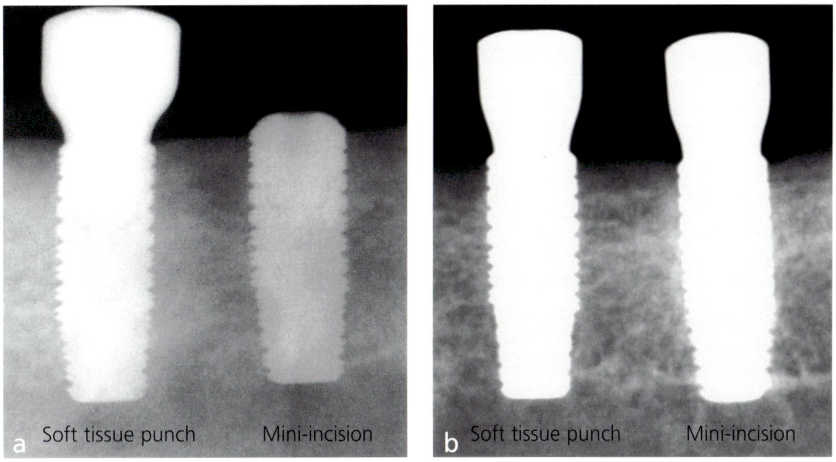

Fig 3-7 Radiographs showing that the soft tissue punch and mini-incision techniques produce similar changes in the peri-implant bone levels during the healing period, from immediately (a) to 5 months (b) after implant placement.

Comparison of peri-implant soft tissue

Experiments were carried out to compare the morphogenesis of the peri-implant mucosa between the soft tissue punch and mini-incision implant surgery using a canine mandible model. A one-stage surgical approach was used for soft tissue punch implant surgery, whereas a two-stage surgical approach was used for mini-incision implant surgery. The results suggest that there were no differences in the morphogenesis of the peri-implant mucosa (Fig 3-8). In addition, these results corroborate the previously reported data generated using the flap procedure in a canine model. In particular, the authors of the aforementioned study reported that there were no differences in histological behavior between the submerged and nonsubmerged implants.[13–16]

Advantages and disadvantages of the two techniques

Soft tissue punch

1. A second surgical procedure is unnecessary, thereby preventing additional patient discomfort.
2. Implants are not submerged at the time of placement.
3. Implants are not protected during the early phase of healing after placement, particularly for patients with poor bone quality and/or low primary implant stability.
4. Soft tissues mature while the bone interface is healing.
5. There exists the risk of loading during initial healing.
6. The soft tissue punch removes some of the keratinized mucosa.

Mini-incision

1. Implants can be either submerged or nonsubmerged at the time of implant placement.
2. The mini-incision can help to save the keratinized mucosa (Fig 3-9).
3. The submerged mini-incision procedure may result in less crestal bone loss during the early phase of healing after implant placement.
4. The submerged mini-incision procedure reduces the risk of early loading during initial healing after implant placement.
5. Primary closure of the soft tissues improves the environment to grow bone into a bone graft site. Hence, the submerged mini-incision procedure is indicated under these conditions.
6. A second surgical procedure is necessary to uncover the implant.
7. When the submerged mini-incision procedure is used, local hygiene issues are not critical factors for the rate of initial healing.
8. Spontaneous exposure of submerged implants to the oral environment after stage I surgery, but before stage II surgery, can be accompanied by early exudate, inflammation, and crestal bone loss.

Implant failure rate and peri-implant bone loss after surgery

Implant failure is commonly classified as either early or late. Early (primary) failures are those where there is an inability to establish osseointegration – all the failures that occur during the period between implant placement to abutment connection of the implant. Late (secondary)

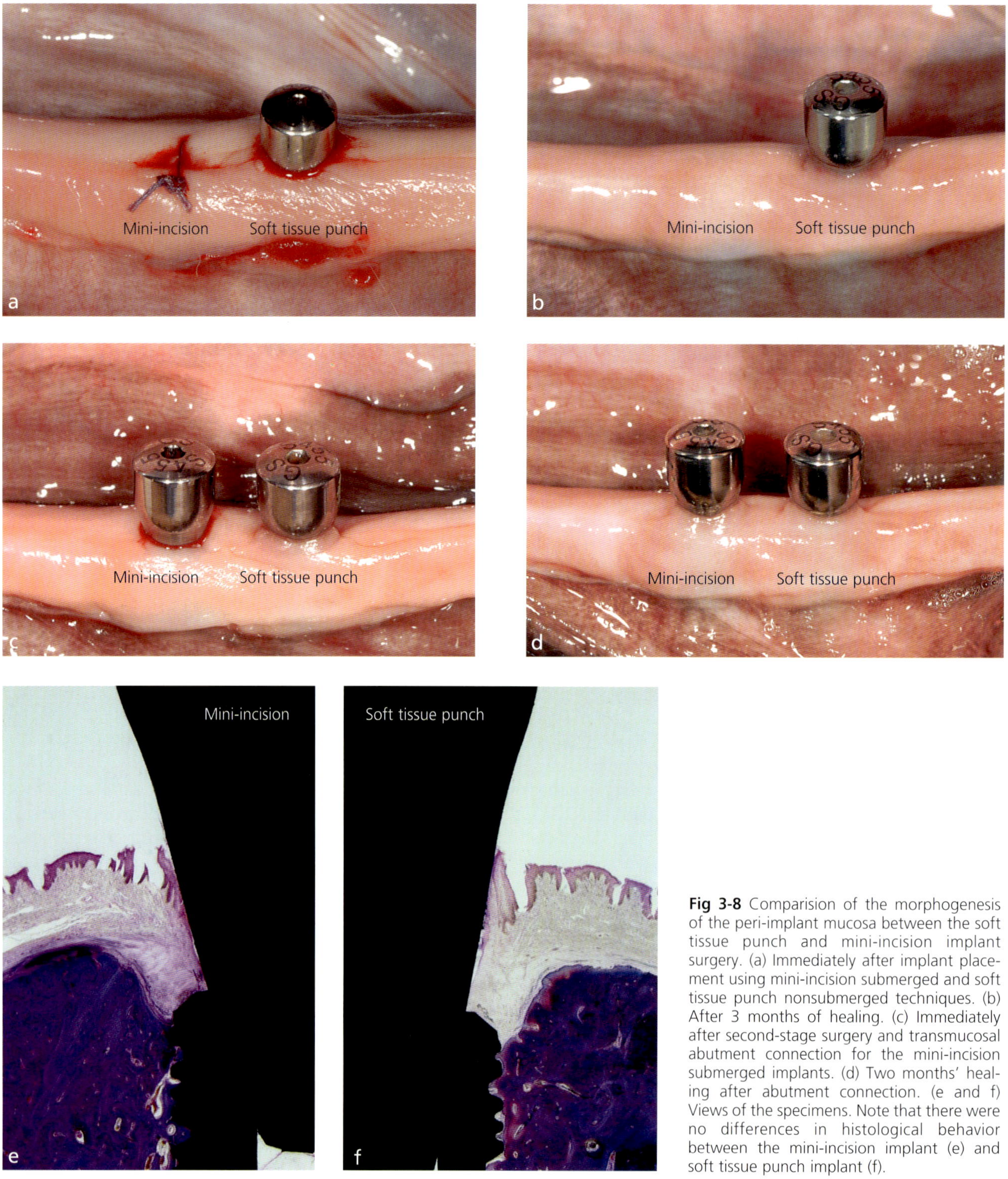

Fig 3-8 Comparision of the morphogenesis of the peri-implant mucosa between the soft tissue punch and mini-incision implant surgery. (a) Immediately after implant placement using mini-incision submerged and soft tissue punch nonsubmerged techniques. (b) After 3 months of healing. (c) Immediately after second-stage surgery and transmucosal abutment connection for the mini-incision submerged implants. (d) Two months' healing after abutment connection. (e and f) Views of the specimens. Note that there were no differences in histological behavior between the mini-incision implant (e) and soft tissue punch implant (f).

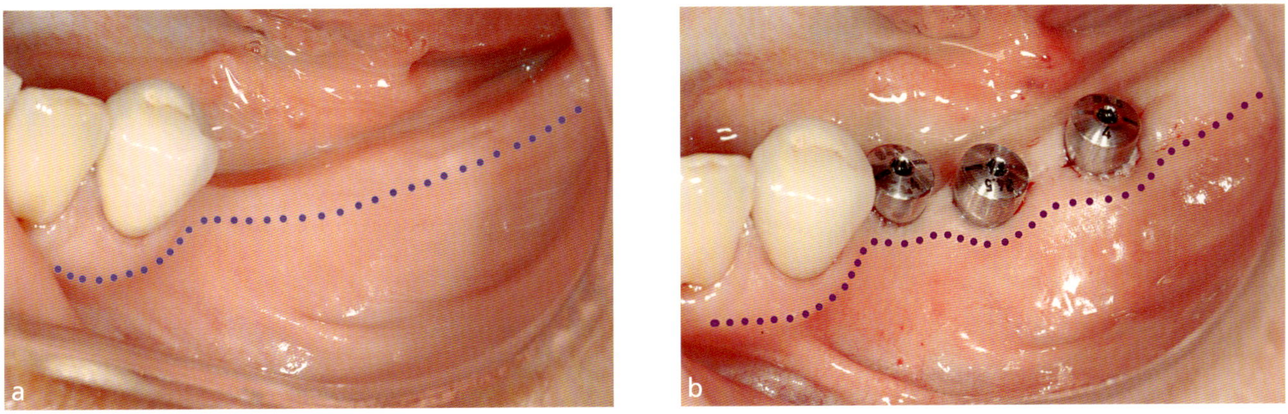

Fig 3-9 (a) Intraoral view of the missing teeth in the left posterior mandible. (b) Intraoral view immediately after implant placement using a mini-incision. The mini-incision technique is beneficial in saving the keratinized mucosa.

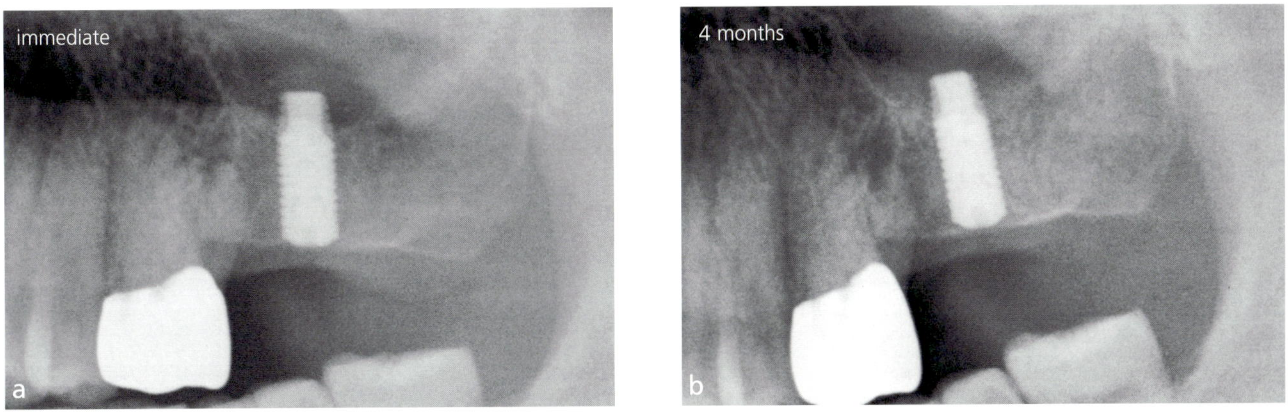

Fig 3-10 There is no bone loss around a mini-incision submerged implant within the osseointegration period between stage I (a) and stage II (b) surgery.

failures are those where there is an inability to maintain the established osseointgration – all the failures that occur after prosthetic rehabilitation.[17]

Failure rate and crestal bone loss in the early phase

A prospective clinical study was carried out to evaluate the implants with respect to failure rates and overall degree of peri-implant bone loss in the early phase after soft tissue punch nonsubmerged and mini-incision submerged implant surgery. Patients who required sinus grafting procedures were also included in this study. All patients were treated at the same university clinic, and all implants were placed by the same surgeon. The secondary procedures were initiated at 3 months (mandible) and 4 months (maxilla) after implant installation. In the second surgery, conventional dental radiographs were taken and the stability of the implant was evaluated. Osseointegration occurred in all 213 patients with 432 implants with no failures (Table 3-2). The average bone loss was 0.4 mm in the soft tissue punch nonsubmerged group and 0.1 mm in the mini-incision submerged group (Figs 3-10 to 3-12). This difference was statistically significant ($P < .05$). The perfect success rate that was achieved in this study confirms the advantages of flapless implant surgery.

Failure rate and crestal bone loss in the late phase

A prospective clinical study was also carried out to determine the late failure rates after soft tissue punch nonsubmerged or mini-incision submerged implant surgery. For all patients in this study, the placement of implants was performed by the same surgeon. For the 2 years after their implant placement, the implants were evaluated with respect to the failure rate and peri-implant bone loss. For an assessment of peri-implant bone loss, conventional dental radiographs were taken immediately after placement and 2 years later. Comparison of the films from these two dates indicated that osseointegration occurred in all 142 implants in 83 patients with no failures (Table 3-3).

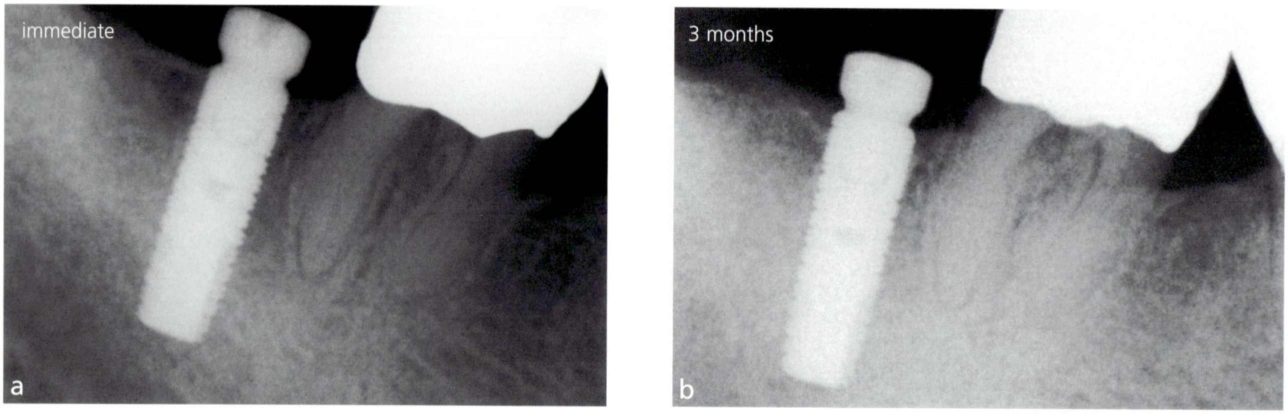

Fig 3-11 A small amount of bone resorption is observed around the soft tissue punch implant within the osseointegration period between stage I (a) and stage II (b) surgery.

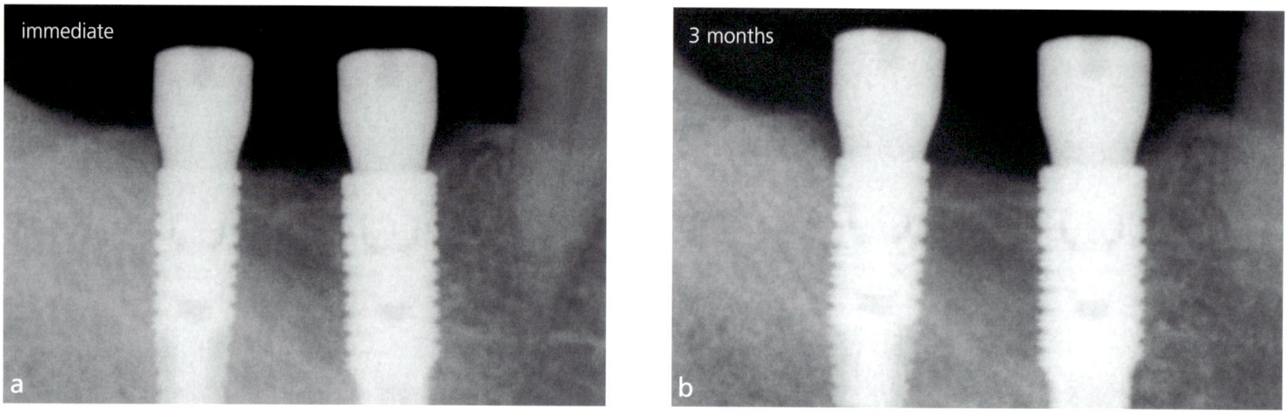

Fig 3-12 A small amount of bone resorption is observed around the soft tissue punch implant within the osseointegration period between (a) stage I and (b) stage II surgery.

Table 3-2 Failure rate and crestal bone loss in the early phase after soft tissue punch nonsubmerged and mini-incision submerged implant surgery.

	Soft tissue punch nonsubmerged group (n = 201)	Mini-incision submerged group (n = 231)	*P* value
Number of failed implants	0	0	
Marginal bone loss (mm ± SD)	0.4 ± 0.2	0.1 ± 0.1	< .05

The average bone loss was 0.4 mm in the soft tissue punch group and 0.3 mm in the mini-incision group (Figs 3-13 and 3-14). This difference was not significant ($P < .05$).

The success criteria for implants proposed by Albrektsson et al.[18] are used widely. Under these criteria, one of the major determinants of implant success is bone loss around the implants as measured annually. According to these success criteria, the average marginal bone loss should be less than 1.5 mm during the first year of function and less than 0.2 mm annually thereafter. The clinical study discussed showed remarkably less bone loss than that proposed as acceptable by Albrektsson et al.[18] Similarly, the failure rate and the rate of bone loss were considerably lower than in other published reports, further confirming the advantages of flapless implant surgery.

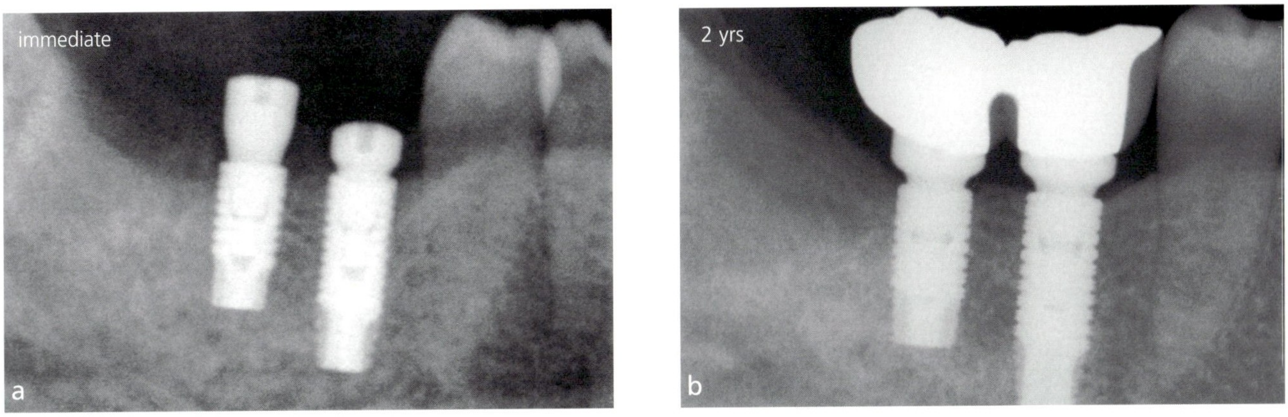

Fig 3-13 Radiographs showing the change in the peri-implant bone-levels from immediately (a) to 2 years (b) after soft tissue punch implant surgery.

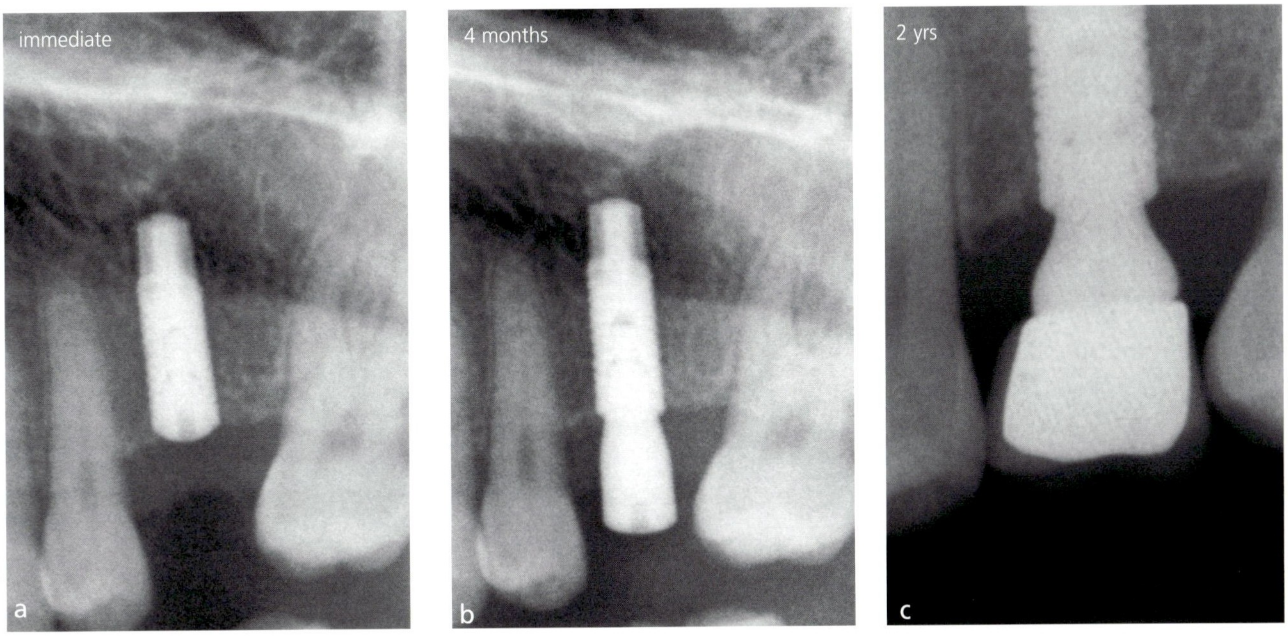

Fig 3-14 Radiographs showing changes in the peri-implant bone levels, immediately (a) 4 months (b) and 2 years (c) after mini-incision submerged implant surgery.

Table 3-3 Failure rate and crestal bone loss two years after soft tissue punch and mini-incision implant surgery.

	Soft tissue punch nonsubmerged group (n = 61)	Mini-incision submerged group (n = 81)	*P* value
Number of failed implants	0	0	
Marginal bone loss (mm ± SD)	0.4 ± 0.3	0.3 ± 0.2	> .05

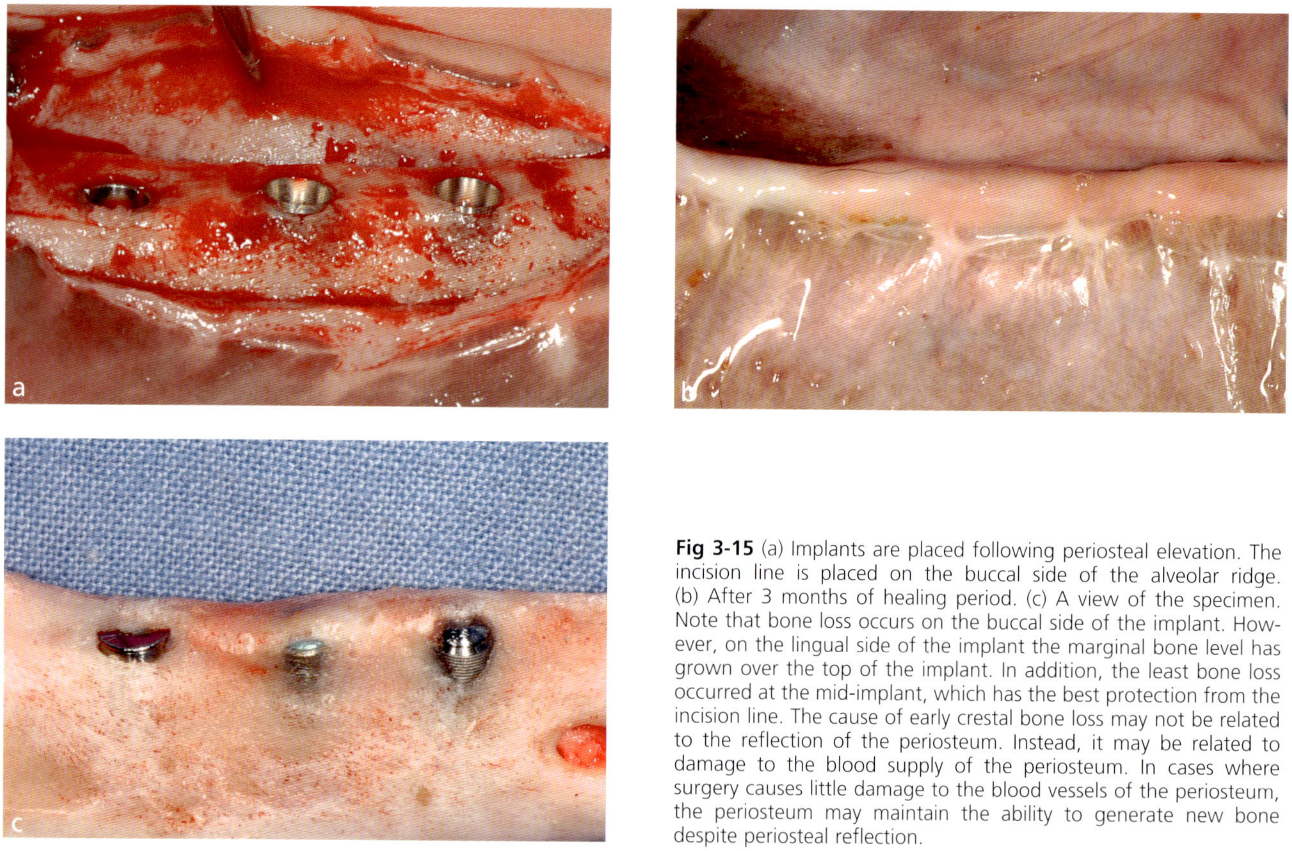

Fig 3-15 (a) Implants are placed following periosteal elevation. The incision line is placed on the buccal side of the alveolar ridge. (b) After 3 months of healing period. (c) A view of the specimen. Note that bone loss occurs on the buccal side of the implant. However, on the lingual side of the implant the marginal bone level has grown over the top of the implant. In addition, the least bone loss occurred at the mid-implant, which has the best protection from the incision line. The cause of early crestal bone loss may not be related to the reflection of the periosteum. Instead, it may be related to damage to the blood supply of the periosteum. In cases where surgery causes little damage to the blood vessels of the periosteum, the periosteum may maintain the ability to generate new bone despite periosteal reflection.

Causes of early bone loss

An understanding of the causes of early crestal bone loss around the dental implants is critical to prevent such occurrences. Several hypotheses have been suggested, ranging from reflection of the periosteum during surgery, preparation of the implant osteotomy, bacterial invasion, the establishment of a biological width, and the presence of stress factors.[19–24]

Periosteal reflection hypothesis

The cortical bone blood supply is affected dramatically when the periosteum is reflected off the crestal bone, resulting in osteoblast death on the surface from both trauma and lack of nutrition. These events support the periosteal reflection theory as a cause for the early bone loss around an implant.[24] The periosteal reflection theory suggests that generalized horizontal bone loss of the entire reflected residual ridge should occur instead of localized ditching around the implant. In addition, this hypothesis suggests that generalized bone loss is already directly noticeable at the second-stage procedure to uncover the implant body, which is generally 4 months after stage I implant placement surgery. However, such generalized bone loss is rarely observed at the second-stage surgery. Instead, new bone can be found on the cover screws of the implants in some cases. Therefore, periosteal reflection does not appear to be the primary causal agent of the marginal crestal bone loss around an implant.

It is believed that the bone loss caused by periosteal reflection may depend on the degree of periosteal vessel breakdown. Bone loss occurs in cases where there is severe damage to the blood supply of the periosteum. However, the periosteum maintains its ability to generate new bone despite periosteal reflection in patients where surgery causes little damage to the blood vessels of the periosteum (Fig 3-15).

Implant osteotomy hypothesis

The bones are sensitive to heat, which has led to the implant osteotomy theory to explain early implant bone loss. Implant osteotomy causes trauma to the bone immediately in contact with the implant, whereby an approximately 1 mm zone of devitalized bone is created around the implant.[25] Therefore, renewed blood supply is necessary to remodel the bone at the interface. The crestal

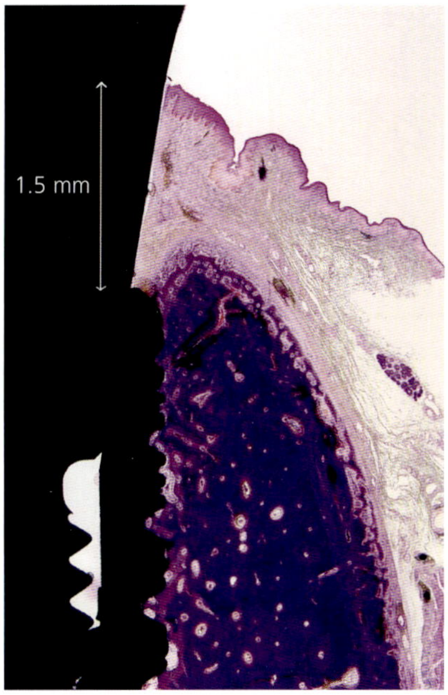

Fig 3-16 For the flapless implant, the implant–mucosa barrier comprises junctional epithelium and a connective tissue, which are less than 2 mm in height, and there is no bone loss around the implant. The biological width hypothesis cannot fully explain the absence of bone loss observed with flapless implant surgery.

region is more susceptible to bone loss during initial repair because of the limited blood supply and relatively greater amount of heat generated at this site owing to the higher bone density.[26,27] These effects should be noticeable during the procedure to uncover the implant body if heat and trauma during implant osteotomy preparation were responsible for the marginal crestal bone loss. However, most implants at the stage II procedure do not demonstrate any bone loss, and may even have new bone growing over the top of the implant. Therefore, it is highly unlikely that implant osteotomy is the primary force behind the early implant bone loss.

Bacteria hypothesis

The bacterial hypothesis suggests that the primary cause of bone loss around implants is bacterially induced. The gingival sulcus, into which the implant is placed, has bacterial flora similar to that of natural teeth. Therefore, a logical assumption is that, if the implants are similar to teeth, the marginal implant bone loss would be caused primarily by bacteria. However, if bacteria were the primary causal agent for initial bone loss, it is unclear why most bone loss occurs during the first year (1.5 mm), with less (0.1 mm) occurring each year thereafter. While the bacteria theory does not adequately explain the marginal crestal bone loss phenomenon, it does not necessarily rule out bacteria as a major contributor to the bone loss around an implant.

Biological width hypothesis

The implant–mucosa barrier comprises a junctional epithelium, approximately 2 mm in length, and a connective tissue compartment that ranges from approximately 1 to 1.5 mm in height. This soft tissue barrier constitutes a biological seal around the dental implants, the dimensions of which are called the biological width. According to the biological width hypothesis, bone loss occurs to create the space necessary for the biological width.[28,29] This theory cannot fully explain the absence of bone loss already observed after flapless implant surgery (Fig 3-16).

Authors' theory: inflammation, infection, and scarring

The major cause of early implant bone loss appears to be closely related to soft tissue wound healing because most early bone loss occurs around the nonsubmerged implants during the first 2 weeks after implant placement (Figs 3-17 to 3-20). The bone loss that occurs during the healing period is closely related to the degree and duration of inflammation and infection as well as the scar volume. In other words, the healing process is slowed if soft tissue wounds around the implants become infected during the period. Inflammation combined with significant scarring results in even more bone loss.

This hypothesis is supported by the results reported by Joly et al.[30] and Weber et al.,[31] who hypothesized that bone loss around nonsubmerged implants is related to connective tissue and is not influenced by the epithelial dimensions. These results also support the theory proposed by Berglund and Lindh,[28] who reported that bone loss occurs to generate the space necessary for the adaptation of the soft tissue zone. Therefore, early implant bone loss can be prevented or minimized if soft tissue wounds around the implants heal quickly with little inflammation and scar tissue formation.

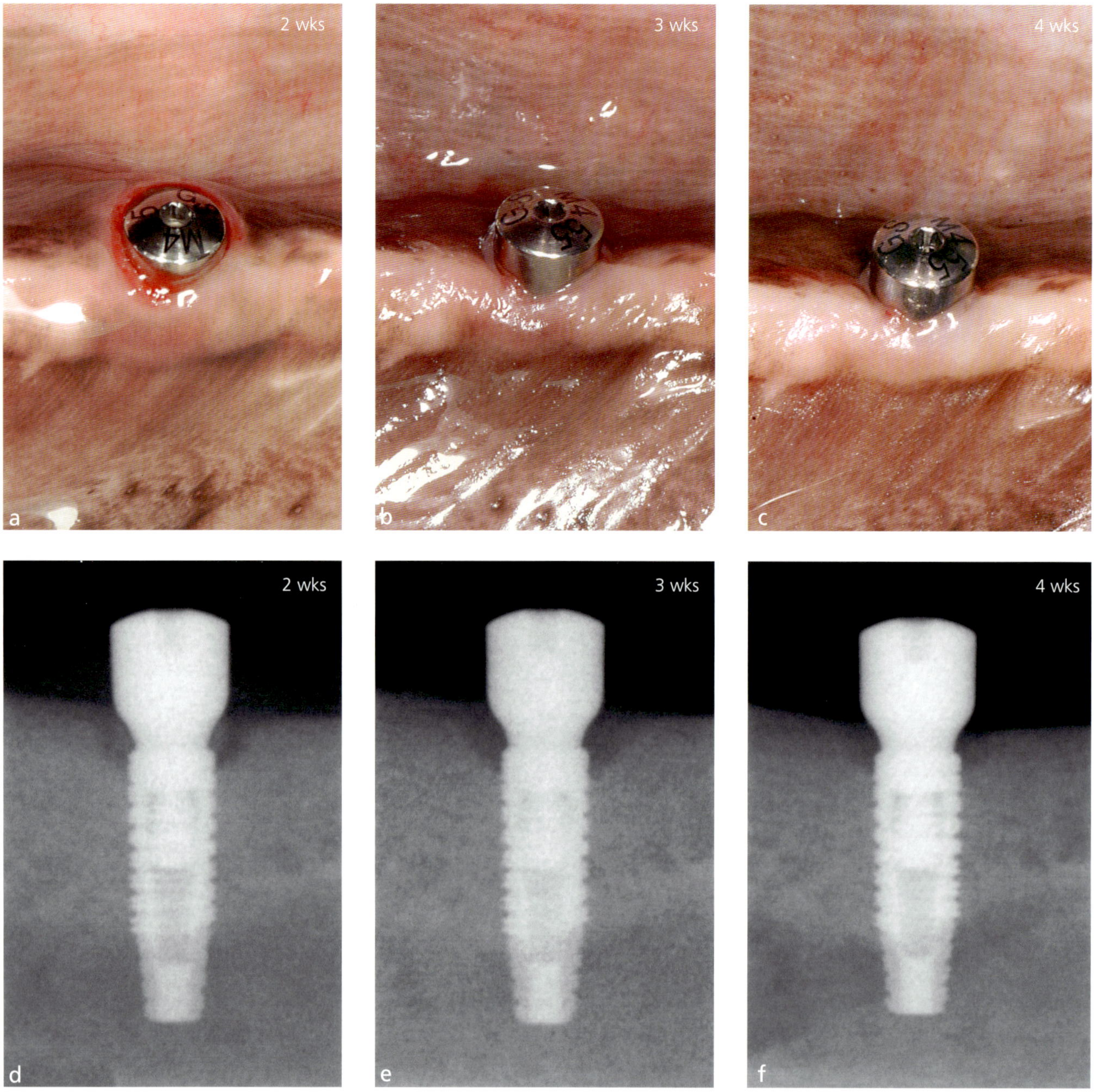

Fig 3-17 (a–f) Soft tissue condition and bone loss at intervals after nonsubmerged flapless implant placement. The soft tissue wound around the implant is in a poor condition during the first 2 weeks. Most bone loss around the implants occurs during the first 2 weeks. After that there is very little bone loss.

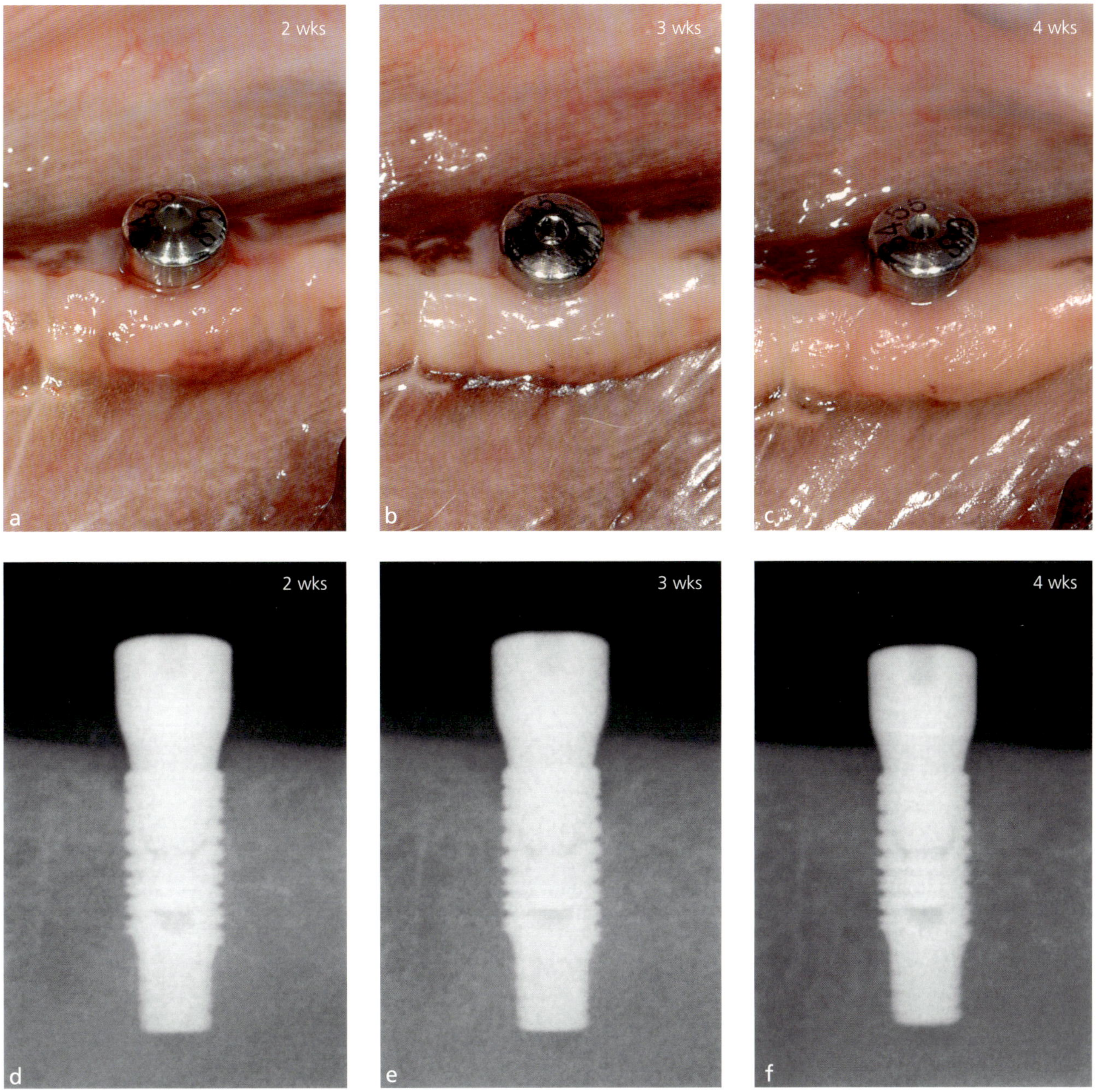

Fig 3-18 (a–f) Soft tissue condition and bone loss at intervals after nonsubmerged flapless implant placement. See also Fig 3-17. The bone loss is closely related to soft tissue healing.

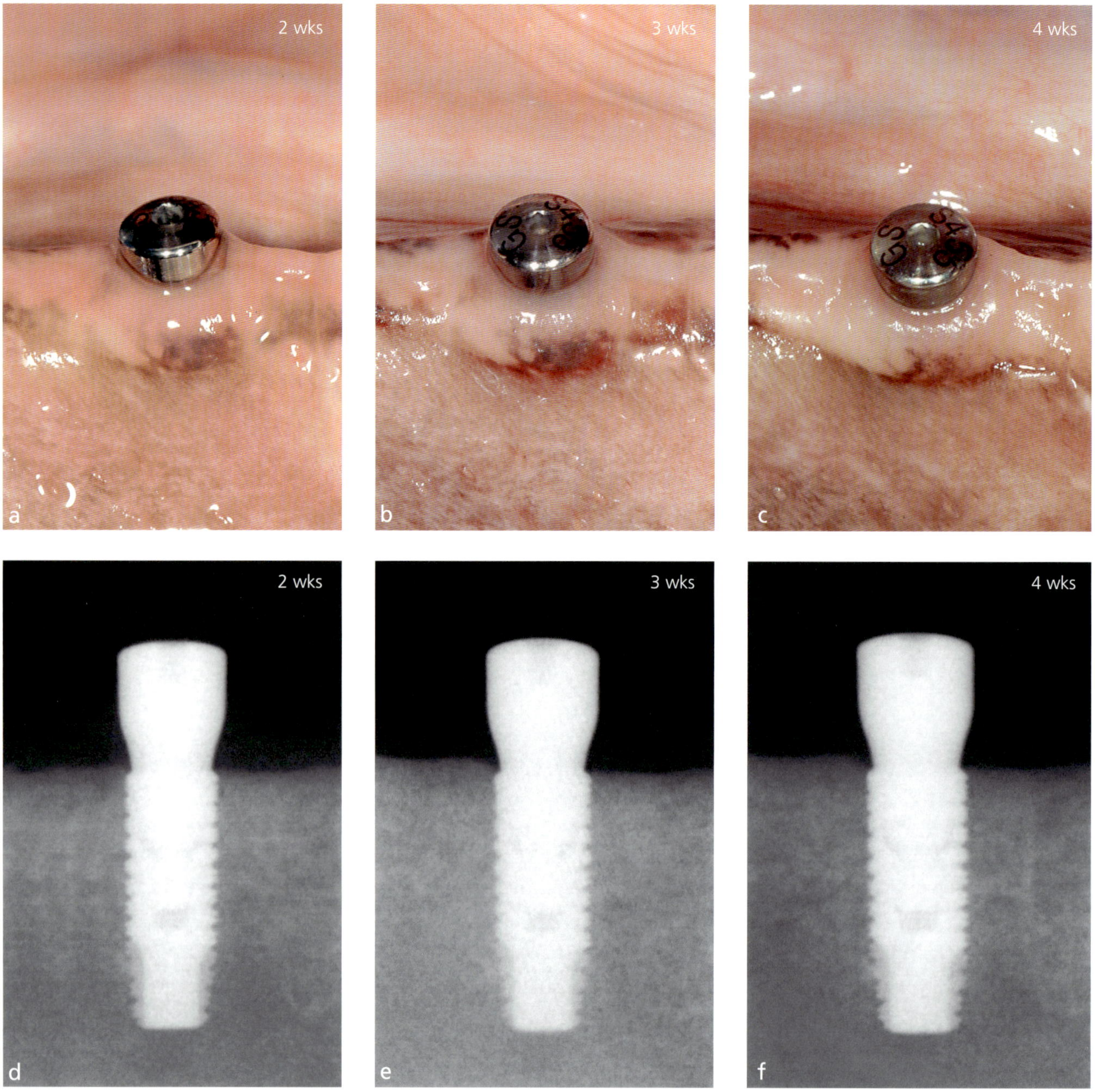

Fig 3-19 (a–f) Soft tissue condition and bone loss at intervals after nonsubmerged flapless implant placement. The soft tissue wound around the implant is in a good condition during the first 2 weeks. There is no bone loss during the first 2 weeks after implant placement. After 2 weeks there is still no bone loss around the implant.

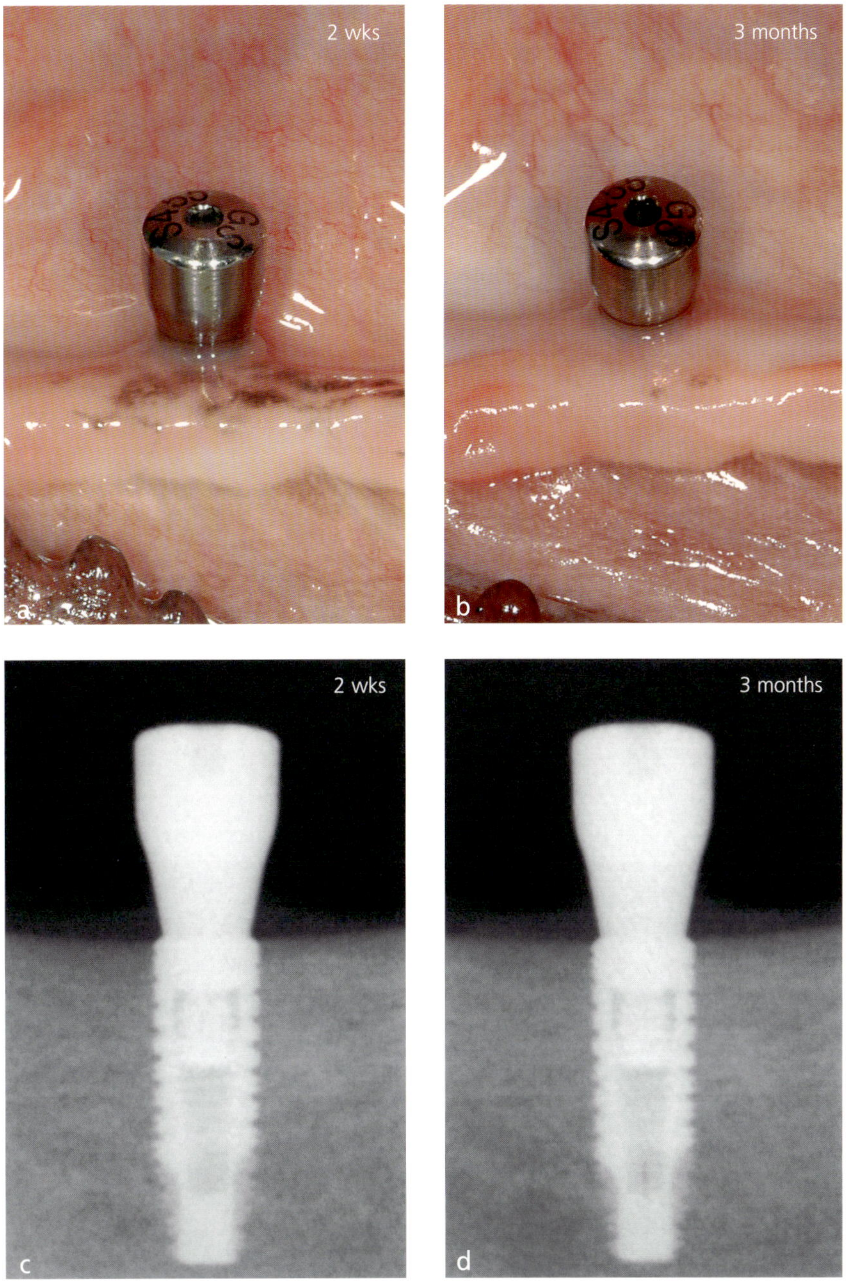

Fig 3-20 (a–d) Soft tissue condition and bone loss at intervals after nonsubmerged flapless implant placement. The soft tissue wound around the implant is in a good condition during the first 2 weeks. There is no bone loss during the first 2 weeks and after 3 months.

Summary

Bone height in the early phase after implant placement is significantly greater around mini-incision submerged implants than around soft tissue punch nonsubmerged implants. However, a small amount of bone resorption occurs in the mini-incision submerged implants after re-entry surgery and attachment of the transmucosal abutment. There were no differences in overall degree of peri-implant bone loss between the soft tissue punch and mini-incision techniques. In addition, there were no differences in the morphogenesis of the peri-implant mucosa between the soft tissue punch and mini-incision techniques.

References

1. Levy D, Deporter DA, Pillar RM, Watson PA, Valiquette N. Initial healing in the dog of submerged versus nonsubmerged porous-coated endosseous dental implants. Clin Oral Implants Res 1996;7:101–110.
2. Abrahamsson I, Berglundh T, Moon I-S, Lindhe J. Peri-implant tissues at submerged and non-submerged titanium implants. J Clin Perio 1999;26:600–607.
3. Ericsson I, Nilner K, Klinge B, Glantz PO. Radiographical and histological characteristics of submerged and non-submerged titanium implants: an experimental study in the Labrador dog. Clin Oral Implants Res 1996;7:20–26.
4. Ericsson I, Randow K, Glantz PO, Lindhe J, Nilner K. Clincal and radiographical features of submerged and non-submerged titanium implants. Clin Oral Implants Res 1994;5:183–189.
5. Ericsson I, Randow K, Nilner K, Petersson A. Some clinical and radiographical features of submerged and non-submerged titanium implants: a 5-year follow-up study. Clin Oral Implants Res 1997;8:422–426.
6. Weber HP, Buser D, Donath K et al. Comparison of healed tissues adjacent to submerged and non-submerged titanium dental implants: a histometric study in beagle dogs. Clin Oral Implants Res 1996;7:11–19.
7. Fiorellini JP, Buser D, Paquette DW, Williams RC, Haghighi D, Weber HP. A radiographic evaluation of bone healing around submerged and non-submerged dental implants in beagle dogs. J Periodontol 1999;70:248–254.
8. Gotfredsen K, Rostrup E, Hjorting-Hansen E, Stoltze K, Budtz-Jorgensen E. Histological and histomorphometrical evaluation of tissue reactions adjacent to endosteal implants in monkeys. Clin Oral Implants Res 1991;2:30–37.
9. Hermann JS, Buser D, Schenk RK, Cochran DL. Crestal bone changes around titanium implants: a histometric evaluation of unloaded non-submerged and submerged implants in the canine mandible. J Periodontol 2000;71:1412–1424.
10. Kohal RJ, LaRosa MD, Patrick D, Huerzeler MB, Caffesse RG. Clinical and histologic evaluation of submerged and nonsubmerged hydroxyapatite-coated implants: a preliminary study in dogs. Int J Oral Maxillofac Implants 1999;14:824–834.
11. Hermann JS, Cochran DL, Nummikoski PV, Buser D. Crestal bone changes around titanium implants: a radiographic evaluation of unloaded nonsubmerged and submerged implants in the canine mandible. J Periodontol 1997;68:1117–1130.
12. Choi BH, Li J, Kim HS, Ko CY, Jeong SM, Xuan F. Comparison of submerged and nonsubmerged implants placed without flap reflection in the canine mandible. Oral Surg Oral Med Oral Pathol Oral Radiol Endod 2008;105:561–565.
13. Buser D, Weber HP, Donath K, Fiorellini JP, Paquette DW, Williams RC. Soft tissue reactions to non-submerged unloaded titanium implants in the beagle dog. J Periodontol 1992;63:226-236.
14. Abrahamsson I, Berglundh T, Wennstrom J, Lindhe J. The peri-implant hard and soft tissues at different implant systems. Clin Oral Implants Res 1996;7:212–219.
15. Abrahamsson I, Berglundh T, Lindhe J. The mucosal barrier following abutment disconnection: an experimental study in dogs. J Clin Periodontol 1997;24:568–572.
16. Cochran DL, Hermann JS, Schenk RK, Higginbottom FL, Buser D. Biologic width around titanium implants: a histometric analysis of the implanto-gingival junction around unloaded and loaded non-submerged implants in the canine mandible. J Periodontol 1997;68:186–198.
17. Esposito M, Hirsch JM, Lekholm U. Thomsen P. Biological factors contributing to failures of osseointegrated oral implants. I: Success criteria and epidemiology. Eur J Oral Sci 1998;106:527–551.
18. Albrektsson T, Zarb GA, Worthington P. The long-term efficacy of currently used dental implants: a review and proposed criteria of success. Int J Oral Maxillofac Implants 1986;1:11–25.
19. Tonetti MS, Schmid J. Pathogenesis of implant failures. Periodontology 2000 1994;4:127–138.
20. Adell R, Lekholm U, Rockler B et al. Marginal tissue reactions at osseointegrated titanium fixtures. 1: A 3-year longitudinal prospective study. Int J Oral Maxillofac Surg 1986;15:39–52.
21. Misch CE, Suzuki JB, Misch-Dietsch FD. A positive correlation between occlusal trauma and peri-implant bone loss: literature support. Implant Dent 2005;14:108–114.
22. Misch CE. Early crestal bone loss: etiology and its effect on treatment planning for implants. Postgrad Dent 1995;2:3–17.
23. Van Steenberghe D. A retrospective multicenter evaluation of the survival rate of osseointegrated fixtures supporting fixed partial prostheses in the treatment of partial edentulism. J Prosthet Dent 1989;61:217–223.
24. Misch CE. Contemporary Implant Dentistry, ed 3. St Louis: Mosby, 2008:68–91.
25. Roberts WE. Osseous adaptation to continuous loading of rigid endosseous implants. Am J Orthodont 1984;86:95–111.
26. Haider R, Watzek G, Plenk H. Effects of drill cooling and bone structure on IMZ implant fixation. Int J Oral Maxillofac Implants 1993;8:83–91.
27. Brisman EL. The effect of speed, pressure and time on bone temperature during the drilling of implant sites. Int J Oral Maxillofac Implants 1996;11:35–37.
28. Berglundh T, Lindhe J. Dimension of the peri-implant mucosa: biological width revisited. J Clin Periodontol 1996;23:971–973.
29. Berglundh T, Lindhe J, Ericsson I, Marinella CP, Liljenberg B, Thomsen P. The soft tissue barrier at implants and teeth. Clin Oral Implants Res 1991;2:81–90.
30. Joly C, de Lima AFM, da Silva RC. Clinical and radiographic evaluation of soft and hard tissue changes around implants: a pilot study. J Periodontol 2003;74:1097–1103.
31. Weber HP, Buser D, Donath K. Comparison of healed tissues adjacent to submerged and non-submerged unloaded titanium dental implants: a histomorphometric study in beagle dogs. Clin Oral Implants Res 1996;7:11–19.

CHAPTER

4

Diagnosis and Treatment Planning

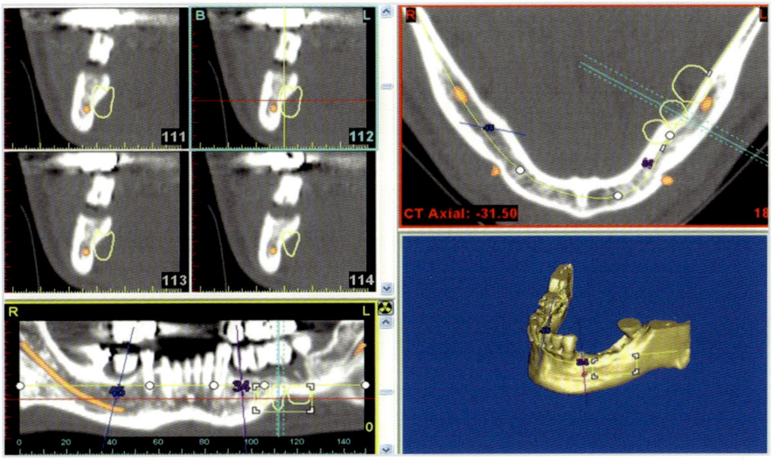

Key point

Planning prevents poor performance.

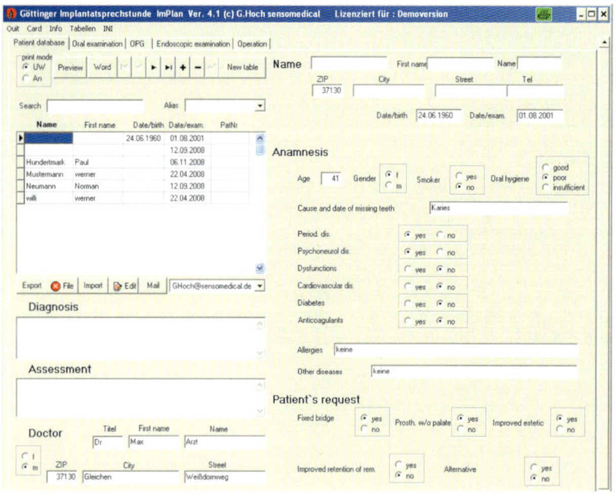

Fig 4-1 Anamnestic screening survey (screenshot of the implant planning program).

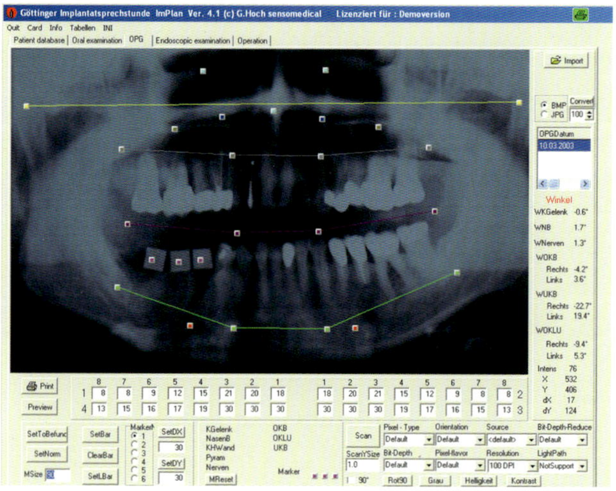

Fig 4-2 Orthopantomogram imported into the implant program.

Overview

This chapter outlines the general concepts of diagnoses and treatment plans for flapless implants. Clinical guidelines are also summarized for both conventional and three-dimensional (3D) virtual planning. After the primary planning phase, there are two options for diagnostics: multiparametric conventional and 3D-image-based planning. Both options may be used successfully for flapless implant placement, but they have different indications. Using flapless implant surgery in ridges with insufficient bone width or height may also achieve excellent results. Guidelines on treatment planning for ridges with insufficient bone width and an edentulous posterior maxilla with insufficient bone height are outlined in this chapter. Finally, this chapter outlines guidelines on the selection of two different options of flapless implant techniques: the soft tissue punch and the mini-incision techniques.

Primary treatment plan

The primary treatment plan is the result of the patient's history, the patient's requests, clinical evaluations, and radiographic diagnoses based on panoramic radiographs. Systematic patient reports include an anamnestic screening, as well as documentation of the patient's requests and the diagnostic summary. A systematic anamnestic evaluation may be supported using an implant planning program, which provides features specially developed for this purpose (Fig 4-1).

The intraoral examination is documented according to the routine dental scheme. A graphic representation of the bony implant site is integrated in the dental scheme. The orthopantomogram may be imported into the planning program as a standard radiographic basis of implant planning. In the orthopantomogram, anatomical structures may be assessed and measured while correcting for distortion factors if a reference marker had been used during the examination (Fig 4-2).

Bone evaluation follows the "cube concept" – bone mapping based on clinical measurements and radiographic evaluations of the orthopantomogram, represented as a column in the dental scheme. According to Misch,[1] a bone volume with 5 mm × 5 mm base and 10 mm height should be provided as a basic need for implant placement prior to further site classification. Engelke[2] developed a bone mapping system (multiple cube concept) for teaching purposes and clinical use. The first step of implant planning with the cube concept is basic site-by-site bone mapping. Using four categories of vertical bone dimension – abundant (>20 mm), sufficient (>15 mm), critical (>10 mm), and insufficient (<10 mm) – and a single additional transverse measurement (I if <5 mm) – primary implant planning is completed. Measurement of the bone width 5 mm below the bony crest is required to classify the transverse bone dimension as "sufficient" or "insufficient (I)". Bone mapping using the cube concept is represented in Figs 4-3 and 4-4.

The goal of the primary treatment plan is to assess the need for prior treatment and to define the general concept of implant reconstructive measures in the patient based on the anamnestic and clinical findings. The number and location of the implants, the prosthetic concept, and the augmentation procedures have to be defined.

After elaboration of the primary treatment plan, two different options may be selected:

- conventional multiparametric planning, or
- 3D-image-based planning.

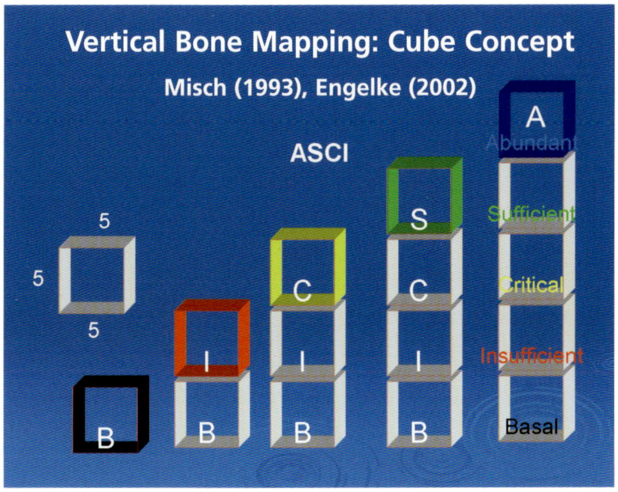

Fig 4-3 Vertical bone mapping: the implant site is represented as a column of 5 mm × 5 mm × 5 mm cubes.[2,3]

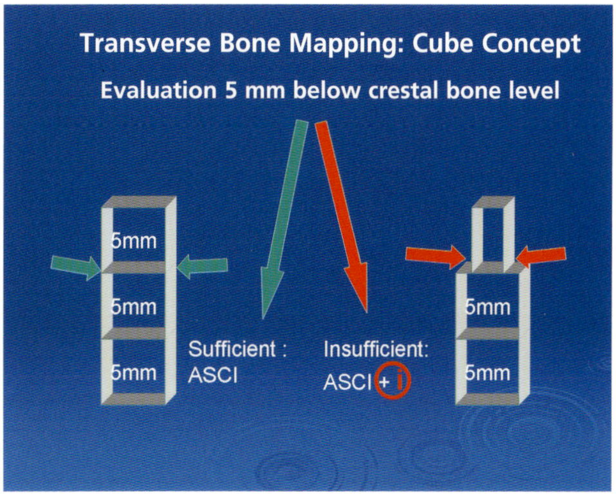

Fig 4-4 Transverse bone mapping: measurement of the bone width 5 mm below the bony crest. Measurements are used to make decisions about sufficient (>5 mm) or insufficient (<5 mm) dimensions.

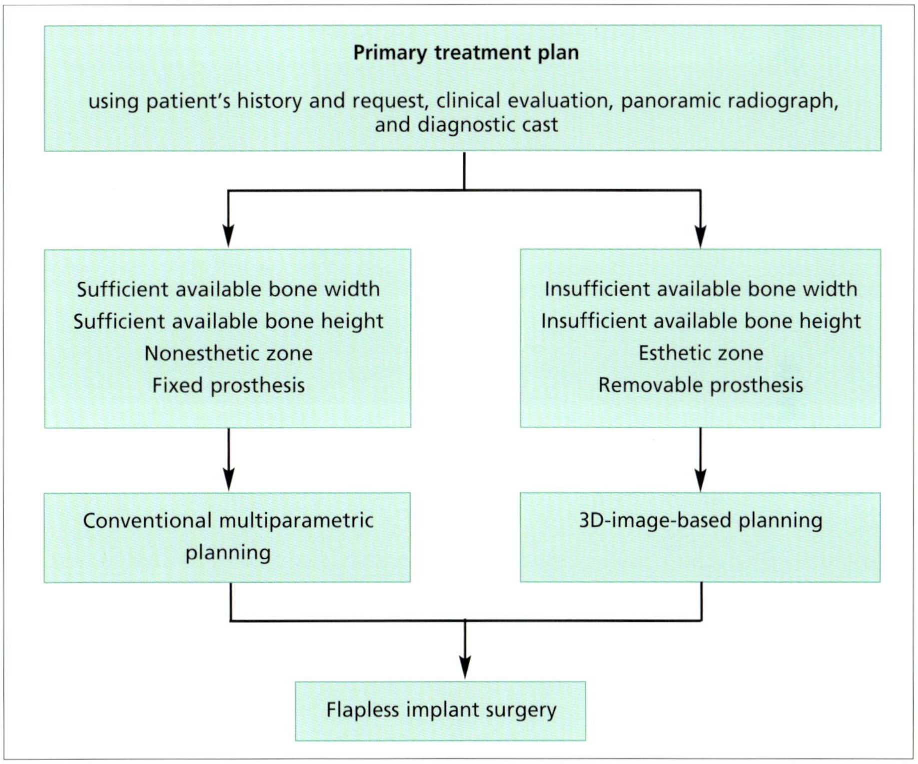

Fig 4-5 After elaboration of the primary treatment plan, two different options may be selected: conventional multiparametric planning or 3D-image-based planning. The selection depends on the resources of both the practitioner and the patient.

The selection depends on the resources of both the dentist and the patients. In general, it should be stressed that proper multiparametric conventional planning may be as effective as 3D planning in cases of uncomplicated implant sites (Fig 4-5).

Conventional multiparametric planning

Conventional multiparametric planning (CMP) makes use of panoramic tomograms, clinical landmarks, and diagnostic casts in conjunction with soft tissue measurement and fabrication of a surgical guide. Generally, five units of information (parameters) are requested to correctly determine

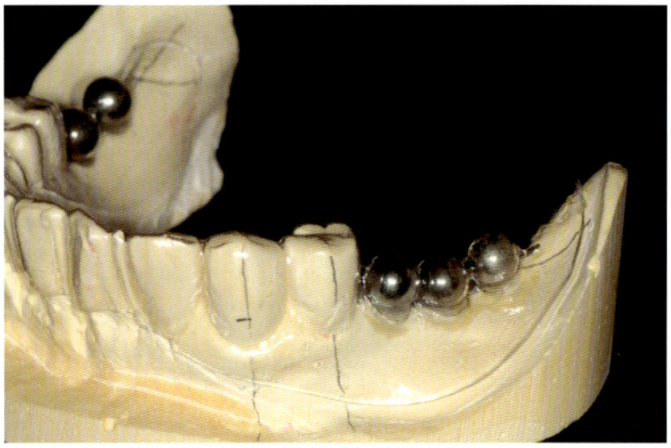

Fig 4-6 Diagnostic template.

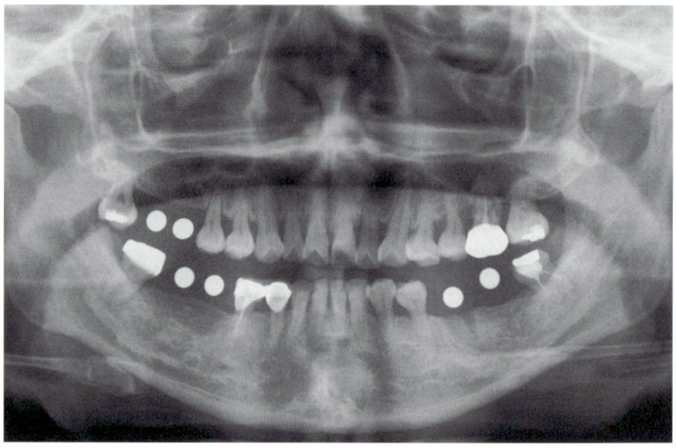

Fig 4-7 Panoramic radiograph with 5 mm ball bearings.

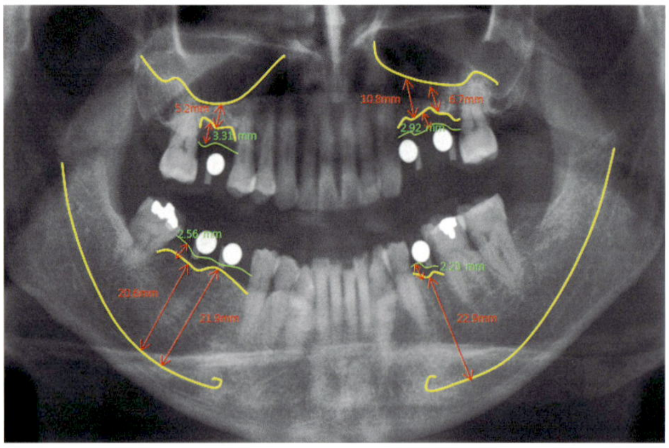

Fig 4-8 The magnification factor is used to assess available bone height at the proposed implant sites, mucosal thickness, and the distance from the alveolar crest to the anatomical landmarks (e.g. the mandibular canal, the mental foramen, and the maxillary sinus).

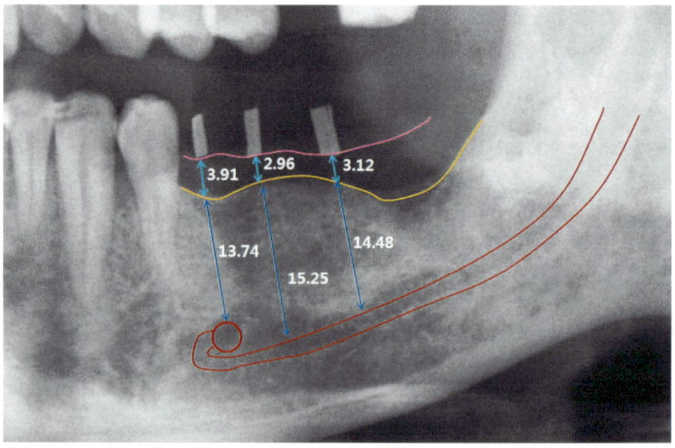

Fig 4-9 In a panoramic view, the thickness of the mucosa covering the alveolar crest can be determined.

the implant position: (1) horizontal location with respect to the bone site; (2) vertical location; (3) direction of insertion; (4) implant length; and (5) implant diameter.

Radiographic evaluation

The goal of presurgical radiographic evaluation is to assess the available bone quality and quantity, the angulation of the bone, and the mucosal thickness, as well as to select potential implant sites and to verify the absence of pathology.

The panoramic radiograph is probably the most used diagnostic modality in implant dentistry. However, this modality has limitations of distortion and magnification. To compensate for its shortcomings, it is necessary to determine the magnification factor by imaging an object of known diameter close to the alveolar ridge. The magnification factor can be calculated at the given site by dividing the actual diameter of the object by the diameter measured on the radiographic image. Diagnostic templates that have 5 mm ball bearings worn by the patient during the panoramic X-ray examination enable the clinician to determine the amounts of magnification or distortion in the radiograph (Figs 4-6 and 4-7). As an alternative, quadrangular markers having a standardized dimension of 5 mm may be used. Therefore, bone mapping can be carried out according to the cube concept. Using the magnification factor, the available bone height at the proposed implant sites and the distance from the alveolar crest to the anatomical landmarks (e.g. the mandibular canal, the mental foramen, and the maxillary sinus) are assessed (Fig 4-8). In a panoramic view, the thickness of the mucosa covering the alveolar crest can also be studied (Fig 4-9).

Diagnostic casts

Diagnostic casts allow dentists to evaluate a patient's intraoral condition and to plan treatment (Fig 4-10). Such casts

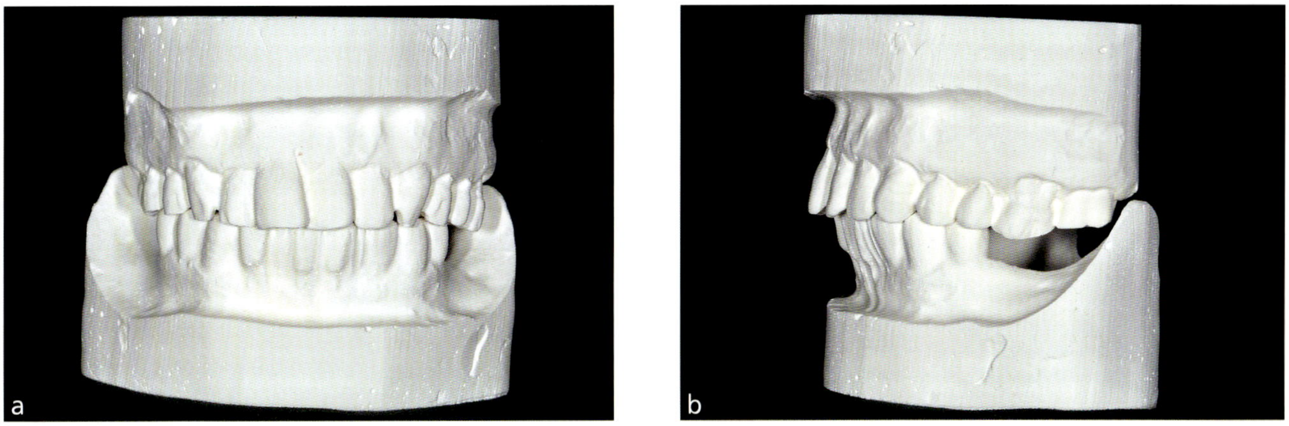

Fig 4-10 (a and b) Diagnostic casts permit evaluation of a patient's intraoral condition and plan of treatment.

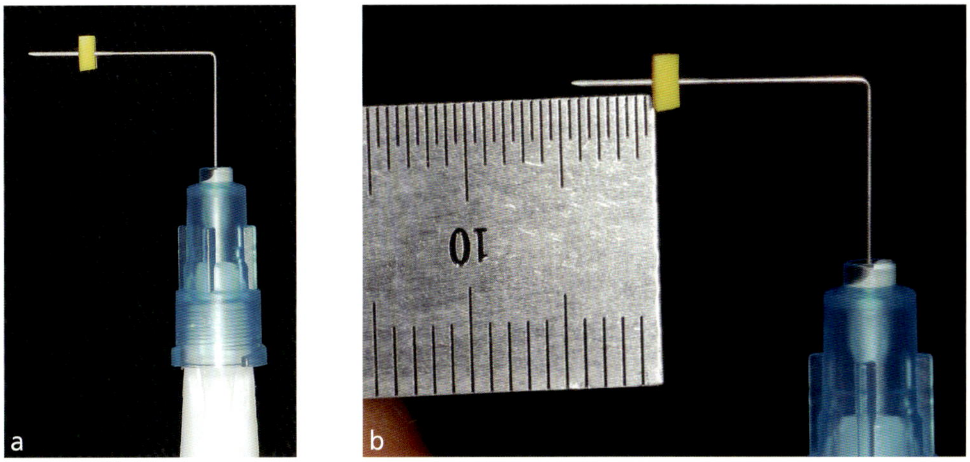

Fig 4-11 (a and b) The simplest method of measuring mucosal thickness is with a needle. The needle is inserted into the bone surface through the mucosa, and the depth is marked with a rubber stop.

mounted using an accurate record of the centric jaw relationship and maxillomandibular occlusion on a semiadjustable articulator provide information related to treatment that influences the final prosthodontic treatment plan. The casts assist in evaluating the vertical and horizontal relationship of the maxilla and the mandible. These casts also influence implant location, size, and angulation. Casts help dentists to determine a prosthetically driven implant placement. Furthermore, they allow dentists to analyze the alveolar ridge condition in the edentulous area, as well as the remaining tooth condition, the occlusal state, and the opposing dentition.

Measurement of mucosal thickness

The third component of multiparametric planning is the measurement of the mucosal thickness at the implant site to control the depth of drilling above the mucosa. In addition, in edentulous sites with an increased soft tissue height, the soft tissue's geometry is an important consideration in the decision for ridge augmentation.

The simplest method of measuring the mucosal thickness is with a needle. The needle is equipped with an endodontic stop and is inserted through the patient's mucosa overlying the implant site. The mucosal thickness is measured on the crest, facial, and lingual areas (Fig 4-11).[4] The clinician can also use a bone caliper that contains sharp beaks penetrating soft tissues at a known height. Sonography can also be used to measure the mucosal thickness.[5]

After obtaining these measurements, the edentulous region of a diagnostic cast is cut perpendicular to the ridge. The marking of the mucosal thickness on the cross-section of the diagnostic cast enables visualization of the mucosal thickness and bone shape (Fig 4-12). In the previously mentioned panoramic view, the thickness of the mucosa covering the alveolar crest can be determined. Prior to drilling, the mucosal thickness at the implant site can be directly measured using a periodontal probe or a depth gauge.

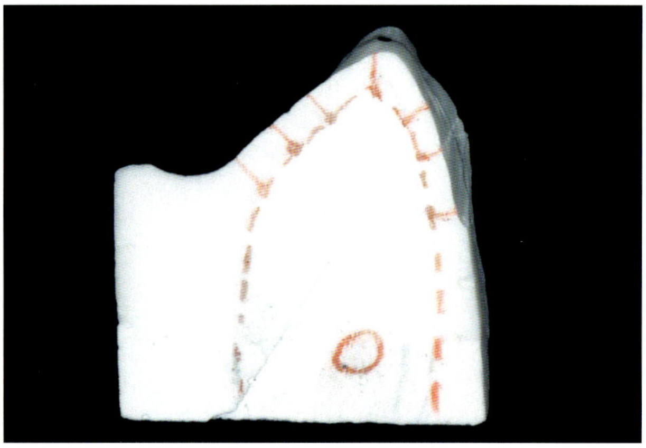

Fig 4-12 Marking of the mucosal thickness on the cross-section of a diagnostic cast enables visualization of the mucosa and the bone shape.

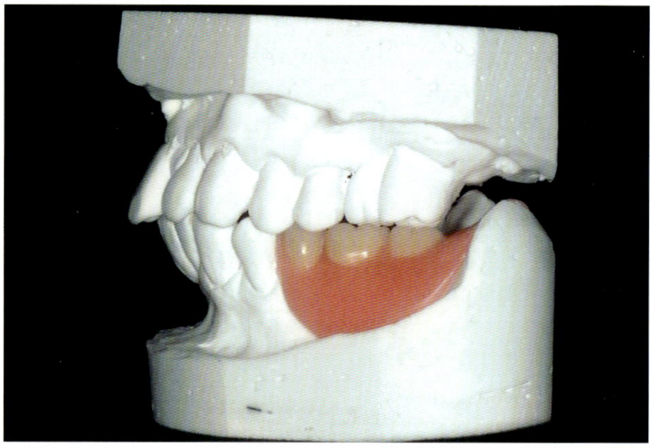

Fig 4-13 A wax-up of the missing teeth in the edentulous region.

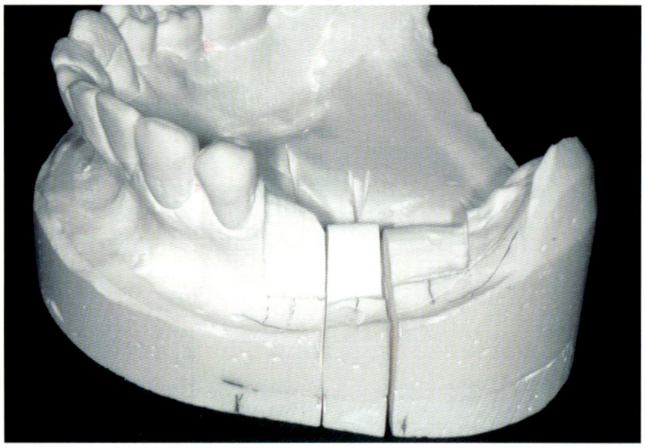

Fig 4-14 The edentulous region of the diagnostic cast is cut perpendicular to the ridge.

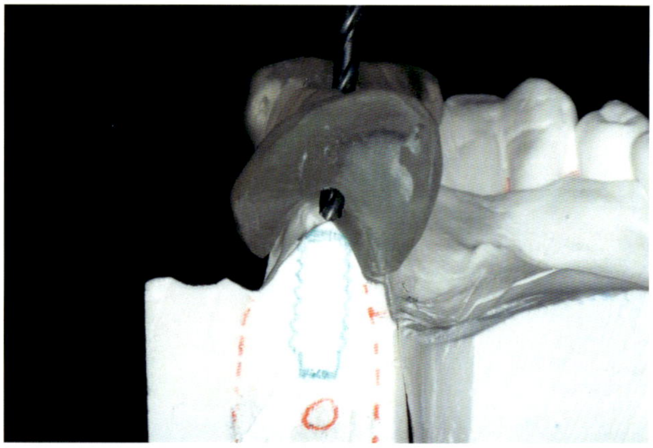

Fig 4-15 The ideal angulation and size for implant insertion is determined based on the bone contour of the diagnostic cast cross-section.

Fabrication of surgical guides using a diagnostic cast

A diagnostic cast can be used to fabricate a surgical guide. The diagnostic wax-up is completed to preview the tooth size, position, contour, and occlusion in the edentulous regions where implants will be inserted (Fig 4-13). After cutting the edentulous region of the diagnostic cast perpendicular to the ridge (Fig 4-14), the diagnostic cast cross-section is shaded with a pencil to represent the mucosal thickness. The remaining cross-section of the cast roughly estimates the bone contours under the soft tissue. The ideal angulation and size for implant insertion are determined based on the bone contours (Fig 4-15). Once implant size and angulation are determined, the implant site is drilled in the template corresponding to the angulation, and then a metal guide is inserted into place (Fig 4-16).

Planning guided by three-dimensional images

Image-guided implant planning and placement reduces pain and blood loss, takes less time, preserves the hard and soft tissue architecture,[6] and improves patient compliance.

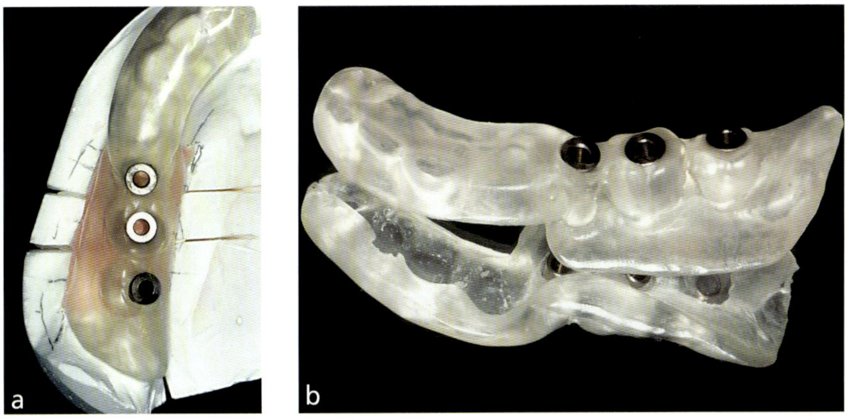

Fig 4-16 (a and b) Once implant size and angulation have been determined, the implant site is drilled into the template corresponding to the angulation, and then a metal tube is placed.

Three-dimensional planning based on CT or DVT

Three-dimensional planning always has to consider the requirements of the final prosthetic restoration as well as the requirements of the anatomical conditions of the implant site. Therefore, at the beginning of the planning phase, a precise diagnostic wax-up is necessary to simulate the patient's final restorative result concerning esthetic and function. The diagnostic wax-up then allows fabrication of a radiographic splint. The diagnostic wax-up of the reconstructed ridge and the restored dentition is advantageous in determining the graft width and position requirements and also for analyzing the occlusion.

Computerized tomography (CT) enables the identification of diseases and of critical structures at the proposed regions, as well as the determination of bone quantity, bone quality, and the position and orientation of the dental implants (Figs 4-17 to 4-21). A cross-sectional view of the CT scan enables the determination of mucosal thickness. Three-dimensional reformatted CT images allow a 360-degree evaluation of the jaw bone (Fig 4-17). Diagnostic templates consist of radiopaque artificial teeth or may have gutta-percha radiopaque cylinders that the patient wears during the CT examination. These templates enable the dentist to evaluate available bone height at the proposed implant sites (Figs 4-18 and 4-19). The cross-sectional view of the CT scan allows the clinician to determine implant size, length, and angulation (Fig 4-20). When bone augmentation in the maxillary sinus is needed to place implants, CT scanning of the sinus may be used to estimate the amount of graft material required for the ideal volume of sinus graft material (Fig 4-21). A 3D evaluation of the implant's proximity to vital structures can also be done.

However, CT scanning is expensive, which can be a disadvantage. The patient radiation level with CT is approximately 200 times higher than with panoramic radiograph. Therefore, CT scanning should be used to obtain additional diagnostic information only if other diagnostic methods are not suitable.

Cone beam tomography (digital volume tomography, DVT) also may be used for 3D imaging. DVT has less radiation exposure than CT. The inherent restriction of DVT for soft tissue imaging does not play a major role in implant planning; resolution of bone structures is usually adequate for judging bone volume as well as the structural aspects of the implant sites.

Radiographic splints serve as a reference while 3D imaging data are being taken. Splints may use reference bodies (like a Lego brick) (Fig 4-22) and provide obligatory radiopaque crowns, which are needed for the alignment of the implants. Radiographic splints do not contain any guiding elements for implants (i.e. tubes). To guarantee a perfect anatomical fit of the splint in situ, radiographic splints are important. This may be difficult in edentulous patients, particularly in the mandible. Therefore, stabilizing pins or temporary implants may be used. Any unintended relative movement of the radiographic splint during the radiographic evaluation can directly lead to erroneous planning and, therefore, counteracts the precision provided by the method.

Planning procedure

Clinicians perform virtual implant placement with the assistance of special planning software according to the systems used. As an alternative, data processing may be provided by planning centers, which also offer suggestions according to the requirements of the practitioner. Planning then can be done interactively online from the office. It must be stressed that the clinician is the person responsible for deciding the implant selection and treatment plan.

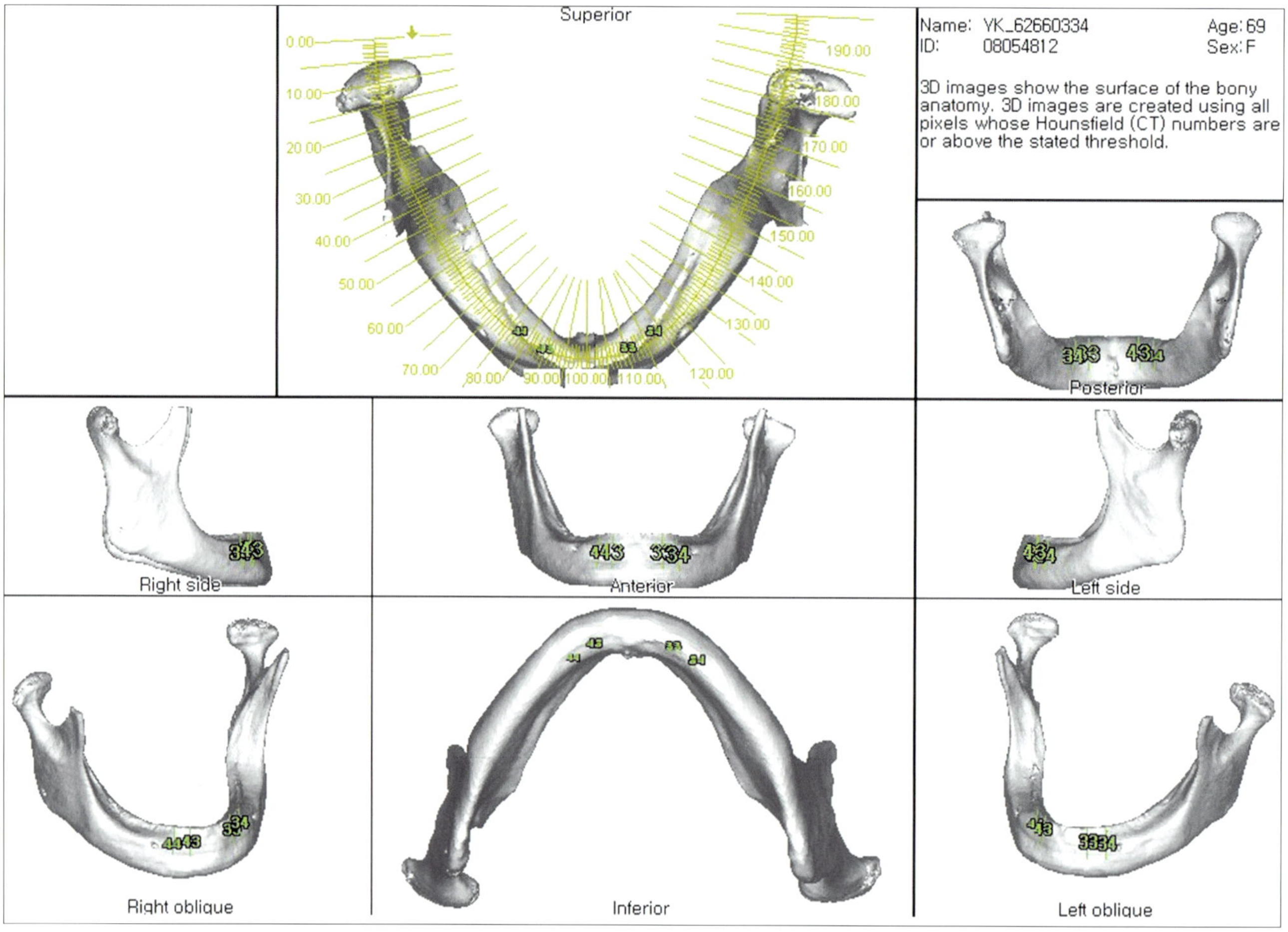

Fig 4-17 Computerized tomography provides a precise view of the actual shape of the jaw bone using 3D osseous images.

Three-dimensional computer-assisted planning is based on reconstructed panoramic, cross-sectional, and horizontal views of the anticipated implant site. Additionally, 3D surface imaging may be provided. Generally, the cross-sectional view is the most informative, and it should be regarded as the standard image for the alignment of implants. Implant location, size, length, and angulation are determined using a 3D image created from CT scan data. The implant axis is aligned with the alveolar process, and an optimum of the crown axis and the implant position can be simulated. Figure 4-23 shows a plan for multiple implants in the maxilla using the med3D system. It depicts implant site 11 with a class C alveolar ridge and the barium-contrasted crown.

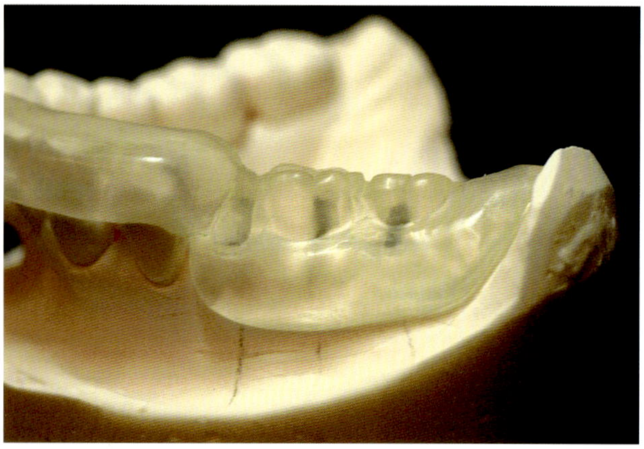

Fig 4-18 Diagnostic templates with gutta-percha radiopaque cylinders.

Contradictory parameters should be considered during planning: the requirements of the crown position, the requirements of the resting bone volume and structure, and the parallelism of adjacent implants that have to be optimized during the planning process. Planning for flapless implantation generally follows the criteria for conventional implant placement.

There are limitations of implant placement precision in edentulous situations with significant mucosal mobility. The patient in Fig 4-23 was operated on without additional fixation of the surgical guide. Figure 4-24 shows that, without screw fixation, repositioning of the splint may lead to errors owing to the mobility of the underlying mucosa. This may be important if narrow ridges require a very high

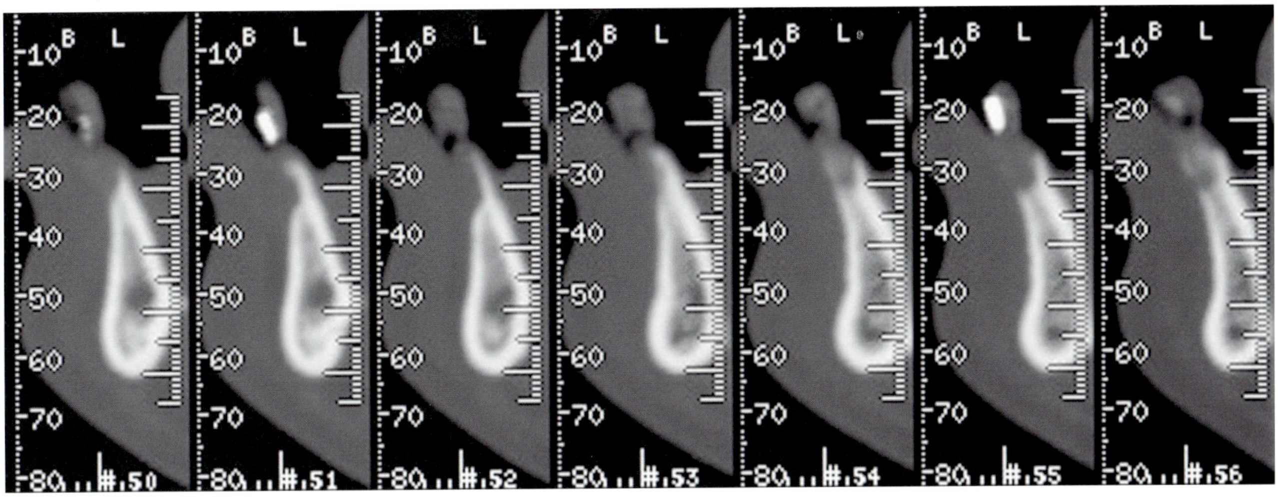

Fig 4-19 Computerized tomography with gutta-percha radiopaque cylinders enables the clinician to evaluate bone quality at prospective implant sites.

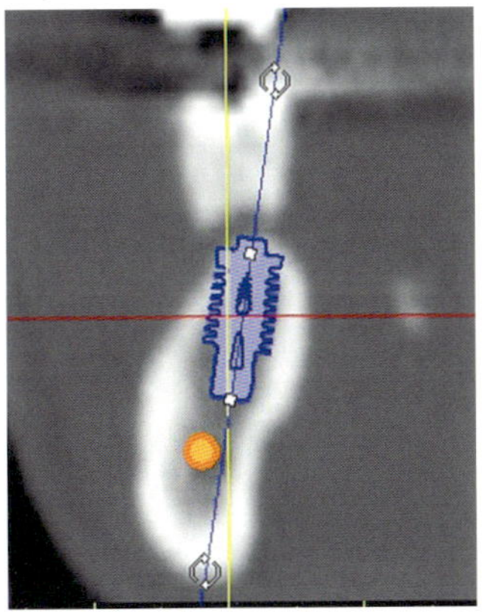

Fig 4-20 A cross-sectional view of the CT scan allows the determination of implant size, length, and angulation.

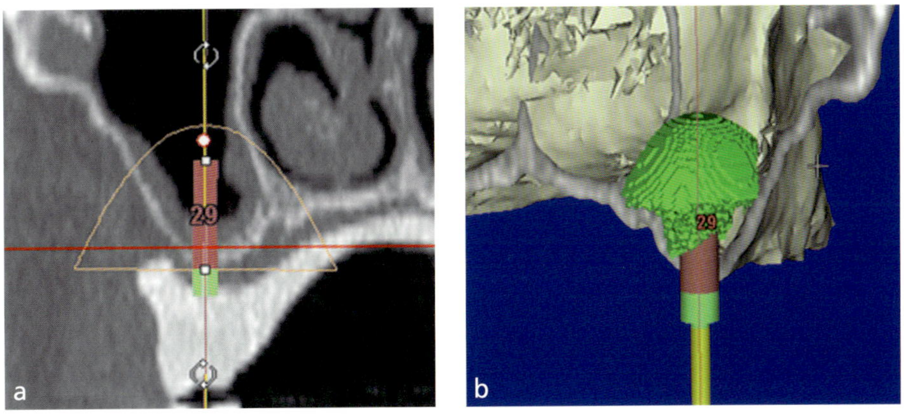

Fig 4-21 (a and b) Computerized tomography of the sinus may be used to estimate the amount of graft material required for the ideal volume of sinus graft material.

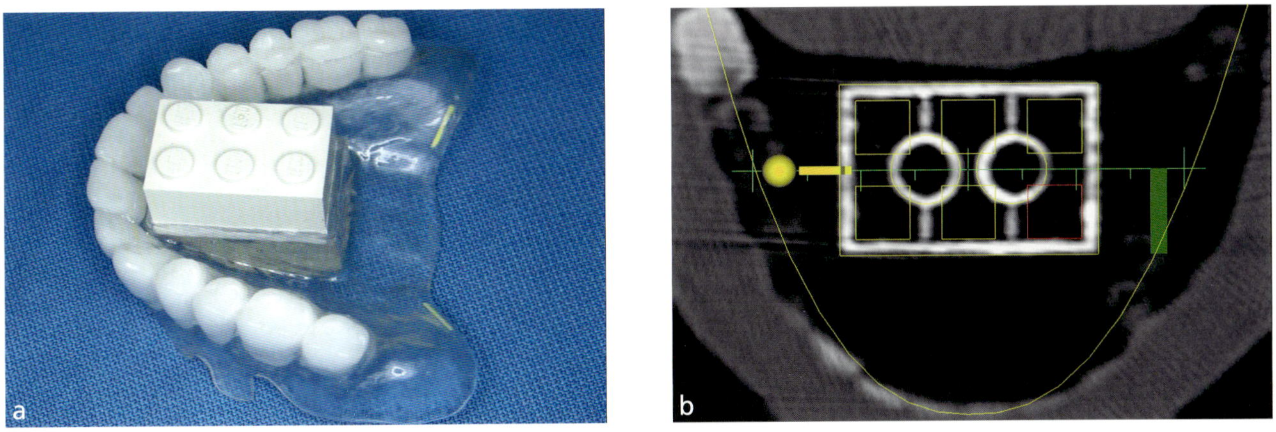

Fig 4-22 (a) Radiographic splint. (b) Radiographic reference (a Lego brick).

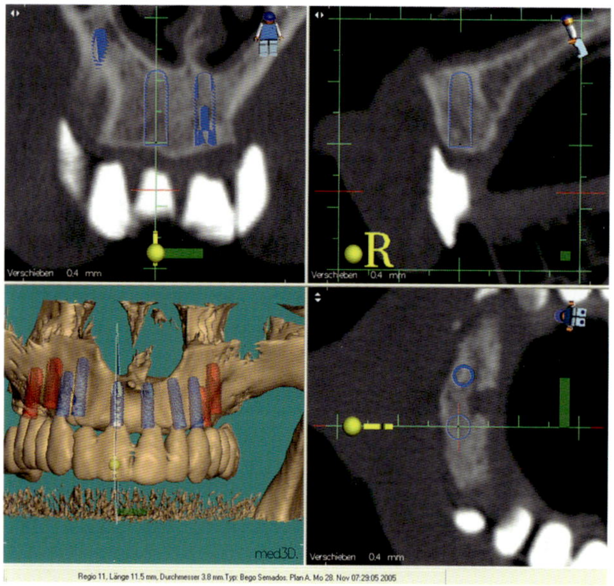

Fig 4-23 Virtual implant planning using the med3D system.

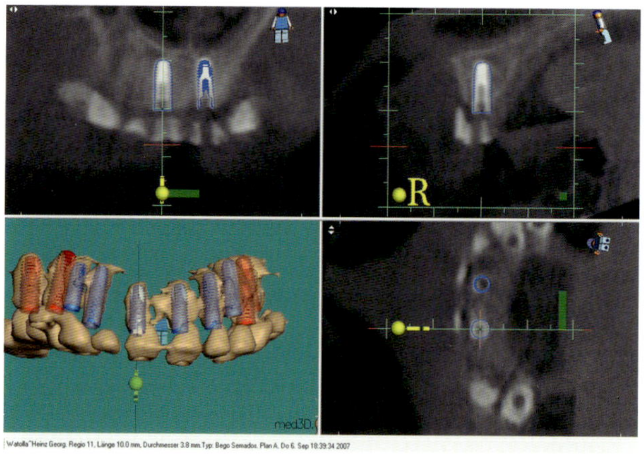

Fig 4-24 Postoperative result of planning of implant site 11.

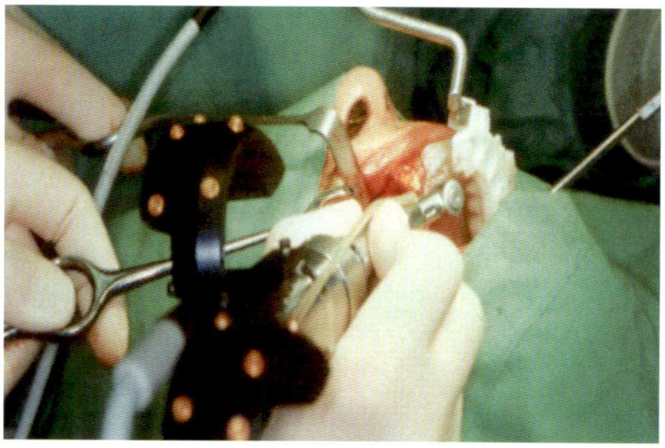

Fig 4-25 Optical tracking system during application (DeneX system).

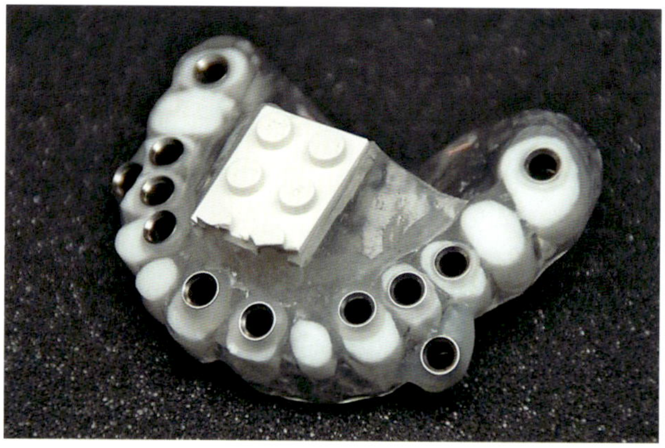

Fig 4-26 Three-dimensional surgical guide (med3D system).

degree of drilling precision, which may occur in cases with a sufficiently broad ridge dependent on the tooth to be reconstructed. Minor deviations below 1 mm may be accepted in the procedure.

Surgical procedures and guidance concepts

Surgical implant placement after 3D planning may be supported online using optical tracking navigation systems, including dynamic computer-assisted guidance[7] (Fig 4-25) and 3D surgical guides (static computer-assisted guidance)[8,9] (Fig 4-26).

Optical tracking system

The use of optical tracking systems requires an online representation of the planned implant position and the actual position of the drilling instrument. After placing the instrument in the patient's mouth, the surgeon guides the instrument via an optical tracking system displayed on a computer screen. The patient's anatomy, as well as the planned implant position, are available online while the cavity is being prepared. Owing to the extensive technical equipment necessary and the time-consuming individual calibration of the systems, optical tracking systems are not being frequently used in routine flapless implant surgery.

Applications of an optical tracking system are shown in Fig 4-27. Various screenshots of the system are displayed. The drilling instrument is displayed virtually online in a

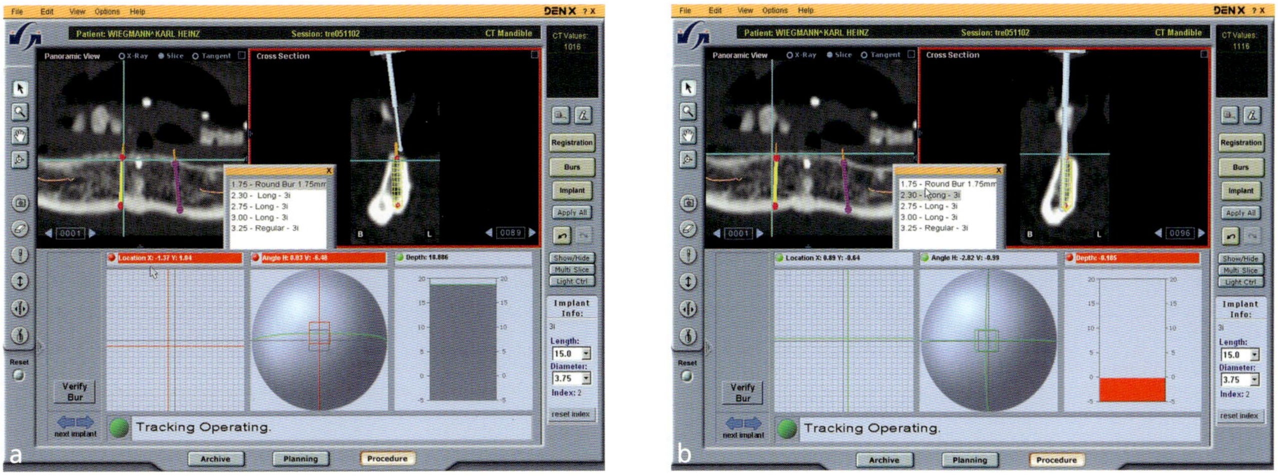

Fig 4-27 Screenshots during insertion of mandibular implants. (a) Alignment of the implant site with the round bur. (b) Final position of the first cylindrical drill.

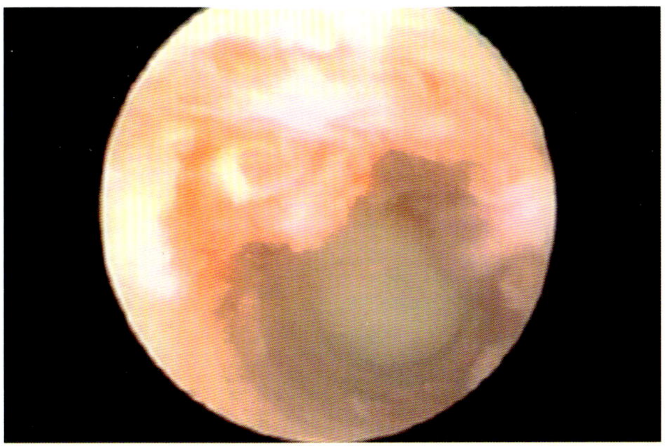

Fig 4-28 Endoscopic control of a transgingivally prepared implant cavity.

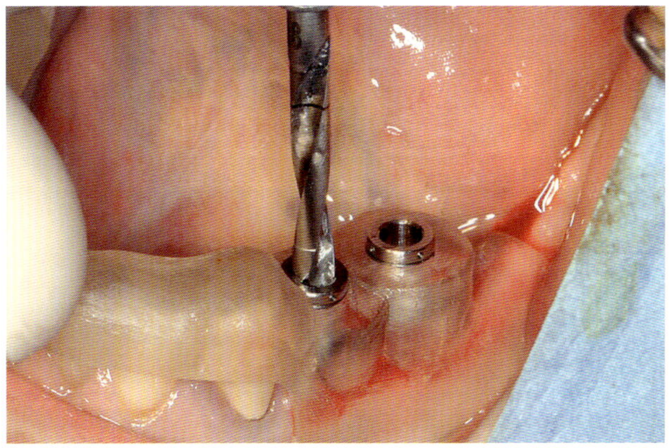

Fig 4-29 The surgical guide containing metal guides.

projection of the 3D cross-sectional image at the implant site. Endoscopic control allows insight into the recently prepared implant cavity, thus providing quality control of transgingival flapless procedures (Fig 4-28).

Static three-dimensional surgical guides

The most common solution for implant placement using a flapless technique is the use of a static 3D surgical guide. After the final decision on the implant position, the radiographic splint is transformed into a surgical guide by integration of the guiding tubes. To facilitate the insertion of the burs, the guiding tubes are placed after removal of the occlusal parts of the crowns directly above the basal surface of the splint. Flapless implant surgery offers ease of use of the surgical guide because the stability of the guide can be secured on the mucosa. The surgical template allows cavity preparation with high accuracy according to the earlier planning. With a telescope tube, a sequence of drilling instruments can be subsequently used to carefully open the bone cavity.

Figure 4-29 shows the intraoral use of the template for transgingival flapless cavity formation. In addition to the surgical guide, the clinician needs information about the depth of the cavity with reference to the tube entrance to choose the adequate bur length. In difficult anatomical situations (including the posterior areas in particular), only a part of the cavity depth can be drilled using the guide, and then apical preparation may be completed using burs with drill stops that are guided by the walls of the crestal cavity.

Treatment planning for ridges with insufficient bone

Implant placement using flapless implant surgery in ridges with insufficient bone width requires greater experience, caution, and training, but excellent results may be achieved. To develop a treatment plan for the ridges, evaluation of the existing bone volume is the primary factor. To assess the amount of labiolingual bone, a CT study is integrated into the pretreatment imaging process. Augmentation procedures also can be planned with 3D assistance. If available bone width or height is inadequate for implants of the proper size, bone grafts with immediate or delayed flapless implant placement are possible (Fig 4-30). Bone grafting is performed using a subperiosteal tunneling procedure (Fig 4-31). The subperiosteal tunnel ensures favorable condi-

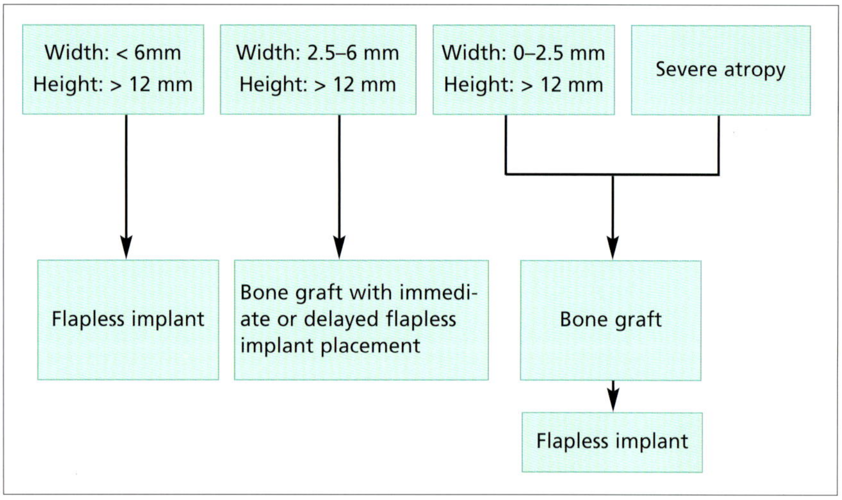

Fig 4-30 Treatment approach for the ridges with insufficient bone is based on the available bone width and height.

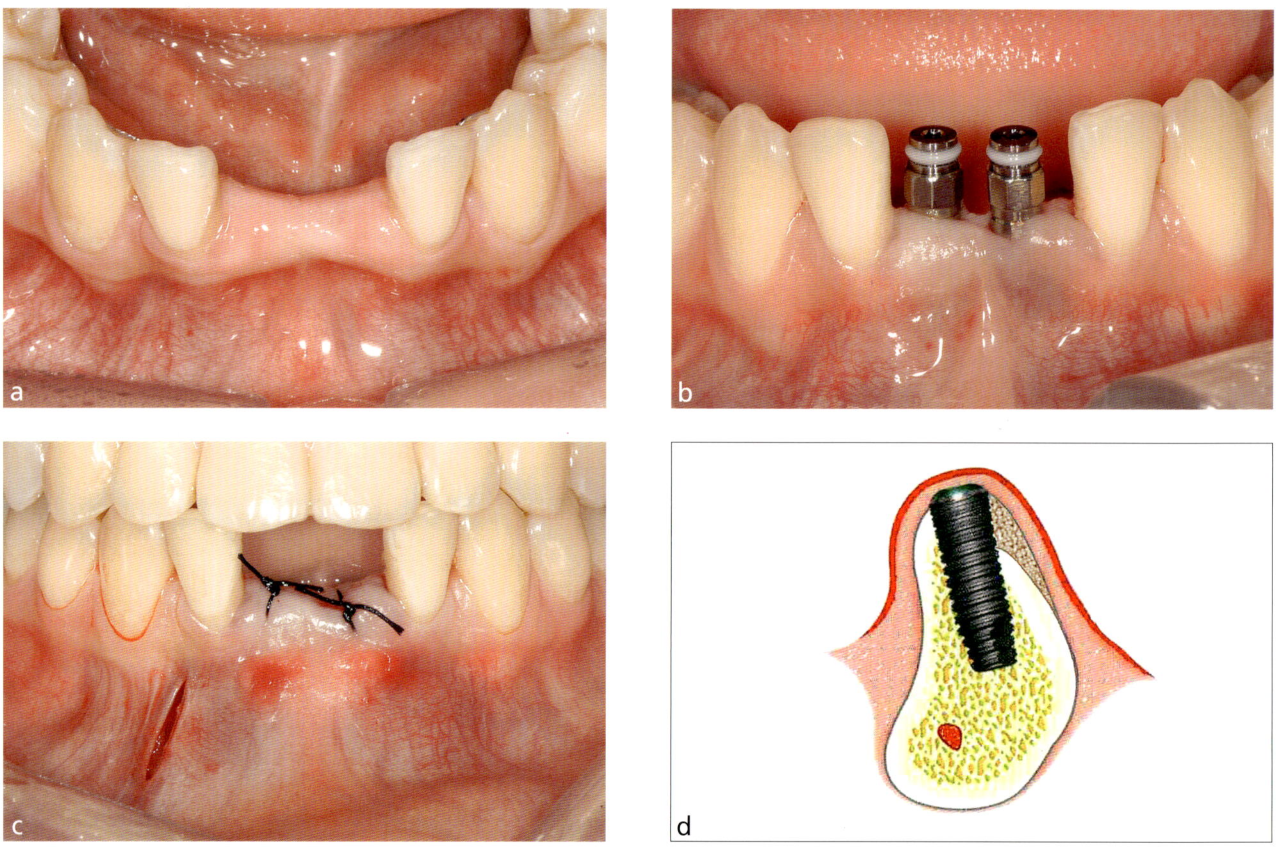

Fig 4-31 (a) Intraoral view before surgery. (b) Two implants were inserted using the mini-incision procedure. (c) The implants were submerged, and the grafting of the Bio-Oss® particles (which had been mixed with autologous fibrin gel to cover the exposed threads) was performed through a subperiosteal tunnel. (d) Illustration of the graft site.

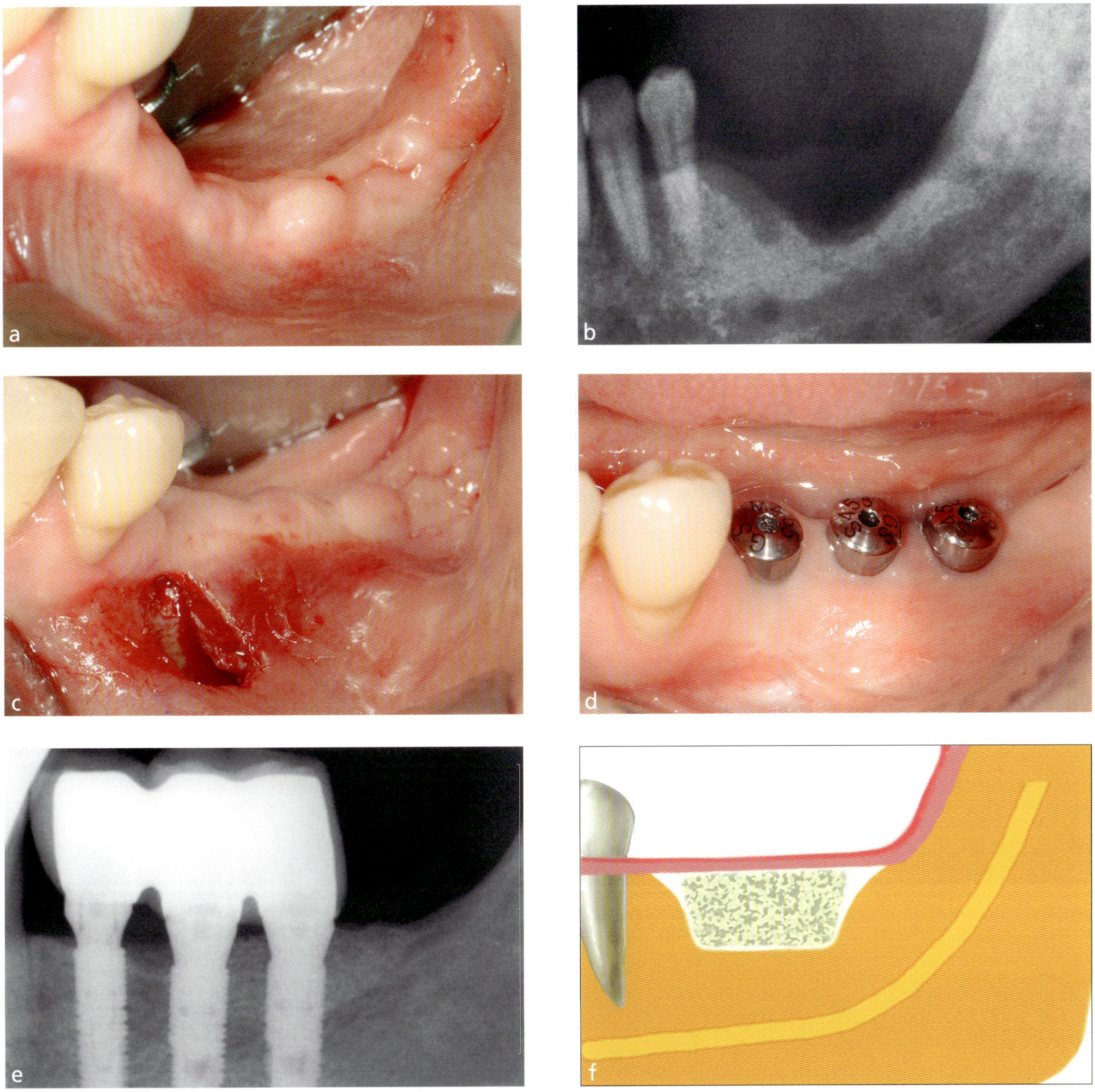

Fig 4-32 (a) Intraoral view before surgery. (b) Radiograph of the mandible before surgery. (c) Intraoral view during surgery. The Bio-Oss® block was placed in a defect area of the mandible through a subperiosteal tunnel. (d) Three implants were inserted using a flapless procedure. (e) Radiograph after 24 months. (f) Illustration of the graft site.

tions for flapless implant surgery and increased healing of soft tissue adjacent to the flapless implant. This procedure also promotes bone generation and reduces the incidence of membrane exposure (see Chapter 12).

If the available bone height of the ridge is insufficient, bone augmentation is performed prior to implant placement. After the ridge is augmented, flapless implant surgery can proceed.

The authors advocate performing a subperiosteal tunneling procedure with Bio-Oss® block onlay grafting. This procedure has several advantages over other bone grafting techniques for vertical bone growth. There is no donor site morbidity, little risk of graft dehiscence and incision-line opening, and less postoperative morbidity. After the ridge is augmented, flapless implant surgery can proceed (Fig 4-32).

Treatment planning for the edentulous posterior maxilla

Implant placement using a flapless procedure in the posterior maxilla with insufficient bone height is one of the most promising procedures in flapless implant surgery. A treatment approach to the posterior maxilla is based on the available bone height between the floor of the antrum and the crest of the residual ridge in the region of the ideal implant locations (Fig 4-33).

Several treatment options are available for an edentulous posterior maxilla. When sufficient bone height (>12 mm) is available, flapless implant surgery using a mini-incision technique is preferred. Socket lift and simultaneous flapless implant placement are selected when 10–12 mm of vertical bone is present. To obtain the 12 mm of vertical bone necessary for improved implant survival, the antral floor is elevated through the implant osteotomy, up to 2 mm (Fig 4-34). Flapless implant surgery reduces the bone loss of the crest during the initial healing period, thus contributing to enhanced implant stability (see Chapter 13).

A particle bone sinus graft with immediate or delayed flapless implant placement is indicated when 5–10 mm of vertical bone are present. The authors advocate Bio-Oss® grafting. Bio-Oss® particle grafting is performed using a small bone window 5 mm in diameter (see Chapter 15). The window is created using a vertical incision approximately 8 mm in length, and it is made on the buccal cortical plate about 8 mm away from the alveolar crest (Fig 4-35). Block or particle bone sinus graft with immediate or delayed flapless implant placement is indicated when less than 5 mm remains between the residual crest of bone and the floor of the maxillary sinus. To access the maxillary sinus, a horizontal incision for the approach is made on the buccal cortical plate of the maxillary sinus horizontally, with the alveolar crest approximately 10 mm away from the crest. These procedures ensure favorable conditions for flapless implant surgery in the alveolar crest. When block autogenous iliac bone is placed, the immediate flapless implant placement in the maxillary sinus may be performed at the same time as the sinus graft (Fig 4-36). The use of the corticocancellous block bone provides initial

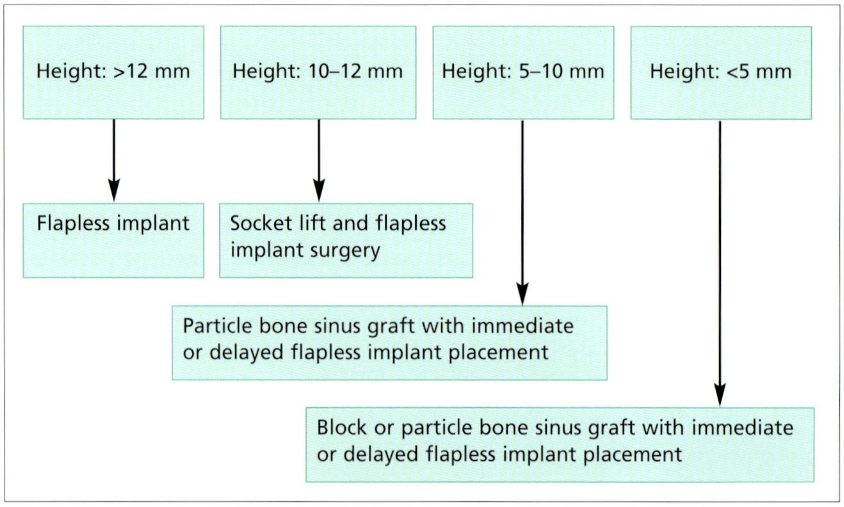

Fig 4-33 Treatment approach to the posterior maxilla is based on the available bone height between the floor of the antrum and the crest of the residual ridge in the region of the ideal implant locations.

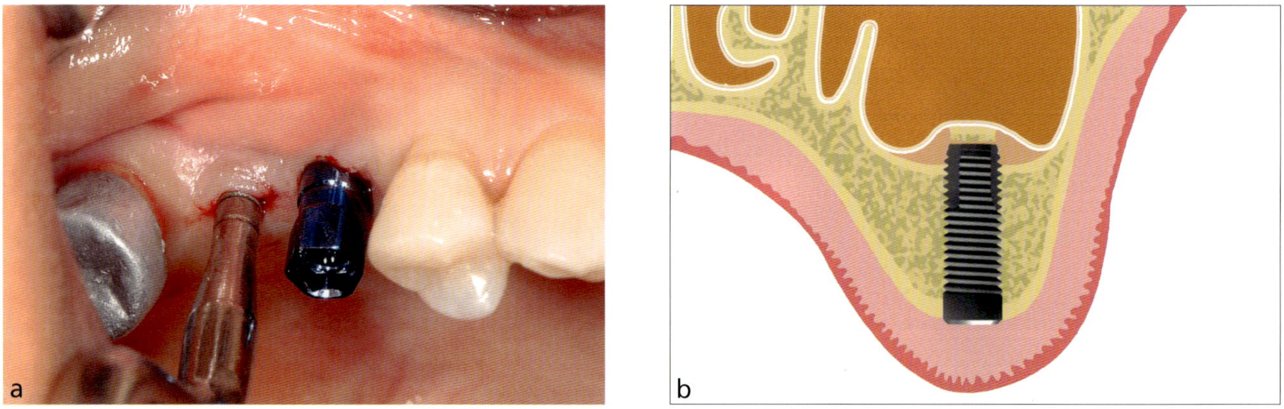

Fig 4-34 When 2 mm of bone augmentation in the maxillary sinus is necessary to place implants, simultaneous socket lift and flapless implant placement procedures are suggested. (a) Intraoral view during surgery. (b) Illustration of the procedures.

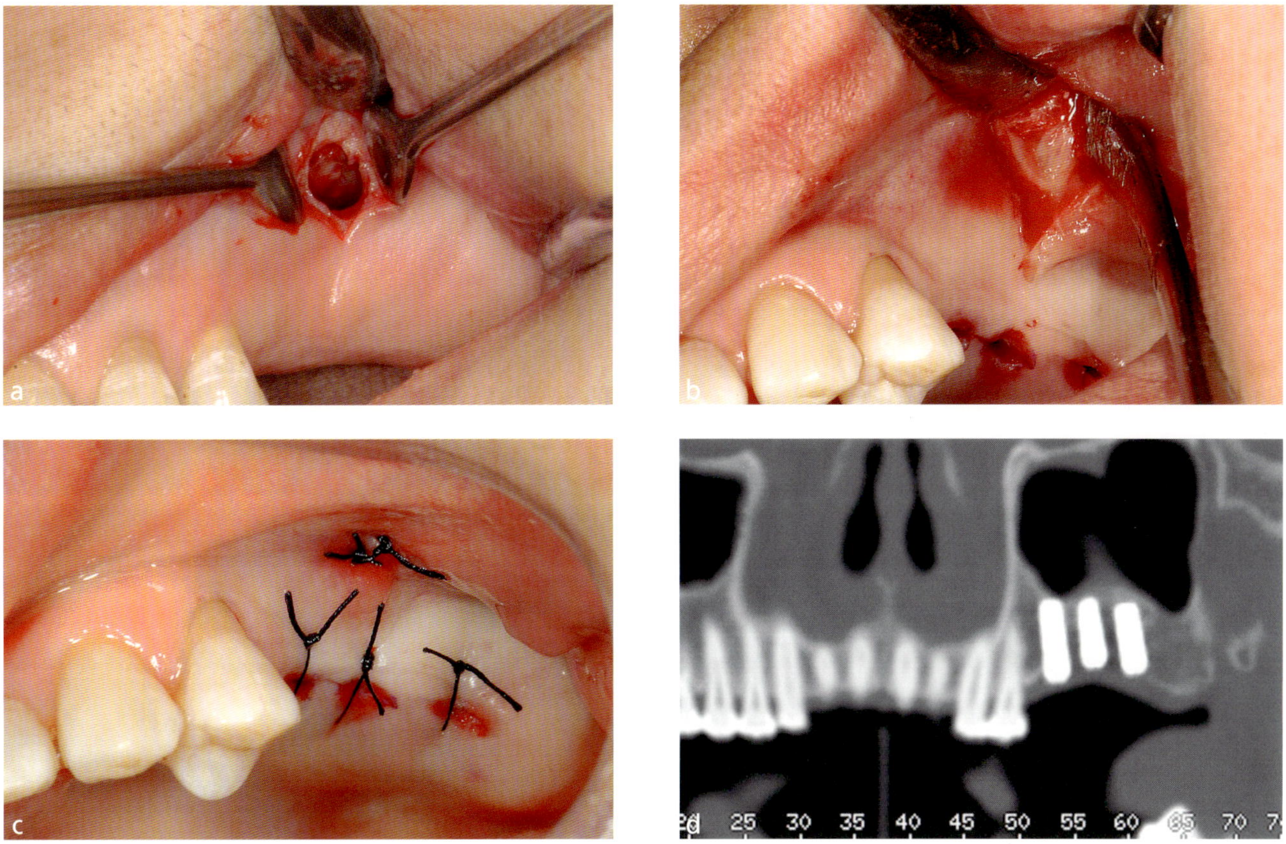

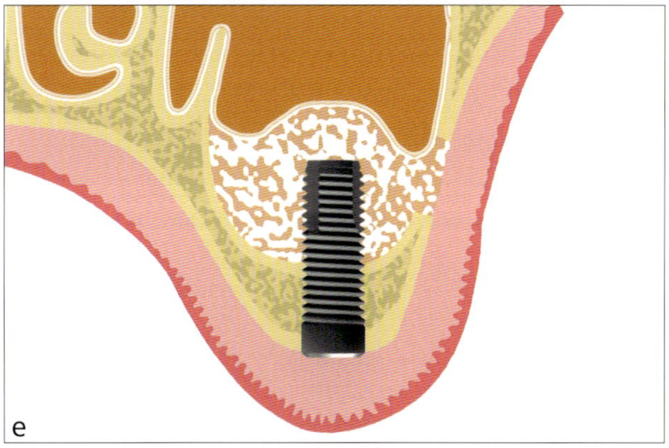

Fig 4-35 (a) A 5 mm diameter hole made in the lateral sinus wall with a round bur. (b) The Bio-Oss® particle/autologous fibrin composite grafting is performed through the small bone window. (c) Intraoral view immediately after surgery. Two implants extend into the graft site. (d) CT image 6 months after surgery. (e) Illustration of the Bio-Oss® particle sinus grafting and simultaneous flapless implant placement.

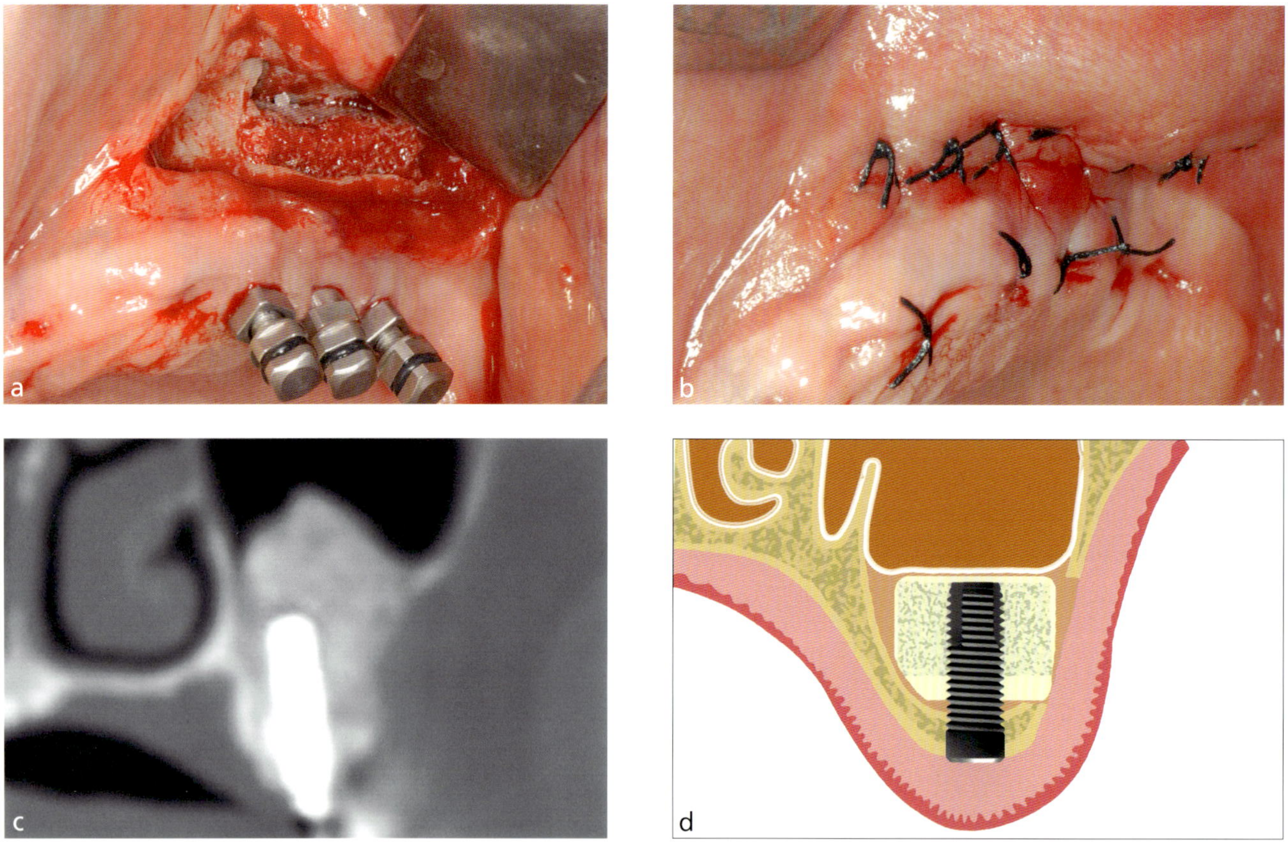

Fig 4-36 (a) Block autogenous iliac bone grafting and simultaneous mini-incision implant placement. (b) Intraoral view immediately after surgery. (c) Postoperative radiographs after 6 months. (d) Illustration of block bone grafting and simultaneous mini-incision implant placement.

mutual graft–implant stability, which facilitates simultaneous implant placement in the posterior atrophic maxilla. When a Bio-Oss® block is required, this is so brittle and weak that it cannot provide sufficient mechanical force for the primary stability of implants. Accordingly, when the remaining bone cannot ensure the primary stability of the implants, flapless implant placement into the Bio-Oss® block should be delayed for 6–10 months.

Guidelines on the selection of technique for flapless implants

The choice of a soft tissue punch technique or a mini-incision technique is dependent on bone quality and primary implant stability. The following guidelines are intended to help clinicians to make the best choice (Fig 4-37).

Guideline 1: Select the soft tissue punch technique for a one-stage approach

The soft tissue punch technique is used for a one-stage surgical approach, whereas the mini-incision technique is used for either a one-stage or a two-stage surgical approach. The two-stage surgical process places the implant body below the soft tissue until bone healing has occurred. It is prudent to use the two-stage surgical approach when implants are not adequately stabilized or if the patient wears a soft tissue-borne partial denture.

Guideline 2: The mini-incision technique is preferred in areas with insufficient amounts of keratinized mucosa

The amount of keratinized tissue should be adequate, and ideally patients need at least 1.5 mm of keratinized tissue to the facial aspect of the healing abutment. The mini-incision technique is beneficial in saving the keratinized mucosa. Therefore, the soft tissue punch technique must be used in cases where at least 1.5 mm of keratinized tissue is left on the buccal side to this incision line of the punch.

Guideline 3: Select the mini-incision technique in the posterior maxilla

On rare occasions, an implant in the maxilla may not remain rigid after implant placement.[10] A nonsubmerged, mobile implant may not heal predictably with a direct

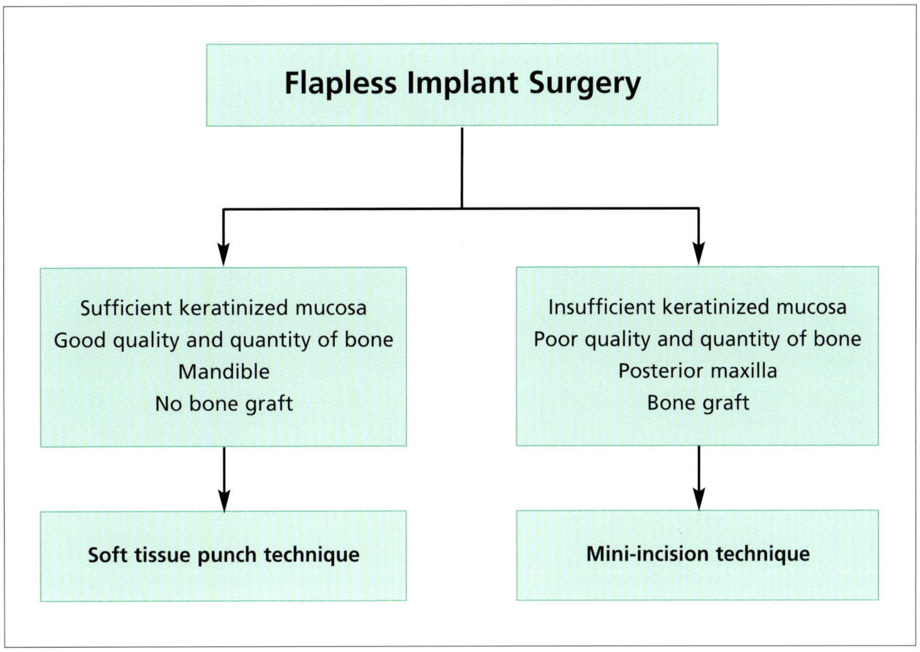

Fig 4-37 Choice of a soft tissue punch technique or a mini-incision technique is dependent on bone quality and primary implant stability.

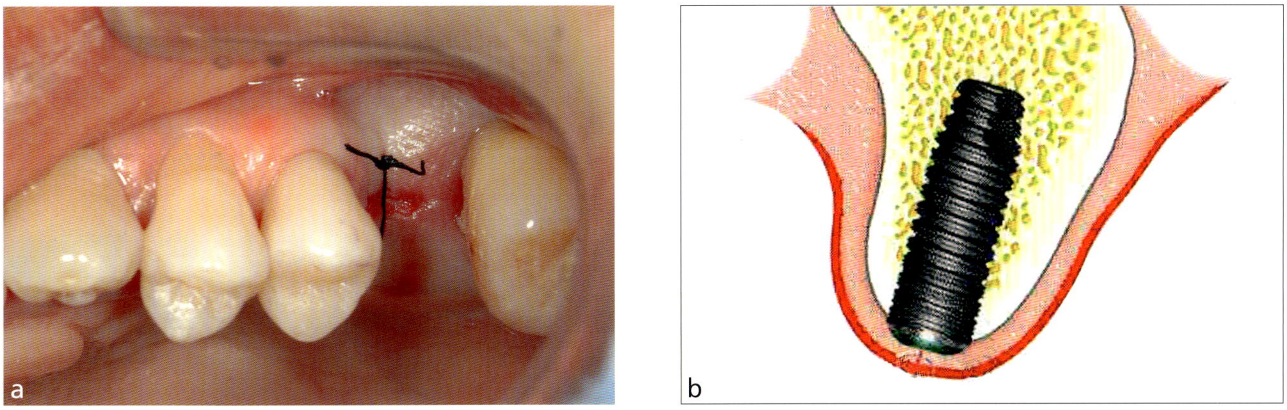

Fig 4-38 (a and b) On rare occasions, the implant in the maxilla may not be rigid after implant placement. Any implant that is not adequately stabilized should be submerged during healing, which reduces the risk of micromovement and early implant failure. Therefore, the mini-incision technique is selected in the maxilla to place the implant body below the soft tissue.

bone interface. Any implant that is not adequately stabilized should be submerged during healing, which reduces the risk of micromovement and early implant failure. Therefore, the mini-incision technique is selected for implants in the posterior maxilla in order to place the implant body below the soft tissue (Fig 4-38). The mini-incision technique is the best approach in the posterior maxilla where deficient osseous structures and an absence of a cortical plate on the crest of the ridge further compromise the initial implant stability at the time of insertion.[11]

Guideline 4: In the mandible, a one-stage approach offers more advantages

The most common complication of a two-stage approach in the mandible is the risk of fistulas or gumboils, which can develop in the mucosa covering the cover screws, because the mandible contains thick cortical bone,[12-14] thin mucosa,[15] and a 1–2 mm wide avascular zone in the crestal area of the edentulous alveolar ridge[16] (Figs 4-39 to 4-41). Fistulas or gumboils that develop in the mandible are dangerous because they can destroy bone (Fig 4-42). Therefore, when the implant is threaded into position with 20 Ncm or more, a one-stage approach is used in the mandible (Fig 4-43). This approach eliminates the risk of postoperative infection and allows the peri-implant soft tissue to be mature at the time of implant placement. When an implant in the mandible is not rigid after implant placement, the implant should be submerged. Periodic, meticulous observation is necessary to check for the formation of a gumboil or fistula.

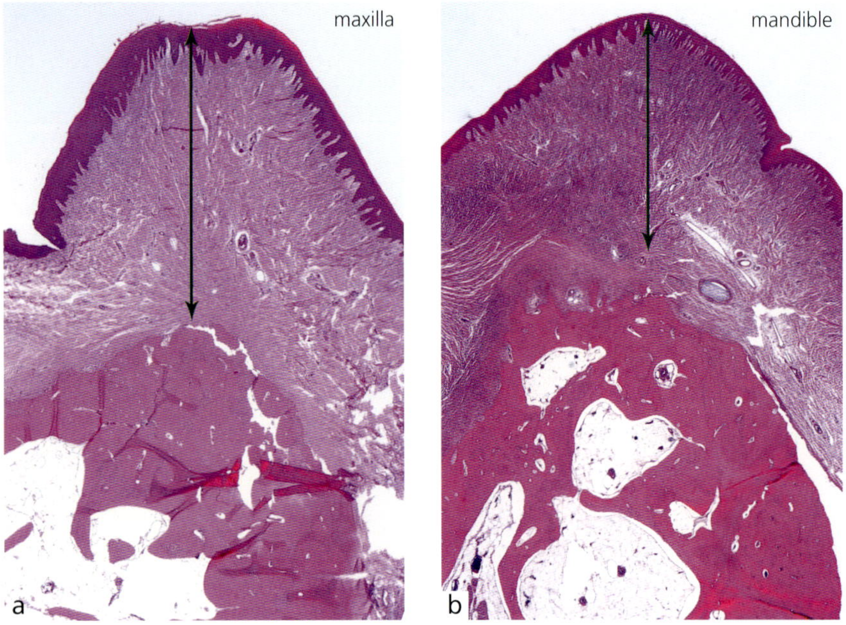

Fig 4-39 (a and b) The maxilla has thicker mucosa than the mandible.

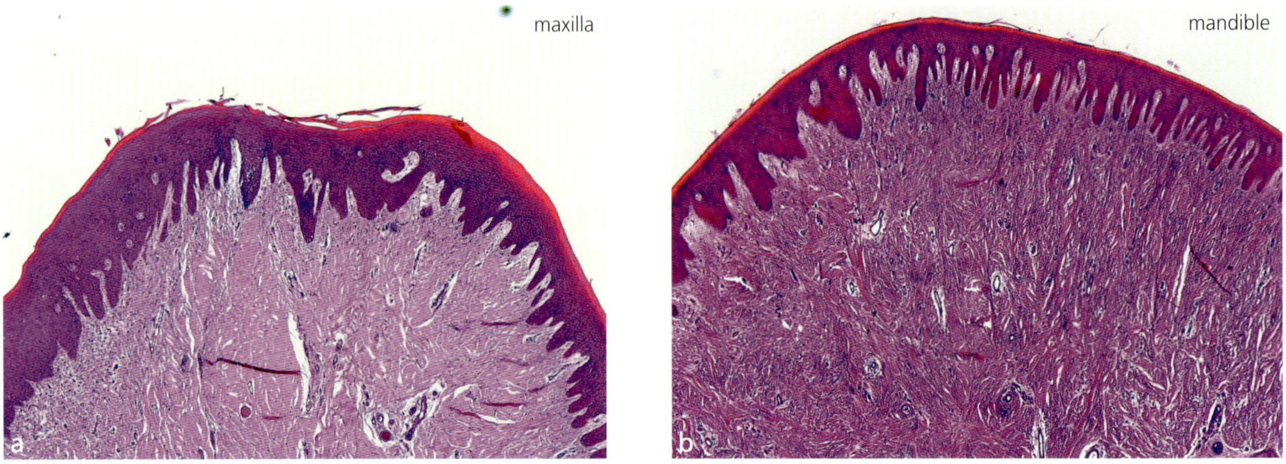

Fig 4-40 (a and b) The maxilla has a thicker epithelial layer than the mandible.

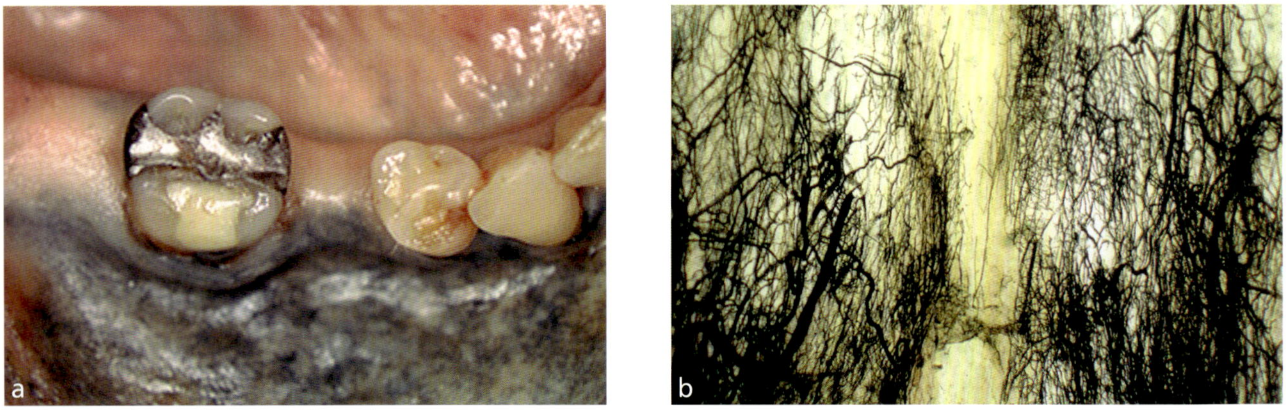

Fig 4-41 (a and b) The mandible has a 1–2 mm wide avascular zone in the crestal area of the edentulous alveolar ridge. (Reproduced from Kleinheinz et al.[16] with permission.)

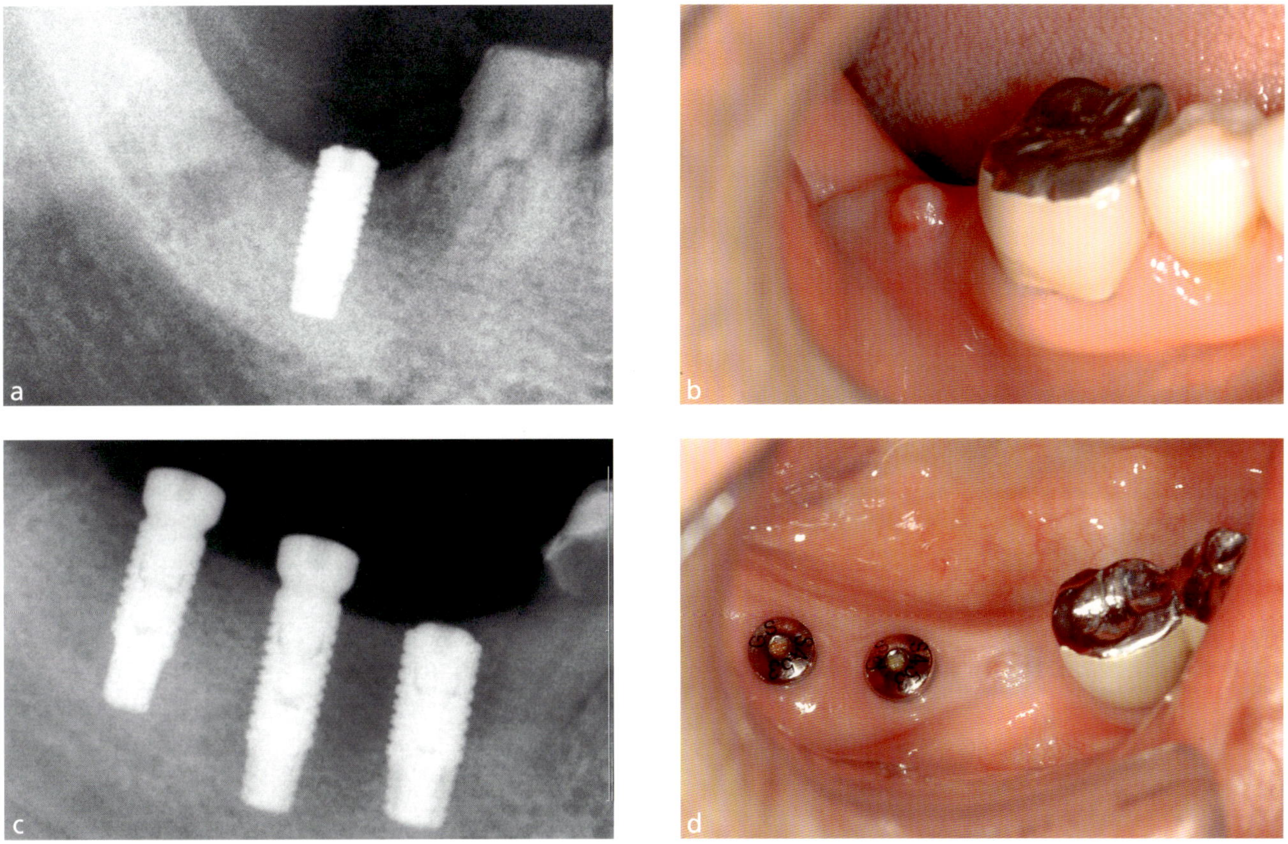

Fig 4-42 (a–d) Radiographs and intraoral views showing fistulas or gumboils developing in the mandible after mini-incision submerged implant placement.

Guideline 5: Select the mini-incision submerged technique in a bone graft

When a bone graft is considered at the time of implant insertion using a subperiosteal tunneling procedure, primary closure of the soft tissues creates a more favorable environment for bone growth. Therefore, the soft tissue punch technique is less indicated under these conditions.

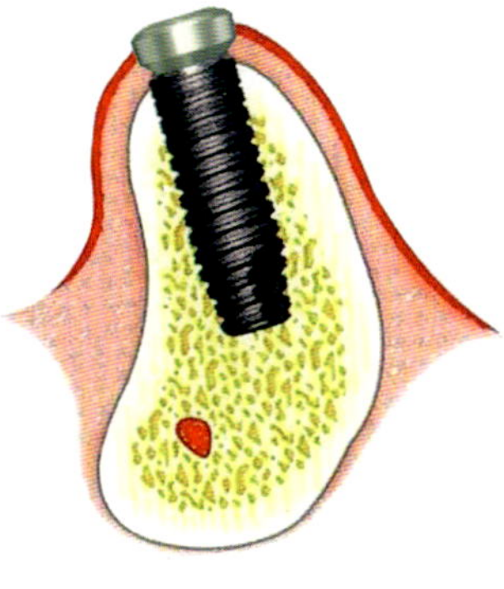

Fig 4-43 When the implant is threaded into position with a torque of 20–Ncm or more, a one-stage approach is used in the mandible. This approach eliminates the risk of postoperative infection.

Summary

To develop an appropriate treatment plan, information on bone quality, mucosal character, narrow and slanted alveolar bone, thick mucosa, and bone height between the sinus floor and the alveolar crest should be acquired from the presurgical evaluation via imaging, casts, and intraoral condition. In areas with insufficient bone width or height, the geometry of soft and hard tissues is an important consideration in the determination of a treatment plan. In the edentulous posterior maxilla, treatment options are chosen based on both the amount of remaining bone and the primary stability of the implants. The choice of a soft tissue punch technique or a mini-incision technique is dependent on both bone quality and primary implant stability. In general, either the soft tissue punch or the mini-incision nonsubmerged procedure is used for mandibles with thick cortical bone and high initial stability of the implant, while the mini-incision submerged procedure is used for maxillae with either poor bone quality or low initial stability of the implant.

References

1. Misch CE. Divisions of available bone in implant dentistry. Int J Oral Implant 1990;7:9–17.
2. Misch CE. Contemporary Implant Dentistry. London: Mosby-Wolfe, 1993.
3. Engelke W. Surgical implantation treatment concept for atrophic upper and lower jaw. Niedersachs Zahnarztebl 1991;26:404–409.
4. Abrahamsson I, Berglundh T, Moon I-S, Lindhe J. Peri-implant tissues at submerged and non-submerged titanium implants. J Clin Periodontol 1999;26:600–607.
5. Jackowski J, Johren P, Muller AM, Kruse A, Dirschka T. Imaging of fibrosis of the oral mucosa by 20 MHz sonography. Dentomaxillofac Radiol 1999;28:290–294.
6. Zeren KJ. Minimally invasive extraction and immediate implant placement: the preservation of esthetics. Int J Periodont Restor Dent 2006;26:171–181.
7. Wittwer G, Adeyemo WL, Schicho K, Figl M, Enislidis G. Navigated flapless transmucosal implant placement in the mandible: a pilot study in 20 patients. Int J Oral Maxillofac Implants 2007;22:801–807.
8. Van Steenberghe D, Glauser R, Blombaeck U et al. A computed tomographic scan-derived customized surgical template and fixed prosthesis for flapless surgery and immediate loading of implants in fully edentulous maxillae: a prospective multicenter study. Clin Implant Dent Relat Res 2005;7:S111–120.
9. Mischkowski RA, Zinser MJ, Neugebauer J, Kuebler AC, Zoeller JE. Comparison of static and dynamic computer-assisted guidance methods in implantology. Int J Comput Dent 2006;9:23–35.
10. Lekholm U, Zarb GA, Albrektsson T. Patient selection and preparation. In: Brånemark PI, Zarb GA, Albrektsson, T (eds). Tissue-integrated Prostheses. Chicago, IL: Quintessence, 1985:199–209.
11. Truhlar RS, Farish SE, Scheitler LE, Morris HF, Ochi S. Bone quality and implant design-related outcomes through stage II surgical uncovering of spectra-system root form implants. J Oral Maxillofac Surg 1997;55:46–54.
12. Friberg B, Jemt T, Lekholm U. Early failures in 4641 consecutively placed Brånemark dental implants: a study from stage I surgery to the connection of completed prostheses. Int J Oral Maxillofac Implants 1991;6:142–146.
13. Orenstein IH, Synan WJ, Truhlar RS, Morris HF, Ochi S. Bone quality in patients receiving endosseous dental implants: DICRG interim Report No. 1. Implant Dent 1994;3:90–94.
14. Friberg B, Sennerby L, Roos J, Lekholm U. Identification of bone quality in conjunction with insertion of titanium implants: a pilot study in jaw autopsy specimens. Clin Oral Implants Res 1995;6:213–219.
15. Vandana KL, Savitha B. Thickness of gingival in association with age, gender and dental arch location. J Clin Periodontol 2005;32:828–830.
16. Kleinheinz J, Büchter A, Kruse-Lösler B, Weingart D, Joos U. Incision design in implant dentistry based on vascularization of the mucosa. Clin Oral Implants Res 2005;16:518–523.

CHAPTER
5

Flapless Implant Surgery Technique

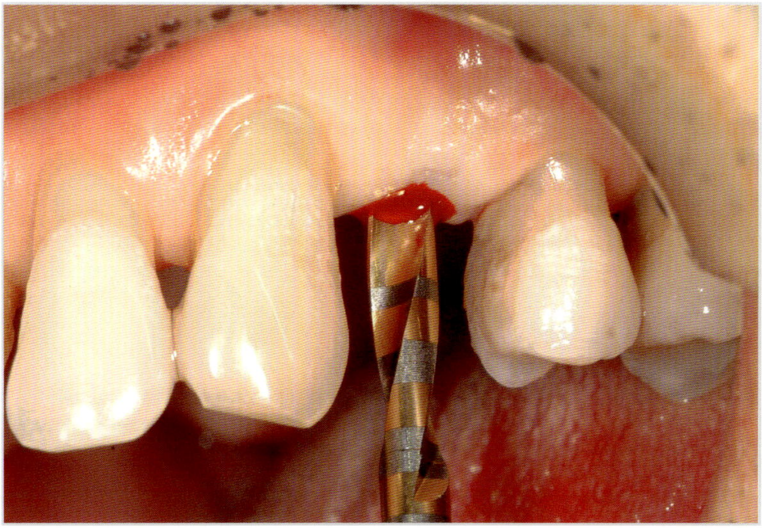

Key point

If we know where the target is, we can hit it without needing to see it.

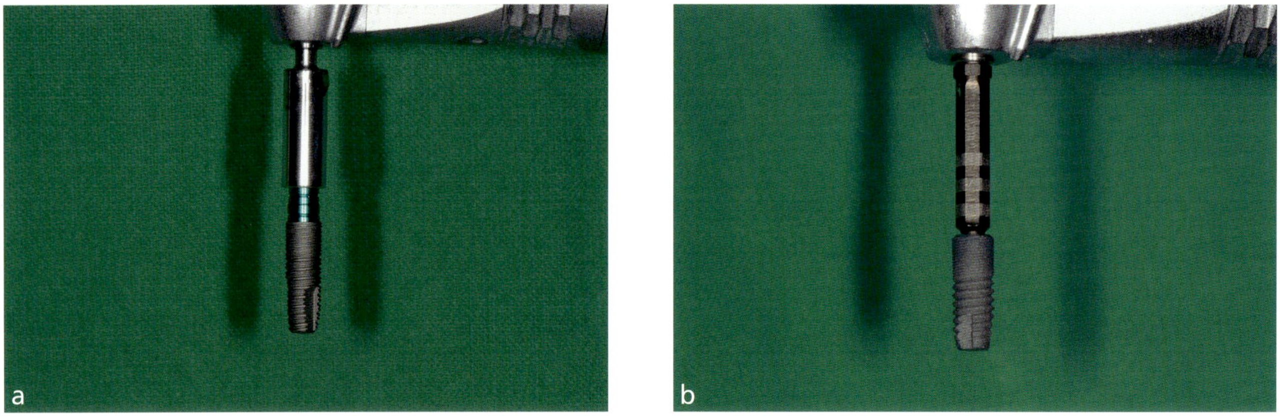

Fig 5-1 (a) Osstem's GS system type, and (b) Astra implant.

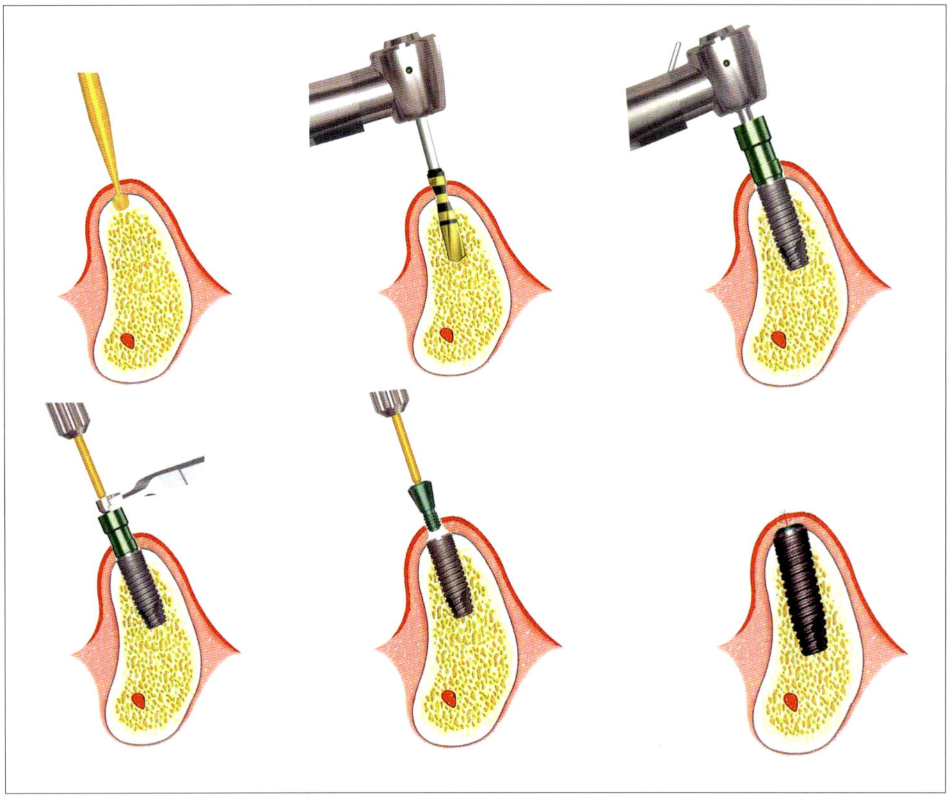

Fig 5-2 Diagram showing flapless submerged implant placement.

Overview

In order to place implants precisely into the bone without directly visualizing the alveolar bone, it is important to have information on the bone and mucosa before, during, and immediately after surgery. This chapter addresses how to perform flapless implant surgery precisely. The method described involves the use of Astra (Mölndal, Sweden) or Osstem (Seoul, Korea) implants (Figs 5-1 and 5-2).

Cleansing and anesthesia

Extraoral and intraoral scrubbing should be performed with iodine, povidone–iodine (Betadine), or 0.12% chlorhexidine, and antibacterial mouth rinses with 0.12% chlorhexidine. Scrubbing around and within the mouth with the agent reduces the risk of a bacterial smear layer resulting from unintentional contamination by direct contact with the implant or indirectly via a glove or instrument. Antibacterial mouth rinses such as chlorhexidine

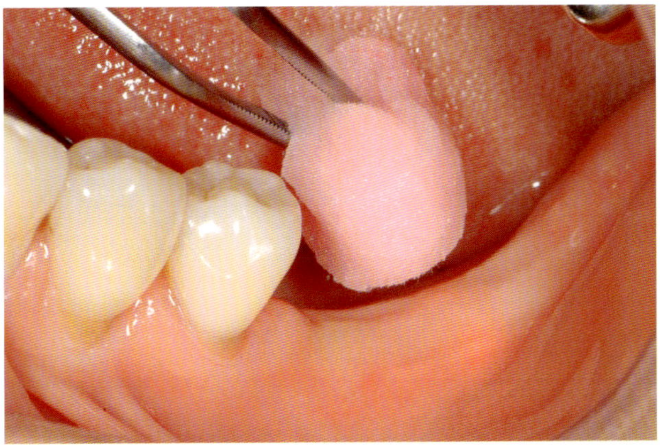

Fig 5-3 Meticulous preoperative disinfection should be performed, particularly in the area of the mucosa through which the implants pass.

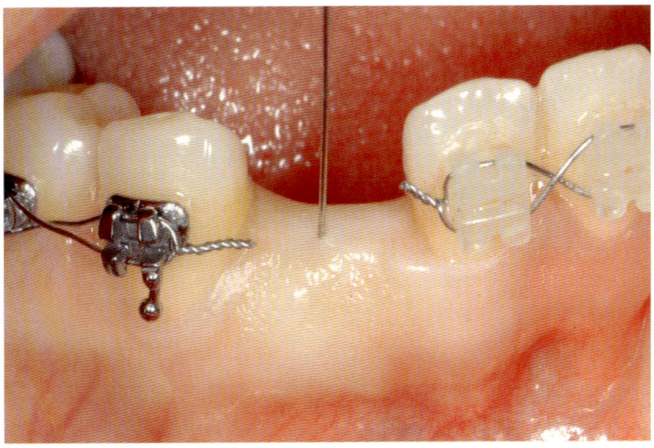

Fig 5-4 Infiltration with 2% lidocaine with 1:100,000 epinephrine is performed at the implant site.

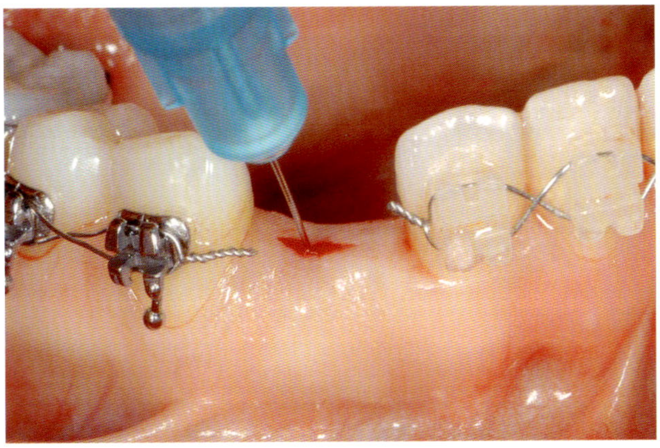

Fig 5-5 Additional infiltration through the osteotomy site into the bone after the initial osteotomy preparation with a pilot drill is required.

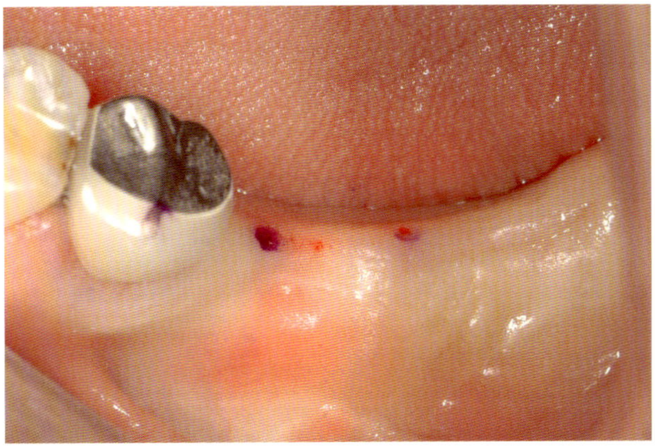

Fig 5-6 The center of the implant site location is marked with gentian violet.

reduce the bacterial count in saliva significantly. It is important to perform meticulous preoperative disinfection, particularly in the area of the mucosa through which the implants pass (Fig 5-3).

Infiltration with 2% lidocaine containing 1:100,000 epinephrine should be performed at the implant site (Fig 5-4). Further infiltration is required through the osteotomy site into the bone after the initial osteotomy preparation with a pilot drill (Fig 5-5).

Surgical preparation of the implant site

Implant site location

The surgical guide template is placed in position, and the center of the implant site location is marked with a surgical pen: gentian violet (GV) or Indian ink (Fig 5-6).

Making the incision

Incision for mini-incision technique

A crestal mini-incision, approximately 5 mm horizontally with the alveolar crest, is made at the center of the implant site (Fig 5-7). It is important that the incision be completed in one pass through the mucosa and periosteum, and the periosteum should be scored precisely. Local undermining of the gingiva is then performed. The amount of undermining of the implant site should not exceed 5 mm, and it should fall within the range of a large-diameter implant (Fig 5-8). During the undermining procedure, the soft tissue on both sides of the incision line is pushed aside to accommodate the drills and implants.

A 5 mm incision is appropriate for 4 mm diameter implants. It is advisable to make a >5 mm incision when a mini-incision technique is used for the placement of 5 mm or larger diameter implants. Drilling through an opening too small using a wide drill can cause significant damage to the adjacent soft tissue. Multiple mini-incisions will be required when more than two implants are placed.

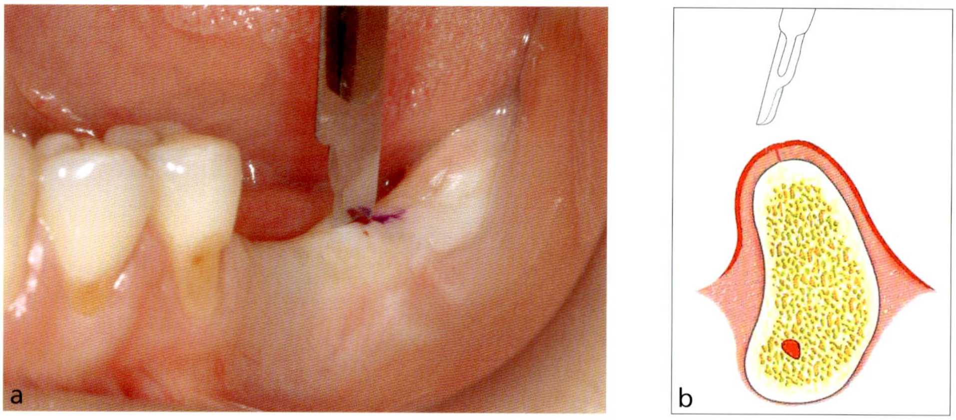

Fig 5-7 (a and b) For mini-incision implant placement, a crestal mini-incision approximately 5 mm long is made at the center of the implant site, parallel to the alveolar crest.

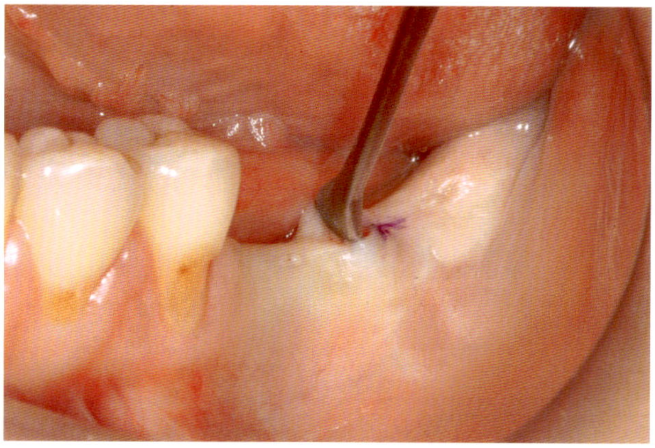

Fig 5-8 Local undermining of the gingiva is performed to allow for the entrance of the drill and implants.

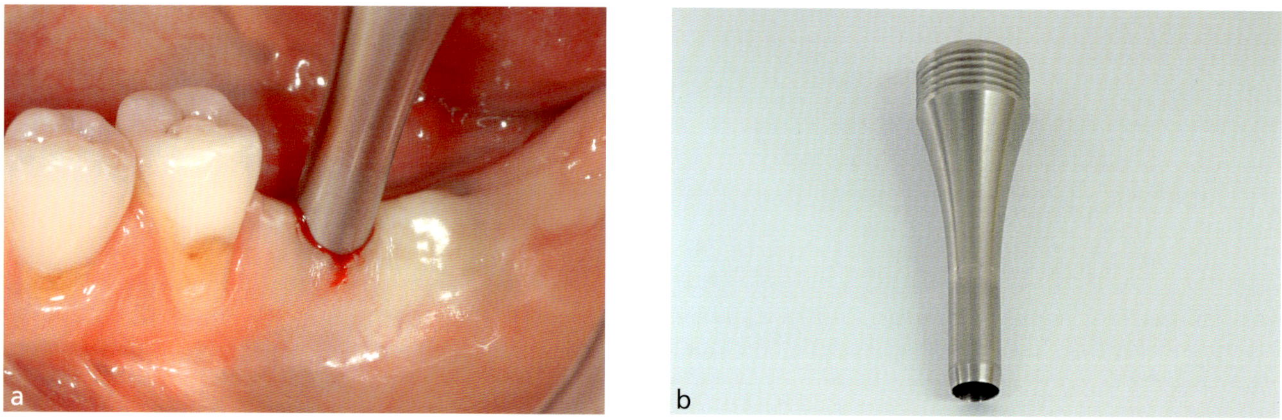

Fig 5-9 (a) A circumferential incision is made in the gingiva at the center of the implant site using a soft tissue punch, and the incised attached gingiva is then removed. (b) The soft tissue punch should be 1.0–1.5 mm narrower than the implant diameter.

Incision for soft tissue punch technique

A circumferential incision is made in the gingiva at the center of the implant site using a soft tissue punch. The incised attached gingiva is then removed (Fig 5-9). A soft tissue punch bur can also be used for the circumferential incision (Fig 5-10). However, a trephine bur should not be used for this purpose because it can tear the soft tissue instead of making an incision (Fig 5-11). The soft tissue punch or bur should be 1.0–1.5 mm narrower than the implant diameter. The peri-implant mucosa is in tight contact with the implant surface after implant placement when the soft tissue punch or bur is 1.0–1.5 mm narrower than the implant. Multiple punches are recommended when more than two implants are to be placed (Fig 5-12).

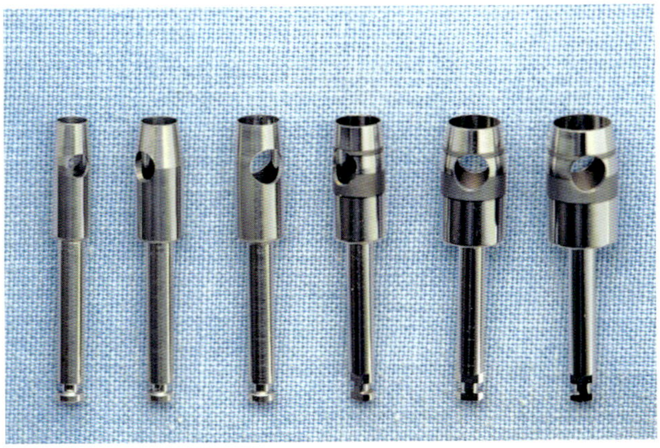

Fig 5-10 Various sizes of soft tissue punch burs. The soft tissue punch burs can be used for circumferential incisions. See also Fig 5-11.

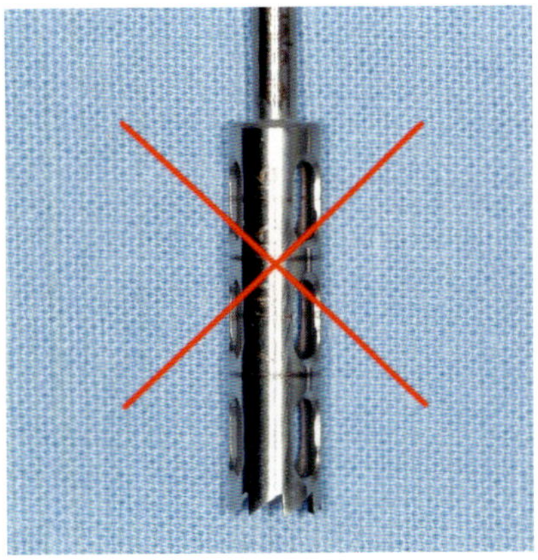

Fig 5-11 A trephine bur should not be used for this purpose because it may tear the soft tissue instead of making an incision.

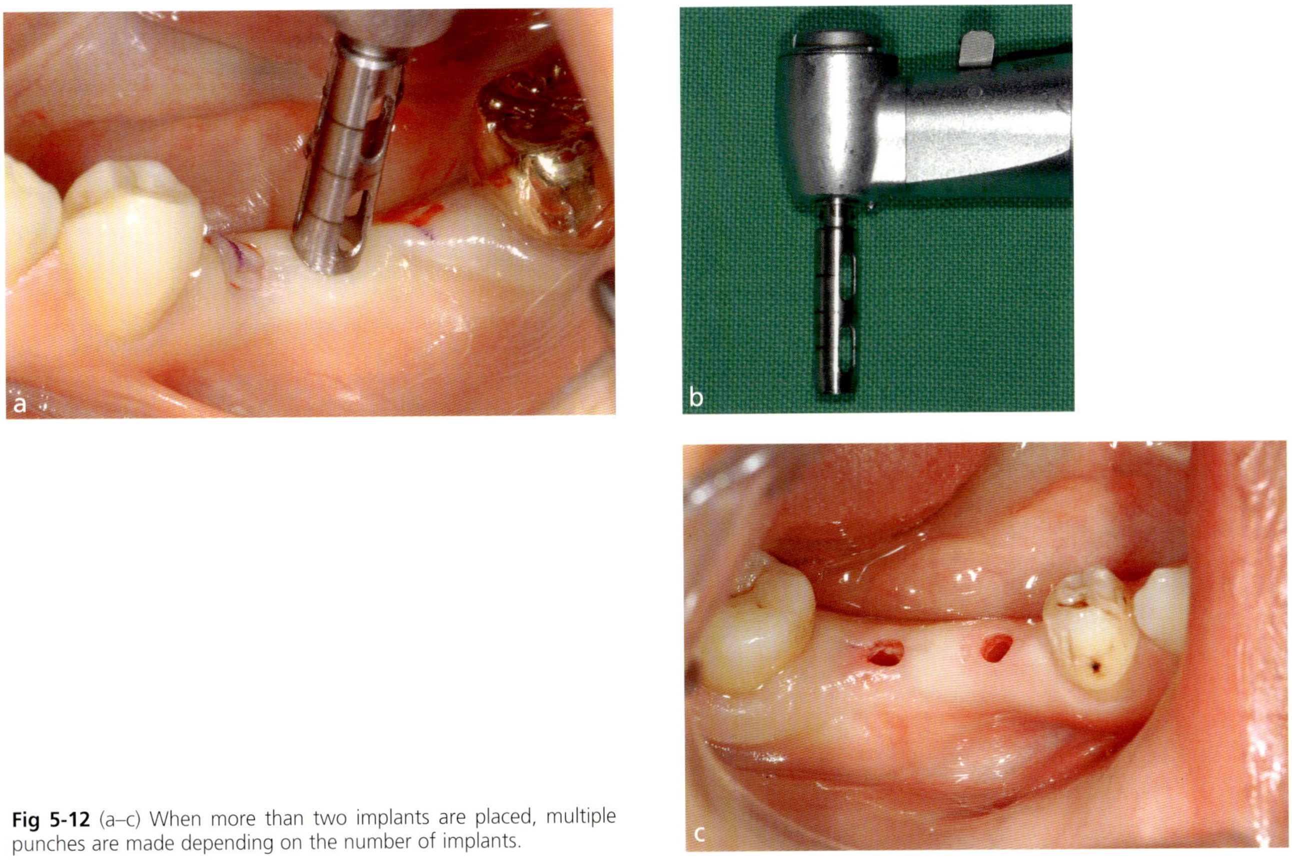

Fig 5-12 (a–c) When more than two implants are placed, multiple punches are made depending on the number of implants.

Measurement of the thickness of soft tissue

Before drilling, the mucosal thickness is measured using a periodontal probe or a depth gauge to verify the height of the mucosa at the implant site (Fig 5-13). The sum of the length of the implant and the thickness of the mucosa is marked on the drill, or stops on the drill can be used for the mark.

Drilling

A pilot hole is made with a No. 6 round bur to prevent the drill from slipping (Fig 5-14). The center implant site is prepared with the pilot drill for the initial depth of bone preparation for the implant length. During the drilling procedure, surgical guides help the surgeon to drill in the precisely planned position and with the desired angulation. The osteotomy preparation proceeds according to the

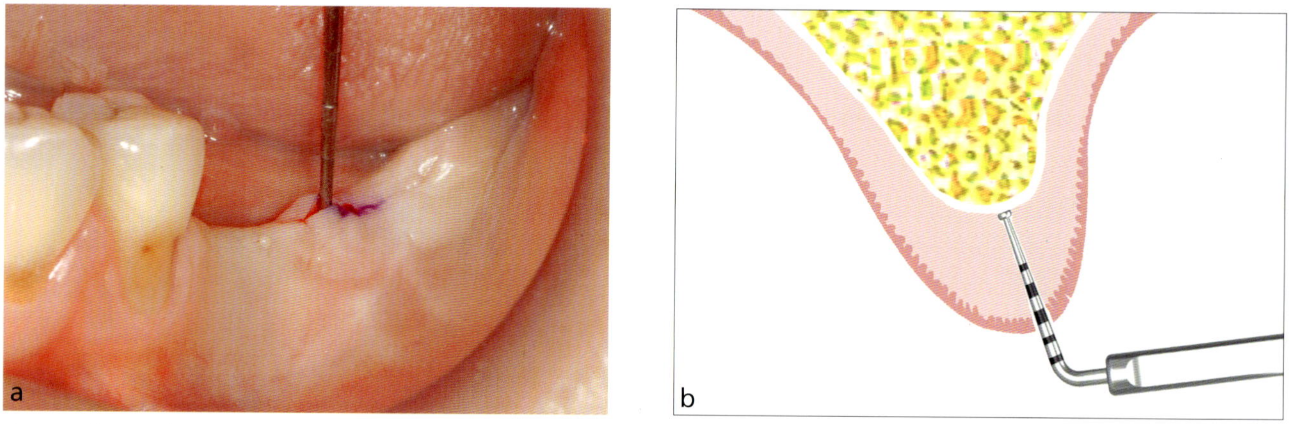

Fig 5-13 (a and b) The mucosal thickness is measured using a periodontal probe or a depth gauge to verify the height of the mucosa at the implant site.

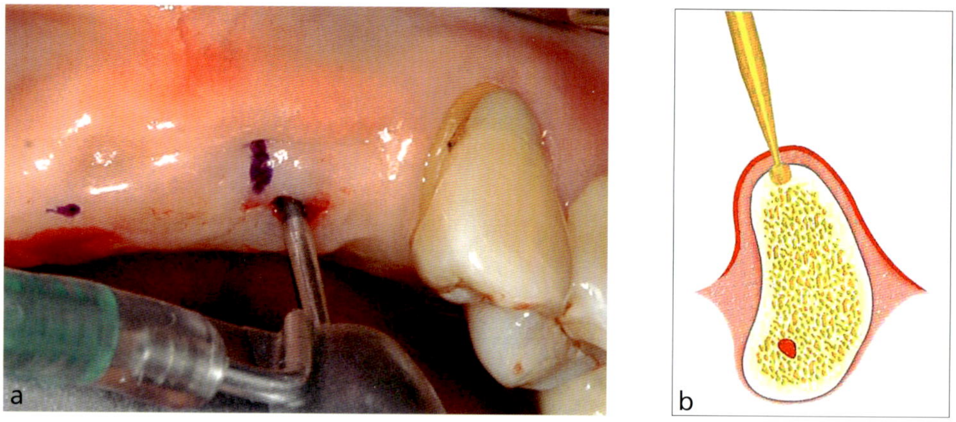

Fig 5-14 (a and b) A pilot hole is made with a No. 6 round bur.

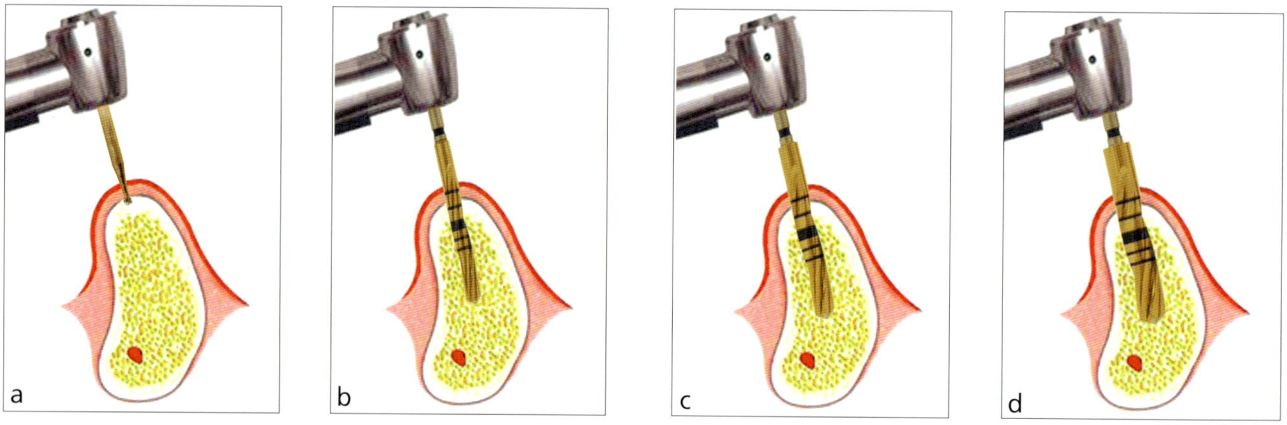

Fig 5-15 (a–d) Drills for osteotomy preparation.

drill sequence (Fig 5-15). It is advisable to use flapless implant drills with cutting surfaces on their tips and rounded surfaces on their other parts (Fig 5-16; see Chapter 6). The drilling depth is controlled above the mucosa by the marks on the drill, which correspond to the sum of the length of the implant and the thickness of the mucosa (Fig 5-17).

The osteotomy site should be irrigated frequently with cooled saline (Fig 5-18). The impact of external irrigation is limited because implant osteotomy is performed below the soft tissue. Therefore, cooled irrigation into the osteotomy site during pauses is essential to reduce the amount of heat generated. Decreasing the mucosal temperature by constant irrigation is also important. Constant irrigation also flushes debris from the osteotomy site.

For the maxilla with less dense bone, osteotomes can be used after the pilot drill to obtain the final osteotomy

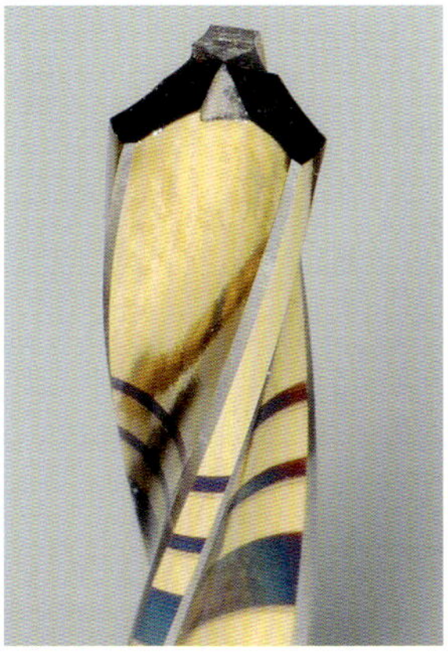

Fig 5-16 A new drill for flapless implant surgery with a cutting surface on the tip and rounded surfaces on all other sides.

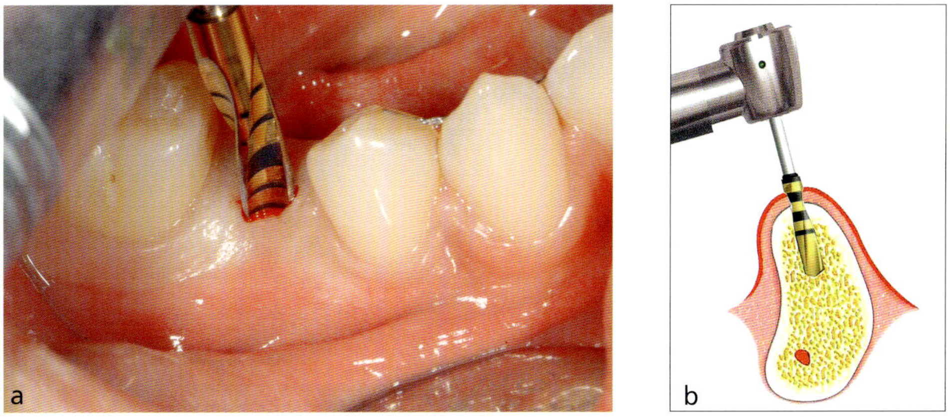

Fig 5-17 (a and b) The depth of drilling is controlled above the mucosa by the mark on the drill corresponding to the sum of the length of the implant and the thickness of the mucosa.

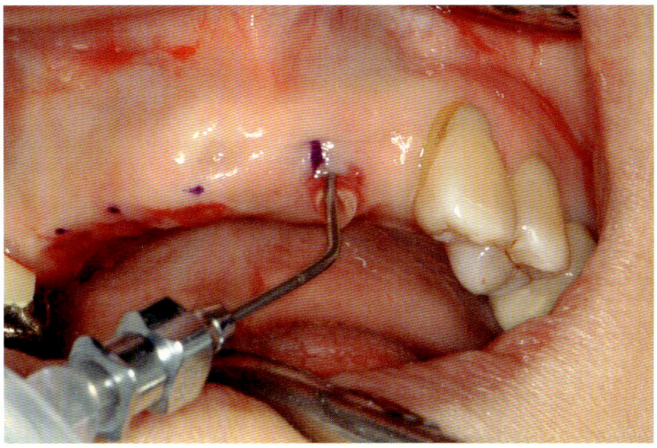

Fig 5-18 The osteotomy site is irrigated frequently with cooled saline.

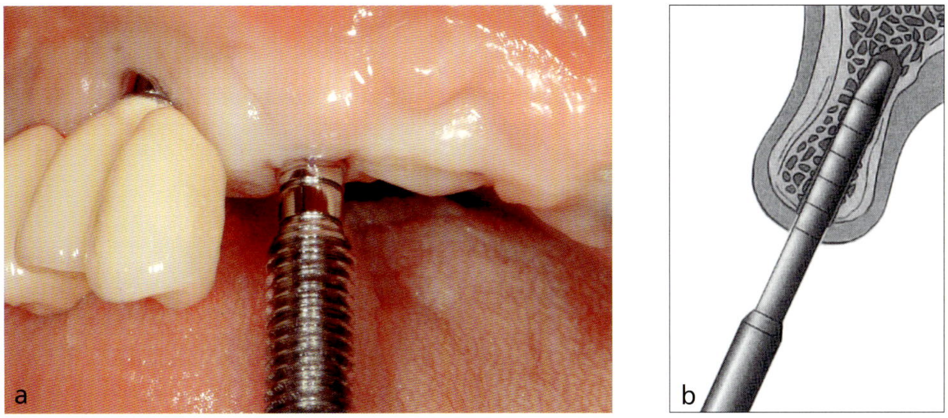

Fig 5-19 (a and b) For the maxilla with less dense bone, osteotomes are used after the pilot drill to obtain the final osteotomy dimension.

dimension (Fig 5-19). Osteotomes both compress the bone trabeculae and expand the osteotomy site. Less dense bone expands easily.

Implant placement

After drilling, the crestal heights in the facial and lingual plates are reassessed by measuring the osteotomy depth and the mucosal thickness around the crest from the mucosal surface (Fig 5-20). This allows an assessment of the crestal bone volume without flap elevation. In addition, a probe is inserted gently along the osteotomy walls, prob-

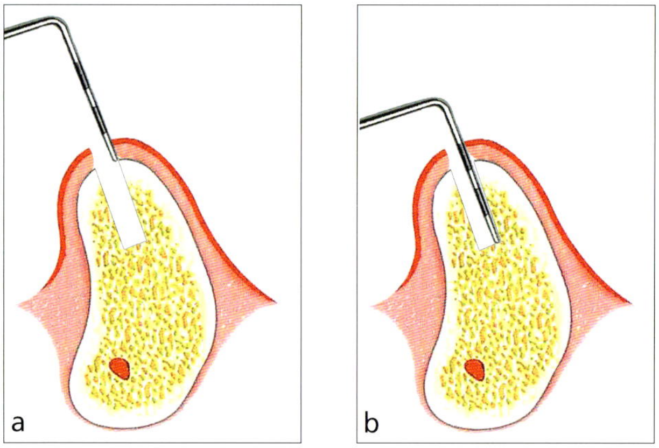

Fig 5-20 (a and b) Crestal heights in the facial and lingual plates are reassessed by measuring the osteotomy depth and the mucosal thickness around the crest from the mucosal surface.

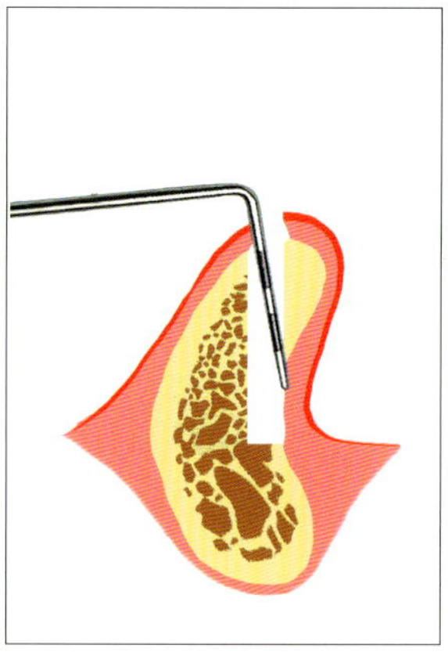

Fig 5-21 After drilling, a probe is gently inserted along the osteotomy walls, probing for any perforation of the cortical plate.

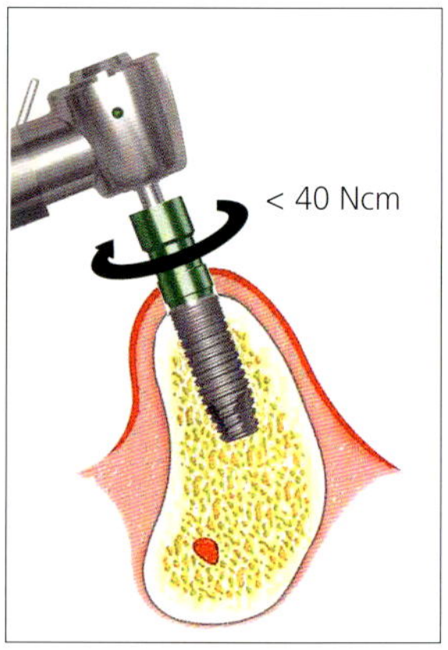

Fig 5-22 Insertion torque should not exceed 40 Nm.

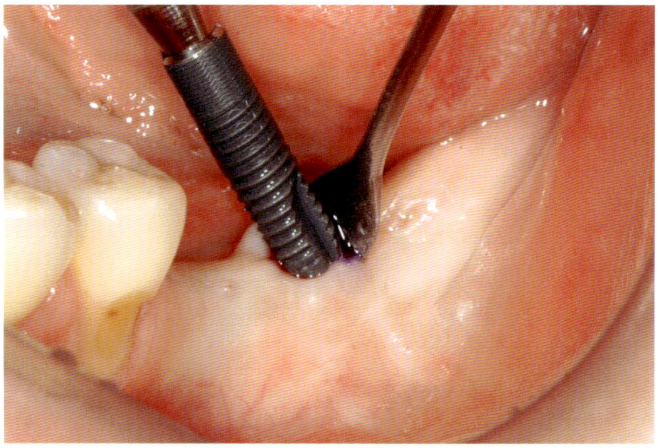

Fig 5-23 When inserting an implant through the mucosa entrance made by a mini-incision technique, the mini-incision is opened using a curette.

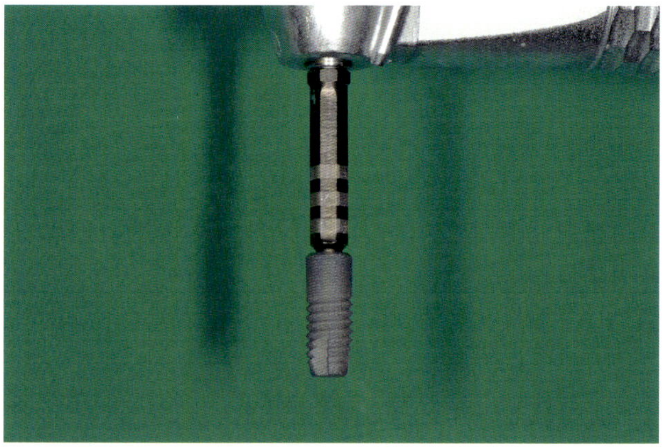

Fig 5-24 To control the depth of the implant fixture above the mucosa, use an implant system with depth lines inscribed on the shank above the mucosa. These lines should include one line that is longer than the sum of the fixture length and mucosal thickness. See also Figs 5-25 and 5-26.

ing for any perforation of the cortical plate (Fig 5-21). If the perforation is palpated, the site can be augmented with graft material using a subperiosteal tunneling procedure (see Chapter 12).

Before inserting the implant, the osteotomy site should be suctioned to remove any bone debris and blood to minimize the hydrostatic pressure during implant insertion. If this is not done, the implant may compress the contents of the site beyond the apex and place pressure on the mandibular nerve.

A low-speed handpiece or a hand wrench is used to place the implants, which allows a more precise implant rotation, and constant pressure ensures that the implant will progress into the site without stripping the bone within the threads. The insertion torque should not exceed 40 Ncm because excessive pressure at the implant–bone interface at insertion can cause bone loss (Fig 5-22).[1]

When inserting an implant through a mucosa entrance made using a mini-incision technique, the mini-incision is opened using a probe or a curette (Fig 5-23). In addition, immediately before engaging the implant in the osteotomy site, peri implant probing is carried out around the implant to confirm that the soft tissue is interposed between the bone and implant. This procedure can prevent soft tissue from infiltrating into the bone holes during implant placement.

Depth lines are inscribed on the shank of the implants above the mucosa (Fig 5-24). These are used to control the

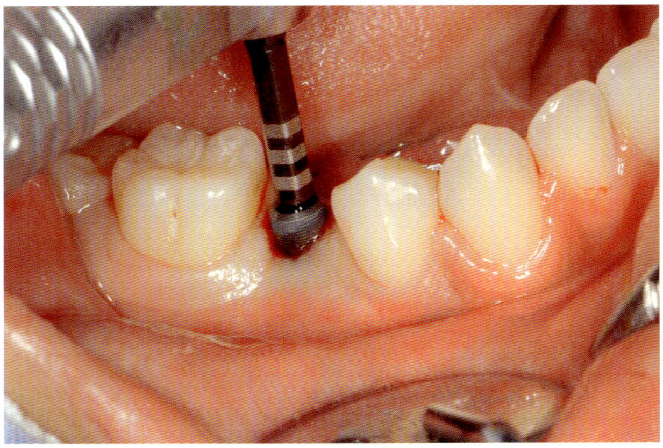

Fig 5-25 The depth of the implant fixture is controlled above the mucosa.

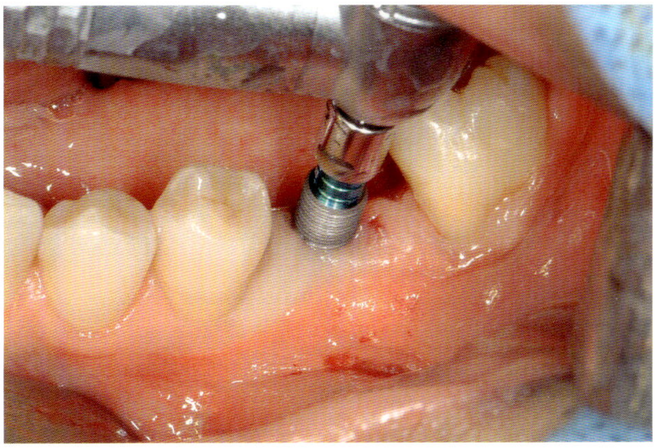

Fig 5-26 The depth of the implant fixture is controlled above the mucosa.

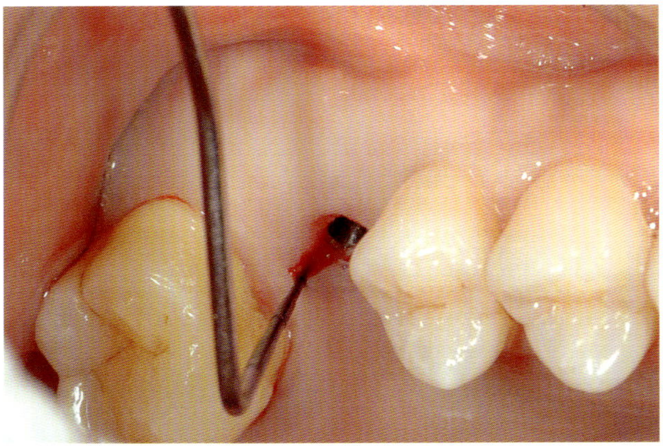

Fig 5-27 Intraoral view showing peri-implant probing around the implant to confirm that the implant crest module is located at the level of the bone crest.

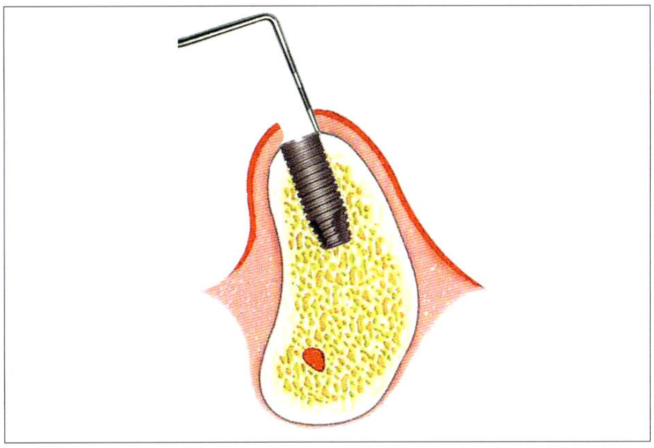

Fig 5-28 Immediately after implant placement, peri-implant probing around the implant is carried out to confirm that the implant crest module is located at the level of the bone crest.

depth of the implant fixture above the mucosa (Fig 5-25). The depth lines should include a line that is longer than the sum of the fixture length and mucosal thickness (Fig 5-26). Immediately after implant placement, peri-implant probing around the implant should be carried out to confirm that the implant crest module is located at the level of the bone crest (Figs 5-27 and 5-28).

Mini-incision technique

After implant placement, either a low-profile cover screw is inserted into the implant body for a two-stage surgical approach (Fig 5-29), or a permucosal healing abutment is inserted for a one-stage approach. For the two-stage approach, the tissues are then approximated over the implant for primary closure (Fig 5-30). One interrupted suture is sufficient to allow primary closure of the soft tissue (Figs 5-31 and 5-32). For the one-stage approach, the procedure is performed in accordance with the soft tissue punch technique.

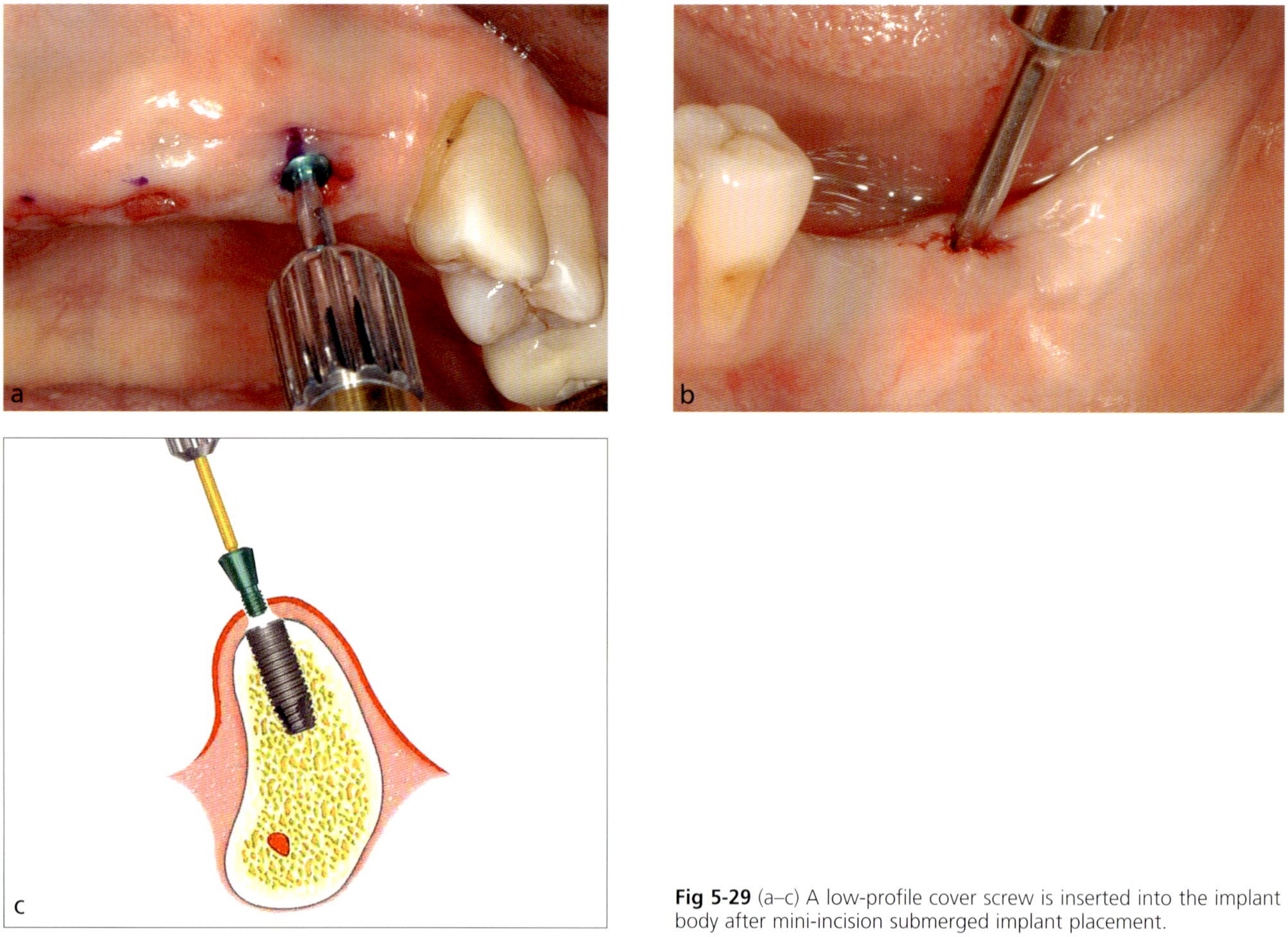

Fig 5-29 (a–c) A low-profile cover screw is inserted into the implant body after mini-incision submerged implant placement.

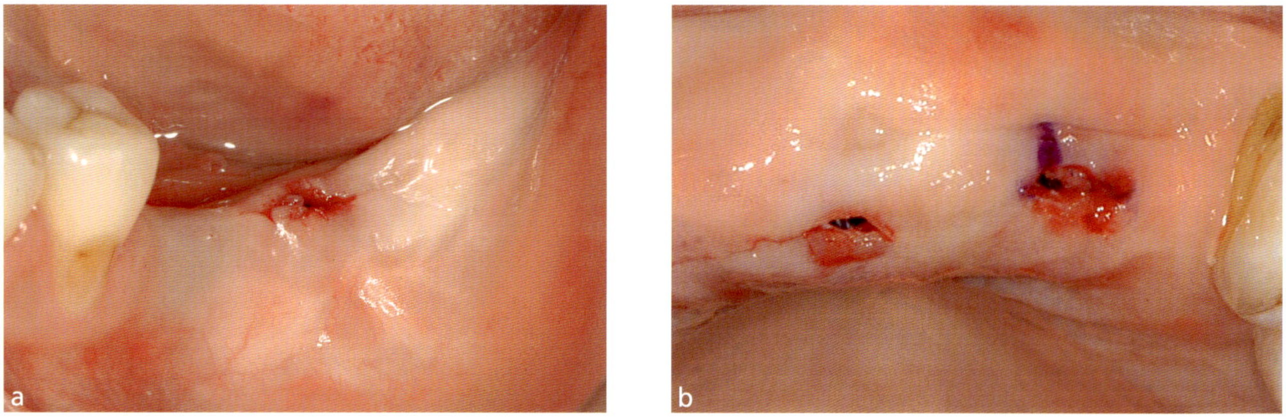

Fig 5-30 (a and b) The soft tissues are approximated over the implant for primary closure.

Soft tissue punch technique

After implant placement, a permucosal healing abutment is inserted for the one-stage surgical approach (Fig 5-33). The permucosal healing abutment should extend 1–2 mm above the adjacent mucosa to help to prevent tissue overgrowth during the healing period (Figs 5-34 and 5-35). This is because the adjacent mucosa swells to approximately 0.7 mm as a result of postoperative edema. The healing abutment should be replaced with a longer one if the implant is covered with tissue overgrowth during the healing period (Fig 5-36). The higher-profile permucosal

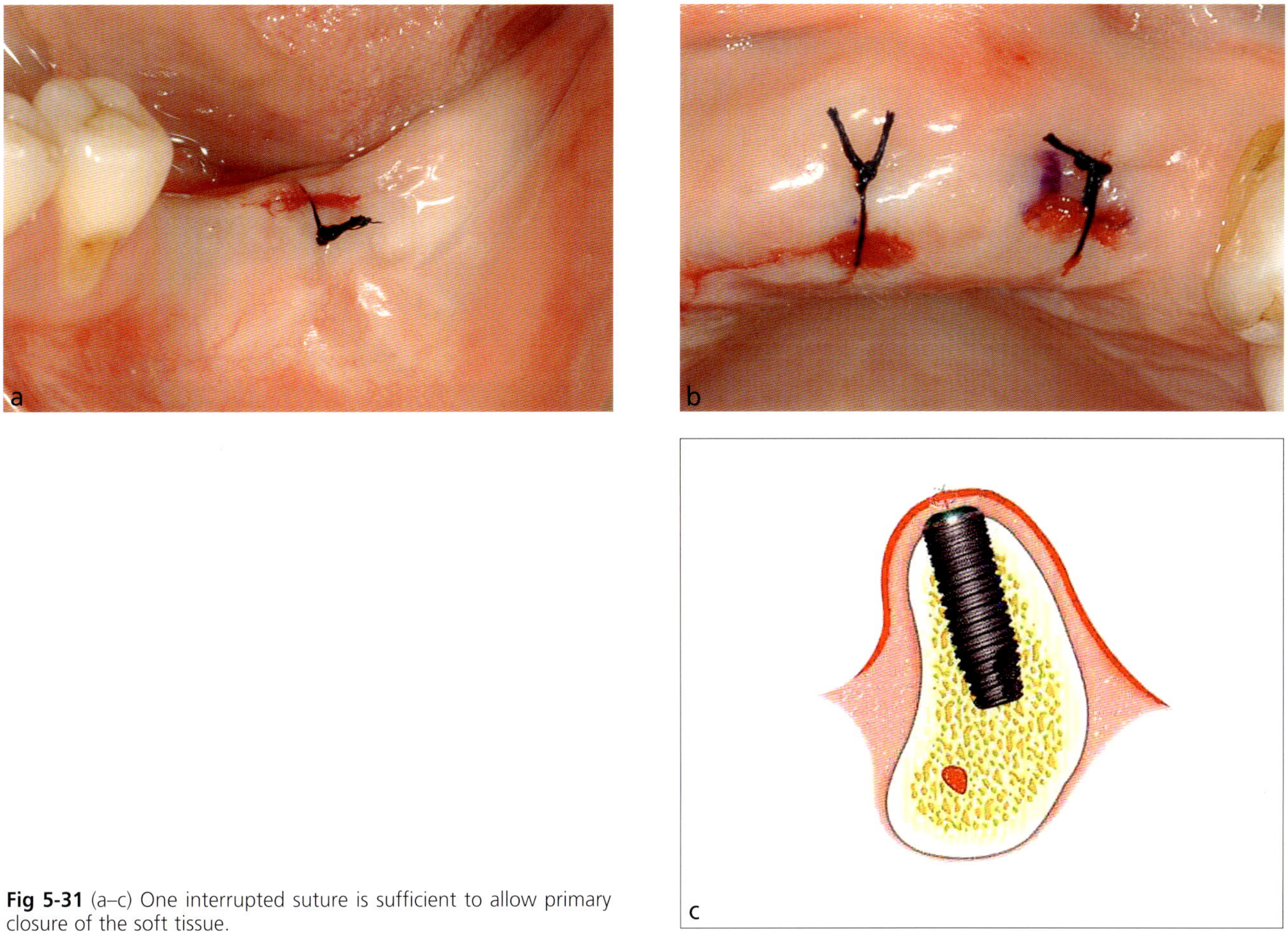

Fig 5-31 (a–c) One interrupted suture is sufficient to allow primary closure of the soft tissue.

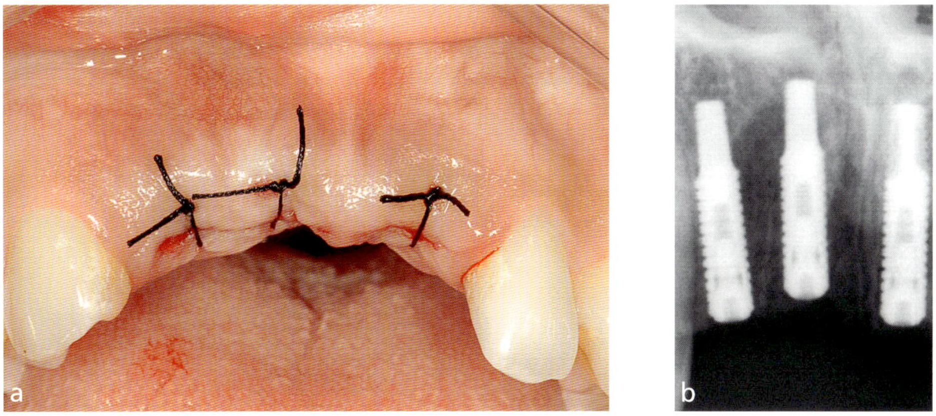

Fig 5-32 (a and b) Intraoral view and radiograph taken immediately after mini-incision submerged implant placement.

healing abutment is more at risk of loading during healing, particularly when an overlying soft tissue-borne transitional restoration is worn (Fig 5-37). The permucosal healing abutment should be 1.0–1.5 mm wider than the soft tissue punch to ensure close contact between the peri-implant mucosa and healing abutment (Figs 5-38 and 5-39). After inserting the healing abutments, the peri-implant mucosa should be evaluated for any irregular edges, which can be cut and removed because the final soft tissue contour depends on the early formation.

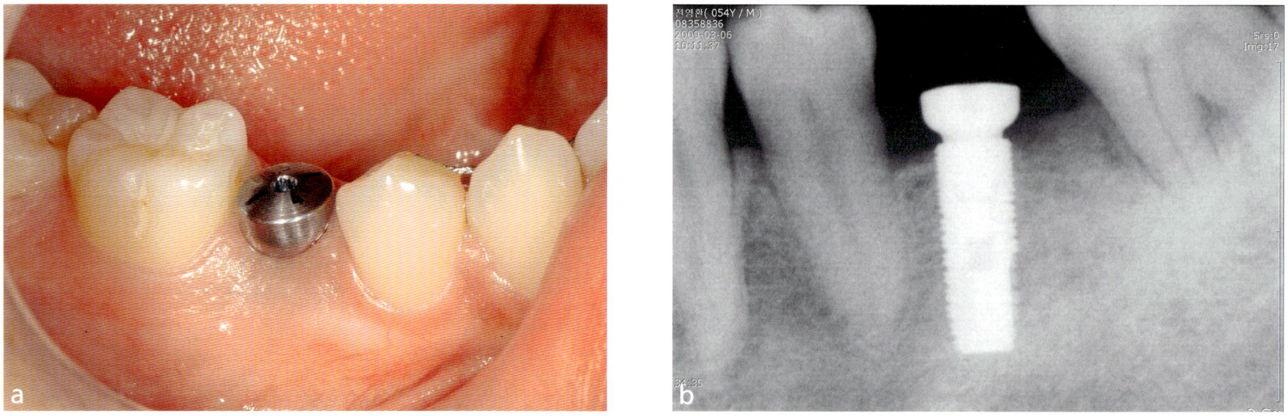

Fig 5-33 (a) Intraoral view showing soft tissue punch implant placement. (b) Radiograph taken immediately after the implant placement.

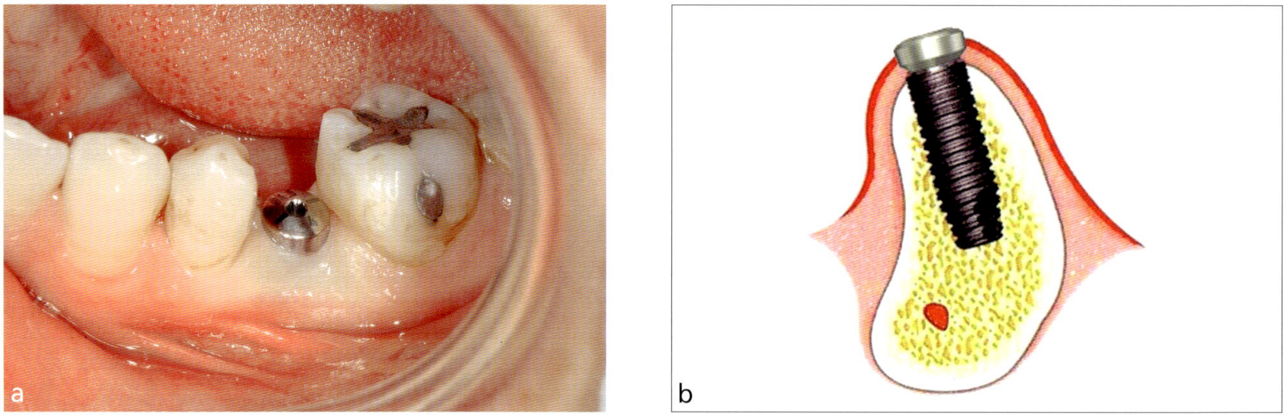

Fig 5-34 (a and b) View immediately after soft tissue punch implant placement. Note that the permucosal healing abutment should extend 1–2 mm above the adjacent mucosa to help prevent tissue overgrowth during the healing period.

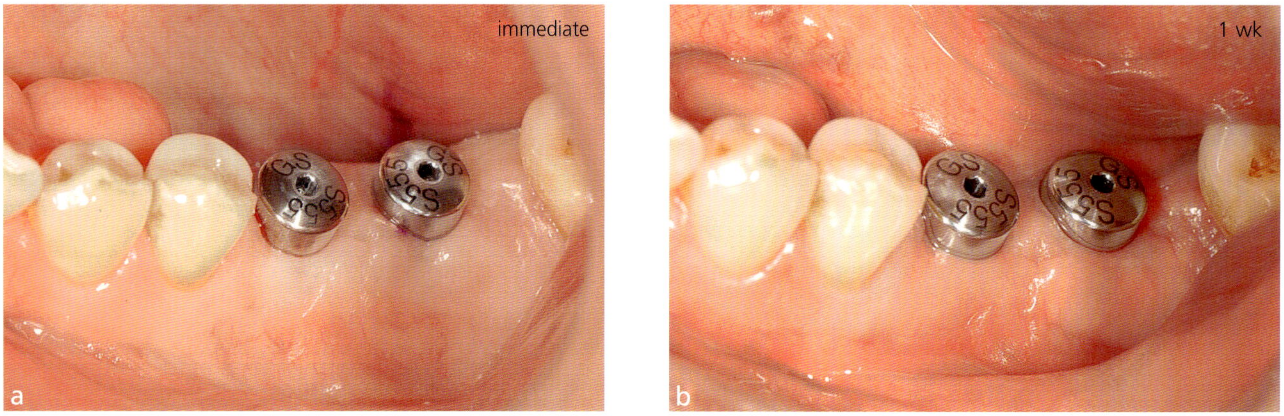

Fig 5-35 (a and b) Views immediately and 1 week after soft tissue punch implant placement. Note that the adjacent mucosa swells to approximately 0.7 mm as a result of edema.

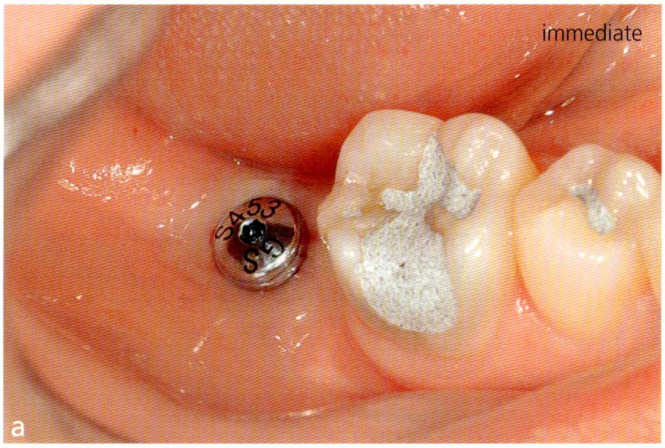

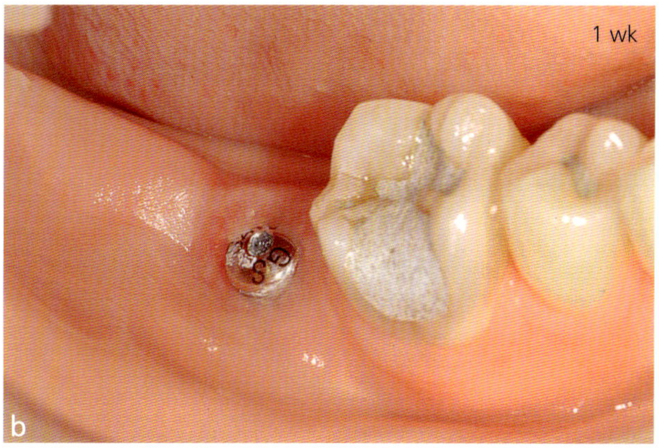

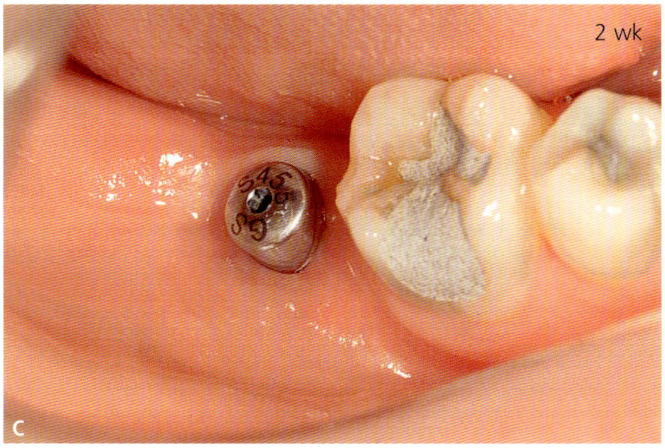

Fig 5-36 (a–c) The healing abutment should be replaced with a higher one if the implant is covered by tissue overgrowth during the healing period.

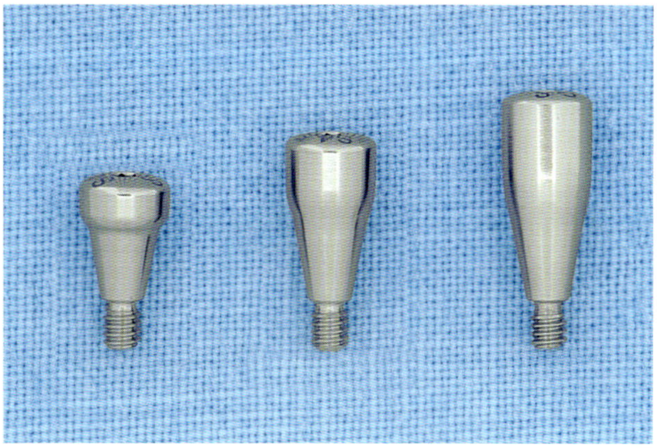

Fig 5-37 Various heights of permucosal healing abutments.

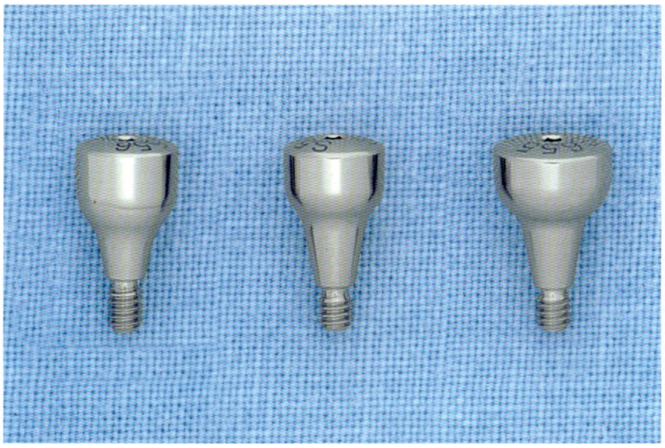

Fig 5-38 Various widths of permucosal healing abutments.

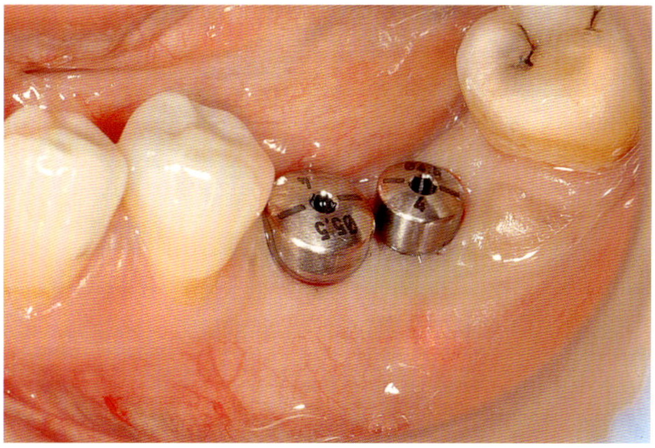

Fig 5-39 The permucosal healing abutment should be 1.0–1.5 mm wider than the soft tissue punch to ensure close contact between the peri-implant mucosa and healing abutment.

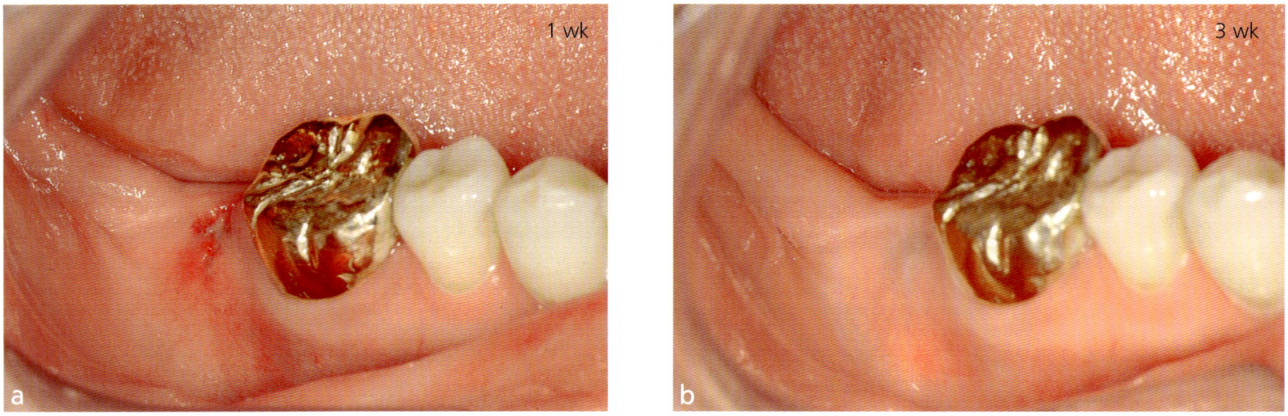

Fig 5-40 (a and b) Intraoral views after mini-incision submerged implant placement. The suture is removed after 1 week.

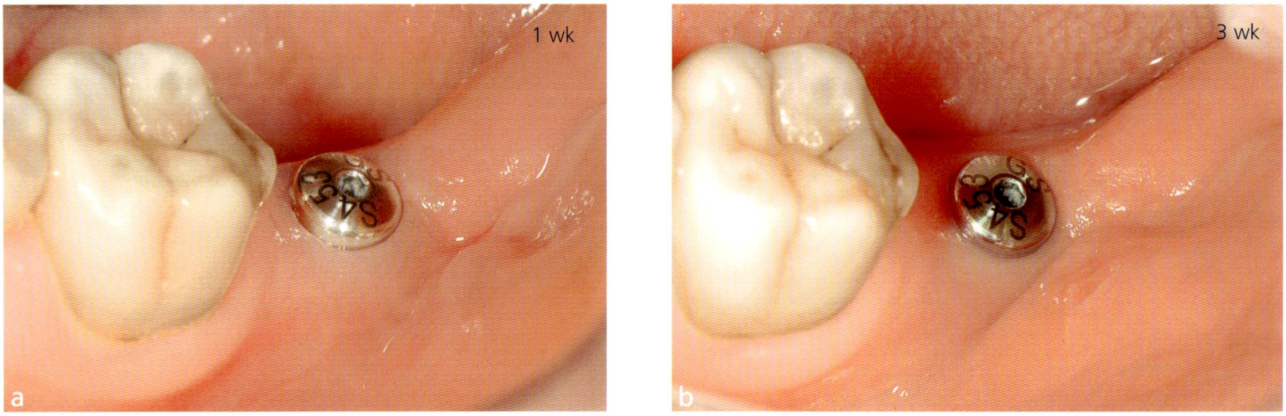

Fig 5-41 (a and b) Intraoral views after soft tissue punch implant placement. The soft tissue punch technique does not require suture removal because it uses no sutures.

Suture removal

The suture is removed 1 week after placing the mini-incision submerged implant (Fig 5-40). The soft tissue punch technique does not use sutures (Fig 5-41).

Choosing the size of the soft tissue punch

An experiment was performed to examine the effect of the size of the gap between implants and surrounding mucosa on the healing of peri-implant tissue. The results show that the size of the gap plays an important role in achieving optimal healing.

The gap between the implants and the peri-implant mucosa was determined from the sizes of the soft tissue punch and permucosal healing abutment. The contact was too tight with a tissue punch up to 2.0 mm in diameter in cases using a 4.5 mm permucosal healing abutment, which can cause pressure necrosis in the adjacent mucosa. There was too much gap created with a tissue punch of 4 mm or more in diameter. The optimal punch was 1.0–1.5 mm narrower than the permucosal healing abutment (Fig 5-42). When the peri-implant mucosa was in tight contact with the implants after implant placement, the peri-implant mucosa healed quickly with little scar formation. For optimal peri-implant mucosa healing, the implant should be in direct contact with the soft tissue, just as the implant needs to be in direct contact with the bone for optimal osseointegration of the implants.

Depth of implant placement

In areas with sufficient crest width, the implant crest module is located at the level of the bone crest. In areas with insufficient crest width, where one marginal crest of

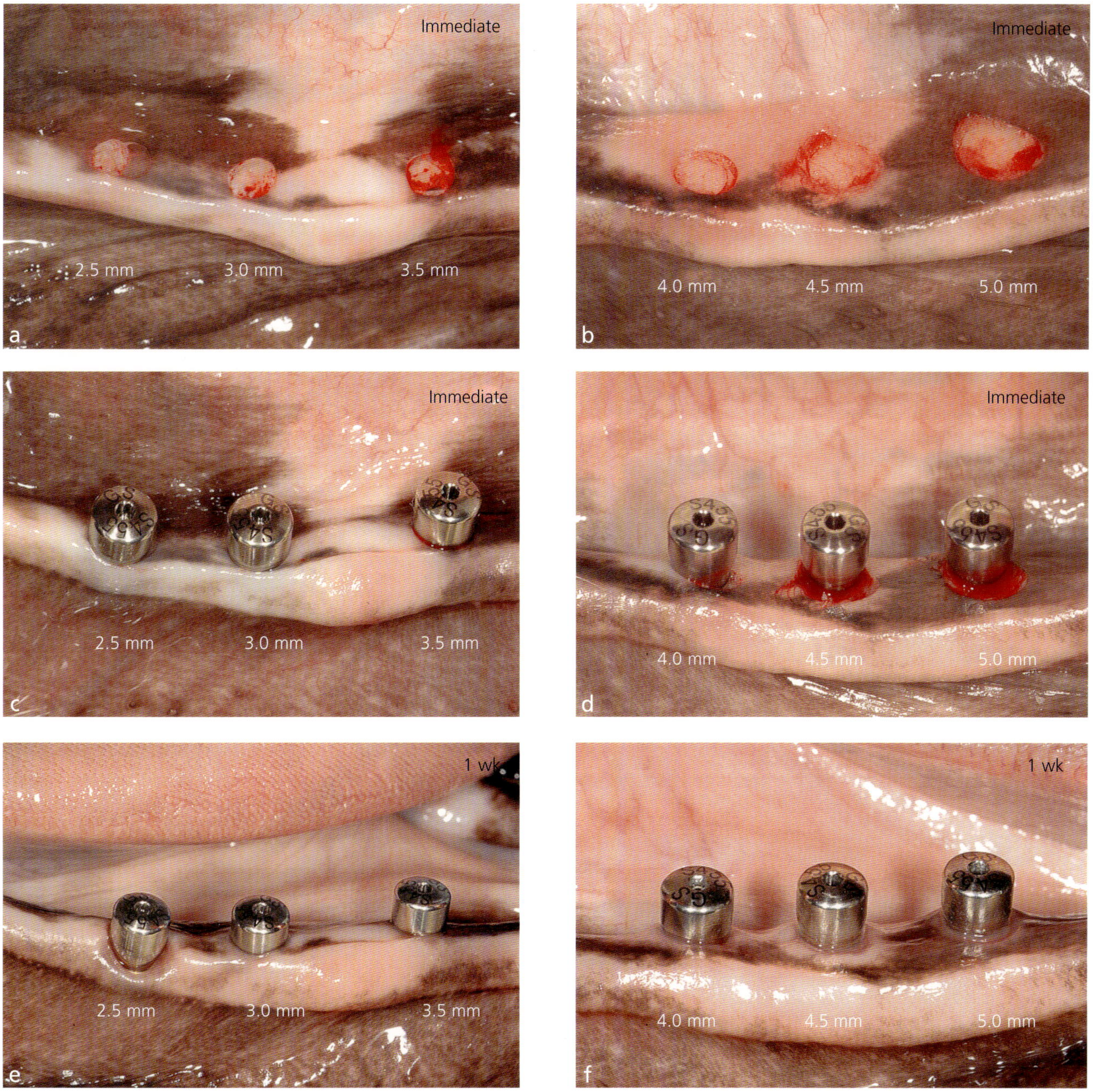

Fig 5-42 (a–f) In cases using a 4.5 mm permucosal healing abutment, the contact is too tight when the mucosa is punched with a tissue punch with a diameter of 2.5 mm or less. Pressure necrosis can occur in the adjacent mucosa. There is too much gap when the mucosa is punched with a tissue punch 4 mm or more in diameter. Therefore, the optimal tissue punch is 1.0–1.5 mm narrower than the permucosal healing abutment.

the bone is higher than the other (usually the lingual), the crest module position of the implant should be selected on an individual basis in relation to the crestal bone.

- If the overlying mucosa is thick for the more dense bone, the crest module can be placed at the level with the most superior edge (lingual crest of the ridge) (Fig 5-43a).
- If the overlying mucosa is thin, the implant should be countersunk below the bone crest so that the entire area of the threads is inside the bone (Fig 5-43b).

Bone grafting to cover the exposed threads is indicated if countersinking the implant below the bone surface is difficult owing to the surrounding anatomical structures. Bone

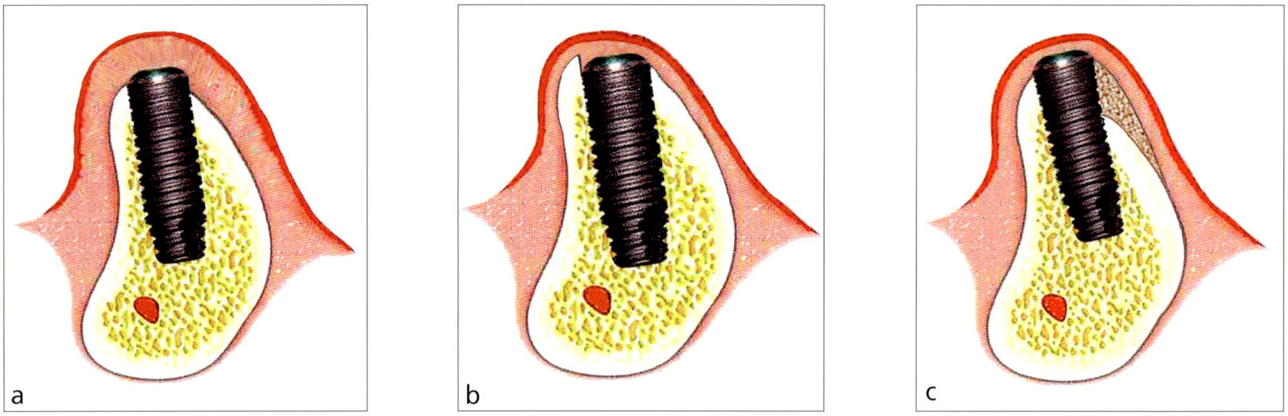

Fig 5-43 (a) If the overlying mucosa in dense bone is thick, the crest module is placed at the level with the most superior edge. (b) If the overlying mucosa is thin, the implant should be countersunk below the bone crest so that the entire area of threads is inside the bone. (c) Bone grafting to cover the exposed threads is indicated using a subperiosteal tunneling procedure if countersinking the implant below the bone surface is difficult owing to the anatomical structures or the mucosa at facial aspects of the anterior esthetic zone is thin.

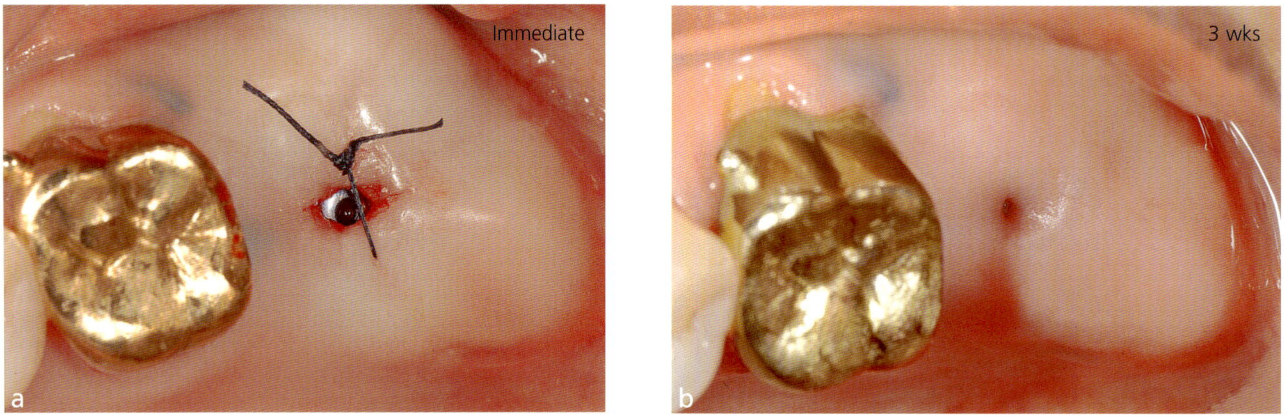

Fig 5-44 (a and b) Intraoral views 1 week and 3 weeks after mini-incision submerged implant placement. The cover screw is only partially covered with soft tissue, but it closed spontaneously 3 weeks later.

grafting is indicated to cover the exposed threads in the anterior esthetic zone too (Fig 5-43c).

Considerations related to flapless implant surgery

- A mini-incision is advisable if an inadequate apicocoronal width of keratinized tissue remains after a soft tissue punch procedure because the mini-incision technique can help to save the keratinized mucosa.
- During mini-incision implant surgery, care should be taken when reflecting the mini-flap. The zone of attached mucosa provides considerable resistance to reflection, which often causes the mucosa to tear. Local undermining of the mucosa should be performed to reflect the periosteum off the alveolar crest.
- Precautions should be taken during the drilling procedure even when surgical guides are used. The surgeon must palpate the cortical plate throughout the procedure to detect any perforation of the cortical plate.
- Care should be taken not to insert soft tissue into the bone holes during implant placement. The implant is inserted through the mucosa while opening the mini-incision with a curette or a probe. Peri-implant probing around the implant should be carried out immediately before engaging the implant in the osteotomy site in order to confirm that the soft tissue is interposed between the bone and the implants.

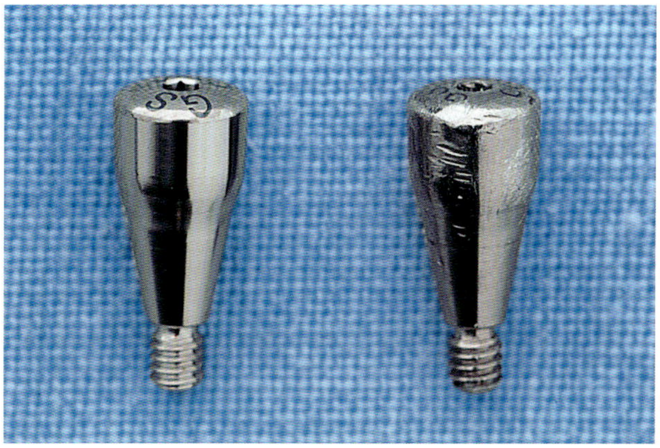

Fig 5-45 Permucosal healing abutments with flawless (left) and flawed (right) surfaces. The flawless one should be used. The smooth surface helps to decrease plaque deposition and facilitates its removal.

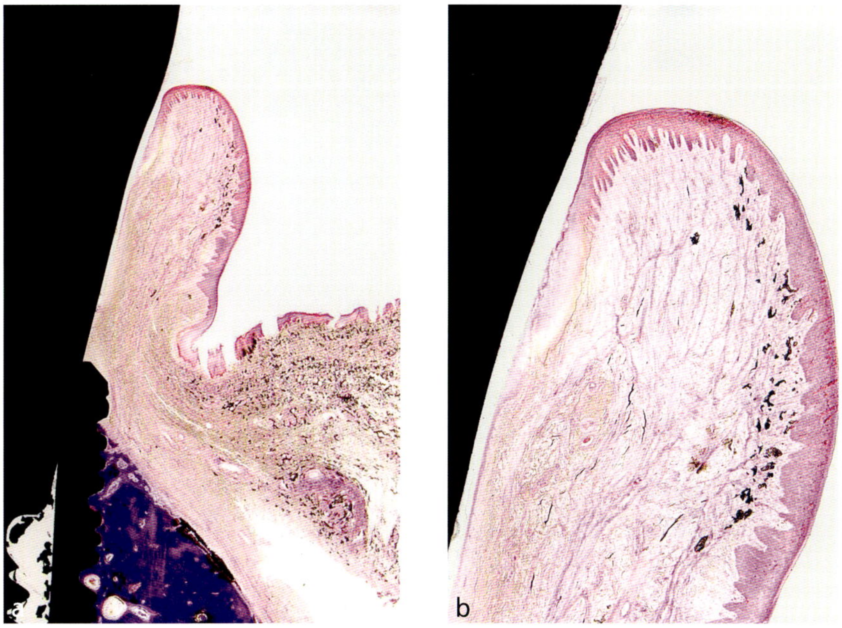

Fig 5-46 (a and b) The soft tissue lifted up around the permucosal healing abutment has a deep sulcus around the implant.

- It is not advisable to close the screws using flap mobilization if the cover screws are covered imperfectly by the soft tissue flap after mini-incision implant placement. Instead, it is prudent to wait for spontaneous closure of the screws during the healing period because the soft tissue can grow into the gap (Fig 5-44).
- In the case of soft tissue punch implant placement, rigid fixation of the implants should always be confirmed at the time of surgery. A mobile implant may not heal predictably with a direct bone interface. The implant should be fixed by inserting it deeper into the osteotomy or by placing an implant with a larger diameter.
- Permucosal healing abutments with flawless surfaces should be used. The smooth surface helps to decrease the level of plaque deposition and facilitates its removal (Fig 5-45).[2]
- After inserting healing abutments following mini-incision nonsubmerged implant placement, the peri-implant mucosa should be evaluated for any lifted-up soft tissue around the permucosal healing abutment. The soft tissue lifted up around the permucosal healing abutment should be cut and removed in order to reduce the sulcus depth around the implant (Figs 5-46 and 5-47).
- Care should be taken to detect loosening of the healing abutments early during the healing period. If it is loosened, bone loss can occur by abutment mobility (Fig 5-48).

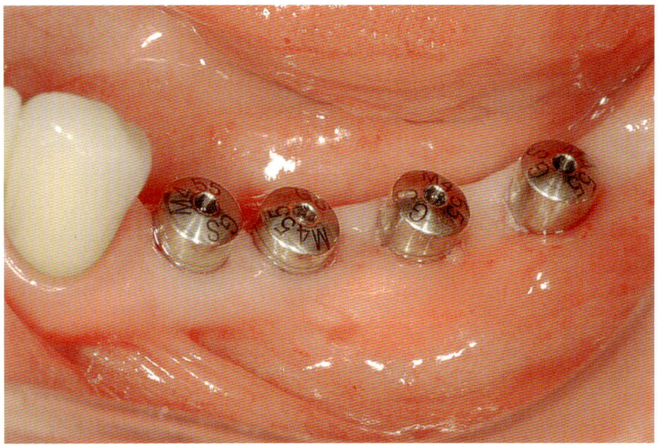

Fig 5-47 Intraoral view after cutting and removing the lifted-up soft tissue around the permucosal healing abutment. After inserting the healing abutments following mini-incision nonsubmerged implant placement, the peri-implant mucosa is evaluated for any lifted-up soft tissue around the permucosal healing abutment. This should be cut and removed to reduce the sulcus depth around the implant.

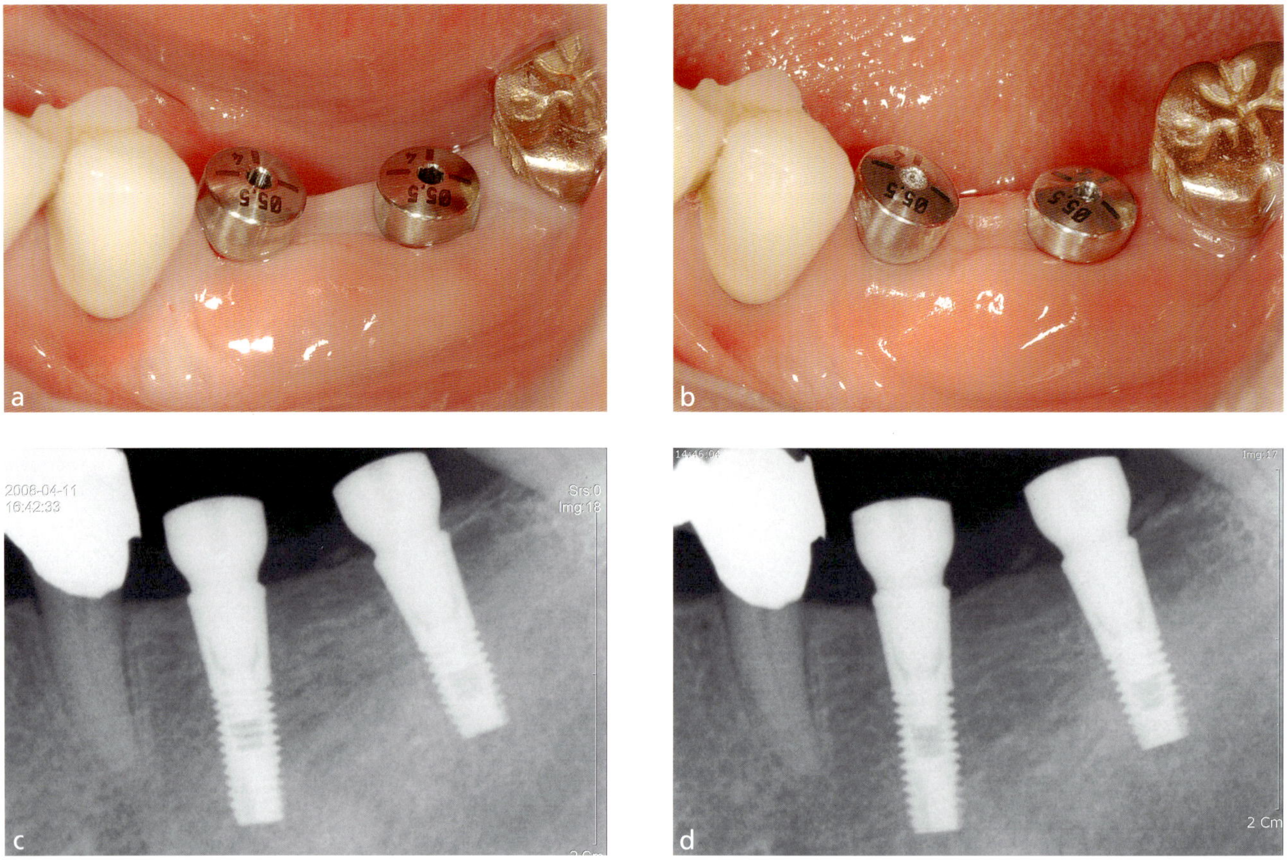

Fig 5-48 (a) Intraoral view immediately after implant placement. (b) Intraoral view 1 month after implant placement. Healing abutments were loosened. (c) Radiograph immediately after implant placement. (d) Radiograph 1 month after implant placement. Crestal bone loss is observed around the implant at the first molar site. The bone loss may be caused by abutment mobility.

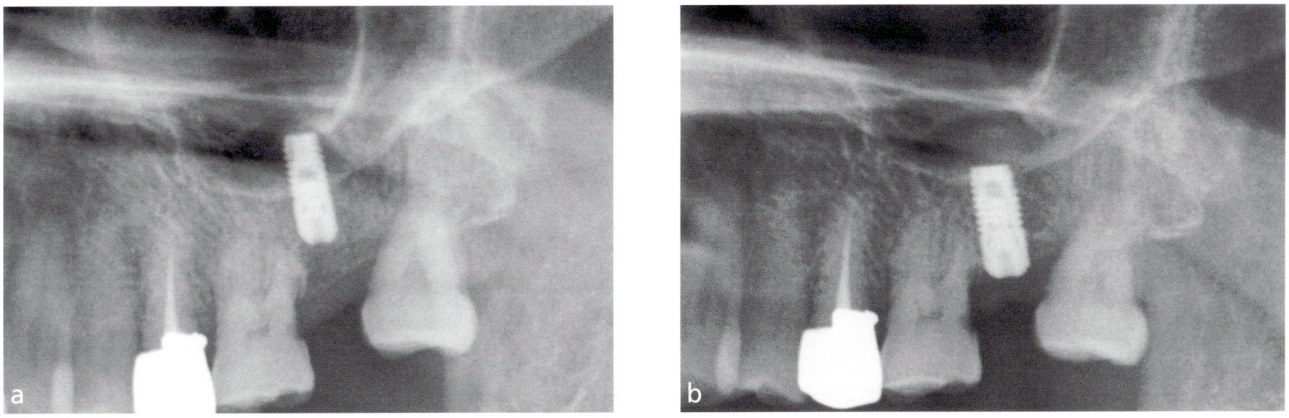

Fig 5-49 If inadequate placement is observed, it should be corrected surgically at the time of implant placement: (a) before correction; (b) after correction.

Immediate postoperative procedures

A postinsertion periapical radiograph should be made once the implant is in its final position in order to identify the implant depth, opposing landmarks, adjacent roots, and position of the crest module and crest of the bone. If inadequate placement is observed, the implant placement should be corrected at this time, rather than modifying the position at a later visit (Fig 5-49). The implant may be unthreaded one to two revolutions in order to lift it away from a neurovascular canal when necessary. It is far better to perform this correction surgery while the patient is still anesthetized, and the surgeon can reuse the tools used for implant placement.

Summary

Precise placement of an implant into bone without direct visualization of the alveolar bone requires information on the bone and mucosa before, during, and immediately after surgery. The shape of the alveolar bone and mucosal thickness should be evaluated before surgery. Before drilling, the mucosal thickness should be measured using a periodontal probe to verify the height of the mucosa at the implant site. During the drilling procedure, the use of surgical guides helps the surgeon to drill precisely in the planned position and with the desired angulation. The depth of drilling is controlled above the mucosa by a mark on the drill that corresponds to the sum of the length of the implant and the thickness of the mucosa. Before inserting the implants, the crestal heights in the facial and lingual plates should be reassessed by measuring the osteotomy depth and the mucosal thickness around the crest from the mucosal surface. Immediately after implant placement, it is important to carry out peri-implant probing around the implant using a probe to confirm that the implant crest module is located at the level of the bone crest. The implant system with a shorter cervical collar should be selected for a mini-incision submerged procedure.

References

1. Bashutski JD, D'Silva NJ, Wang HL. Implant compression necrosis: current understanding and case report. J Periodontol 2009;80: 700–704.
2. Briner WW, Grossman E, Buckner RY. Effect of chlorhexidine gluconate mouth rinse on plaque bacteria. J Periodont Res 1986;16: 44–52.

CHAPTER

6

Drilling in Flapless Implant Surgery

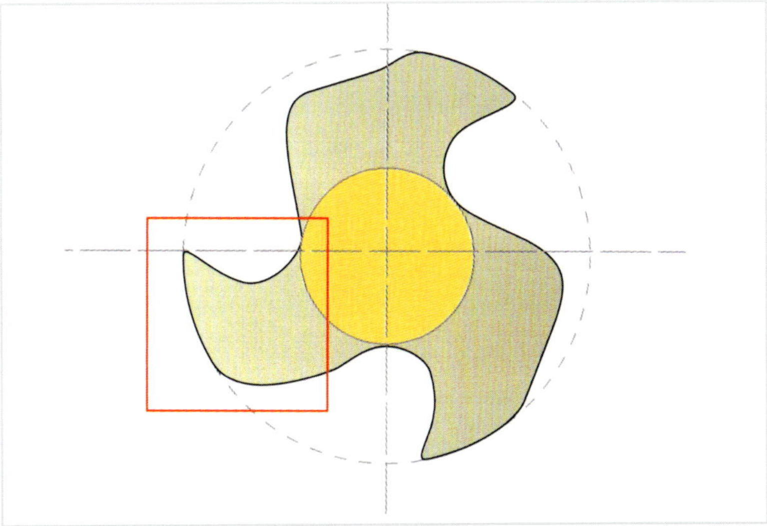

Key point

Care should be taken to avoid damaging the mucosa when cutting bone during flapless implant surgery.

Overview

Flapless implant surgery must be performed in a way to protect soft tissues and produce favorable conditions for the healing of soft tissue adjacent to the implant. Since the procedure is performed without reflecting the soft tissues, a good drilling process is essential for protecting the soft tissue at the implant placement site. However, contact between the soft tissue and the rotating drill is unavoidable (Fig 6-1). In particular, the drill can damage the soft tissue adjacent to the cutting blades when a mini-incision technique is used. It is critical to choose a drilling method and type of drill that can minimize the damage to soft tissues. This chapter addresses the drilling methods and drill types that can protect the mucosa.

Drill types

Commercially available implant drills have two or three blades and grooves (Fig 6-2). A groove is the indented part between the blades. The blades cut the bone, and the grooves help to remove bone debris. Removing the debris generated while preparing the osteotomy is very important. If the grooves are full of debris, the spinning of the drill may be compromised, resulting in drill fracture.

The three basic drill types are straight, tapered, and side-cutting (Fig 6-3). The side-cutting drill (e.g. Lindemann) has more cutting blades on the sides. However, side-cutting drills can cause more damage to the soft tissue when in contact with it.

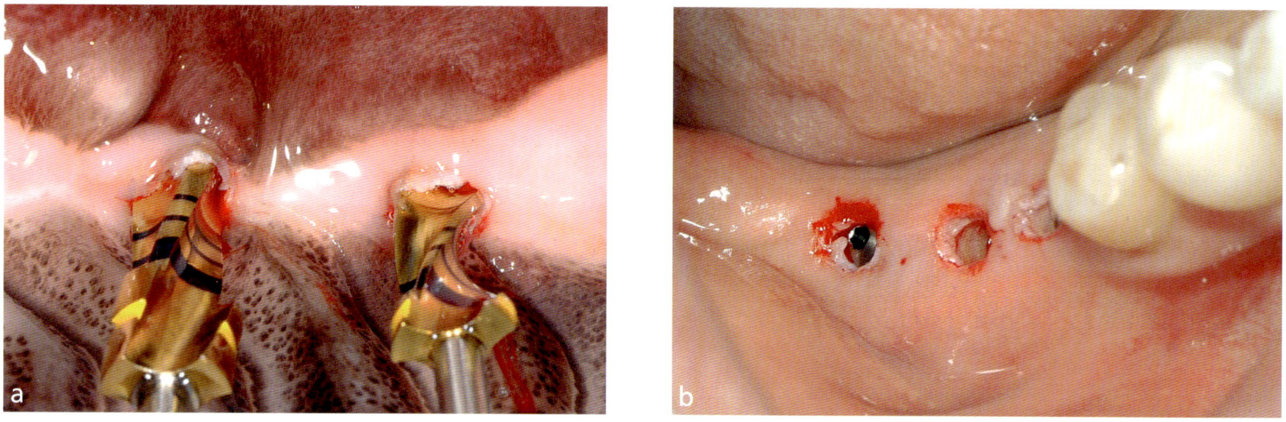

Fig 6-1 (a and b) When a flapless method is used for the implant placement, the drills can damage soft tissue adjacent to the cutting blades.

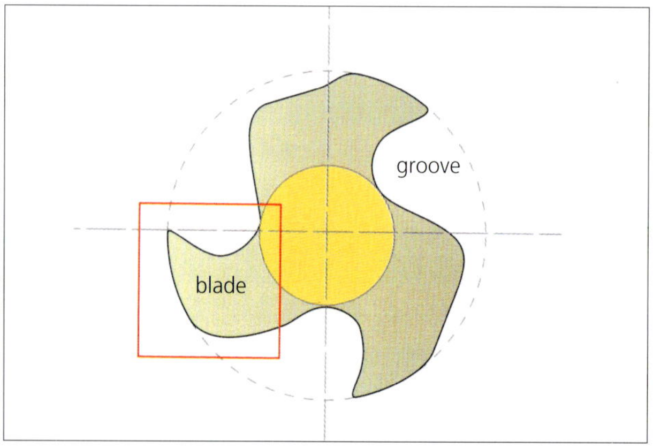

Fig 6-2 Cross-section view of the implant drill.

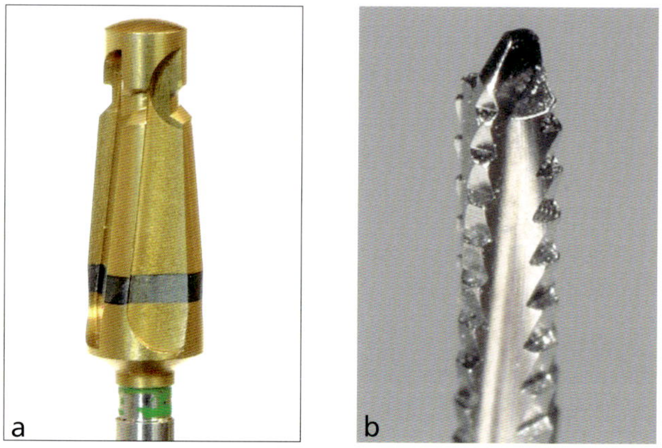

Fig 6-3 Tapered (a) and side-cutting (b) drills.

Soft tissue damage

Effect of the number of blades

Depending on the number of blades, there is a difference in terms of the drill stability, cutting efficiency, and ability to remove the debris. A three-blade drill is superior to a two-blade one in terms of drilling stability and cutting efficiency, but inferior in terms of debris removal and bone collection owing to its narrower grooves (Fig 6-4). However, a three-blade drill can cause more damage to the soft tissues (Fig 6-5).

Effect of blade thickness

The thickness of the blades can affect the extent of soft tissue damage.[1] The use of a thinner drill blade causes more damage to the soft tissue when the drill is in contact. A thick-bladed drill is advantageous in terms of decreasing the level of soft tissue damage during drilling (Figs 6-6 and 6-7).

Effect of drill size

The amount of soft tissue damage in flapless implant surgery is related directly to the drill diameter. When a mini-incision technique is performed through a 5.0 mm incision, the use of drills 3.5 mm in diameter or larger is likely to cut the soft tissue (Fig 6-8). Accordingly, when the mini-incision technique is performed, the use of these larger drills requires special attention in order to protect the soft tissue (Fig 6-9).

Effect of soft tissue characteristics

Since the gingiva in the maxillary alveolar crest is thick and is characterized by little movement, it is likely to be damaged when the rotating blades come in contact with it. In contrast, the gingiva in the mandibular alveolar crest is thin and flexible, so it sustains less damage than the gingiva in the maxilla (Fig 6-10). Accordingly, extra care should be taken to minimize damage to the soft tissue while drilling in the maxilla.

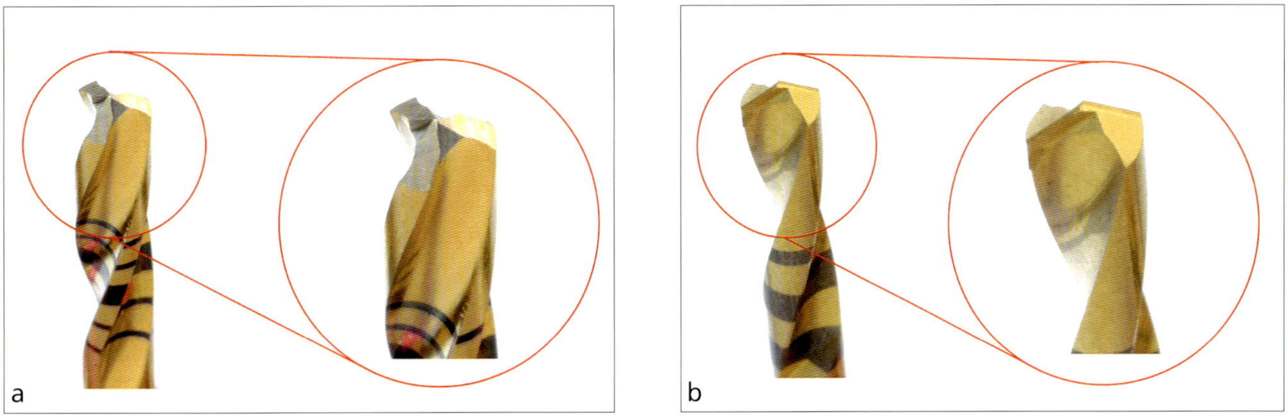

Fig 6-4 A three-bladed drill (a) is superior to a two-bladed one (b) in terms of the drilling stability and cutting efficiency, but inferior in terms of debris removal and bone collection owing to its narrow grooves.

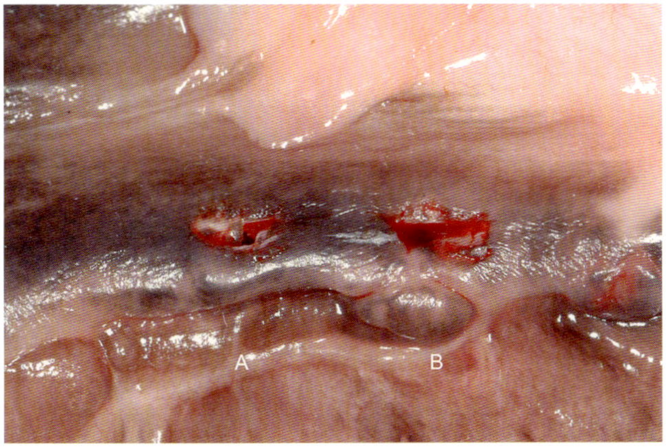

Fig 6-5 A three-bladed drill (right, B) can cause more damage to the soft tissue than a two-bladed drill (left, A) when the drill is in contact with the soft tissue.

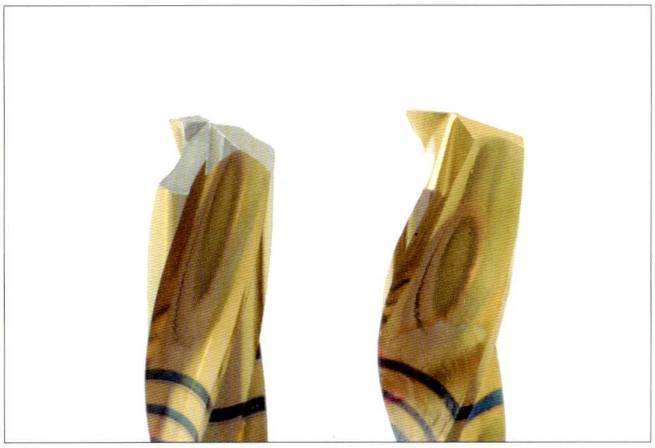

Fig 6-6 Thick-bladed and thin-bladed drills.

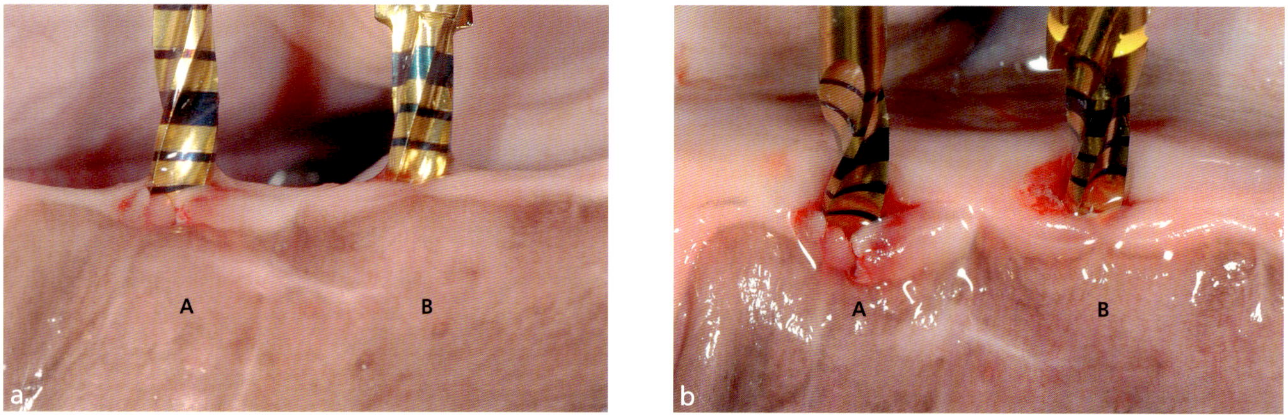

Fig 6-7 (a and b) The thinner the drill blade, the more potential damage can occur to the soft tissue in contact with the blades. A thin-bladed (A) and a thick-bladed (B) drill.

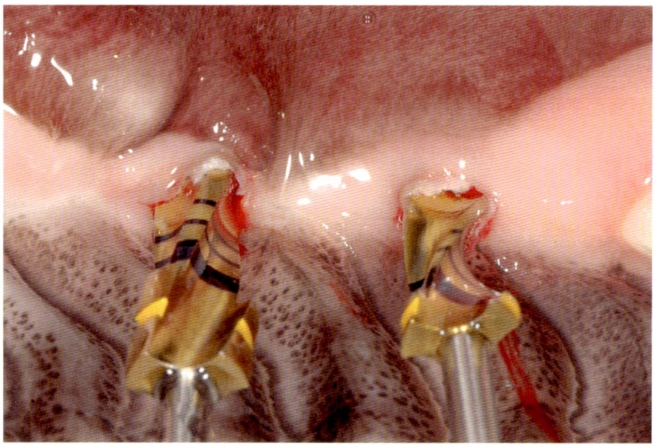

Fig 6-8 Drilling through a small opening using a wide drill can cause significant damage to the adjacent soft tissue.

Effect of drill speed

The rotation speed of the drill during implant site preparation in the mandible should be approximately 2500 rpm. A lower speed (1000 rpm) should be used for the maxilla. A higher speed carries a higher risk of damaging the soft tissues during drilling in flapless implant surgery (Fig 6-11). Soft tissue punch techniques are more advantageous in minimizing the level of soft tissue damage during drilling than mini-incision techniques because there is less contact between the soft tissue and drill in the soft tissue punch technique (Figs 6-12 and 6-13).

The importance of irrigation

Copious cooled saline irrigation is needed during drilling. This also acts as a lubricant to reduce the level of mechanical trauma to the soft tissue adjacent to the cutting blade of the drill.

Dense cortical bone is more difficult to prepare for implants than any other bone owing to its density.[2–5] The most common cause of implant failure in cortical bone is the surgical trauma resulting from the bone overheating during an implant osteotomy procedure, because rotary drills progress with greater difficulty in dense bone. The surgeon must take steps to minimize the thermal trauma. The heat generated during an implant osteotomy is related to the presence and temperature of irrigation,[2,6] the amount of bone being prepared,[3,7] drill sharpness and design,[1,4,8] time of preparation,[9] depth of the osteotomy,[6,8] pressure on the drill,[4] drill speed,[5,7,10] and variation in cortical thickness.[2,11] Eriksson and Albrektsson reported that, in rabbits, a bone temperature as low as 3°C above normal (40°C) can cause bone cell necrosis.[12]

In flapless implant surgery, the impact of external irrigation is limited because the osteotomy is performed below the soft tissue, so conscious effort is needed to control temperature elevation each time a rotary instrument is placed in contact with the bone. Cooled irrigation into the osteotomy site during pauses is critical. Constant irrigation also flushes

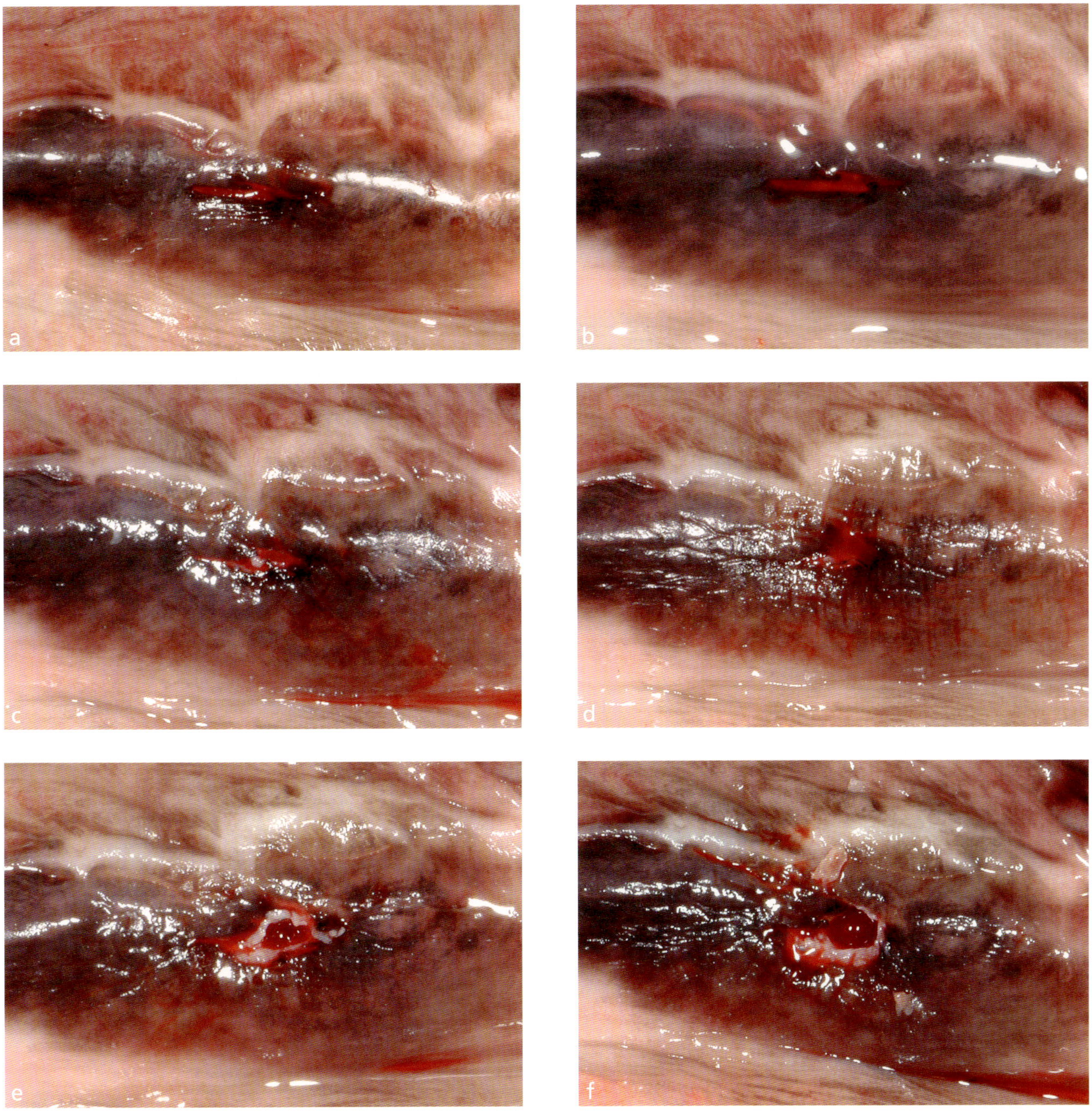

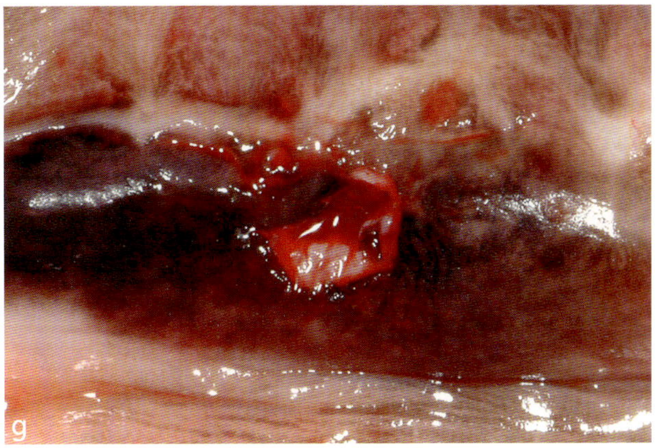

Fig 6-9 When a mini-incision technique is performed through a 5.0 mm incision (a), the use of a 2.0 mm (b), 2.5 mm (c), or 3.0 mm (d) wide drill is unlikely to cut the adjacent soft tissue; the use of a 3.5 mm (e) or more than 3.5 mm (f and g) drill is likely to cut the soft tissue.

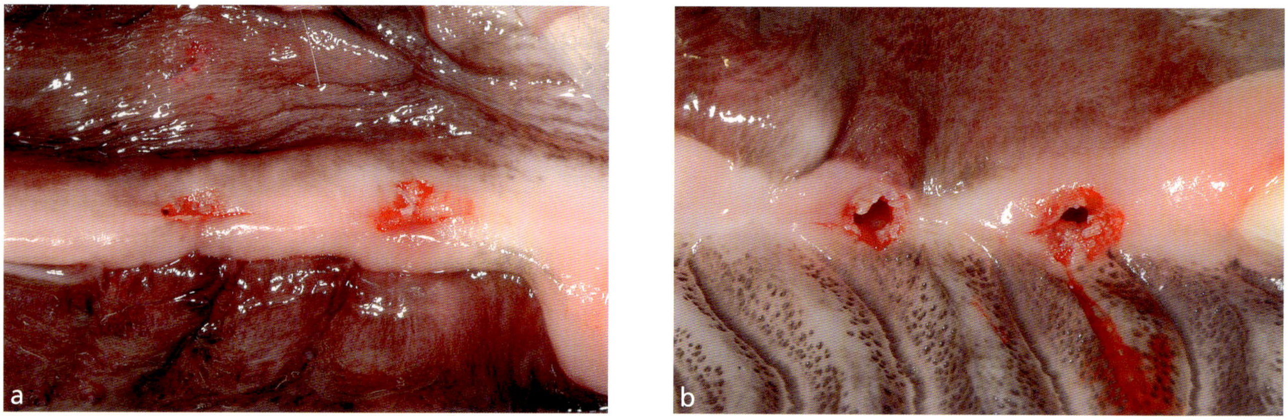

Fig 6-10 When the drill blades are in contact with the soft tissue, the gingiva in the mandibular alveolar crest (a) sustains less damage compared with the gingiva in the maxilla (b).

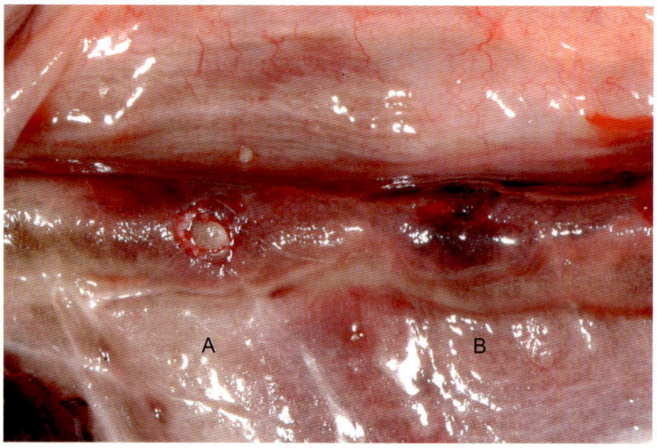

Fig 6-11 A view showing the mucosa after implant site preparation using either a 2500 rpm (left, A) or 1000 rpm (right, B) drill speed. Note that the risk of damage to the soft tissue during drilling in flapless implant surgery increases with increasing drill speed.

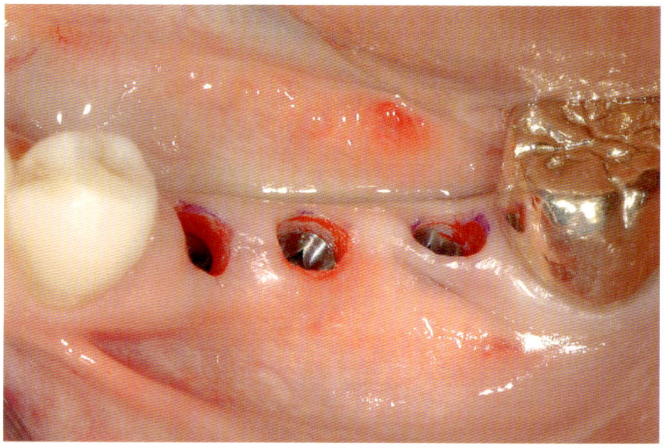

Fig 6-12 Mucosa after implant site preparation using the soft tissue punch technique.

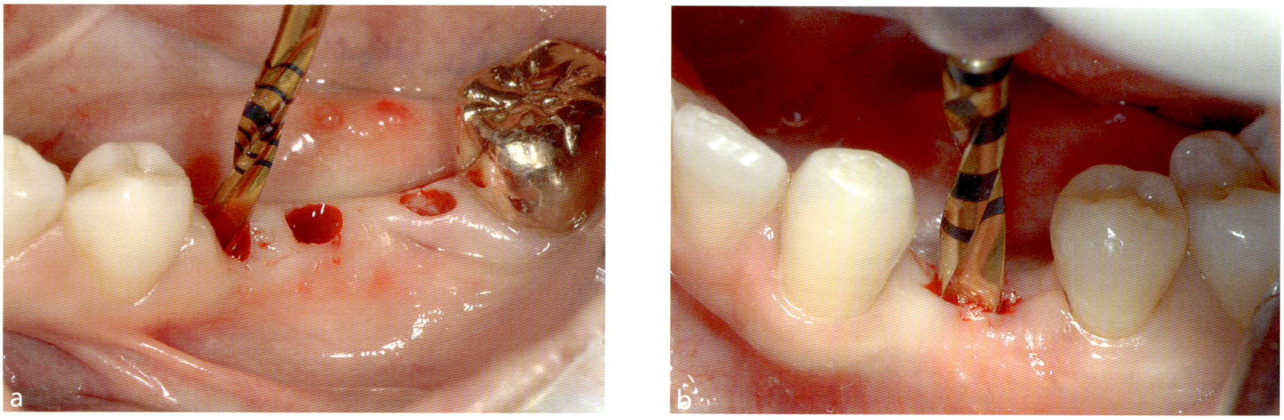

Fig 6-13 Soft tissue punch techniques (a) are more advantageous than mini-incision techniques (b) in terms of minimizing soft tissue damage during drilling.

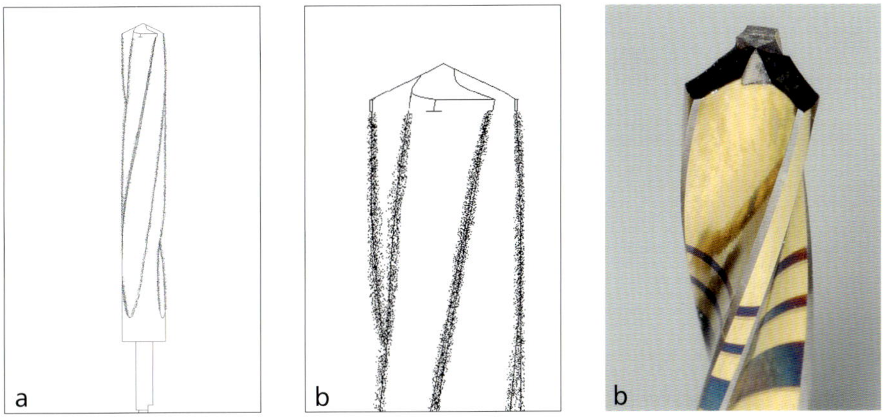

Fig 6-14 (a–c) A new drill for flapless implant surgery has a cutting surface on the tip and rounded surfaces on the other sides.

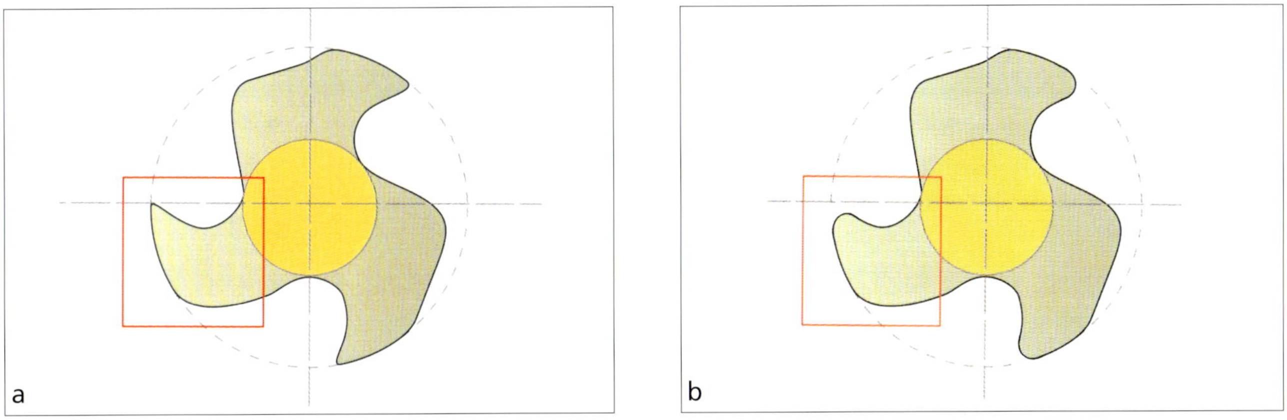

Fig 6-15 Cross-sectional views of the flapless implant drill on the tip (a) and the other sides (b) .

debris out of the osteotomy site. An up-and-down pumping motion is used to prepare the osteotomy and to provide constant irrigation to the drill cutting surface.

Special drill for flapless implant surgery

A drill has been developed for flapless implant surgery (Figs 6-14 and 6-15). The drill has a cutting surface on its tip and rounded surfaces on all other sides. This can protect the soft tissue adjacent to the blades when the rotating blades come in contact with it. The effect of the drill in terms of soft tissue damage and cutting efficiency has been evaluated in animal experiments. The results showed that the drill is considerably better at protecting the soft tissue (Figs 6-16 and 6-17). It has the same cutting efficiency as a conventional drill. In addition, the new drill helps to maintain a consistent drilling direction because it does not cut any parts of the bone wall except for the site that is in contact with the drill tip.

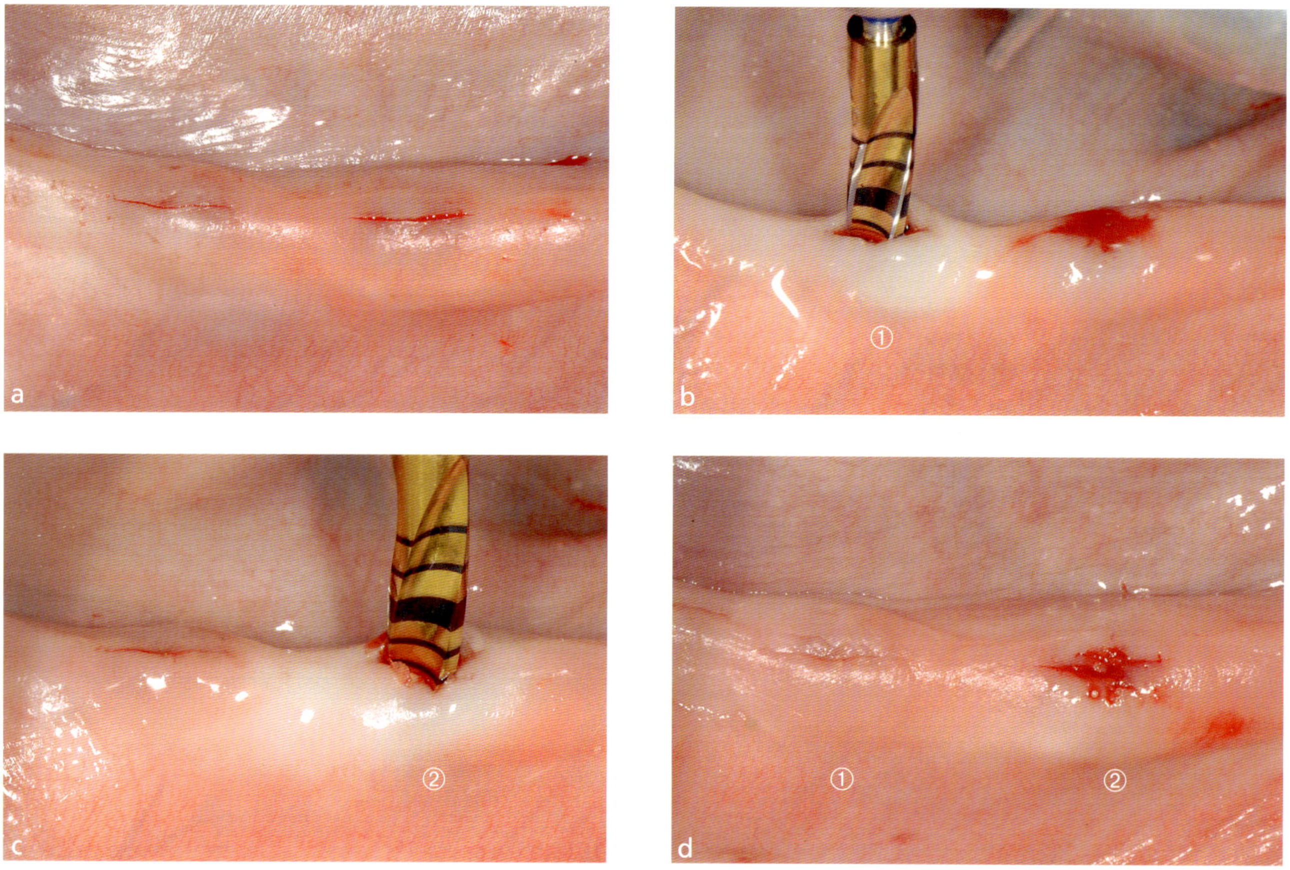

Fig 6-16 Comparison of soft tissue damage between the flapless implant drill (1) and conventional drill (2). (a) View after a crestal mini-incision incision. (b) Drilling with a flapless implant drill. (c) Drilling with a conventional drill. (d) View after drilling. Note that the flapless implant drill is considerably more advantageous in terms of protecting the soft tissue.

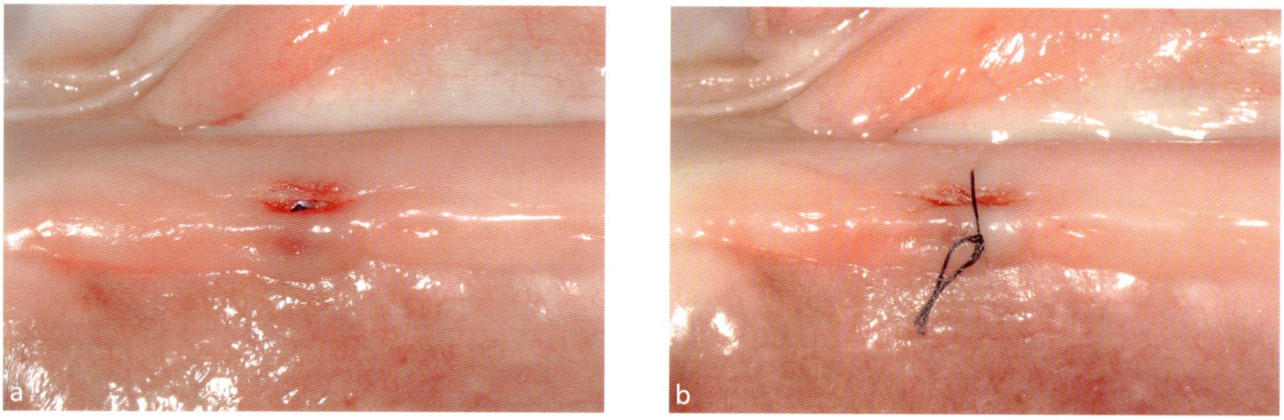

Fig 6-17 Intraoral views showing the mucosa after mini-incision submerged implant placement using a flapless implant drill: (a) before and (b) after closure of the soft tissue.

Considerations related to drilling for flapless implant surgery

- Most commercially available implant systems are designed for flap implant surgery and may be unsuitable for flapless surgery. The drills for flapless surgery require a sufficient length to allow for the cutting of bone through the soft tissue. To control the depth of drilling above the mucosa, the drills need to have stops or depth lines inscribed on their shanks (Figs 6-18 and 6-19). These depth lines should include a line that is longer than the sum of the fixture length and mucosal thickness. Short-step drills do not allow deep drilling in bone through the soft tissue (Fig 6-20).
- Straight drills are the most suitable for flapless implant surgery (Fig 6-21). A tapered drill can damage the soft tissue in deeper preparations because of the wide diameter at the top.
- It is advisable to use special drills for flapless implant surgery that have cutting surfaces on their tips and rounded surfaces on their other parts (Fig 6-22).
- Drill rotation should be started only after the cutting edge has been placed in contact with bone, because soft tissue can be damaged more severely by the cutting edge than the blades on the sides (Fig 6-23).
- In the maxilla, the use of an osteotome is advantageous in terms of protecting the soft tissue (Fig 6-24).

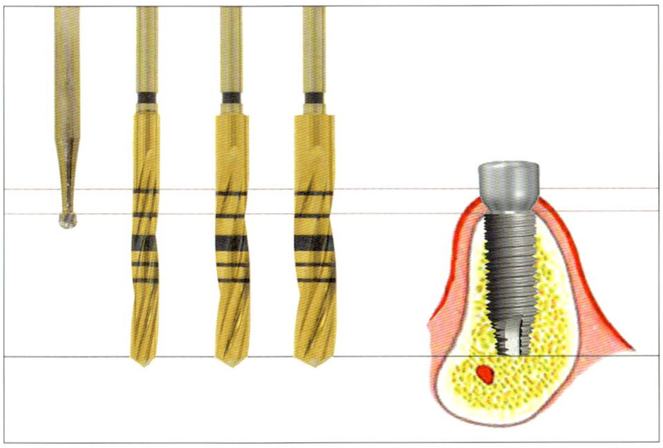

Fig 6-18 Drills for flapless surgery in the mandible. To control the depth of drilling above the mucosa, the drills require depth lines inscribed on their shanks.

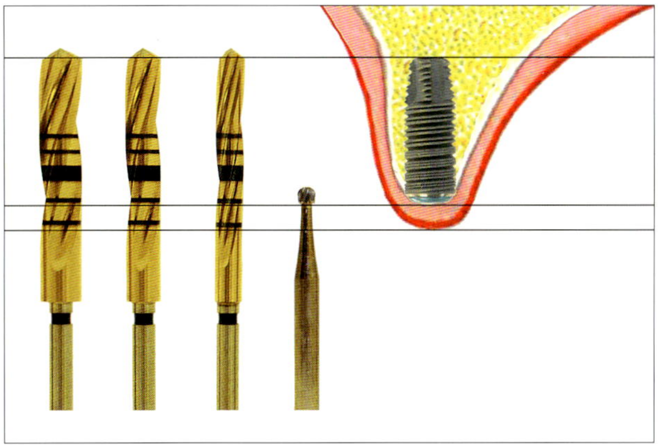

Fig 6-19 Drills for flapless surgery in the maxilla. To control the depth of drilling above the mucosa, the drills require depth lines inscribed on their shanks.

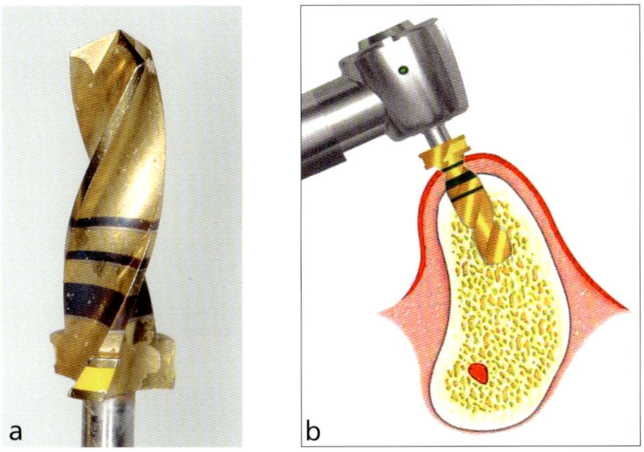

Fig 6-20 (a and b) Short-step drills do not allow deep drilling through soft tissue.

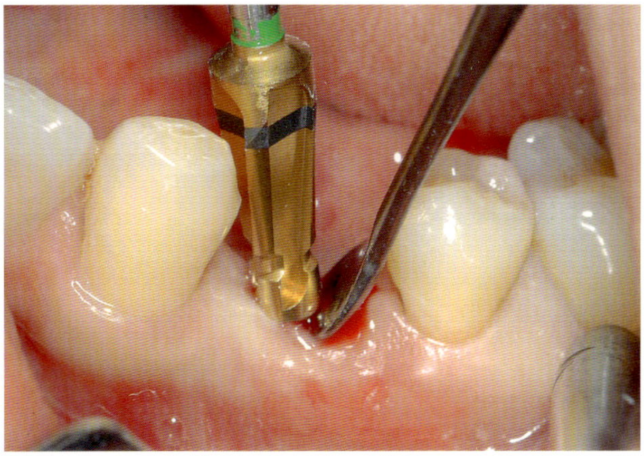

Fig 6-21 A tapered drill can cause damage to the soft tissue in deeper preparations because of its wide diameter at the top.

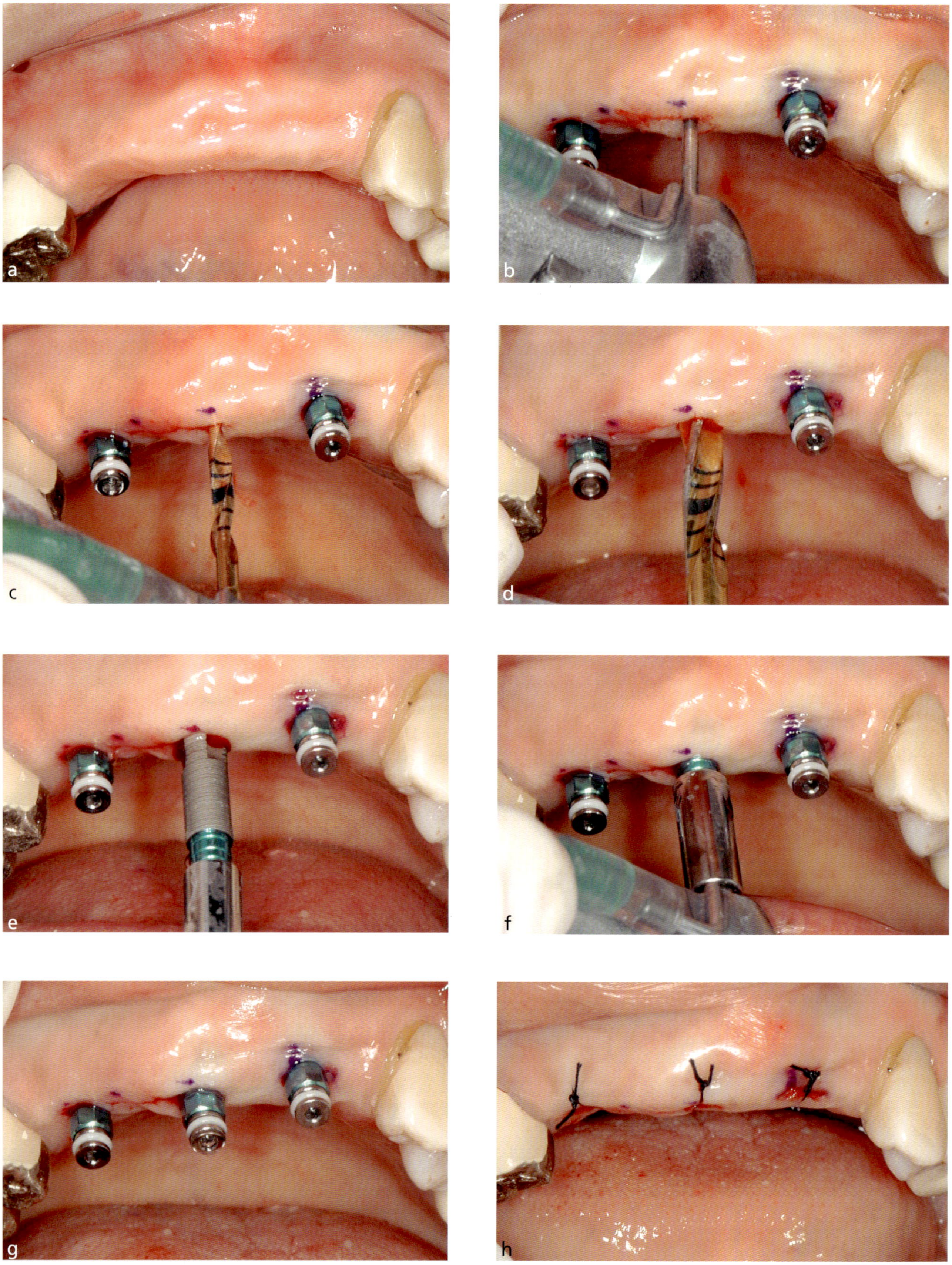

Fig 6-22 (a–h) Intraoral views showing implant site preparation and implant placement using the mini-incision submerged technique. It is advisable to use a special drill.

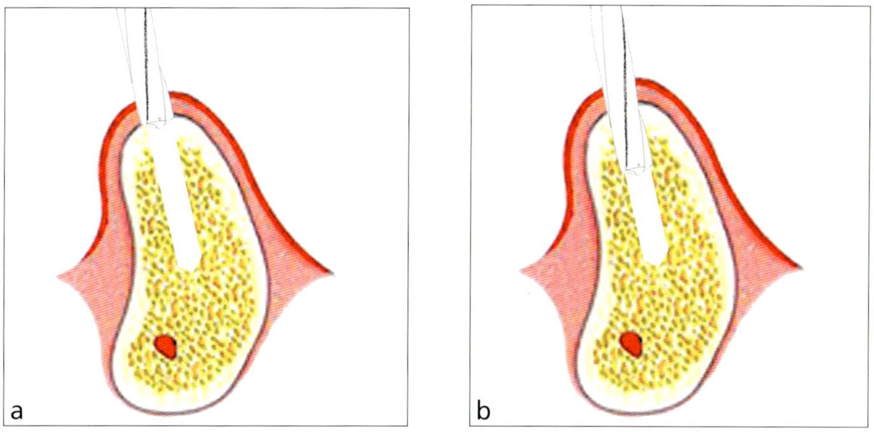

Fig 6-23 (a and b) Drill rotation should be started only after the cutting edge of the drill has been placed in contact with the bone, because soft tissue can be damaged severely by the cutting edge.

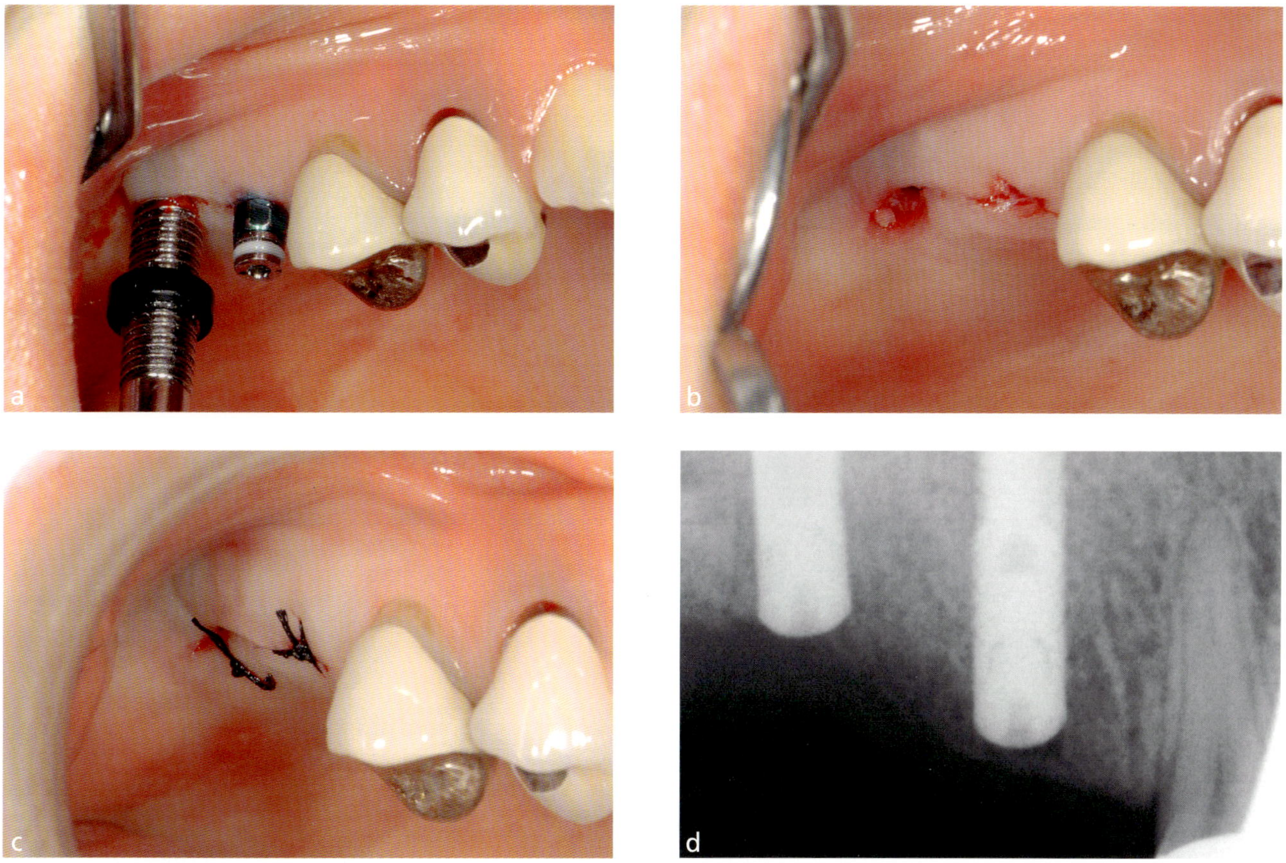

Fig 6-24 (a–d) In the maxilla, the use of an osteotome is advantageous in protecting the soft tissue.

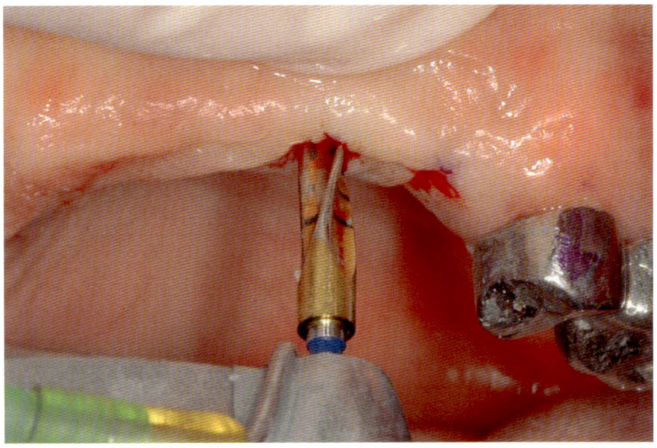

Fig 6-25 Throughout the drilling procedure in the maxilla, the surgeon must palpate the cortical plate on the anterior labial side to detect a perforation of the cortical plate.

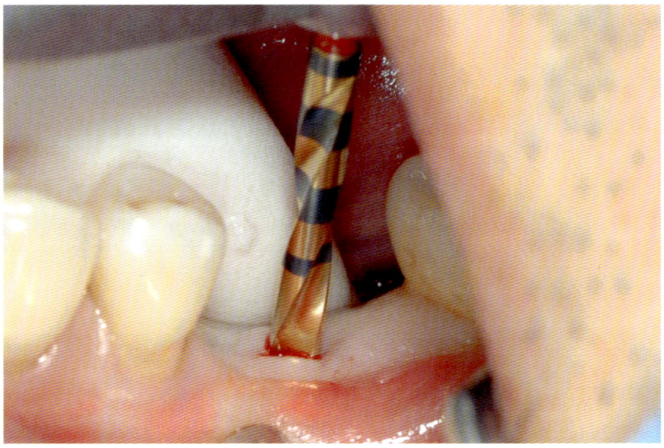

Fig 6-26 Throughout the drilling procedure in the mandible, the surgeon must palpate the cortical plate in the lingual fossa to detect a perforation of the cortical plate.

- A deep undercut is present in the sublingual fossa on the lingual aspect of the mandible. For the maxillae, the undercuts are present on the anterior labial side. While drilling these undercut sites, care should be taken not to perforate the outer surface of the bone with the drill. The use of a precisely planned surgical guide helps the surgeon to drill in the precisely planned position in flapless implant surgery. Computerized tomography or computer imaging software can help to increase the precision of the surgical templates in guiding the direction of the implant drilling. Even with a surgical guide, precautions should be taken during the drilling procedure. Throughout, the surgeon must palpate the cortical plate to detect perforations of the cortical plate. Incorrect angulation of the implant drill can result in such perforation, usually on the buccal aspect. Perforation of the buccal plate is generally detected by palpation (Figs 6-25 and 6-26).
- If a bone drill becomes locked in the bone, the handpiece should not be wiggled back and forth to disengage the drill. This can increase the size of the bone preparation or cause injury and necrosis to the bone. Instead, the rotation of the drill in the handpiece should be reversed or the drill disengaged from the engine and rotated counterclockwise with forceps.

Summary

In order to protect the soft tissue it is essential to use a drilling method and a type of drill that can cause minimal damage. The use of flapless implant drills with cutting surfaces on their tips and rounded surfaces on their other parts is advisable. Copious cooled saline irrigation should be used. Irrigation reduces the mechanical trauma to the soft tissue adjacent to the drill and decreases the heat in the osteotomy site.

References

1. Chacon GE, Bower DL, Larsen PE, McGlumphy EA, Beck FM. Heat production by 3 implant drill systems after repeated drilling and sterilization. J Oral Maxillofac Surg 2006;64:265–269.
2. Eriksson AR, Albrektsson T, Albrektsson B. Heat caused by drilling in cortical bone: temperature measured in vivo in patients and animals. Acta Orthop Scand 1984;55:629–631.
3. Eriksson R, Adell R. Temperatures during drilling for the placement of implants using the osseointegration technique. J Oral Maxillofac Surg 1986;44:4–7.
4. Matthews J, Hirsch C. Temperatures measured in human cortical bone when drilling. J Bone Joint Surg 1972;45A:297–308.
5. Brisman DL. The effect of speed, pressure, and time on bone temperature during the drilling of implant sites. Int J Oral Maxillofac Implants 1996;11:35–37.
6. Ercoli C, Funkenbusch PD, Lee HJ. The influence of drill wear on cutting efficiency and heat production during osteotomy preparation for dental implants: a study of drill durability. Int J Oral Maxillofac Implants 2004;19:335–349.
7. Sharawy M, Misch CE, Weller N. Heat generation during implant drilling: the significance of motor speed. Oral Maxillofac Surg 2002;60:1160–1169.
8. Wiggins KL, Malkin S. Drilling of bone. J Biomech 1976;9:553–559.
9. Adell R, Lekholm U, Brånemark PI. Surgical procedures. In Brånemark PI, Zarb GA, Albrektsson T (eds). Tissue-integrated Prosthesis Osseointegration in Clinical Dentistry. Chicago, IL: Quintessence, 1985.
10. Rafel SS. Temperature changes during high-speed drilling on bone. J Oral Surg Anesth Hosp Dent Serv 1962;20:475–477.
11. Hobkirk J, Rusiniak K. Investigation of variable factors in drilling bone. J Oral Surg 1977;35:968–973.
12. Eriksson RA, Albrektsson T. Temperature threshold levels for heat-induced bone tissue injury: a vital microscopic study in the rabbit. J Prosthet Dent 1983;50:101–107.

CHAPTER

7

Stage II Surgery

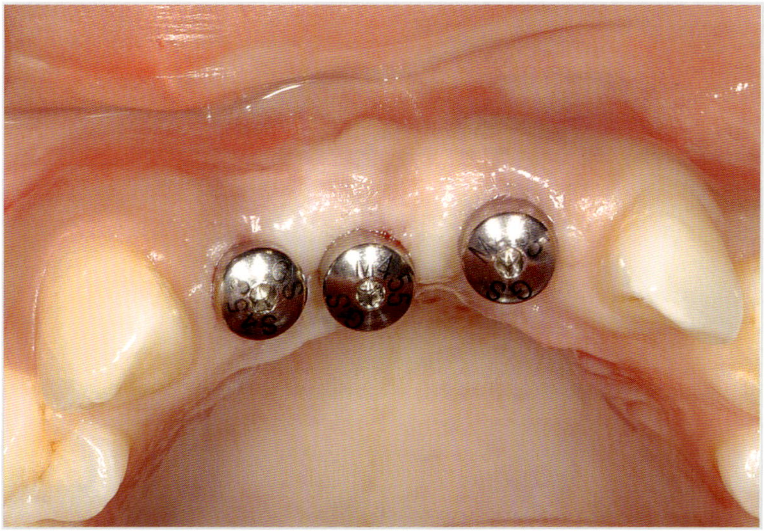

Key point

Second-stage surgery in flapless implantology is performed using a flapless technique.

Overview

Stage II surgery is necessary to uncover implants when they are submerged using a mini-incision technique. A clear understanding of the advantages of the flapless procedure also includes its application in stage II surgery. This chapter addresses stage II surgery using the flapless technique.

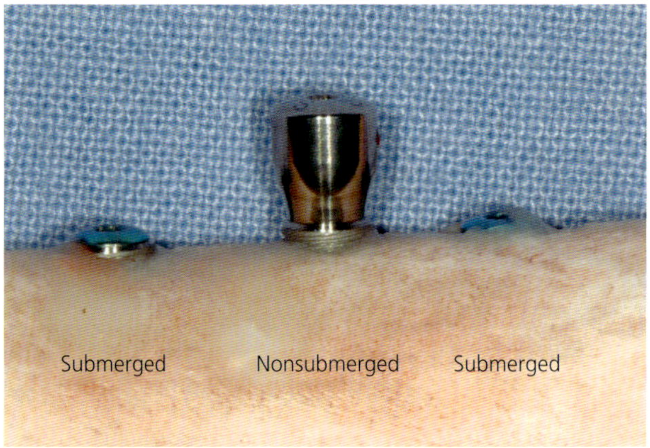

Fig 7-1 Mini-incision submerged implant (left); soft tissue punch nonsubmerged implant (middle); mini-incision submerged implant (right). There is no crestal bone loss at stage II uncovering after mini-incision submerged implant placement.

Challenges for the flapless technique in stage II surgery, and solutions

Misch[1] recommended reflection of a full-thickness flap for stage II surgery to identify and correct any bone defects around an implant, to reposition keratinized tissue, and to decrease the amount of thick mucosa. However, the necessity of using flap reflection in stage II surgery appears to be questionable after flapless implant placement, based on the following considerations.

Identifying and correcting peri-implant bone defects

Peri-implant defects can be identified without flap elevation. Radiographs are used to closely evaluate the crestal, mesial, and distal bone–implant interfaces before the stage II uncovering procedure. Probing is used to evaluate the facial and palatal conditions. Reflection of a full-thickness flap is unnecessary to identify these defects.

In animal and clinical studies by the authors, there was little or no crestal bone loss identified at stage II uncovering after the mini-incision submerged procedure (Figs 7-1 and 7-2). Indeed, there were no bony defects around the mini-incision submerged implants that required treatment (Fig 7-3). Therefore, there is no need to reflect a mucoperiosteal flap in order to identify a defect after the mini-incision submerged procedure. It should be noted that additional surgery can lead to additional bone loss when a full-thickness flap is reflected. If a bone defect around the implant at stage II uncovering requires a bone graft, it can instead be reconstructed using a subperiosteal tunneling procedure (Fig 7-4). This procedure is described in Chapter 12.

Repositioning of the keratinized tissue

Although keratinized tissue cannot be repositioned without flap elevation, it can be saved using a mini-incision technique. Conflicting results regarding the necessity of having keratinized mucosa around implants have been reported. Krekeler et al.[2] suggested that implants placed in keratinized gingiva had a more stable interface between the

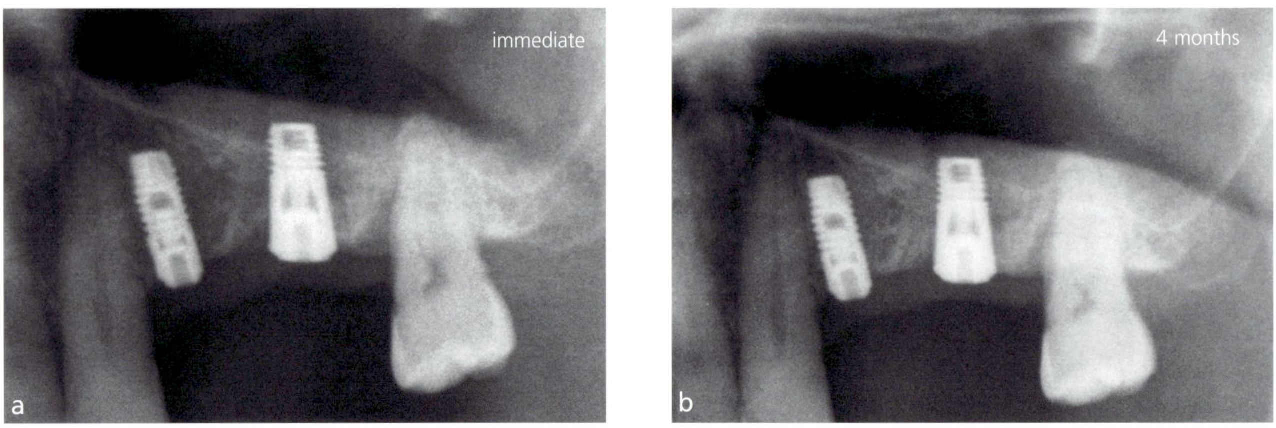

Fig 7-2 In a patient who underwent the mini-incision submerged implant placement, there is no crestal bone loss at stage II uncovering: (a) immediately after the implant placement; (b) 4 months later.

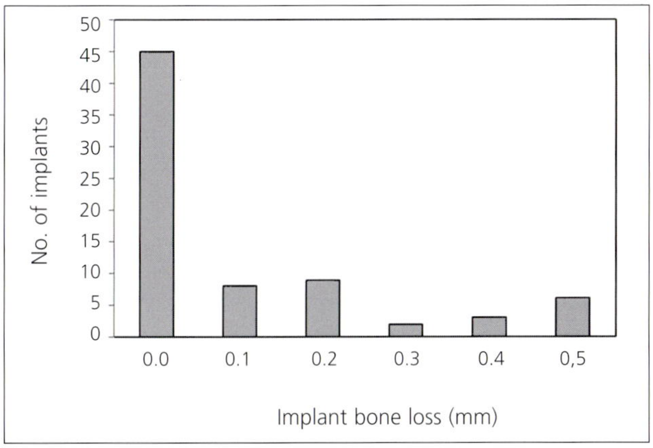

Fig 7-3 Bar chart showing the implants that exhibit varying amounts of bone loss during the healing period after first-stage surgery using the mini-incision submerged procedure.

soft tissue and implant than did implants in the movable soft gingiva, and the latter were more likely to cause soft tissue problems such as infection. However, the presence or absence of a zone of keratinized gingiva around implants remains a controversial issue.[3–6] Several reports have demonstrated long-term implant survival in the absence of keratinized tissue.[5–7] They suggest that keratinized tissue is not essential for the success of an implant. The necessity of keratinized tissue around flapless implants should be reevaluated.

Following flapless implant surgery, the peri-implant mucosa heals with little scar formation, and there is an increase in blood vessels and a decrease in peri-implant bone loss resulting in the soft tissue health around the implant. When a full-thickness flap is reflected to reposition keratinized tissue, this additional surgery can cause scar formation in the adjacent soft tissue, infection, and bone loss around the implant (Fig 7-5). Considering all

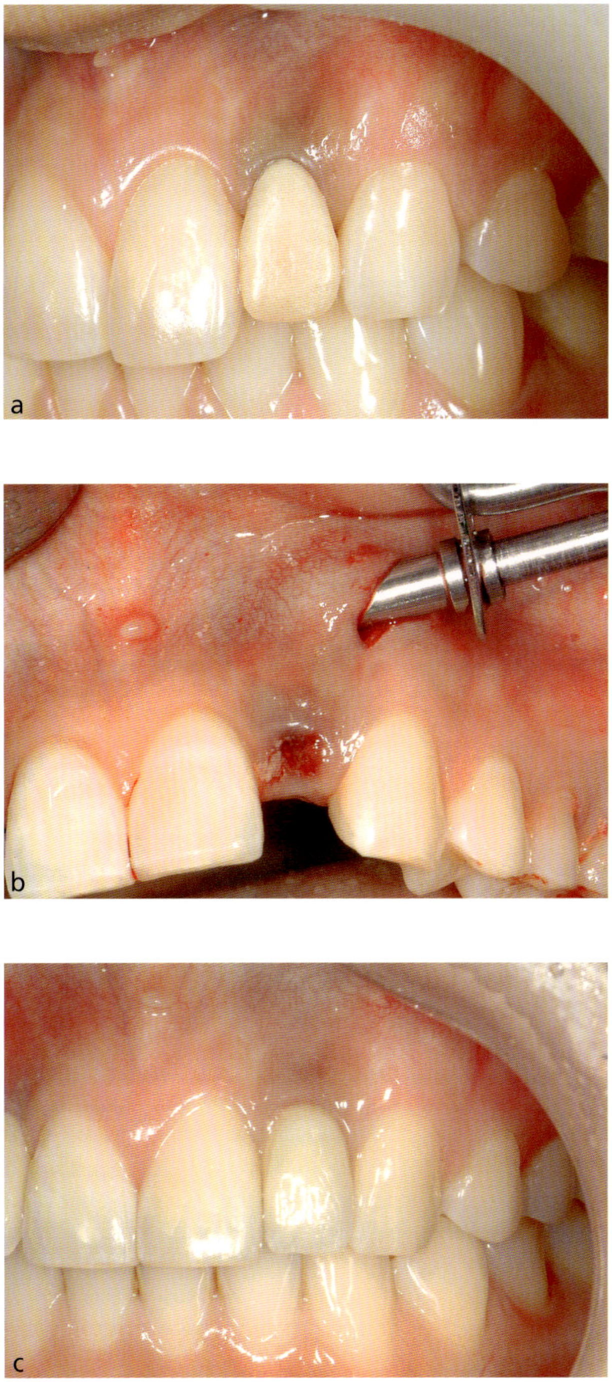

Fig 7-4 The bone defect in the facial region of the upper left lateral incisor implant (a) is reconstructed by a subperiosteal tunneling procedure (b) instead of reflecting a full-thickness flap. Bio-Oss® particles mixed with autologous fibrin gel are grafted. (c) Intraoral view 3 months after surgery. Note that the increased tissue thickness from augmentation prevents the grayish hue of the titanium implant body from being observed through the labial mucosa.

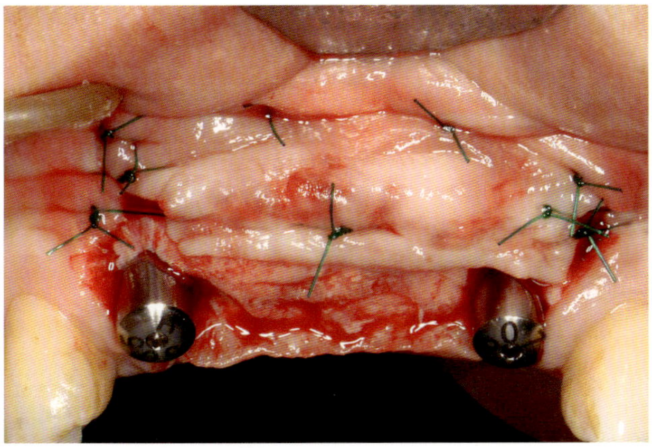

Fig 7-5 When a full-thickness flap is reflected to reposition keratinized tissue, the additional surgery can cause complications such as scar formation in the adjacent soft tissue, infection, and bone loss.

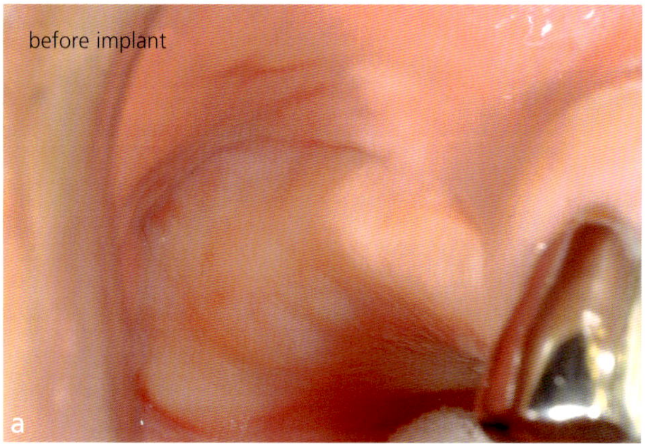

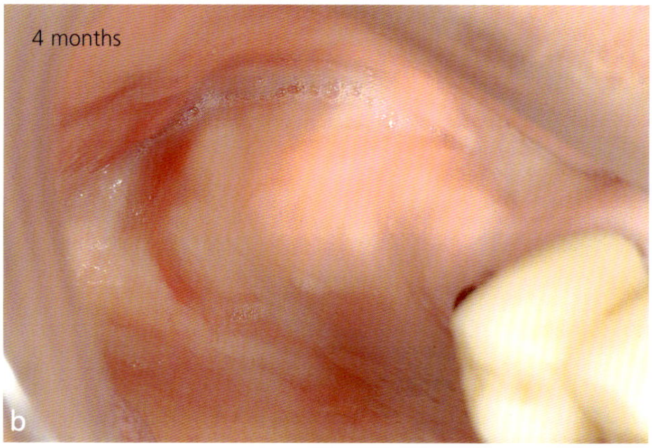

Fig 7-6 The original thickness of the mucosa surrounding the implants is maintained after placement of a mini-incision submerged implant: (a) before placement; (b) four months later.

these points, it is advisable to consider flapless implants without a correction of the absence of keratinized mucosa. In specific clinical cases where keratinzed mucosa is desirable – as in a fixed prosthesis restoration in the esthetic zone or a mandibular overdenture – the absence of keratinized mucosa can be corrected using a tissue graft at another appointment.

Correction of the thickness of mucosa

Misch[1] recommended that the correction of soft tissue thicker than 4 mm should have an ideal pocket depth around the implant. However, the desirability of the presence or absence of thick mucosa around implants is controversial.

Kan et al.[8] measured the mucosal thickness around anterior maxillary implants that had shown successful functioning: at least 70% had a mucosal thickness between 5 and 7 mm. Lekholm et al.[9] evaluated the sulcus depth and marginal bone loss around implants. They reported that the deep pockets were not accompanied by accelerated marginal bone loss around implants. These findings prompted the present authors to question the necessity of correction of thick mucosa as a precondition for implant success.

Complications associated with procedures to reduce the mucosal thickness must be considered. Gingivoplasty can cause infection, bone loss, or implant failure. Thinning the soft tissue can damage the blood vessels in the peri-implant tissue. The surgical process can cause extensive scar formation with a reduction in the number of blood vessels around implants, resulting in impaired healing and reduced defensive ability.[10] When these factors are considered, it is advisable to consider flapless implants without a correction of the thick mucosa in regions with a thick soft tissue bulk. When flapless implant surgery is performed in areas with a thick mucosa, it has the advantage of reducing the peri-implant sulcus depth, thereby ensuring favorable conditions for healing of soft tissue adjacent to the implant and avoiding complications associated with gingivoplasty (Figs 7-6 and 7-7).

Flapless implants in regions with a thick mucosa are described in more detail in Chapter 11.

Stage II uncovering procedure using a flapless technique

The stage II procedure is as critical as the stage I procedure with regard to protecting soft tissue and ensuring favorable conditions for healing around the implant. The soft tissue incision for stage II flapless surgery is similar to that used in stage I flapless surgery. A mini-incision or a soft tissue punch is used to uncover the implant (Fig 7-8). This procedure is performed under local anesthesia via infiltration of the implant sites.

Uncovering procedure using a mini-incision

The position of an implant is evaluated in radiographic views (Fig 7-9). On the alveolar ridge, the mucosal color or the scar line of the incision from stage I surgery can also provide useful information (Fig 7-10). The surgical splints used for the original surgery can also help to identify the implant position. The first-stage cover screws are located using an explorer (Fig 7-11). The sound of the metal explorer striking on the metal screws is different from the striking sound on the bone surface.

After the screws have been identified, a crestal mini-incision is made at the center of the implant site, approximately 4 mm horizontally with the alveolar crest (Fig 7-12). When more than two implants are uncovered,

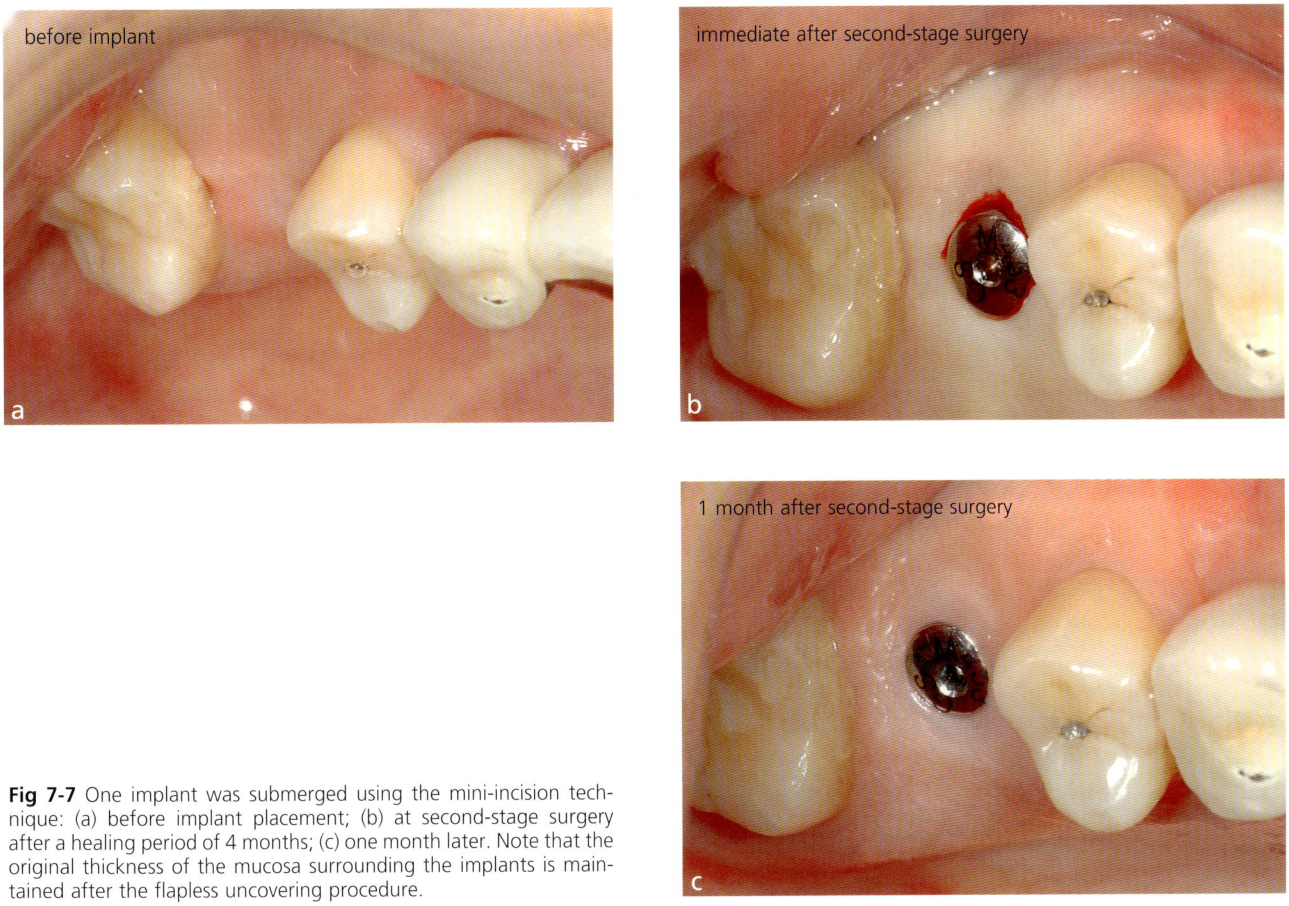

Fig 7-7 One implant was submerged using the mini-incision technique: (a) before implant placement; (b) at second-stage surgery after a healing period of 4 months; (c) one month later. Note that the original thickness of the mucosa surrounding the implants is maintained after the flapless uncovering procedure.

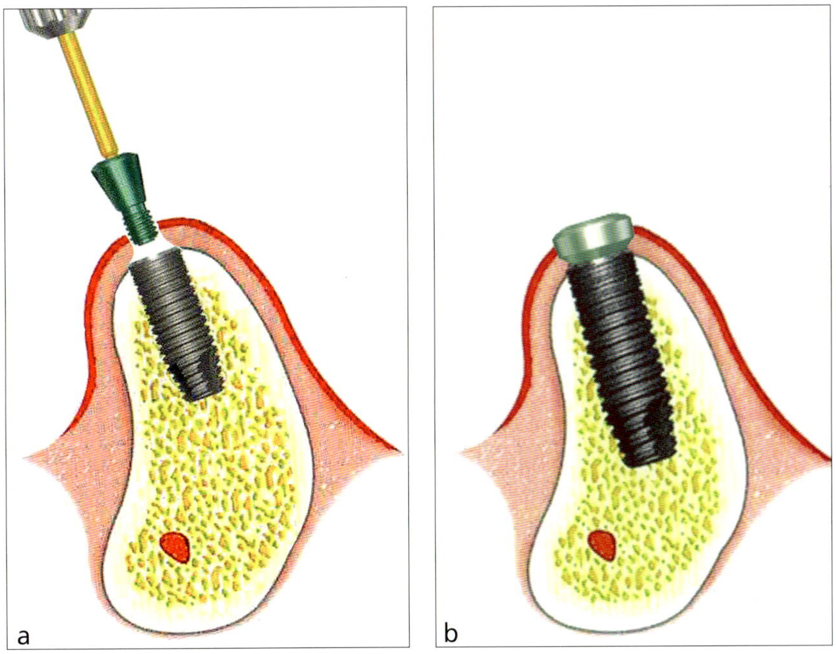

Fig 7-8 (a and b) A soft tissue punch or a mini-incision is used to uncover the submerged implant.

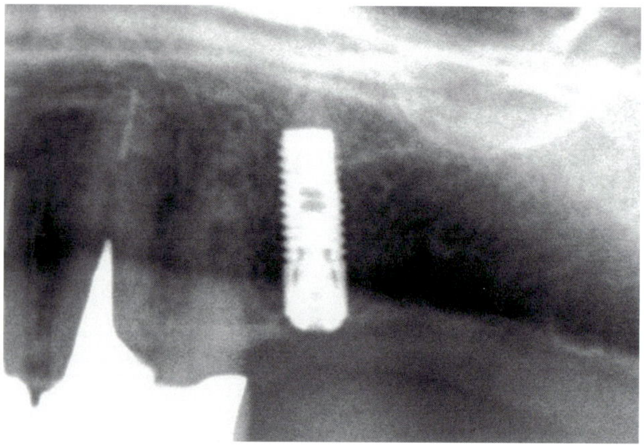

Fig 7-9 The position of the implants is evaluated radiographically before the flapless uncovering procedure.

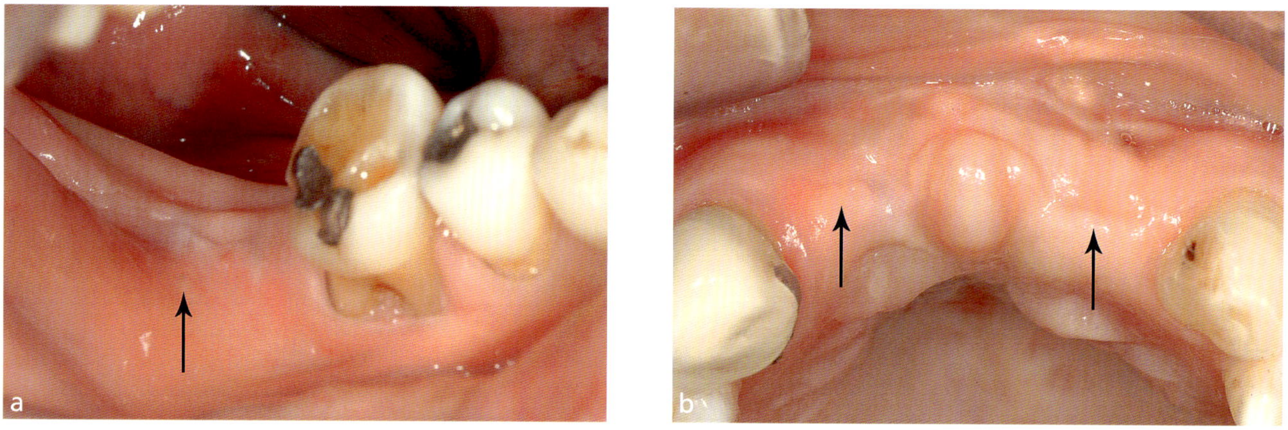

Fig 7-10 (a and b) Mucosal color or the scar line of the incision from the original stage I surgery can provide relevant information regarding the position of the implants.

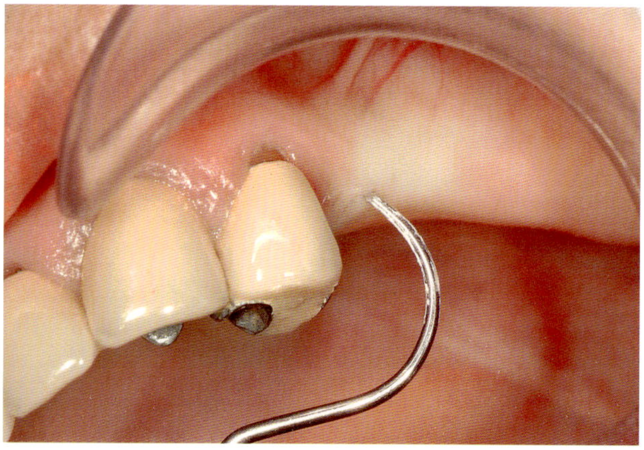

Fig 7-11 The first-stage cover screws are identified using an explorer.

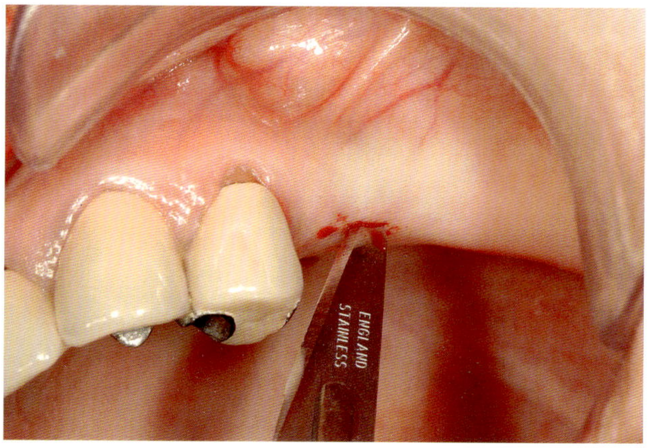

Fig 7-12 A crestal mini-incision is made, approximately 4 mm horizontally with the alveolar crest at the center of the implant site.

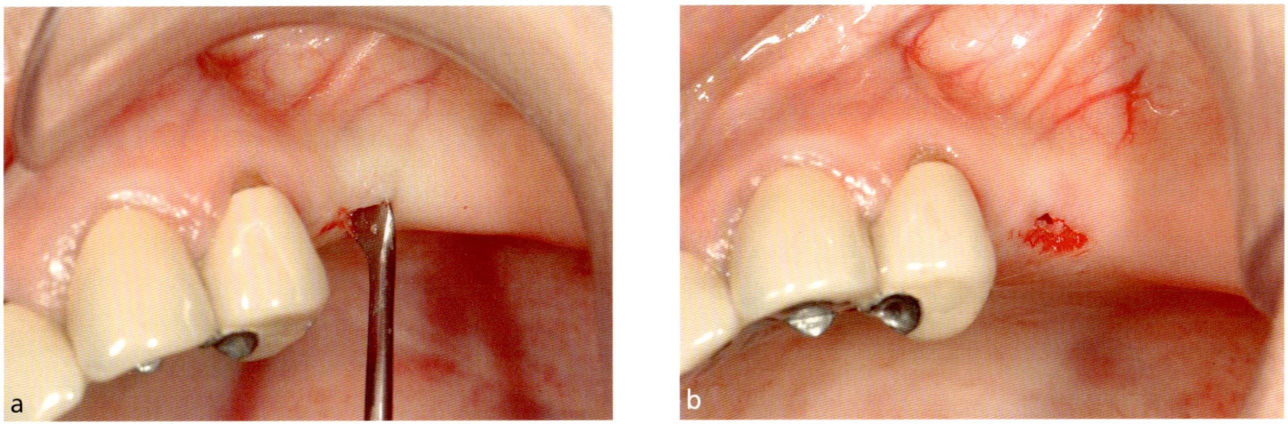

Fig 7-13 (a and b) The soft tissue above the cover screws is pushed aside.

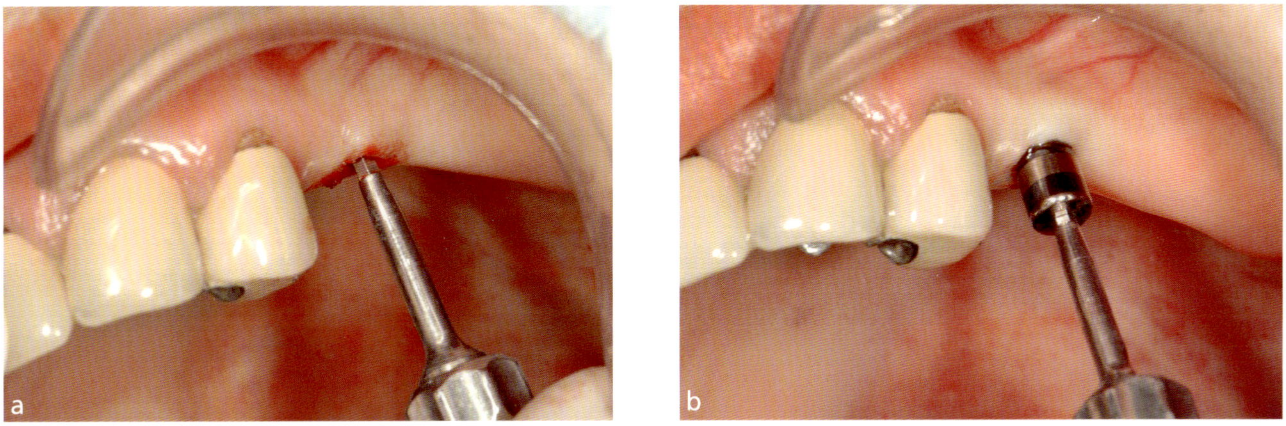

Fig 7-14 (a and b) After removing the first-stage cover screws, a permucosal healing abutment is seated into the implant body.

multiple mini-incisions are made in the alveolar crest depending on the number of implants. Local undermining at the implant site can be performed until the first-stage cover screw is exposed. During the procedure, the soft tissue above the cover screw is pushed aside within the range of the implant diameter (Fig 7-13). Any bone growth on the cover screw is removed using surgical curettes.

After removal of the first-stage cover screw, the internal chamber of the implant body is flushed thoroughly with 0.12% chlorhexidine. A permucosal healing abutment is then seated into the implant body using finger pressure (Fig 7-14). The connection of healing abutments is evaluated closely to ensure that the soft tissue is not interposed into the space between the implant and healing abutment. The presence of soft tissue in this space impedes the perfect connection of healing abutments. When in doubt, a periapical radiograph of the abutment connection region is taken to ensure proper component fit (Fig 7-15). The permucosal healing abutment should extend at least 1 mm above the adjacent mucosa to help to prevent tissue overgrowth during the healing period (Fig 7-16). This is because the adjacent mucosa swells by approximately 0.7 mm owing to postoperative edema.

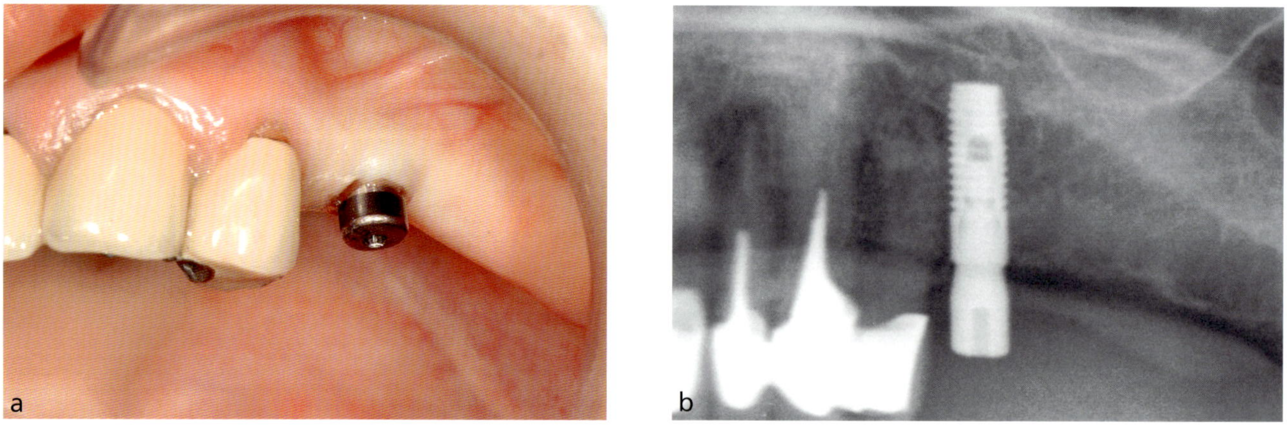

Fig 7-15 (a and b) After connecting the healing abutments, a periapical radiograph is taken to ensure proper component fit.

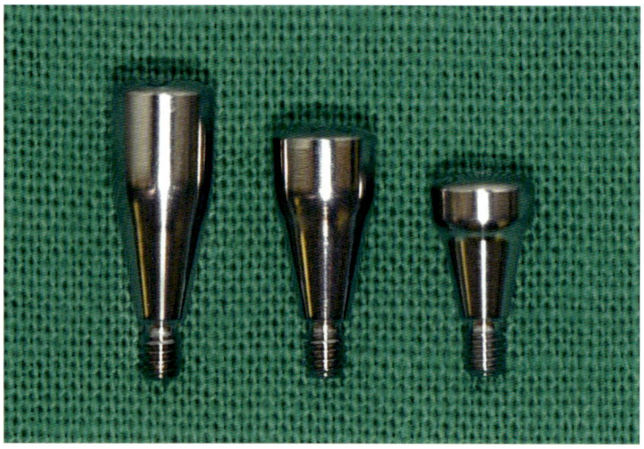

Fig 7-16 The permucosal healing abutment should be chosen to extend at least 1 mm above the adjacent mucosa.

Uncovering procedure using a soft tissue punch

A soft tissue punch can be used to uncover the implant when 1.5 mm or more of keratinized tissue remains buccal to the incision of the punch (Fig 7-17). A mini-incision procedure can be used to uncover the implant when there is a lack of attached keratinized tissue on the facial aspect of the implant. The mini-incision technique is beneficial for preserving the keratinized mucosa.

The soft tissue punch should be 1.0–1.5 mm narrower than the permucosal healing abutment (Figs 7-18 to 7-20). The peri-implant mucosa is in tight contact with the healing abutment when the permucosal healing abutment is 1.0–1.5 mm wider than the punch (see Figs 7-18 and 7-19). Multiple punches are made in the alveolar crest when there are more than two implants.

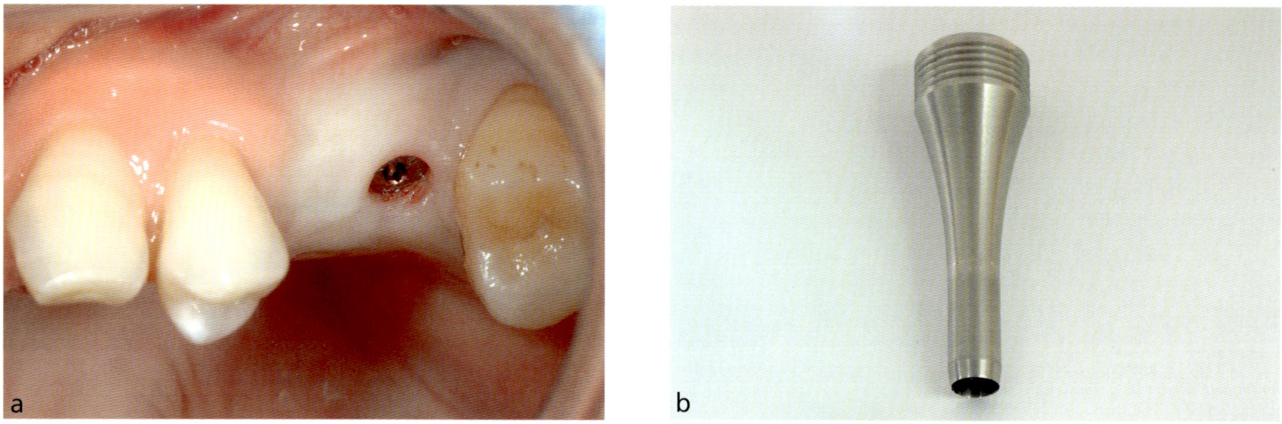

Fig 7-17 (a and b) A soft tissue punch with a diameter between 3 and 3.5 mm is used to uncover the implant. A soft tissue punch is used when there is 1.5 mm or more of keratinized facial tissue attached to the implant site.

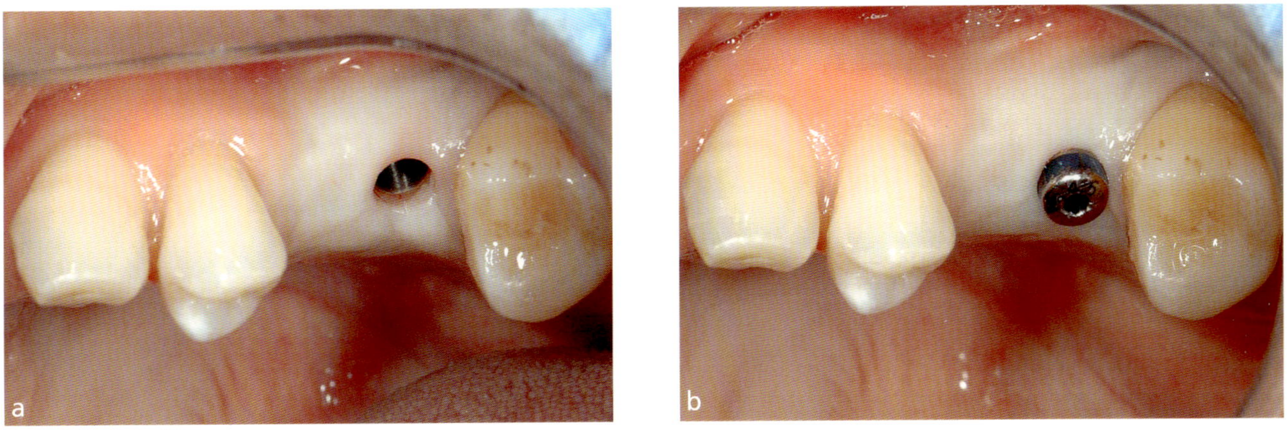

Fig 7-18 (a and b) After uncovering the implant using a soft tissue punch, a permucosal healing abutment is seated into the implant body. See also Fig 7-19.

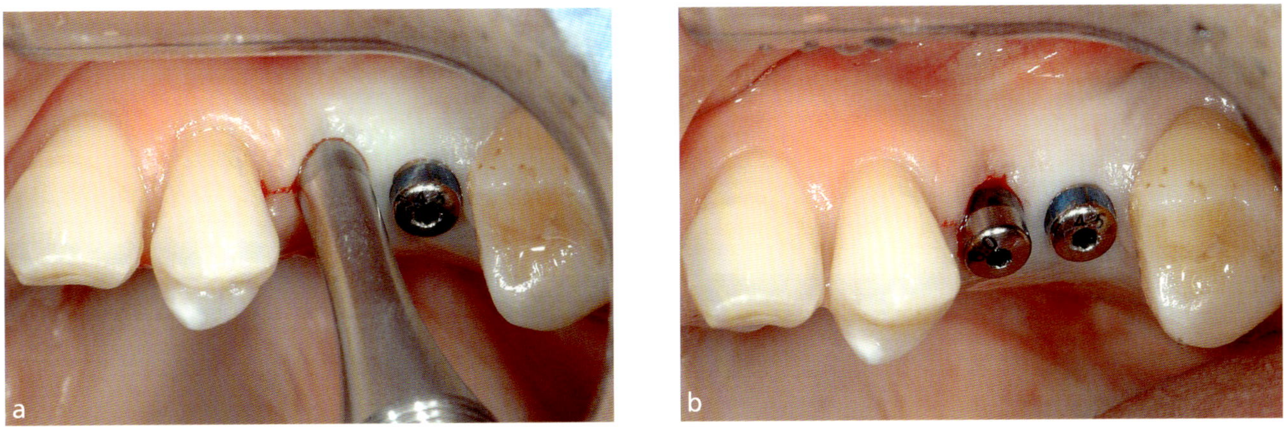

Fig 7-19 (a and b) After uncovering the implant using a soft tissue punch, a permucosal healing abutment is seated into the implant body. See also Fig 7-18.

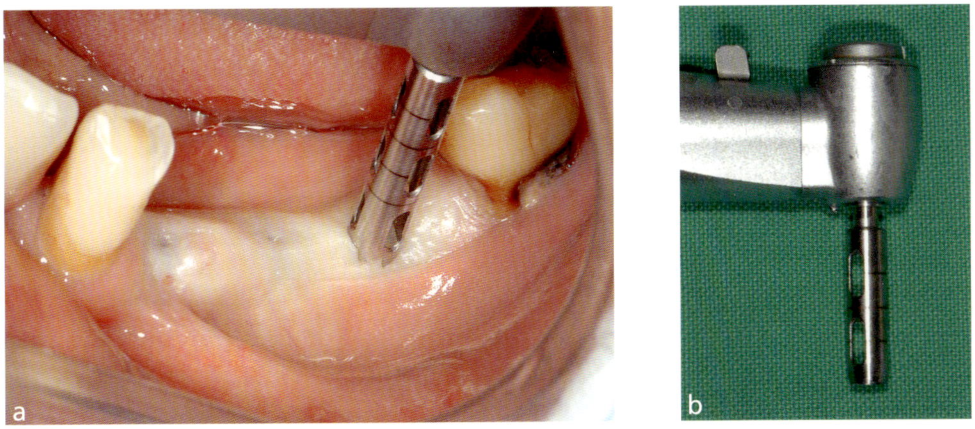

Fig 7-20 A soft tissue punch bur with a diameter between 3.0 and 3.5 mm is used to uncover the implant.

Uncovering procedure using both a mini-incision and soft tissue punch

When implant fixtures are placed below a thick mucosa, it may be difficult to make a circumferential incision in the gingiva at the center of the implant using a soft tissue punch. In this case, the soft tissue punch is used in combination with a crestal mini-incision. A crestal mini-incision is made approximately 3 mm horizontally with the alveolar crest at the center of the implant site. Local undermining at the implant site is then performed until the first-stage cover screw is exposed. After removing the first-stage cover screws, a guide pin is connected to the implant body. A soft tissue punch with a diameter between 3.0 and 3.5 mm is used to uncover the implant using the guide pin (Figs 7-21 and 7-22). This procedure ensures that the peri-implant mucosa is in tight contact with the healing abutment around the implant.

Considerations related to the uncovering procedure

- Care should be taken to incise and undermine only the soft tissue above the cover screw when uncovering implants using a mini-incision. During the procedure, the implant surface should not be scratched or contaminated.
- Care should be taken to make a circumferential incision in the gingiva at the center of the implant using a soft tissue punch to allow close contact between the peri-implant mucosa and the healing abutment around the implant.
- Any bone growth on the cover screws should be removed with surgical curettes (Fig 7-23). A drill is not used to remove bone growth on the cover screws because it can damage the implant surface. The implant surface should not be scratched during this procedure.
- The size and shape of the permucosal healing abutment should be smaller than the cervical contour of the final crown (Fig 7-24). A wide-profile permucosal healing abutment should not be used because it can cause gingival shrinkage and limit the ability of the restoring surgeon to shape it into its desired form.
- The permucosal healing abutment should extend through the soft tissue at least 1 mm above the adjacent mucosa to help to prevent tissue overgrowth during the healing period.
- The soft tissue punch should be 1.0–1.5 mm narrower than the permucosal healing abutment to ensure close contact between the peri-implant mucosa and the healing abutment.

Fig 7-21 *(Facing page)* The uncovering procedure using both a crestal mini-incision and a soft tissue punch. A crestal mini-incision of approximately 3 mm horizontally with the alveolar crest at the center of the implant site is made. Local undermining at the implant site is then performed until the first-stage cover screw is exposed. After removing the first-stage cover screws (a), a guide pin is connected to the implant body (b). Using the guide pin, a soft tissue punch with a diameter between 3.0 and 3.5 mm is used to uncover the implant (c–e). After uncovering the implant, a permucosal healing abutment is seated into the implant body (f and g). (h) A periapical radiograph is taken to ensure proper component fit.

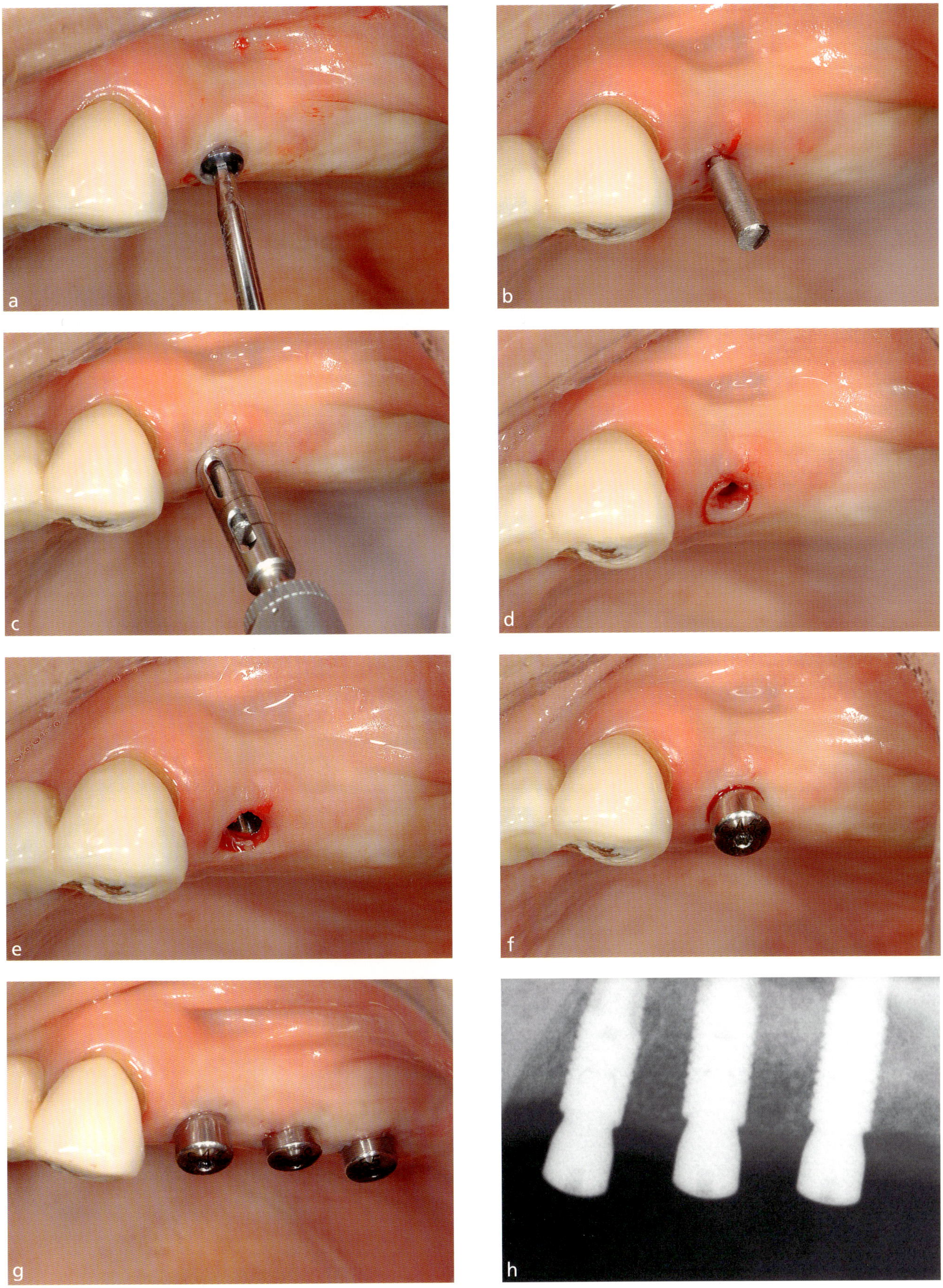
a
b
c
d
e
f
g
h

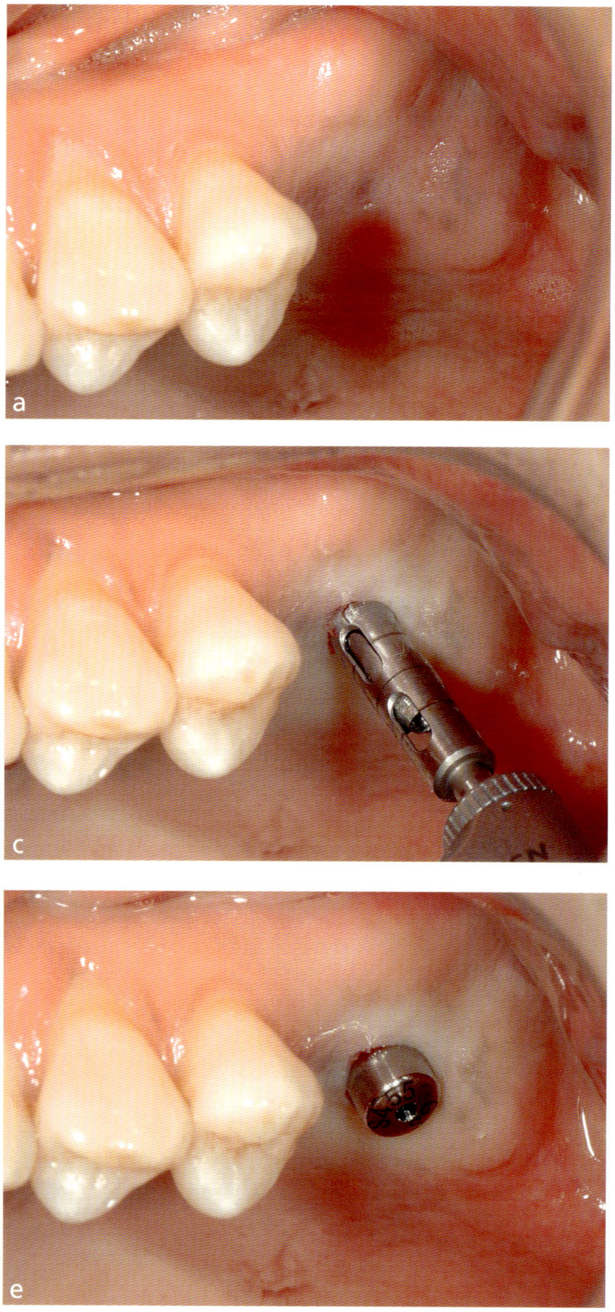

Fig 7-22 Intraoral views showing the uncovering procedure using both a crestal mini-incision and a soft tissue punch: (a) before the procedure; (b) after connecting a guide pin to the implant body; (c) uncovering the implant using a soft tissue punch bur; (d) after uncovering the implant; (e) after connecting a permucosal healing abutment.

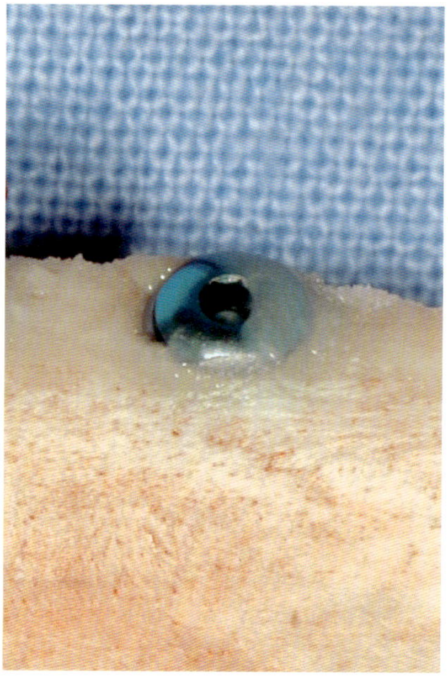

Fig 7-23 A specimen showing bone growth on the cover screw.

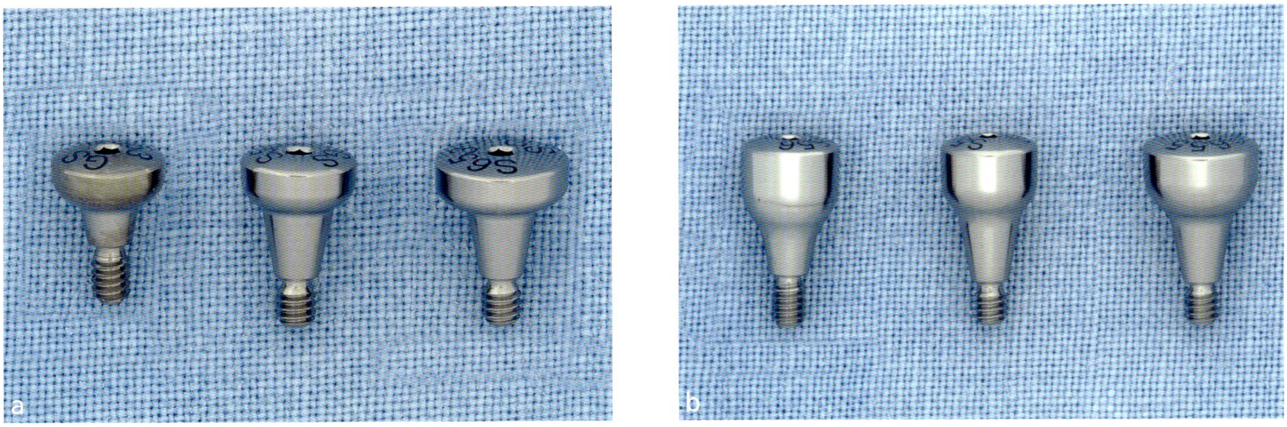

Fig 7-24 (a and b) Various sizes of permucosal healing abutments.

Soft tissue emergence contours

At the stage II uncovering procedure, exposure of the implant body should be accomplished considering the final architecture of the soft tissue. Gingivoplasty at the uncovering procedure is performed to achieve the proper soft tissue architecture when excess tissue forms on the facial and interproximal regions. When the soft tissue along the edentulous crest is at the level of the desired interdental papillae, gingivoplasty is performed to sculpt the crest of the ridge and form a scalloped emergence profile around the abutment (Fig 7-25). The contour of the midfacial position of the gingival margin is 1 mm more incisal than the contour of the adjacent teeth in order to

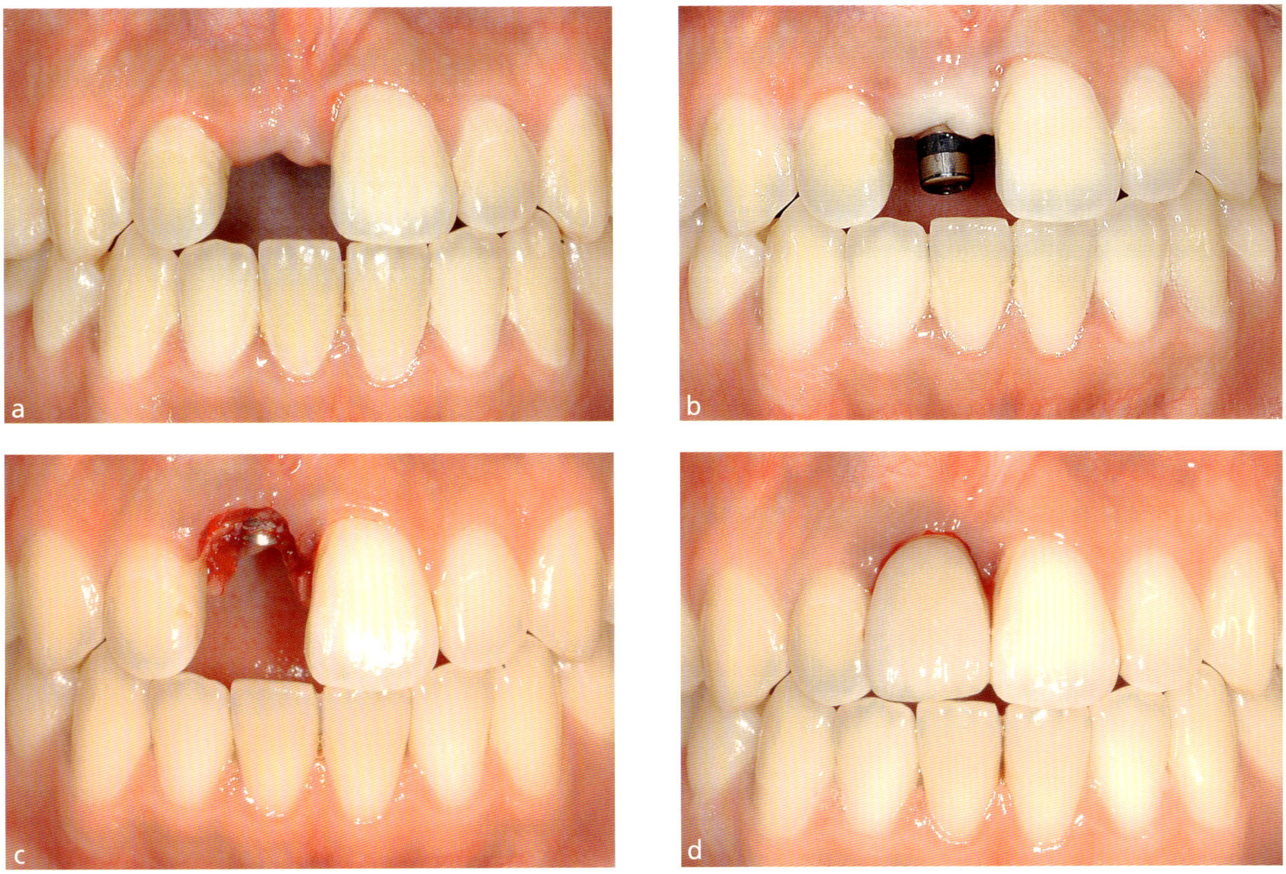

Fig 7-25 (a–d) When the soft tissue along the edentulous crest is at the level of the desired interdental papillae, gingivoplasty is performed to sculpt the crest of the ridge and form a scalloped emergence profile around the abutment.

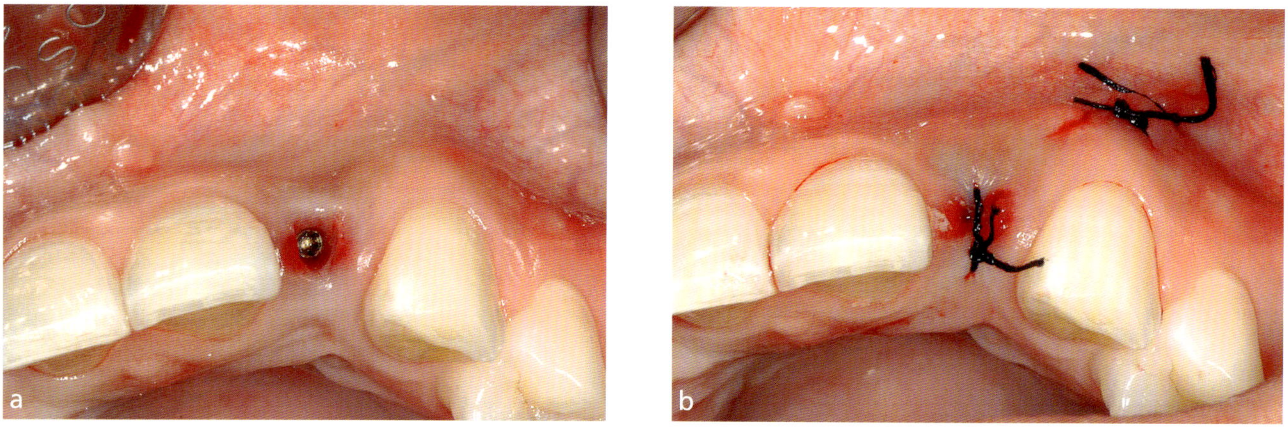

Fig 7-26 The gingival contour can be corrected for esthetic purposes with graft material using a subperiosteal tunneling procedure: (a) the thin labial plate; (b) after grafting Bio-Oss® particles mixed with autologous fibrin gel through a subperiosteal tunnel.

allow for the gingival shrinkage commonly observed during the first year of implant loading. The interdental papilla zones are also made slightly larger than the final desired form to accommodate possible shrinkage.

Further surgery can be performed to gain additional height if the gingival contour at stage II uncovering is insufficient for a good esthetic result. Several techniques have been proposed.[11–14] We normally graft Bio-Oss® particles mixed with autologous fibrin gel on the facial or interproximal regions through a subperiosteal tunnel, as described in Chapter 12. The gingival contour can be corrected with graft material using a subperiosteal tunneling procedure to meet esthetic demands (Fig 7-26). This does not increase the volume of the soft tissue alone. Augmentation consists of a zone of dense connective tissue interposed between the particles. However, augmentation provides an improved esthetic result and limited long-term tissue shrinkage. The increased tissue thickness from augmentation prevents the grayish hue of the titanium implant body from being observed through the labial mucosa. The most significant advantage of the procedure is that the minimally invasive technique using a small incision offers less postoperative morbidity.

Final prosthesis

Four weeks after the stage II uncovering procedure, the permucosal healing abutments are removed and replaced with the final abutment for screw retention or cement retention. In the esthetic regions, a transitional prosthesis is worn until the final prosthesis is fabricated. The transitional prosthesis is relieved over the permucosal healing abutments and in any region of desired secondary soft tissue healing.

Peri-implant bone loss

Several studies have reported crestal bone loss around the implants related to stage II surgery performed using full-thickness flap elevation. Engquist et al.[15] examined the marginal bone changes around submerged implants and reported that the mean bone losses in the maxilla between the abutment connection and crown placement were 0.82 mm and 1.58 mm for Astra Tech and Brånemark System® implants, respectively. The corresponding figures for the mandible were 0.48 mm and 1.23 mm. Cardaropoli et al.[16] reported a mean loss of 0.9 mm between the abutment connection and crown placement. In all these studies, the implants were uncovered with flap elevations.

However, in the authors' clinical study, the implants were uncovered without flap elevation. The study evaluated 104 maxillary implants in 50 patients. When the implants were uncovered without flap elevation, there was only a small amount of bone loss (0.11 ± 0.14 mm) between the abutment connection and crown placement (Table 7-1; Fig 7-27). These results suggest that the flapless procedure can reduce crestal bone loss related to stage II surgery (Figs 7-28 to 7-30). One interesting finding is that no implants failed during the healing process after stage II surgery. This total success rate is in stark contrast to other previously published reports,[17–19] which demonstrated higher failure rates (1.3–5.9%) after performing stage II surgery using full-thickness flap elevation.

An understanding of the cause of crestal bone loss around dental implants after flapless stage II surgery is essential for preventing such occurrences. The cause of such bone loss is the same as after flapless stage I surgery, because stage II surgery is similar in terms of the manipulation of soft tissue. The major cause of early implant bone loss appears to be closely related to soft tissue wound healing after the procedures. Bone loss that occurs during the healing period is closely related to the degree and duration

Table 7-1 Marginal bone loss and number of failed implants during the healing period after stage II surgery (n = 104).

Marginal bone loss	0.1 ± 0.1 mm
Number of failed implants	0

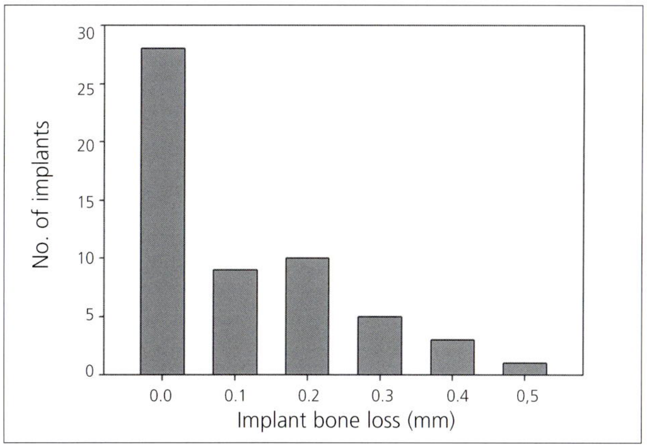

Fig 7-27 Bar chart showing the implants with various amounts of bone loss during the healing period after stage II surgery.

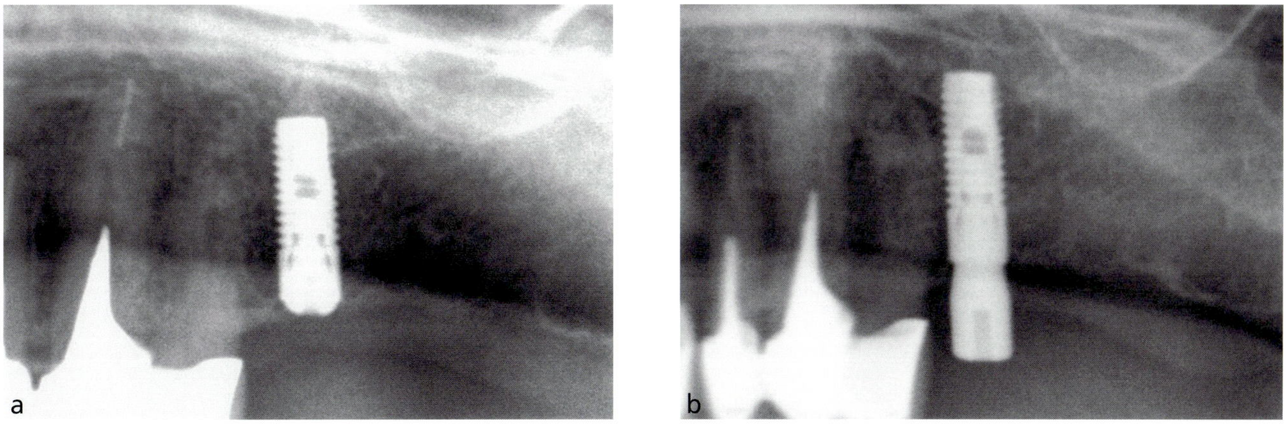

Fig 7-28 Radiographs taken (a) before flapless stage II surgery and (b) 1 month postoperatively. See also Figs 7-29 and 7-30.

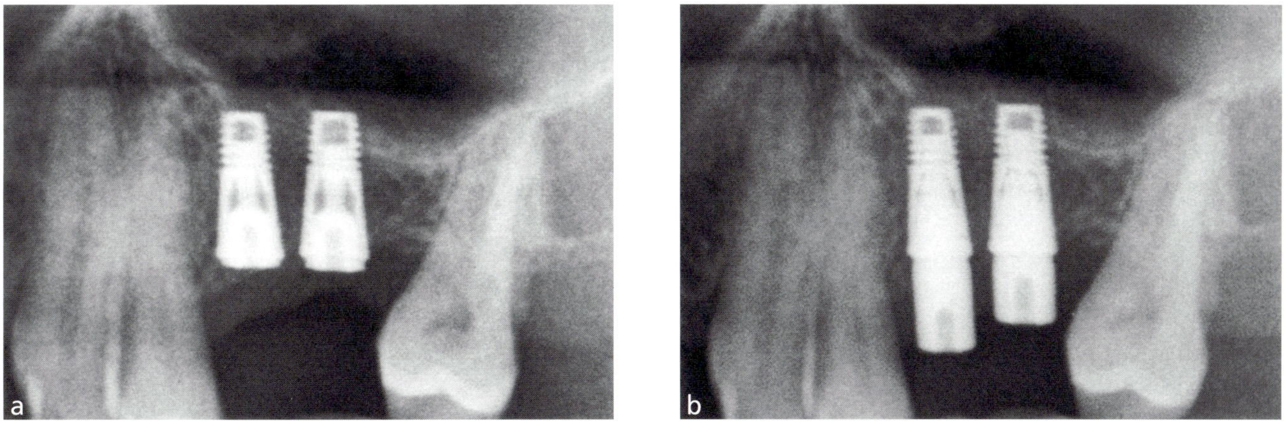

Fig 7-29 Radiographs taken (a) before flapless stage II surgery and (b) 1 month postoperatively. See also Figs 7-28 and 7-30.

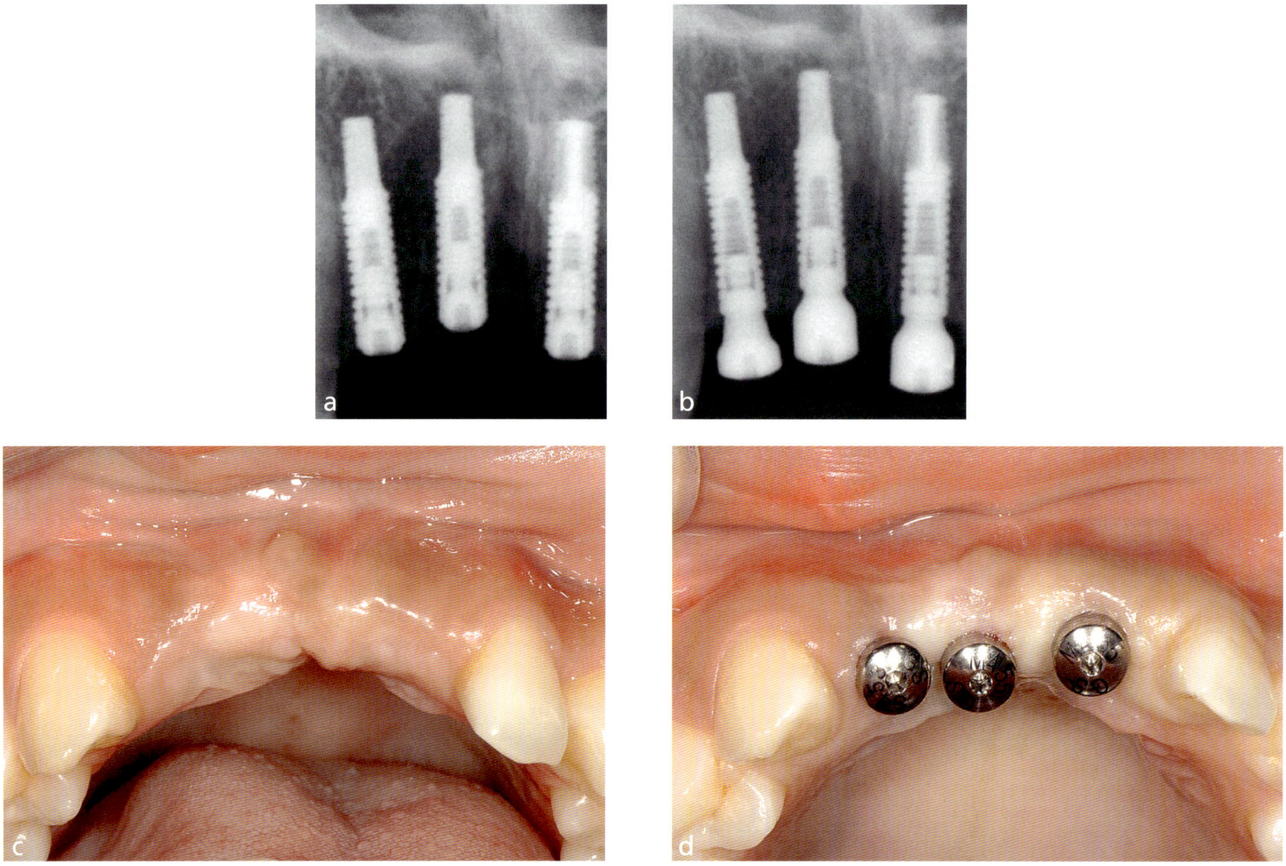

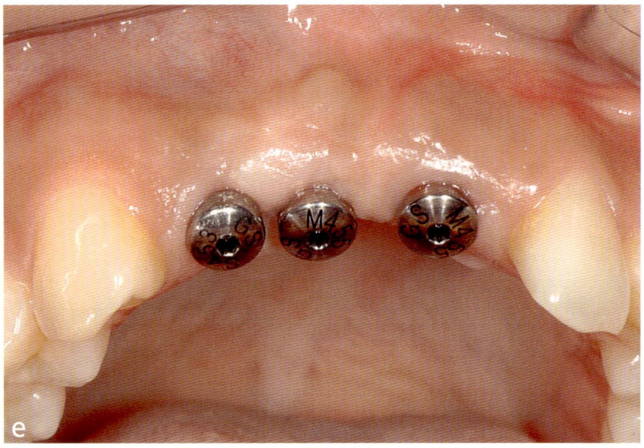

Fig 7-30 Radiographs taken (a) before flapless stage II surgery and (b) 1 month postoperatively. Intraoral views (c) before surgery, (d) immediately after surgery, and (e) 1 month later.

of inflammation and infection as well as the scar volume. This means that the healing process is slowed if soft tissue wounds around implants are infected during the postoperative period. Inflammation combined with significant scarring results in even more bone loss. These findings suggest that peri-implant bone loss after flapless stage II surgery can be prevented or minimized if the soft tissue wounds around the implants heal quickly with little inflammation or scar formation. It is advisable to have small, clean, closed wounds around the implants after a flapless uncovering procedure and to perform meticulous early plaque control to prevent or minimize peri-implant bone loss.

Summary

Stage II surgery is necessary if flapless implant placement is performed via a mini-incision technique and is then submerged. The stage II procedure is as important as the stage I procedure in terms of protecting the soft tissue and ensuring favorable conditions for the healing of soft tissue adjacent to the implant. It is advisable to perform a stage II procedure using a flapless technique, have small, clean, closed wounds around the implants, have the peri-implant mucosa in tight contact with the healing abutment around the implant, and perform meticulous early plaque control after the procedure.

References

1. Misch CE. Contemporary Implant Dentistry, ed 3. St Louis, MO: Mosby, 2008:720–738.
2. Krekeler G, Schilli W, Diemer J. Should the exit of the artificial abutment tooth be positioned in the region of the attached gingiva? Int J Oral Surg 1985;14:504–508.
3. Adell R, Lekholm U, Rockler B et al. Marginal tissue reactions at osseointegrated titanium fixtures: a 3-year longitudinal prospective study. Int J Oral Maxillofac Implants 1986;15:39–52.
4. Lekholm U, Adell R, Lindhe J et al. Marginal tissue reactions at osseointegrated titanium fixtures. II: A cross-sectional respective study. Int J Oral Maxillofac Surg 1986;15:53–61.
5. Wennström JL, Bengazi F, Lekholm U. The influence of the masticatory mucosa on the peri-implant soft tissue condition. Clin Oral Implants Res 1994;5:1–8.
6. Warrer K, Buser D, Lang NP, Karring T. Plaque-induced peri-implantitis in the presence or absence of keratinized mucosa. Clin Oral Implants Res 1995;6:131–138.
7. Esposito M, Hirsch J-M, Lekholm U, Thomsen P. Biological factors contributing to failures of osseointegrated oral implants. I: Success criteria and epidemiology. Eur J Oral Sci 1998;106:527–551.
8. Kan JYK, Rungcharassaeng K, Umezu K, Kois JC. Dimensions of peri-implant mucosa: an evaluation of maxillary anterior single implants in humans. J Periodontol 2003;74:557–565.
9. Lekholm U, Adell R, Lindhe J et al. Marginal tissue reactions at osseointegrated titanium fixtures. II: A cross-sectional retrospective study. Int J Oral Maxillofac Surg 1986;15:53–61.
10. Berglundh T, Lindhe J, Jonsson K. The topography of the vascular systems in the periodontal and peri-implant tissues in the dog. J Clin Periodontol 1994;21:189–193.
11. Salama H, Salama M, Garber DA, Adar P. Developing optimal peri-implant papillae within the esthetic zone: Part I: Guided soft tissue augmentation: the three-stage approach. J Esthet Dent 1995;7:125–129.
12. Salama H, Salama M, Garber DA, Adar P. The interproximal height of bone: a guidepost to predictable aesthetic strategies and soft tissue contours in anterior tooth replacement. Pract Periodontics Aesthet Dent 1998;10:1131–1141.
13. Becker W, Becker B. Flap designs for minimization of recession adjacent to maxillary anterior sites: a clinical study. Int J Oral Maxillofac Implants 1996;11:46–54.
14. Misch CE, Al-Shammari KF, Wang HI. Creation of interimplant papillae through a split-finger technique. Implant Dent 2004;13:20–27.
15. Engquist B, Åstrand P, Dahlgren S, Engquist E, Feldmann H, Gröndahl K. Marginal bone reaction to oral implants: a prospective comparative study of Astra Tech and Brånemark System® implants. Clin Oral Implants Res 2002;13:30–37.
16. Cardaropoli G, Lekholm U, Wennström JL. Tissue alterations at implant supported single tooth replacement: a 1-year prospective clinical study. Clin Oral Implants Res 2006;17:165–171.
17. Kraut RA. Clean operating conditions for the placement of intraoral implants. J Oral Maxillofac Surg 1996;54:1337–1338.
18. Zarb GA, Schmitt A. The longitudinal clinical effectiveness of osseointegrated dental implants (the Toronto study). I: Surgical results. J Prosthet Dent 1990;63:451–457.
19. Naert I, Quirynen M. A six-year prosthodontic study of 509 consecutively inserted implants for the treatment of partial edentulism. J Prosthet Dent 1992;67:236–245.

CHAPTER

8

Spontaneous Early Exposure of Flapless Submerged Implants

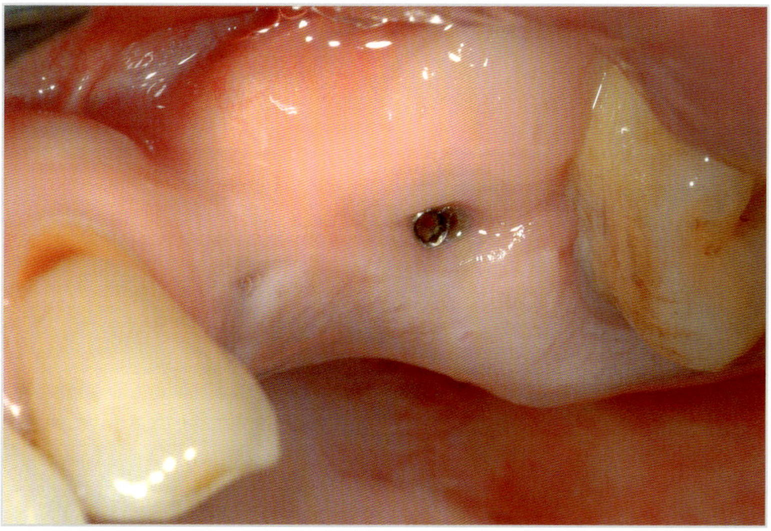

Key point

Prevention is better than cure.

Overview

When implants are submerged using a mini-incision technique, they become covered with mucosa after implant placement. Favorable conditions for osseointegration are established by complete mucosal coverage during the healing phase. However, an implant covered with soft tissue at the first-stage procedure can sometimes become exposed early before stage II uncovering (Fig 8-1). This can result in direct communication between the implant surface and the oral environment. Plaque accumulation on the exposed implant can lead to a soft tissue inflammatory lesion, which, if left untreated, can initiate peri-implantitis. This chapter addresses the causes of early exposure of submerged implants after flapless submerged implant surgery as well as its effect on the peri-implant tissues. The management of prematurely exposed implants is also discussed.

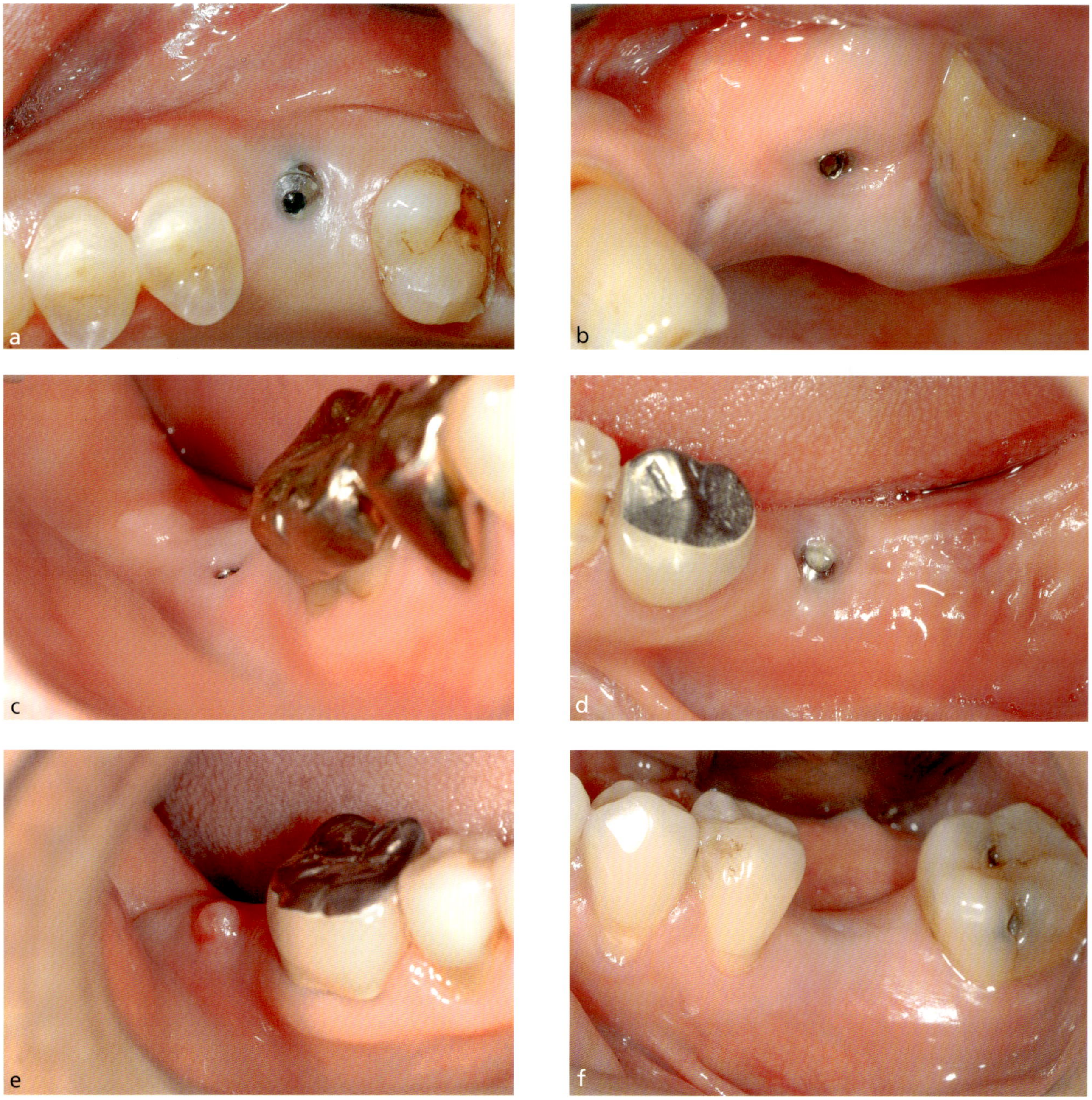

Fig 8-1 (a–f) Various exposures of submerged implants after flapless implant surgery.

Causes of spontaneous early exposure

Damage to soft tissue

When flapless implant surgery is performed using a mini-incision technique, drills can damage the adjacent soft tissue. In particular, the soft tissue is likely to be cut if the size of the drill is 3.5 mm or more. When the soft tissue is damaged, implant exposure can occur.

Soft tissue condition

An avascular zone 1–2 mm wide is created in the crestal area of the edentulous alveolar ridge.[1] Further, the mucosa covering the cover screws receives no blood supply from underneath. As a result, the cover screws are likely to be exposed. The mucosal thickness is another factor involved in prematurely exposed implants. A thick mucosa is more resistant to trauma than a thin mucosa, so implant exposure is more likely to occur with a thinner mucosa. For this reason, exposure occurs more frequently in the mandible than in the maxilla (Fig 8-2).

Bone tissue condition

In the maxilla, early exposure of submerged implants occurs less frequently with fine trabecular bone and a good blood supply. In the mandible, exposure occurs more frequently with a thick cortical plate and reduced blood supply.

Implant design

When a long, smooth metal collar is placed above the alveolar crest, it is difficult to submerge implants using a mini-incision. The risk of implant exposure is greater when the implant is extended further above the bone crest. Therefore, it is prudent to select an implant system for a mini-incision technique in which the top of the implants can be placed at the same level as the alveolar crest (Fig 8-3).

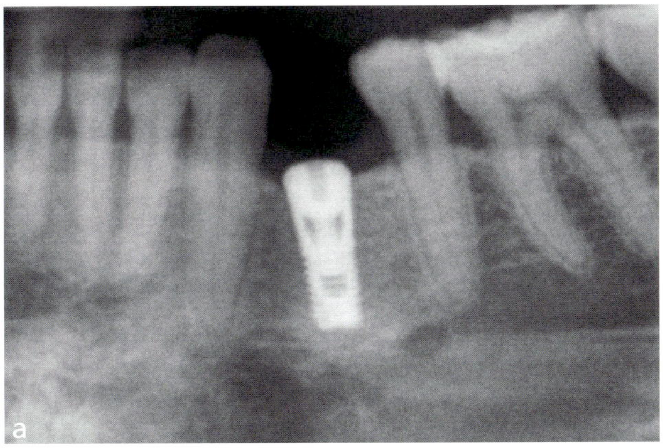

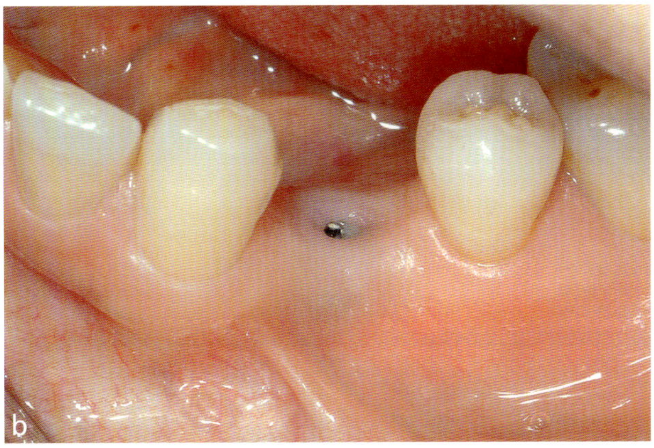

Fig 8-2 (a and b) In the mandible, the cover screw is likely to be exposed after implant placement because of the thin mucosa.

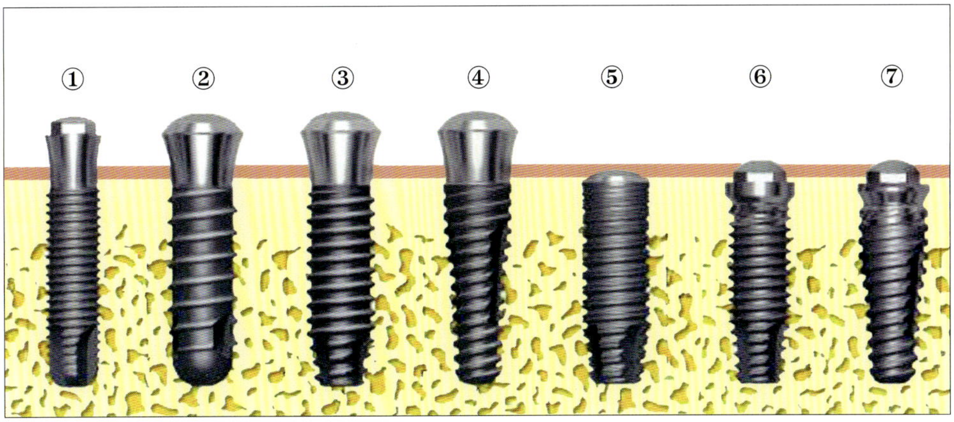

Fig 8-3 Implant no. 5 among various types is optimal for a mini-incision technique. When a long, smooth metal collar is placed above the alveolar crest, submerging implants after a mini-incision technique is difficult.

Effects of spontaneous early exposure

Effect on the morphogenesis of peri-implant mucosa

If early implant exposure occurs, the peri-implant soft tissue zone, which is analogous to the biological width associated with natural teeth, does not develop, and epithelial invagination and inflammatory infiltration at the implant surface occurs, resulting in the formation of a deep sulcus (Fig 8-4). The pathological structure of the perforated mucosa can act as a plaque-retentive site, which can increase the amount of bone loss. Plaque accumulation generally results in peri-implant mucositis.

Effect on crestal bone loss

Spontaneous early exposure is associated with an increased incidence of crestal bone loss. Tal et al.[2] reported a significant difference between the bone loss associated with implants covered with intact mucosa and that associated with implants that experienced spontaneous early exposure. According to Toljanic et al.,[3] the overall mean crestal bone losses after flap implant surgery were 2.71 mm and 0.43 mm for early exposed and unexposed implants, respectively. Exposed sites were 3.9 times more likely to develop bone loss than unexposed sites. Tal et al.[2] showed also that the amount of peri-implant bone loss differs according to the degree of exposure. The rates of spontaneous exposure reported in a series of clinical observations are between 5% and 15%.[2,4-8]

A total of 144 implants were placed by the present authors in 71 patients using a mini-incision submerged procedure. The implants were evaluated radiographically for changes in the crestal bone level from the time of placement to the time of exposure (3–4 months later). The overall mean crestal bone losses after flapless implant surgery were 0.43 mm and 0.12 mm for early exposed and unexposed implants, respectively (Table 8-1; Fig 8-5). Bone loss was three times higher in the exposed implants than in the unexposed implants. Interestingly, there was a significant difference in crestal bone loss between the maxilla (0.27 mm) and mandible (0.56 mm) (Figs 8-6 to 8-8). The reason is that the thick mucosa in the maxilla has a protective role for the exposed implants, and relatively less bone resorption occurs after implant exposure.

Mechanism of bone loss around early exposed implants

The bone loss around early exposed implants has a close association with wound healing. If spontaneous early implant exposure occurs, the mucosa around the exposed implants fails to form a stable attachment and the spread of the inflammatory reaction can be more extensive. The unstable attachment of the soft tissue lengthens the inflammatory phase of repair. In addition, epithelial invagination and inflammatory infiltration at the implant surface occur, forming a deep sulcus. The structure acts as a plaque-retentive site, making it difficult to access for plaque control. Subsequently, inflammation is likely to occur and is more extensive around the implants,[9] possibly developing downward along the implant surface[8,10-12] and leading to bone loss.

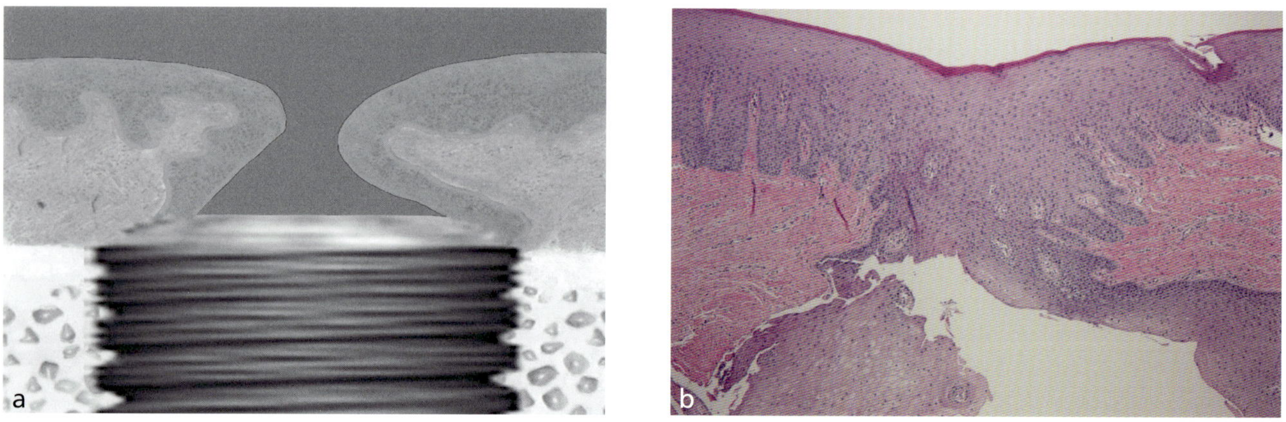

Fig 8-4 (a and b) The perforated mucosa at the early exposed implant site shows epithelial invagination and inflammatory infiltration at the implant surface.

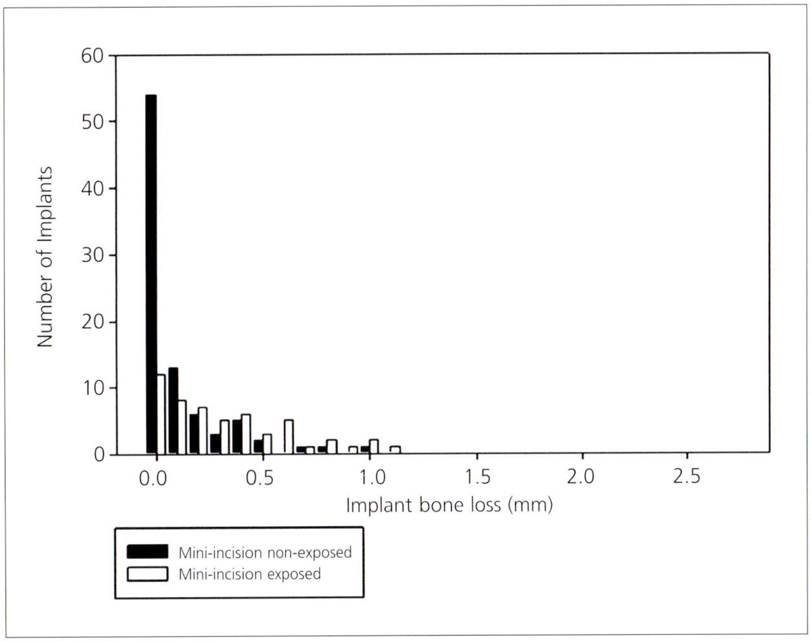

Fig 8-5 Bar chart showing the number of implants that exhibited loss of peri-implant bone height during the healing period in the early exposed implant and unexposed implant groups after mini-incision submerged implant surgery.

Table 8-1 Effect of spontaneous early exposure on crestal bone loss after mini-incision submerged implant surgery.

	Non-exposed (n = 104)	Exposed (n = 44)	*P* value
Mean bone loss (mm)	0.12	0.43	< .05
Maxilla/mandible (mm)	0.10/0.23	0.27/0.56	< .05

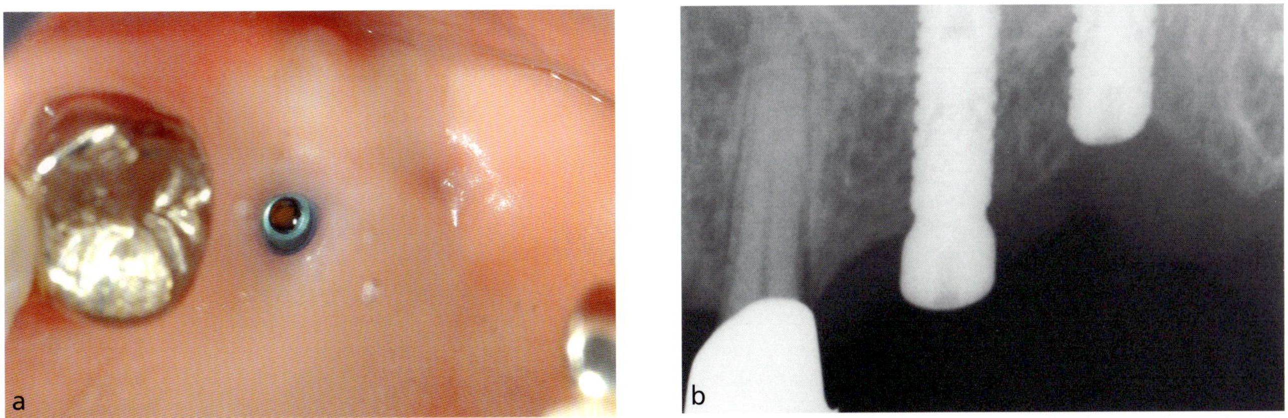

Fig 8-6 (a) Two implants were placed in the maxillary left first and second molar sites using a mini-incision submerged technique. The implant in the first molar site was exposed early during the healing period. (b) Radiographic examination performed 4 months after surgery revealed no crestal bone loss in either implant site.

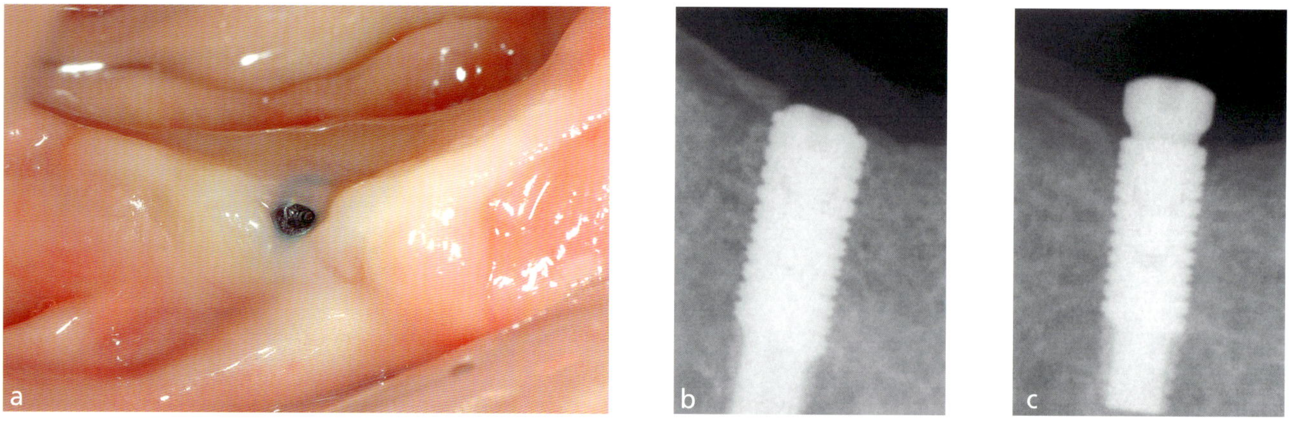

Fig 8-7 (a and b) An implant was placed in the mandibular right second molar site using a mini-incision submerged technique. The implant was exposed early during the healing period. (c) Radiographic examination performed 3 months after surgery revealed a 0.7 mm loss of crestal bone.

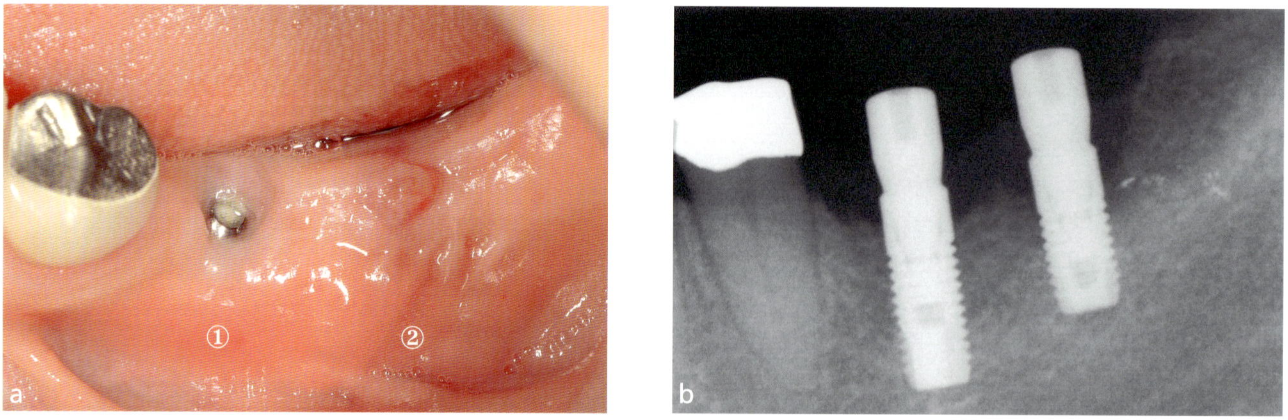

Fig 8-8 (a) Intraoral view of early exposure of the implant (1) and gumboil (2). (b) Radiograph taken 1 month after mini-incision submerged implant placement shows bone loss around the implants.

Initial healing of prematurely exposed implants

Effect of abutment connections

To obtain data on the most appropriate management of prematurely exposed implants, an animal experiment was performed to determine the influence of abutment connections on initial healing. Crestal bone loss was greater at partially exposed implant sites than at abutment-connected implant sites (Table 8-2). This suggests that the placement of transmucosal abutments on exposed implants will help to prevent more bone loss in prematurely exposed implants.

This has implications for patient management between the stage I and II procedures with regard to the frequency of follow-up and the management of prematurely exposed implants. After two-stage implant surgery, asymptomatic patients do not typically return until implant uncovering. However, more frequent follow-up between the stages will be needed to identify and address implant exposure. When implant exposure is detected, placement of healing abutments can help to limit bone loss and avoid complications resulting from that loss (Figs 8-9 and 8-10). These abutments can help to develop a stable soft tissue attachment, which is a biologically beneficial condition for the peri-implant tissues.[13-16] Soft tissue cannot form a stable attachment around partially exposed implants.

Effect of plaque control

To obtain data on the most appropriate management of prematurely exposed implants, an animal experiment was performed to determine the effect of plaque control on initial healing.[17,18] When meticulous plaque control was performed, a noninflammatory peri-implant mucosa could be established for abutment-connected implants, whereas for partially exposed implants the peri-implant mucosa responded with an inflammatory reaction and crestal bone loss. One explanation for this observation may be

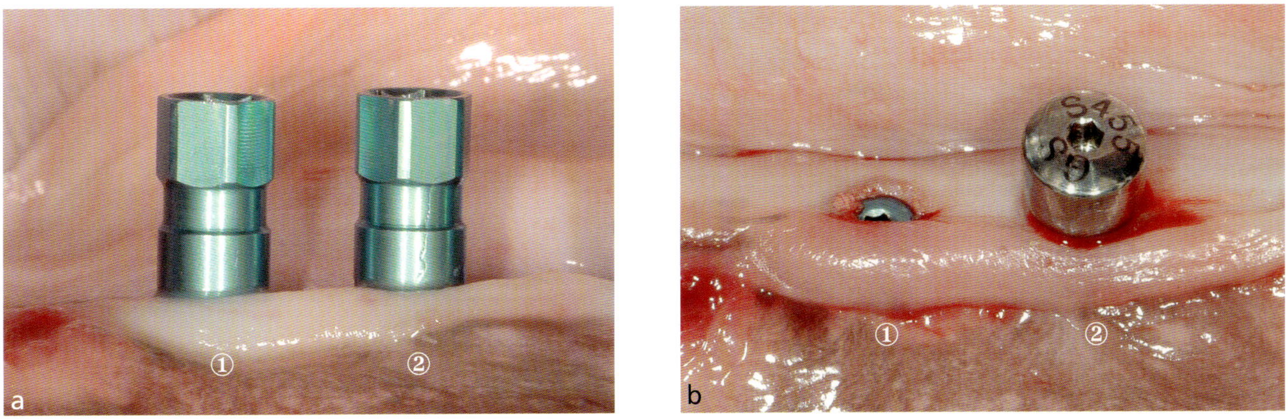

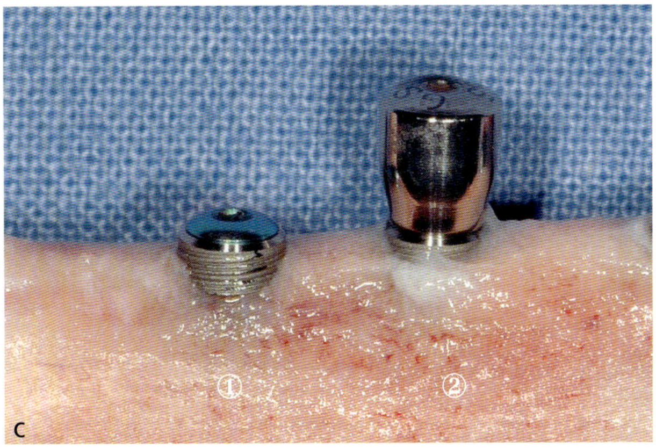

Fig 8-9 (a) Clinical features after implant placement using a mini-incision technique. (b) For the first implant, a cover screw was connected to the fixture and the incised gingiva was partially removed to expose the implant. For the second implant, a healing abutment was connected to the fixture so that the coronal portion of the abutment could remain exposed to the oral cavity. (c) The mandible, showing bone height around the implants. 1. partially exposed implant; 2. abutment-connected implant.

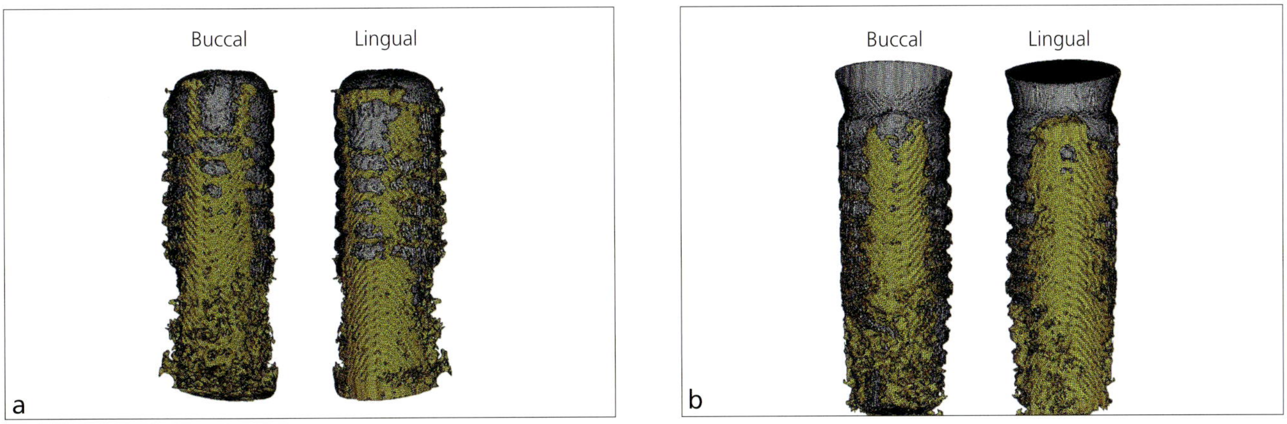

Fig 8-10 Three-dimensional micro-CT showing the bone (yellow) around implants (gray), for (a) partially exposed implant, and (b) abutment-connected implant. Buccal – buccal side of the alveolus; lingual – lingual side of the alveolus.

Table 8-2 Parameters of the bone height around implants in the abutment-connected and partially exposed groups during the healing period for prematurely exposed implants.

	Abutment-connected group (n = 12)	Partially exposed group (n = 12)	*P* value
Mean bone height (mm ± SD)	9.8 ± 0.5	9.3 ± 0.5	< .05

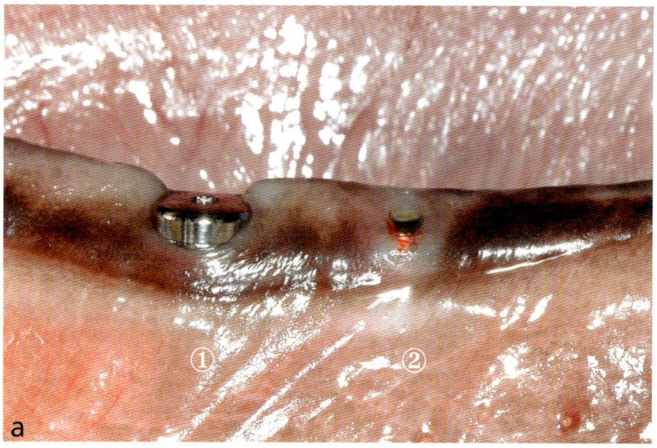

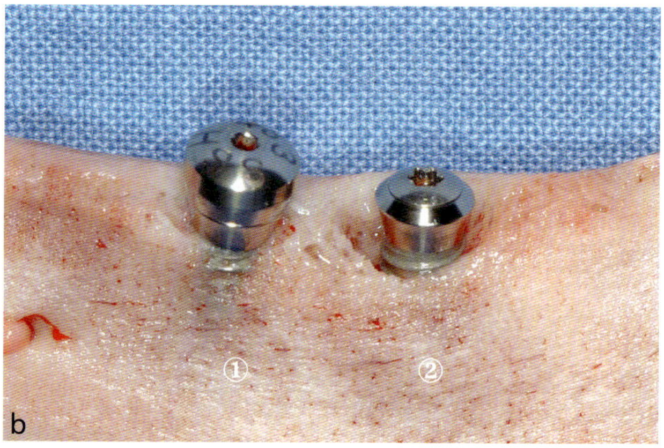

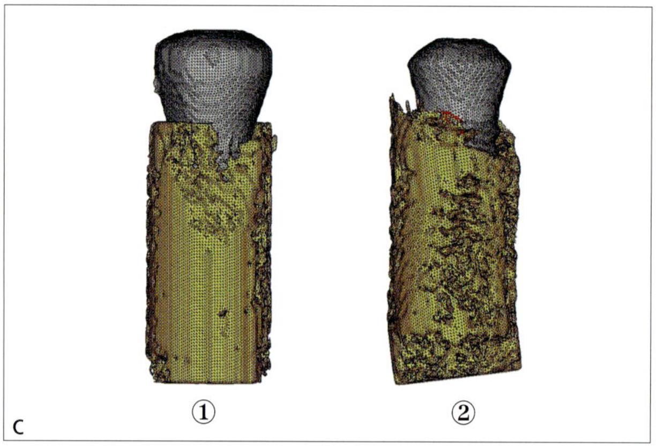

Fig 8-11 (a) Clinical features in the plaque control group 8 weeks after implant placement using a mini-incision technique. (b) The mandible, demonstrating the bone height around the implants. (c) Three-dimensional micro-CT demonstrating bone (yellow) around the implants (gray). The results suggest that meticulous plaque control alone does not appear to prevent inflammatory reactions in partially exposed implants. 1 – abutment-connected implant; 2 – partially exposed implant.

that the perforated mucosa of partially exposed implants acted as a plaque-retentive site, making it difficult to access for plaque control. The results suggest that meticulous plaque control alone does not prevent inflammatory reactions in partially exposed implants (Fig 8-11).

When plaque was allowed to form at both abutment-connected and partially exposed implants, the peri-implant bone showed more bone loss around the former. This greater bone loss is believed to be caused by the greater amount of inflammation, which suggests that the spread of the inflammatory reaction may be more extensive in abutment-connected implants than in partially exposed implants when a healthy soft tissue barrier has not formed around implants. This observation demonstrates the importance of proper plaque control in the establishment and maintenance of healthy barrier tissue at implants (Table 8-3; Fig 8-12).

Management of spontaneous early exposure

Various methods for managing the spontaneous early exposure of submerged implants after flap implant surgery have been proposed. Adell et al.[4] suggested that any communication with the oral cavity observed during the first 6 weeks after surgery should be treated with an excision of the perforated site, flap mobilization, re-suturing, and appropriate adjustment of the denture. Kim[19] recommends cleaning exposed implants using chlorhexidine. Covering exposed implants with a polytetrafluoroethylene membrane has also been proposed.

For managing the spontaneous early exposure of submerged implants after flapless implant surgery, closing the exposed implants using either barrier membranes or re-suturing is not advisable because this may aggravate the problem. First, it is prudent to wait 3 weeks because inadequately stabilized implants were submerged at the first-stage surgery. During the observation period, the exposed

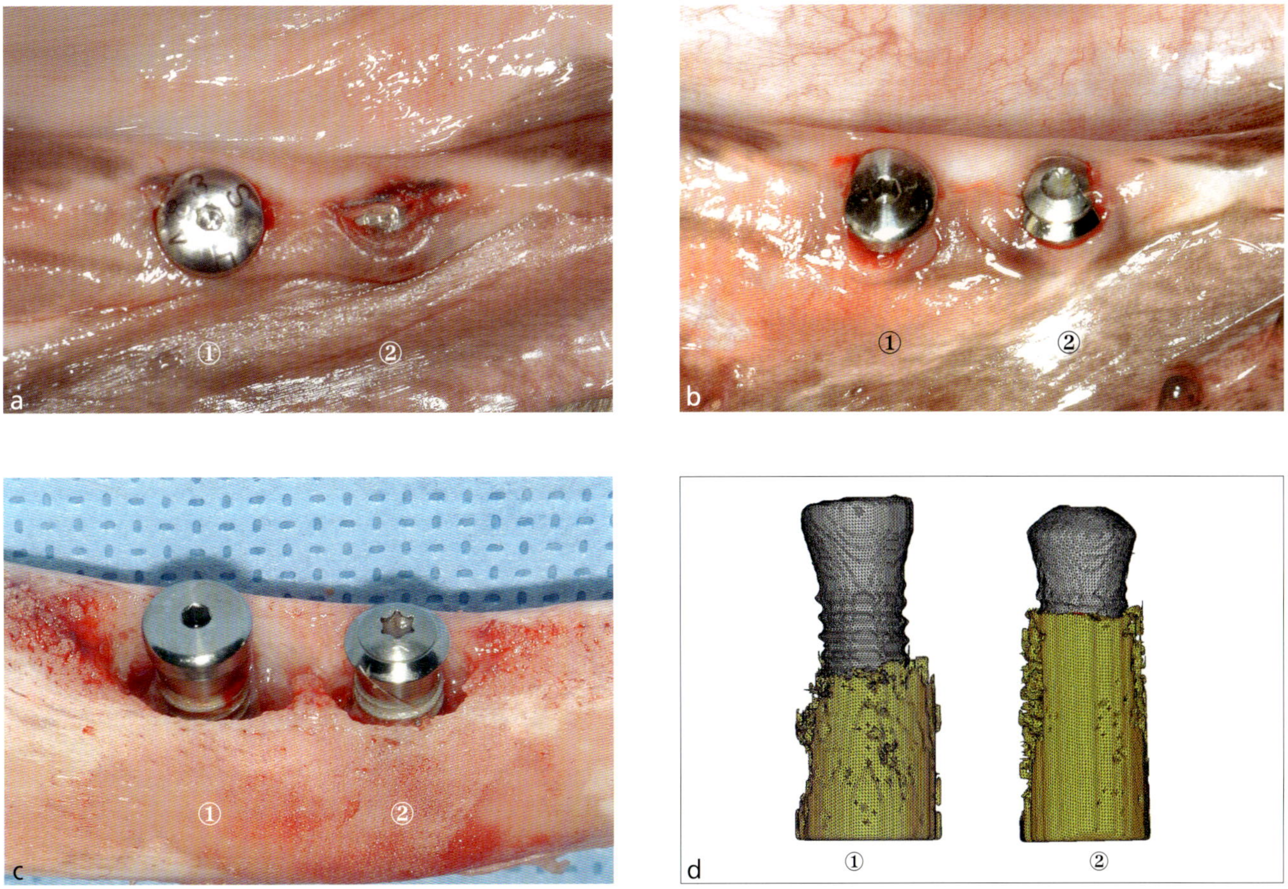

Fig 8-12 (a) Clinical features in the group without plaque control immediately after implant placement using a mini-incision technique. A healing abutment was connected to the implant to allow the coronal portion of the abutment to remain exposed to the oral cavity (1). A cover screw was connected to the implant and the incised gingiva was partially removed to expose the implant (2). (b) Clinical features 8 weeks after implant placement. (c) The mandible, demonstrating the bone height around the implants. (d) Three-dimensional micro-CT demonstrating bone (yellow) around the implants (gray). The results demonstrate the importance of proper plaque control for the establishment and maintenance of healthy barrier tissue at implants.

Table 8-3 Parameters (mean values) of the bone height during the healing period in the abutment-connected and partially exposed dental implant groups, with and without plaque control.

	Abutment-connected group	Partially exposed group	*P* values
Plaque control (mm ± SD)	10.1 ± 0.5	9.3 ± 0.5	< .05
No plaque control (mm ± SD)	6.5 ± 0.7	8.2 ± 0.6	< .05

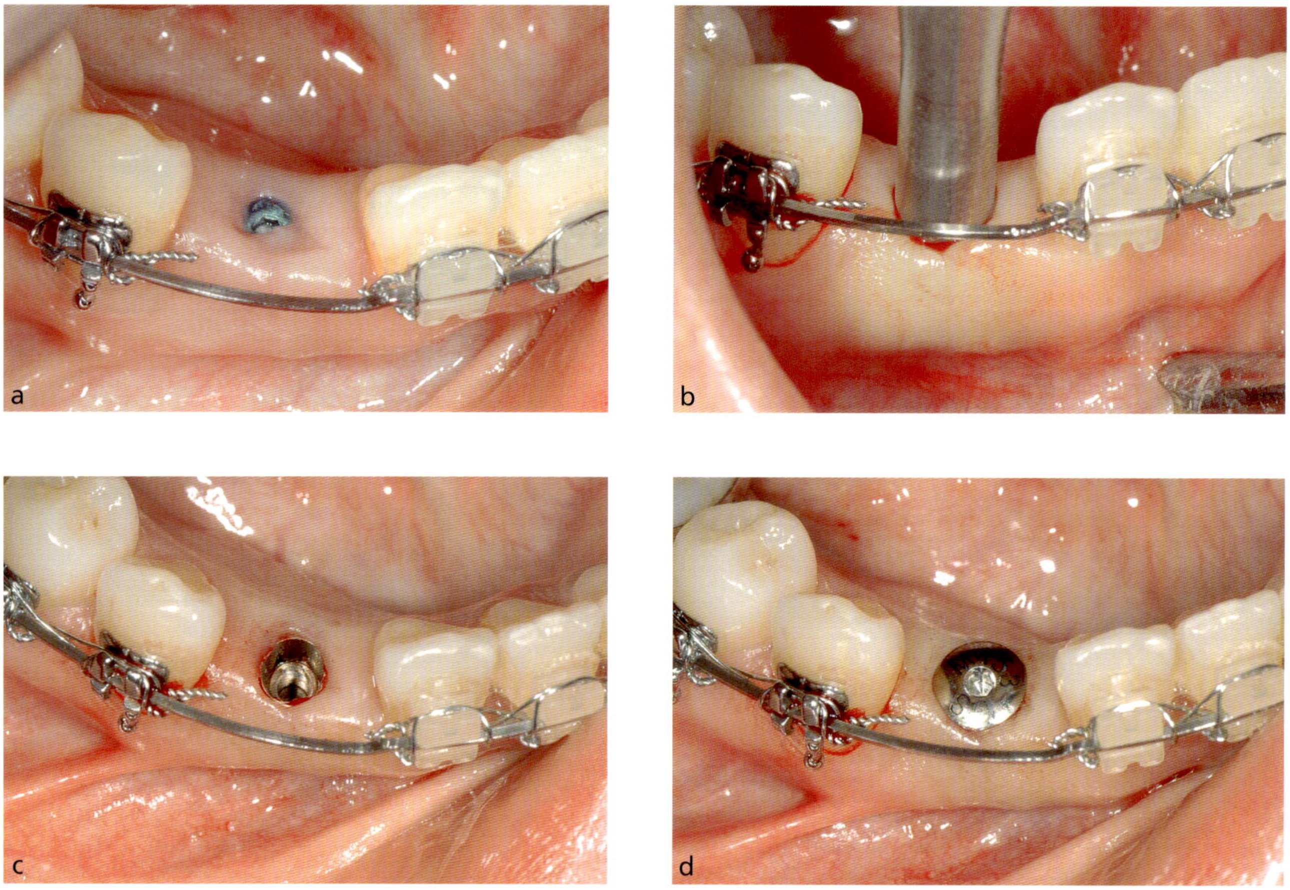

Fig 8-13 (a–d) The implant at the mandibular right lateral incisor site is exposed early during the healing period. Three weeks later, the marginal mucosa is excised around the exposed implants and a healing abutment is connected.

site should be cleaned with chlorhexidine. Three weeks later, it is advisable to manage the partially exposed implants with the placement of healing abutments and meticulous plaque control (Fig 8-13), which is described in Chapter 9. When placing healing abutments, it is advisable to excise the marginal mucosa around the exposed implants to induce new soft tissue attachment (Figs 8-14 and 8-15).

Management of fistulas and gumboils

Fistulas and gumboils are further examples of spontaneous early exposure of implants, and are more likely to develop in the mandible than in the maxilla after flapless implant surgery using a mini-incision submerged technique, because the mandible has a 1–2 mm wide avascular zone in the crestal area of the edentulous alveolar ridge as well as a thin mucosa (Fig 8-16).

Fistulas or gumboils that develop in the mandible are dangerous because they can rapidly destroy bone (Fig 8-17). Implant failure can occur if treatment is delayed. Fistulas often have minimal mucosal perforations and cannot be seen easily. In addition, patients are often asymptomatic. Therefore, periodic, meticulous observation is essential when flapless implant placement is performed in the mandible using a mini-incision submerged technique (Fig 8-18). If a gumboil or fistula is confirmed, immediate excision of the soft tissue on top of the implants is recommended in order to expose the cover screw completely (Fig 8-19). Three weeks after stage I surgery, healing abutments are connected to the fixtures.

Prevention of spontaneous early exposure

Preventing spontaneous early exposure of submerged implants is clearly better than managing the problem after-

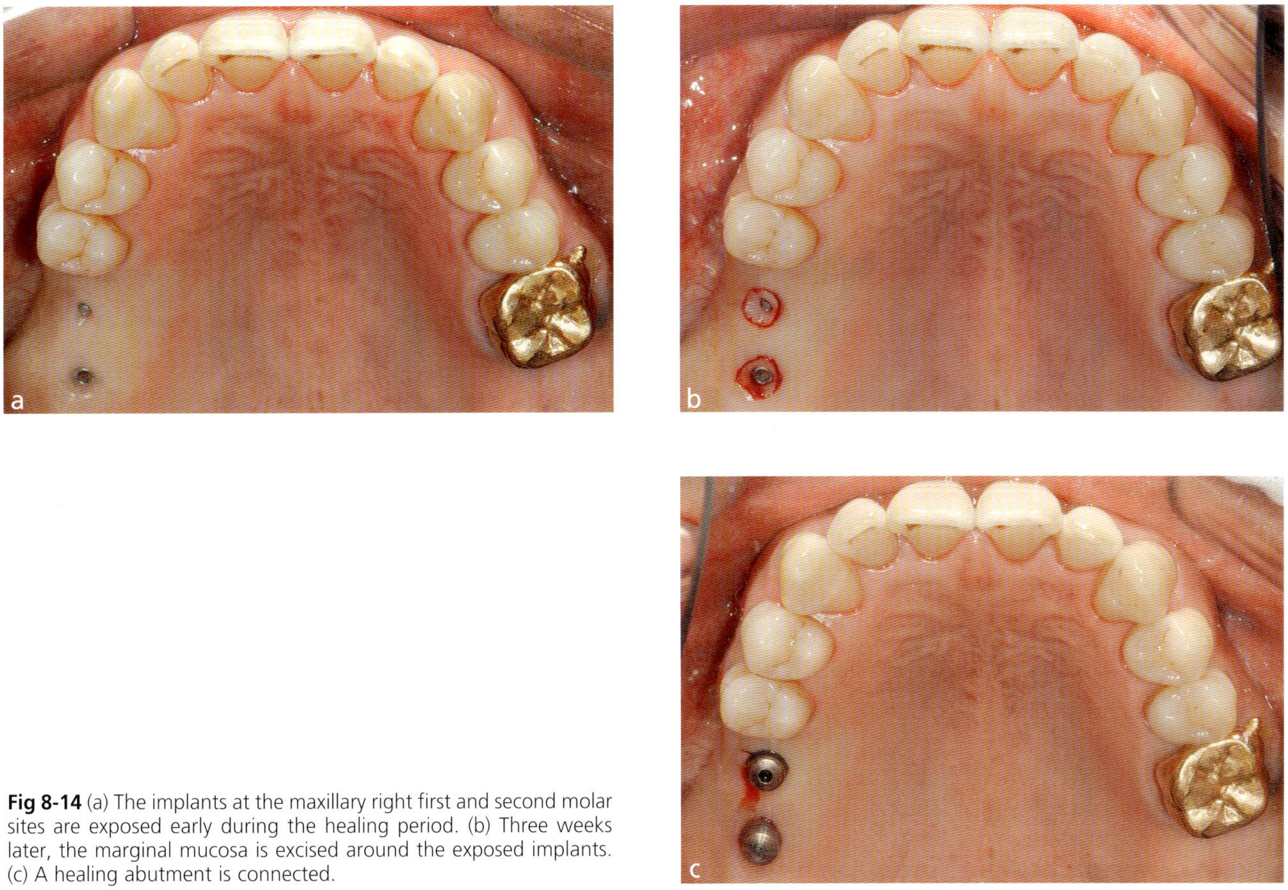

Fig 8-14 (a) The implants at the maxillary right first and second molar sites are exposed early during the healing period. (b) Three weeks later, the marginal mucosa is excised around the exposed implants. (c) A healing abutment is connected.

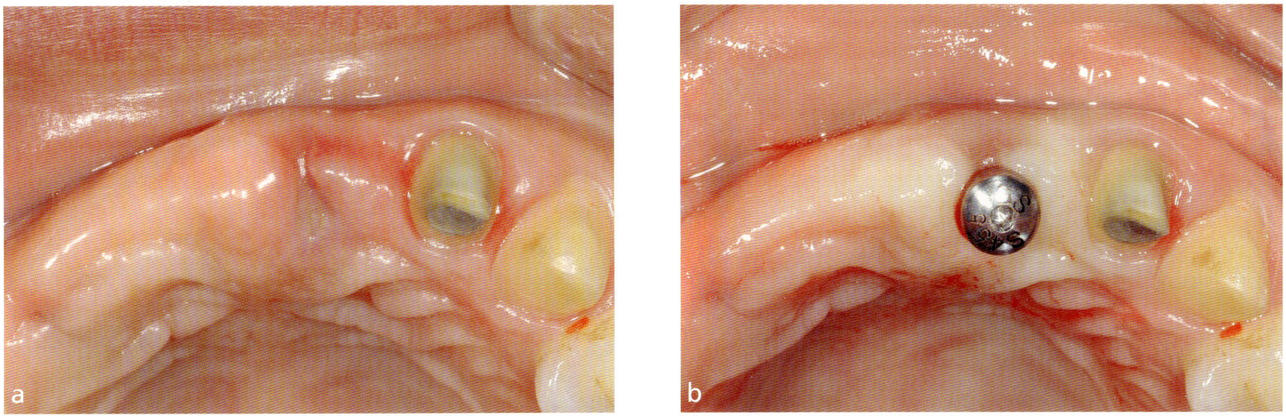

Fig 8-15 (a and b) The implant at the maxillary left lateral incisor site was exposed early during the healing period. Inflammation persisted at the exposed site and, therefore, replacement with healing abutments was performed.

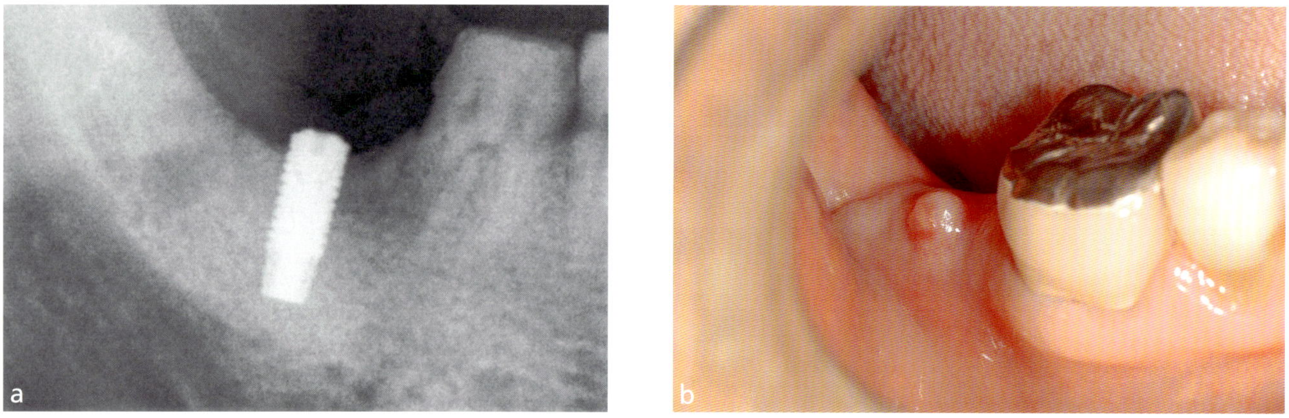

Fig 8-16 (a and b) A gumboil developed after mini-incision submerged implant placement at the mandibular right second molar site.

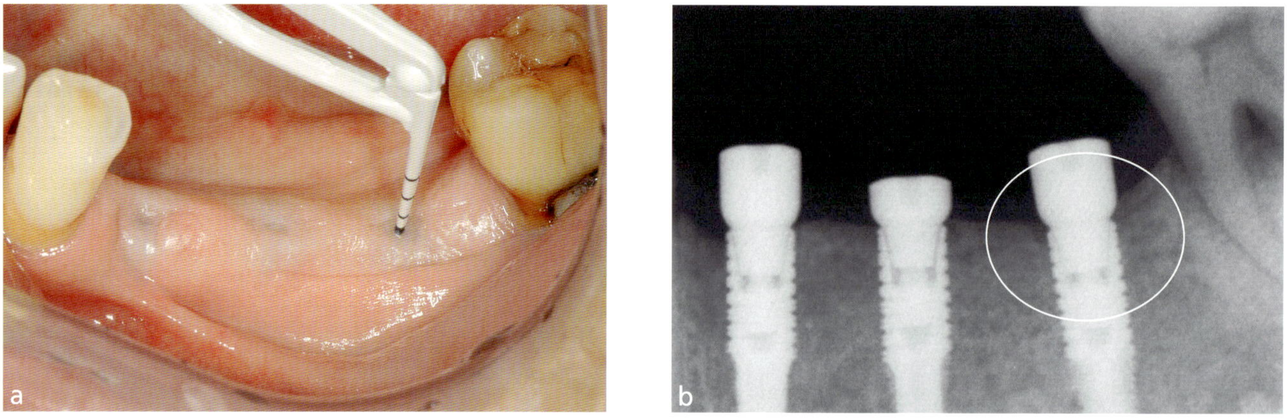

Fig 8-17 (a) Intraoral view showing a fistula with a periodontal probe. (b) Radiograph 3 months after mini-incision submerged implant placement showing bone loss around the implant.

wards. The best method is to use a one-stage approach when the implant is adequately stabilized. In other words, implants are exposed completely using a permucosal healing abutment at the time of implant placement if the bone can ensure primary stability of the implant. This approach eliminates spontaneous early exposure and allows the peri-implant soft tissue to be mature at the time of implant placement.

Another approach is to protect the mucosa during implant placement surgery. The methods that can be used include a reduced drill speed, use of flapless implant drills, use of an impactor, choice of an implant system with a short and smooth metal collar and short cover screws, and slightly deeper placement of implants.

Because postoperative smoking causes wound opening in the incision area,[20] it is advisable for the patient to stop smoking from at least 1 day before surgery until after the incision has healed.

Summary

When implants are submerged using a mini-incision technique, the implant may spontaneously become exposed early before stage II uncovering. Plaque accumulation on the exposed implant surface can lead to a soft tissue inflammatory lesion, which, if untreated, can progress and initiate peri-implantitis. It is prudent to wait 3 weeks when implants are exposed after a mini-incision submerged technique. After 3 weeks, it is advisable to manage the partially exposed implants with placement of healing abutments and meticulous plaque control. Immediate excision of the soft tissue on top of the implants is recommended if the occurrence of a gumboil or fistula is confirmed. More frequent follow-up visits will be needed to identify and manage implant exposure as soon as possible when flapless implant surgery is performed using a mini-incision submerged technique.

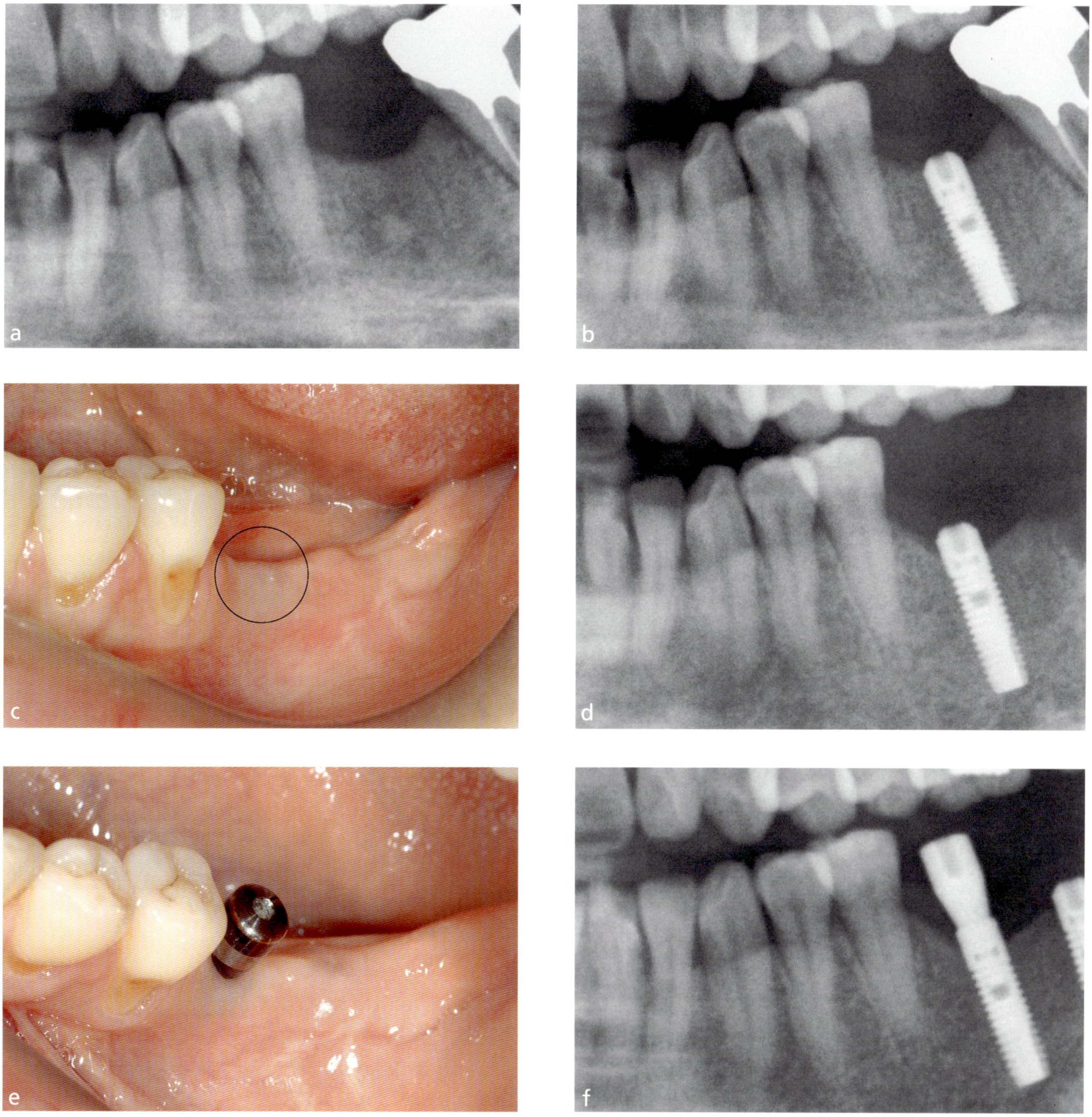

Fig 8-18 (a) Radiograph before implant placement and (b) immediately after mini-incision submerged implant placement. (c) Intraoral view of a fistula 3 months after implant placement. (d) Three months after implant placement, showing bone loss around the implant. (e) One month after the connection of a healing abutment. (f) One month after connecting the healing abutment, showing an absence of additional bone loss after connecting the healing abutment. Periodic, meticulous observation is necessary to check for the formation of a gumboil or fistula when flapless implant surgery is performed in the mandible using a mini-incision submerged technique.

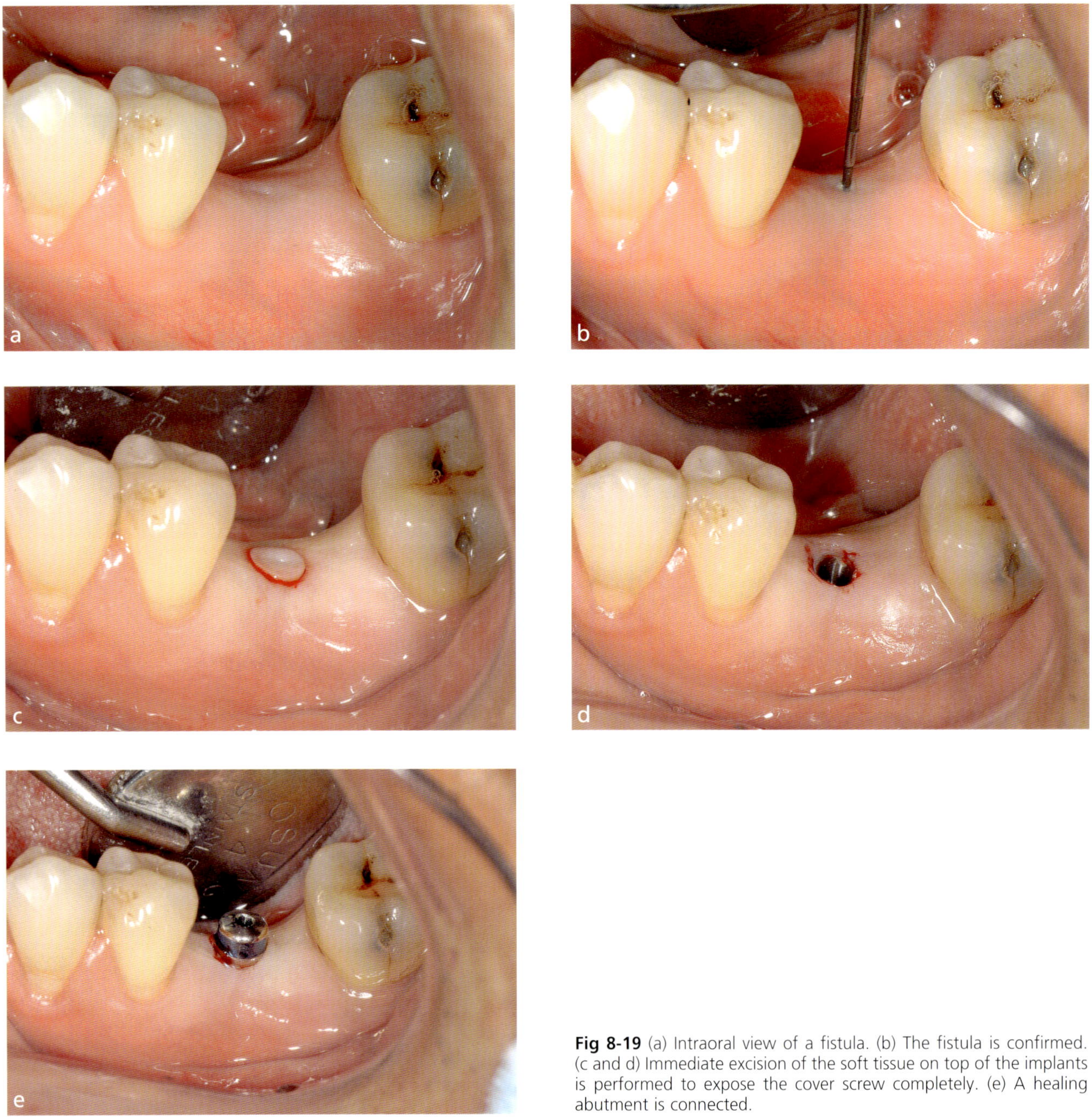

Fig 8-19 (a) Intraoral view of a fistula. (b) The fistula is confirmed. (c and d) Immediate excision of the soft tissue on top of the implants is performed to expose the cover screw completely. (e) A healing abutment is connected.

References

1. Kleinheinz J, Büchter A, Kruse-Lösler B, Weingart D, Joos U. Incision design in implant dentistry based on vascularization of the mucosa. Clin Oral Implants Res 2005;16:518–523.
2. Tal H, Moses O, Nemcovsky CE, Kozlovsky A. Spontaneous early exposure of submerged endosseous implants resulting in crestal bone loss: a clinical evaluation between stage I and stage II surgery. Int J Oral Maxillofac Implants 2001;16:514–521.
3. Toljanic JA, Banakis ML, Willes LAK, Graham L. Soft tissue exposure of endosseous implants between stage I and stage II surgery as a potential indicator of early crestal bone loss. Int J Oral Maxillofac Implants 1999;14:436–441.
4. Adell R, Lekholm U, Rockler B, Brånemark P-I. A 15-year study of osseointegrated implants in the treatment of edentulous jaws. J Oral Surg 1981;10:387–415.
5. Rosenquist B, Grenthe B. Immediate placement of implants into extraction sockets: implant survival. Int J Oral Maxillofac Implants 1996;11:205–209.
6. Tal H. Spontaneous early exposure of submerged implants: classification and clinical observations. J Periodontol 1999;70:213–219.
7. Tal H, Dayan D. Spontaneous early exposure of submerged implants: histopathology and histomorphometry of non-perforated mucosa covering submerged implants. J Periodontol 2000;71:1224–1230.
8. Tal H, Dayan D. Spontaneous early exposure of submerged implants. III: Histopathology of perforated mucosa covering submerged implants. J Periodontol 2000;71:1231–1235.
9. Barboza EP, Caula AL, Carvalho WR. Crestal bone loss around submerged and exposed unloaded dental implants: a radiographic and microbiological descriptive study. Implant Dent 2002;11:162–169.
10. Berglundh T, Lindhe J, Marinello C, Ericsson I, Liljenberg B. Soft tissue reaction to de-novo plaque formation on implants and teeth: an experimental study in the dog. Clin Oral Implants Res 1992;3:1–8.
11. Ericsson I, Berglundh T, Marinello CP, Liljenberg B, Lindhe J. Long-standing plaque and gingivitis at implants and teeth in the dog. Clin Oral Implants Res 1992;3:99–103.
12. Pontoriero R, Tonelli MP, Cornevale G, Mobelli A, Nyman S, Lang NP. Experimentally induced peri-implant mucositis: a clinical study in humans. Clin Oral Implants Res 1994;5:254–259.
13. Buser D, Weber HP, Donath K, Fiorellini JP, Paquette DW, Williams RC. Soft tissue reactions to non-submerged unloaded titanium implants in the beagle dog. J Periodontol 1992;63:226–236.
14. Abrahamsson I, Berglundh T, Wennström J, Lindhe J. The peri-implant hard and soft tissues at different implant systems. Clin Oral Implants Res 1996;7:212–219.
15. Abrahamsson I, Berglundh T, Lindhe J. The mucosal barrier following abutment disconnection: an experimental study in dogs. J Clin Periodontol 1997;24:568–572.
16. Cochran DL, Hermann JS, Schenk RK, Higginbottom FL, Buser D. Biologic width around titanium implants: a histometric analysis of the implanto-gingival junction around unloaded and loaded non-submerged implants in the canine mandible. J Periodontol 1997;68:186–198.
17. Yoo JH, Choi BH, Li J et al. Influence of premature exposure of implants on early crestal bone loss: an experimental study in dogs. Oral Surg Oral Med Oral Pathol Oral Radiol Endod 2008;105:702–706.
18. Jeong SM, Choi BH, Li J, Kim HS, Ko CY, Lee SH. Influence of abutment connections and plaque control on the initial healing of prematurely exposed implants: an experimental study in dogs. J Periodontol 2008;79:1070–1074.
19. Kim SG. Sinus Bone Grafts. Seoul: Daehan Publishing, 2004:181–211.
20. Jones JK, Triplett RG. The relationship of smoking to impaired intraoral wound healing. J Oral Maxillofac Surg 1992;50:237–239.

CHAPTER

9

Early Plaque Control Following Flapless Implant Surgery

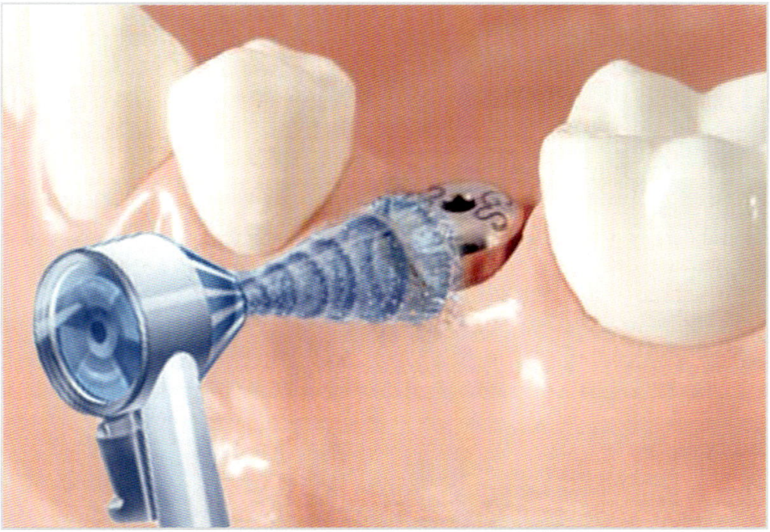

Key point

The value of plaque control after implant placement cannot be over-emphasized.

Overview

For a submerged implant, plaque control immediately after implant surgery is considered to be of little importance. In contrast, early plaque control is very important after a nonsubmerged implant installation because peri-implant wounds are vulnerable to bacterial infections in the first 2 weeks before a biological seal forms (Fig 9-1). One way of limiting bacterial invasion into the deeper layers of the surrounding tissue is to remove plaque in the postoperative period. This chapter addresses a method for early plaque control and its effect on the initial healing of nonsubmerged implants.

Influence of early plaque control on initial healing

When a permucosal healing abutment is placed into the implant body at the time of implant insertion or during the uncovering procedure, a wound repair process consisting of inflammatory, proliferative, and remodeling phases occurs in the peri-implant wound. If bacterial plaque accumulates at the wound site, each of the healing phases takes considerably longer (particularly the inflammatory and proliferative stages) and there is much more granulation tissue formation. As a result the scar is more extensive. The bacteria can cause bone loss around the implants.[1–3] Early plaque control is, therefore, crucial.

The present authors examined the effect of early plaque control on the initial healing of nonsubmerged implants in the canine mandible. Bilateral, edentulated, flat alveolar ridges were created in the mandibles of 10 mongrel dogs. After 3 months of healing, two implants were placed on each side of the mandible employing a common, one-stage surgical protocol. In five dogs, meticulous plaque control was carried out immediately after surgery. Plaque was allowed to accumulate in the other five dogs. Clinical examinations after a 2-month period showed that in the dogs with plaque control the soft tissue around the implants appeared free of inflammation. In the other five dogs, the gingiva around the implants was red and edematous, and bled when probed gently (Fig 9-2). The group with plaque control had greater vertical alveolar ridge height (9.7 ± 0.5 mm) than the others (7.4 ± 0.7 mm; $P < .05$). This suggests that early plaque control plays a key role in the initial healing, consistent with previously published reports.[4–7]

Methods of early plaque control

Cleaning implants immediately after flap surgery can be difficult because a long sutured wound in the incision area is vulnerable to mechanical irritation. After flapless surgery, the implant surface is in close contact with the surrounding mucosa without sutures around a permucosal healing abutment, which allows effective cleaning immediately after implant placement. The inflammatory phase has been observed at the wound approximately 1–6 days after implant surgery.[8] During this period, implants should be cleaned without irritating the wounds.

Chlorhexidine oral rinse

Chlorhexidine gluconate is a potent antibacterial agent that causes bacterial cell lysis by binding to bacterial cell membranes (Fig 9-3). A 30-second rinse with a 0.12% concentrate of chlorhexidine can totally eliminate bacteria in the oral cavity for up to 5 hours.[9,10] However, this antibac-

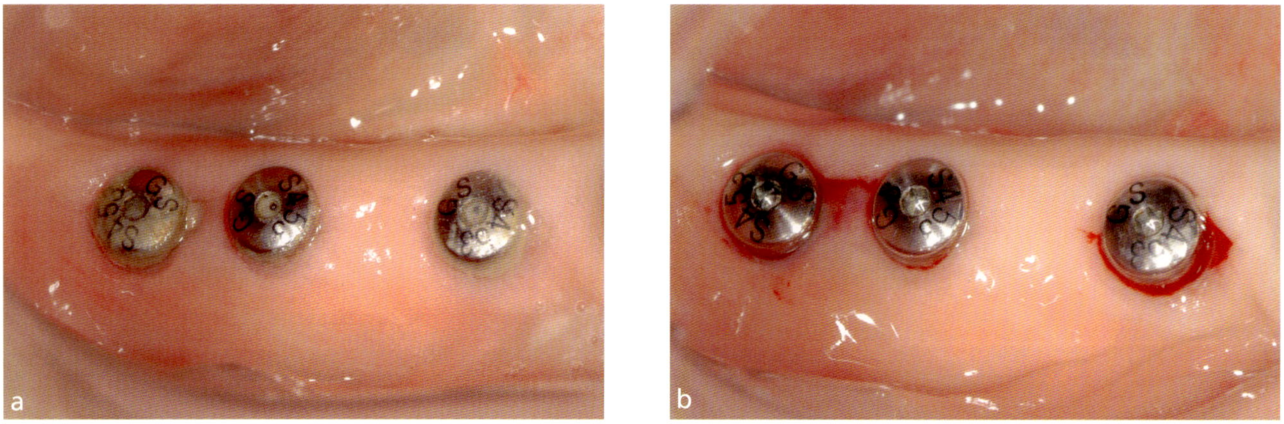

Fig 9-1 (a and b) The gum around the implants bleeds easily and shows inflammation in the marginal portion of the peri-implant mucosa when implants are not cleaned for early plaque control.

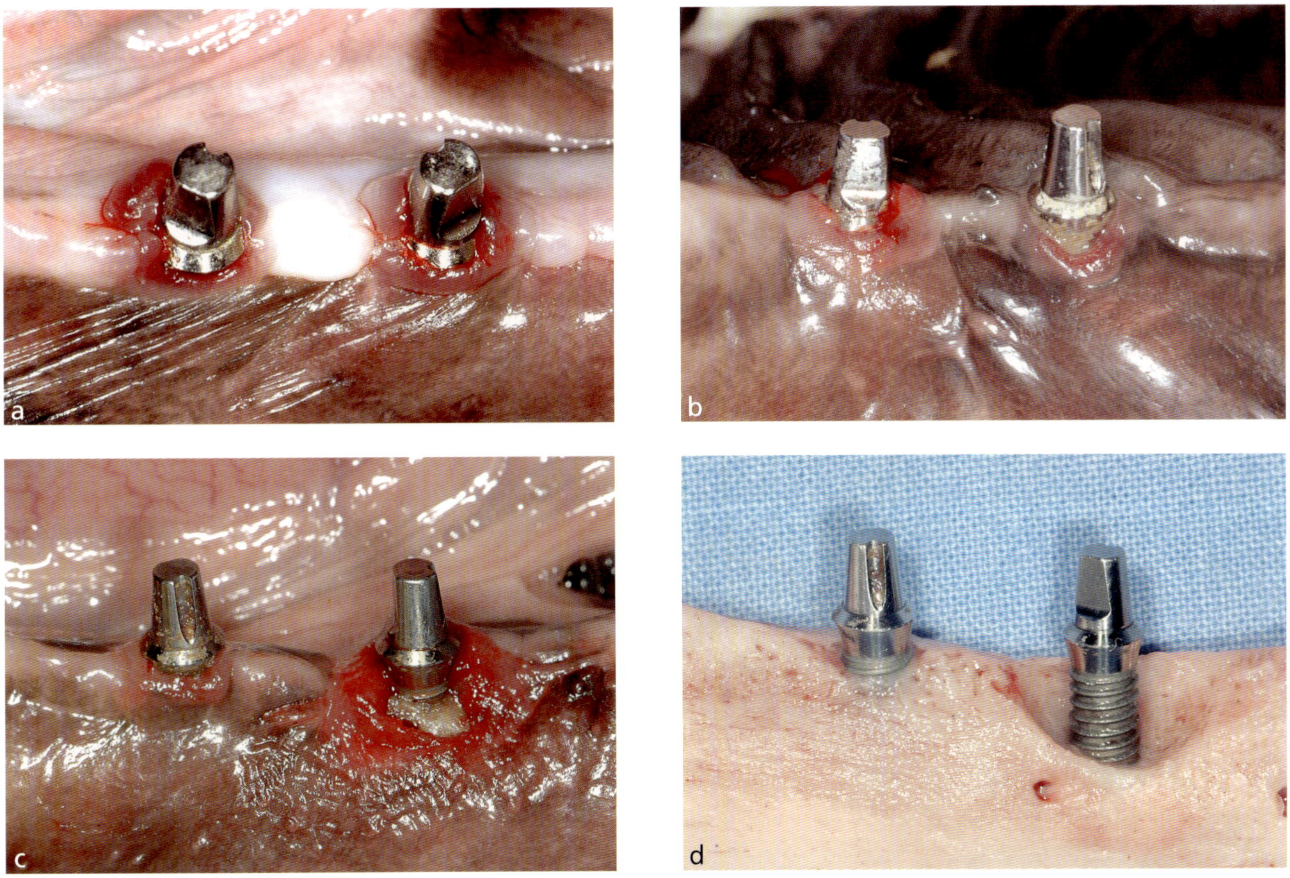

Fig 9-2 (a and b) Plaque was allowed to accumulate on implants after flapless implant placement in a canine model. (c and d) Clinical examinations after a 2-month healing period showed that the gingiva around implants was red and edematous, with peri-implant bone loss.

terial mouth wash fails to remove plaque deposited on the permucosal healing abutment surface (Figs 9-4 and 9-5). Plaque is the primary causative factor of periodontal disease processes. When a permucosal healing abutment is placed into the implant body at the time of implant insertion, or during the uncovering procedure, a chlorhexidine oral rinse should be used as an adjuvant to removing plaque accumulation.

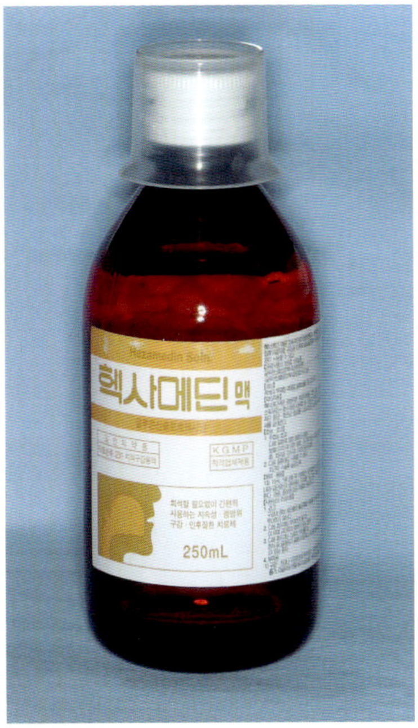

Fig 9-3 A 0.12% solution of chlorhexidine.

Toothbrush

A toothbrush is effective in removing plaque: a 20-second brushing guarantees 85% plaque removal from the implant surface (Figs 9-6 and 9-7). Brushing is more effective on the buccal and lingual sides of the implants than on the proximal side. During the initial phase after implant placement, the adherence and tenacity of plaque around the implants is usually low. Therefore, a toothbrush can easily remove plaque from the smooth surface of titanium.

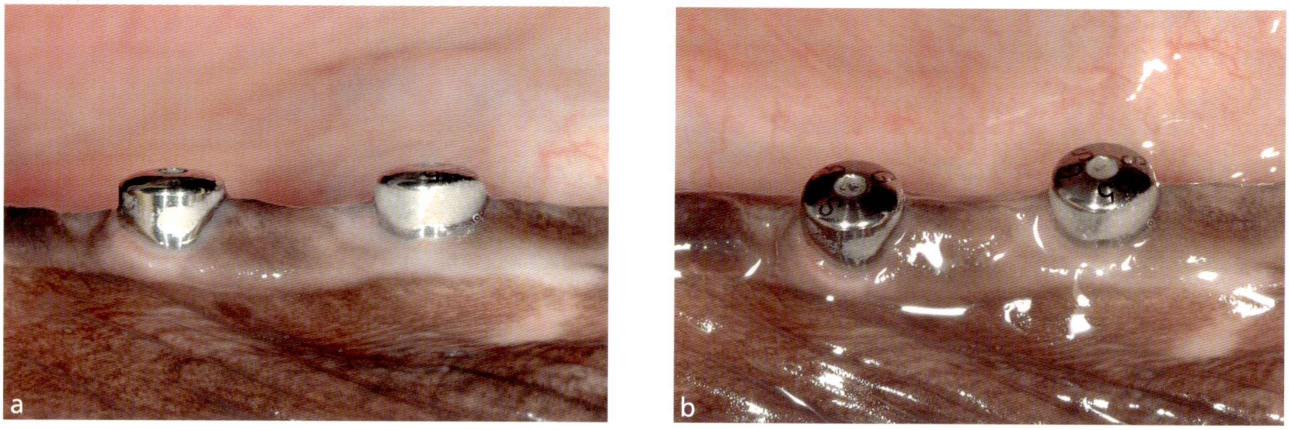

Fig 9-4 (a and b) Intraoral views of implants after local irrigation with chlorhexidine for 1 week. Note that plaque builds up on the surface of the implants.

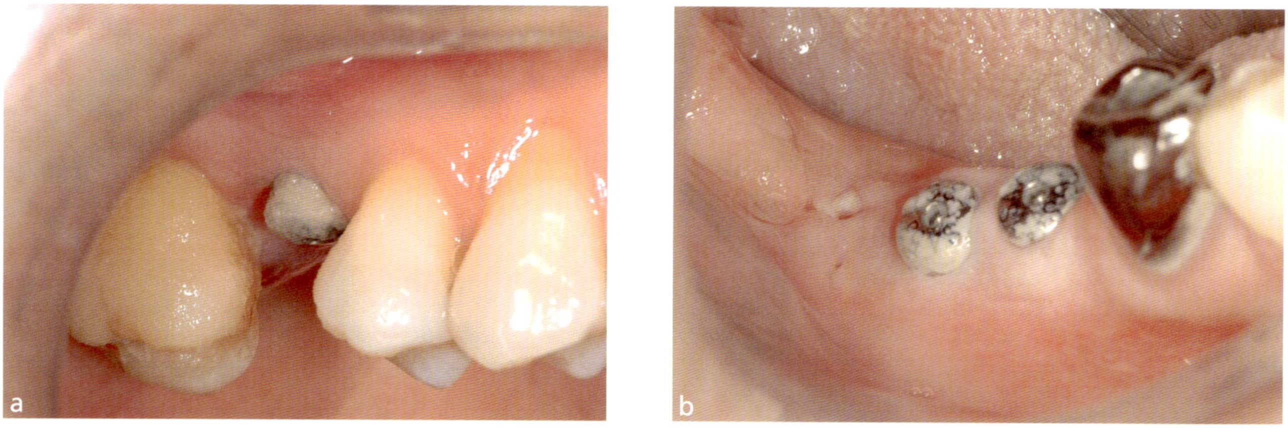

Fig 9-5 (a and b) Intraoral views of implants after mouth washing with chlorhexidine for 2 weeks. The antibacterial mouthwash fails to remove plaque deposited on the permucosal healing abutment surface.

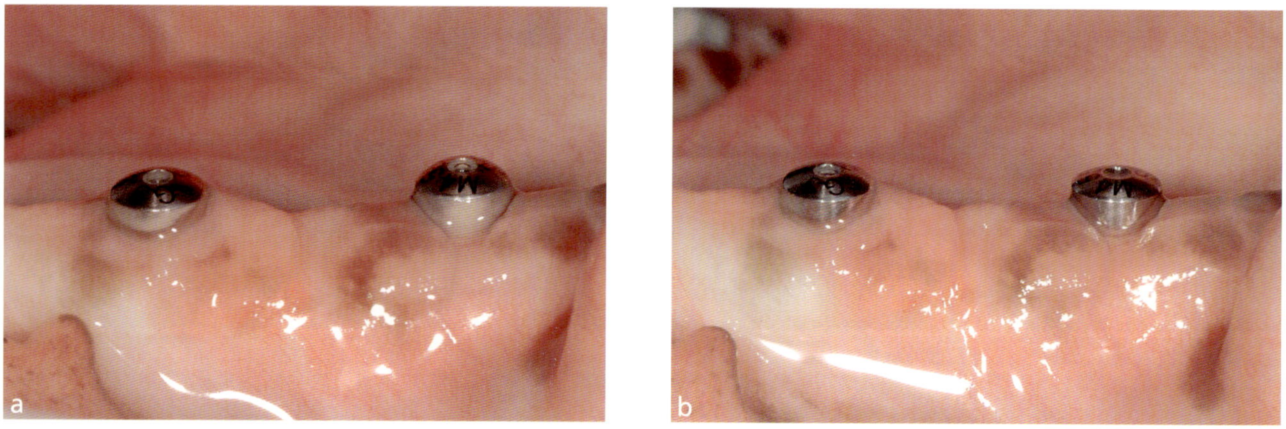

Fig 9-6 Intraoral views of implants (a) before and (b) after the use of a toothbrush. This is an effective means of removing plaque.

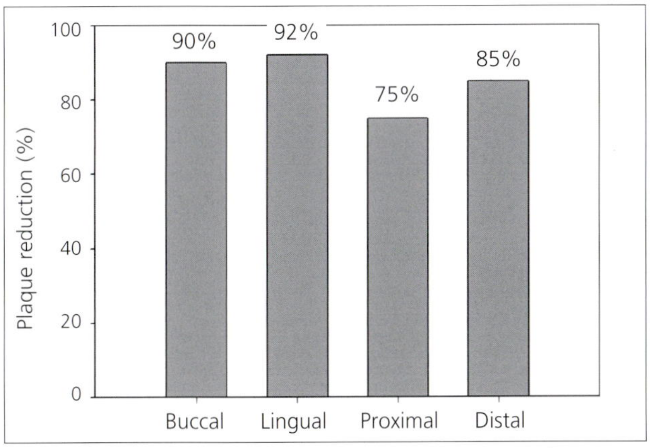

Fig 9-7 Percentage of plaque reduction with a toothbrush. A 20-second use guarantees 85% plaque removal. It is more effective on the buccal and lingual sides than on the proximal side of the implants.

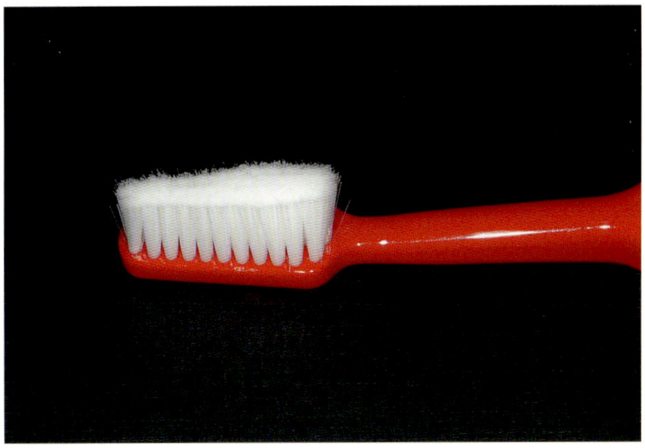

Fig 9-8 A soft toothbrush (TePe Special Care).

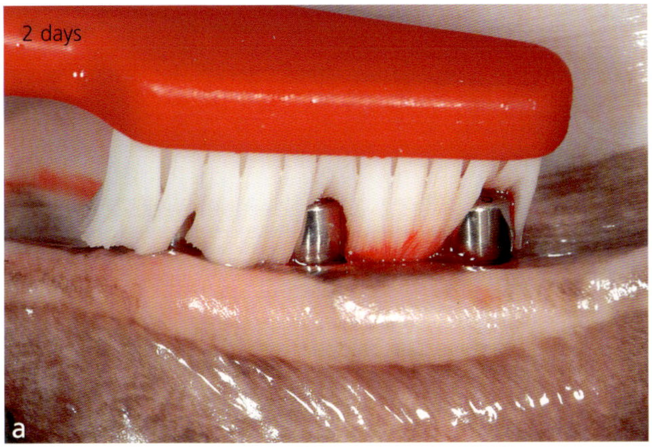

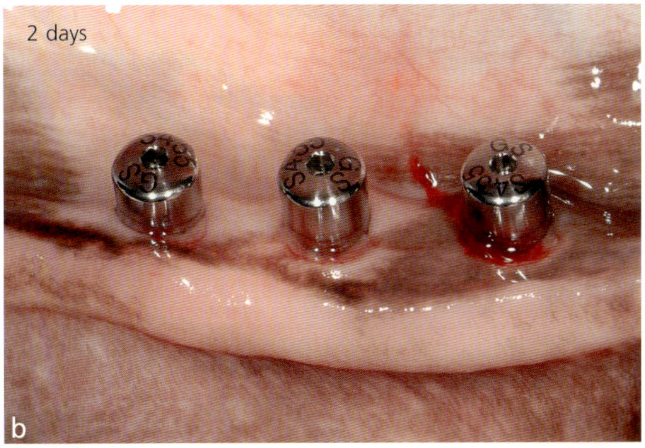

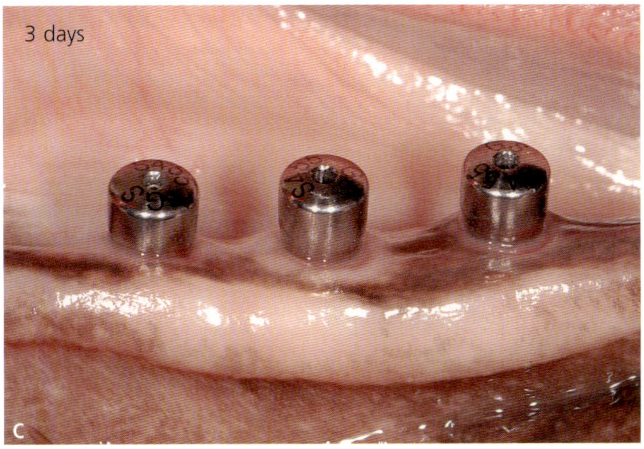

Fig 9-9 (a–c) Canine gum after using a soft toothbrush. The gum bleeds on the second day but does not bleed on the third day after flapless implant placement.

A soft brush should be used during the early phase to avoid irritating the wounds (Fig 9-8). The gum will bleed with a soft toothbrush on the second day but not on the third day after implant placement (Fig 9-9).

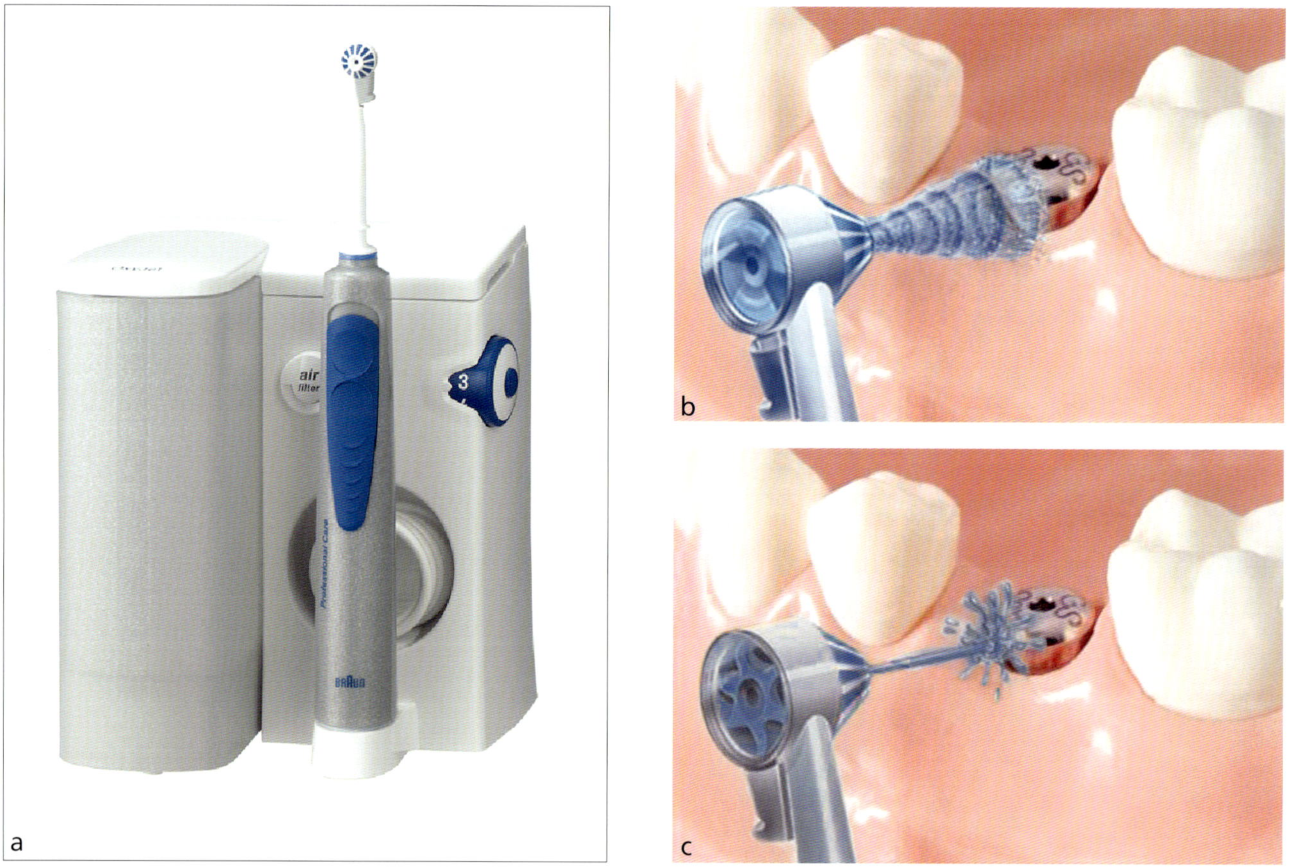

Fig 9-10 (a) The OxyJet system, (b) rotation spray and (c) concentrated spray.

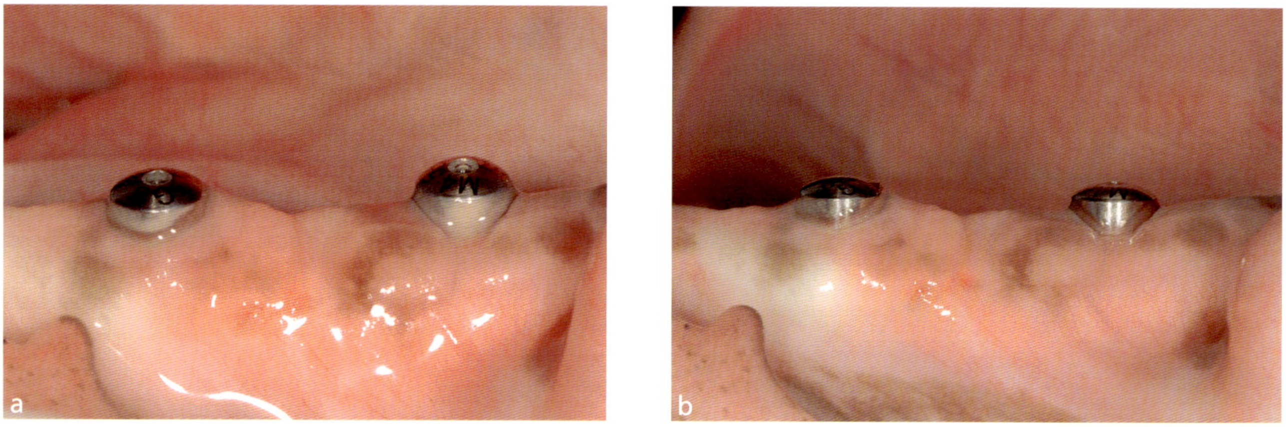

Fig 9-11 Intraoral views of implants (a) before and (b) after use of an OxyJet.

Oral irrigator

Since the development of Waterpik® in the 1960s, several oral irrigators have been produced by various manufacturers – including OxyJet (Oral B, Germany), Water Jet (Conair, USA), Oral Irrigator (Panasonic, Japan), and AquaJet (Self Dr. Medical Instrument Co., South Korea). Oral irrigators use strong hydraulic pressure to remove plaque and employ various spray styles: concentrated, rotation, and pulse. Approximately 60% of plaque is cleared from the implant surface after a 20-second use of the OxyJet (Figs 9-10 to 9-12). Oral irrigators have been

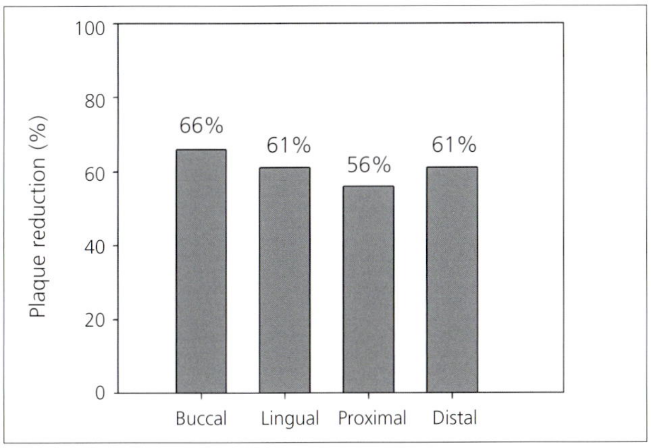

Fig 9-12 Percentage plaque reduction with an OxyJet. Approximately 61% of plaque is cleared from the implant surface after a 20-second use.

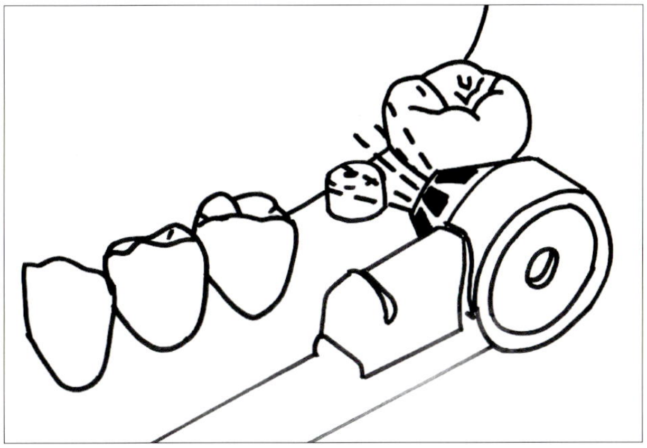

Fig 9-13 The oral irrigator should be used during the early phase with the lowest setting and the irrigation flow direction to prevent damage to the peri-implant wounds by hydraulic pressure.

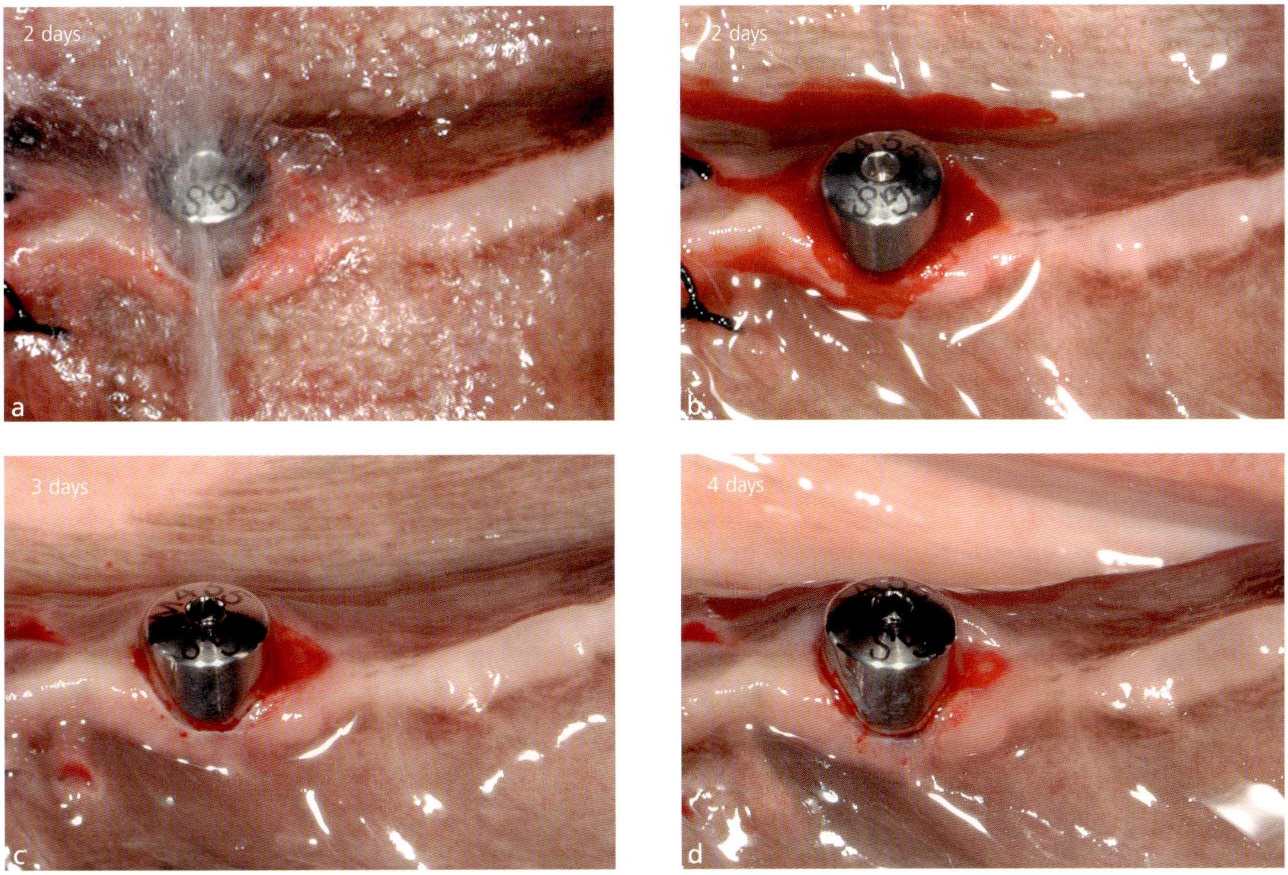

Fig 9-14 (a–d) Intraoral views showing that the gums bleed when using an oral irrigator on the second, third, and fourth days after flapless implant placement. The irrigator should be used from the sixth day to prevent wound damage.

found to reduce plaque less than toothbrushing. Therefore, the use of an oral irrigator combined with toothbrushing is recommended.

An oral irrigator can be used during the early phase with the lowest setting and irrigation flow direction, to prevent damage to the peri-implant wounds by hydraulic pressure (Fig 9-13). The gum bleeds with the oral irrigator during the first few days but not on the sixth day (Fig 9-14). If an oral irrigator is used immediately after flapless implant placement, it can influence the formation of the attachment structures of peri-implant soft tissues and lead to a soft tissue inflammatory lesion (Fig 9-15).

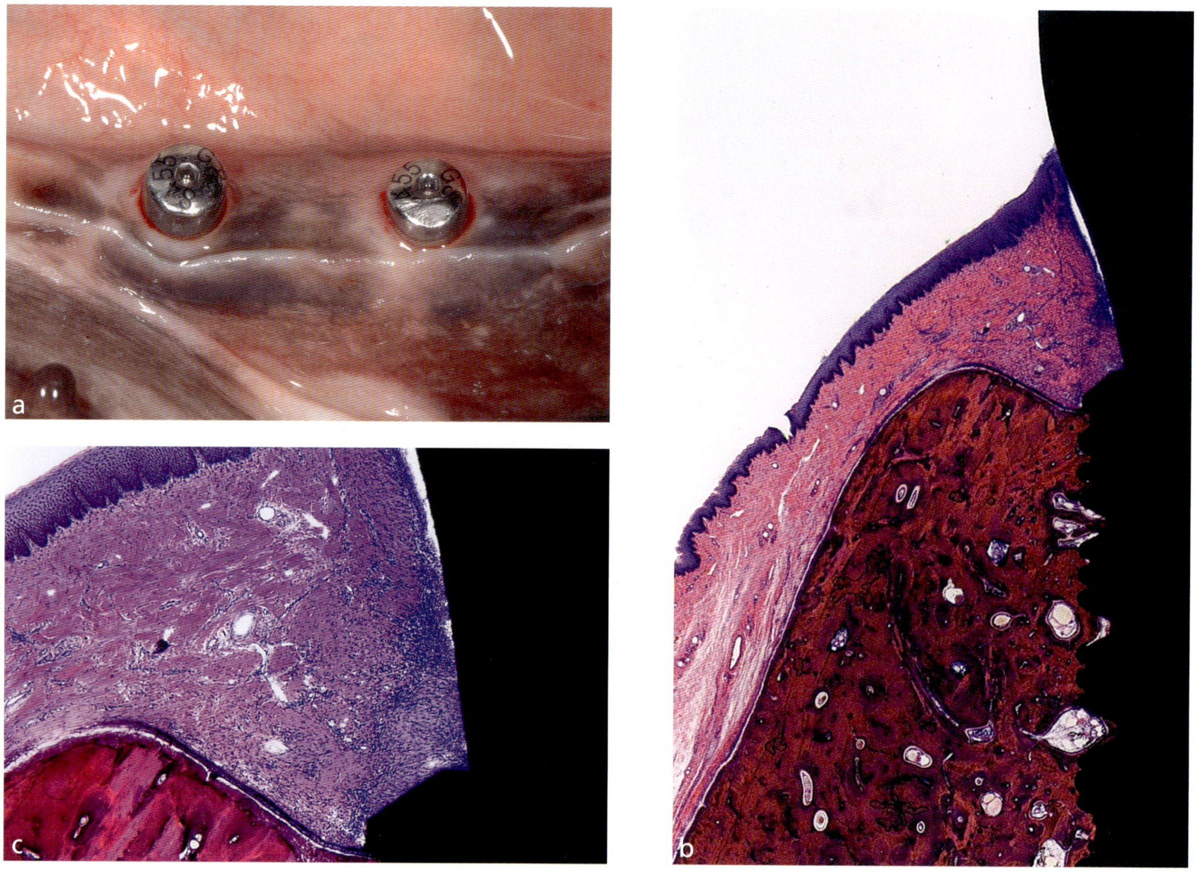

Fig 9-15 Oral irrigators were used immediately after flapless implant placement in a canine model. (a) Three months after implant placement. (b and c) Histological studies of the implants. The attachment structures of peri-implant soft tissues were not well formed and a soft tissue inflammatory lesion was observed around the implant.

Toothbrush and oral irrigator

The use of a toothbrush combined with an oral irrigator can remove more plaque than brushing alone (Fig 9-16).[11,12] The plaque remaining in areas not accessible to the brush can be removed by the irrigator. Using the toothbrush first is more effective than using the irrigator first (Figs 9-17 and 9-18). Using an oral irrigator after toothbrushing ensures >95% plaque reduction.

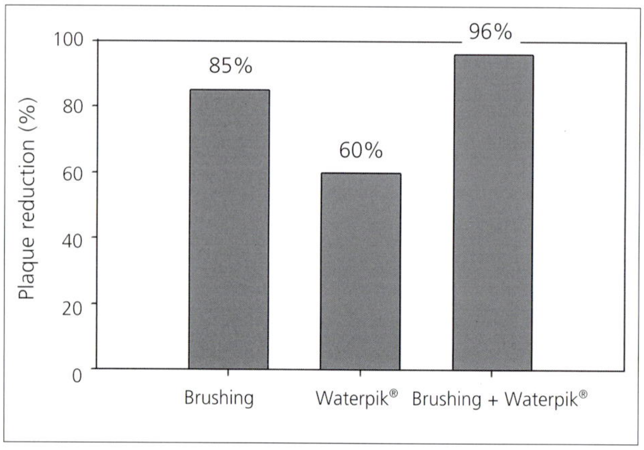

Fig 9-16 The use of a toothbrush, combined with oral irrigation, can reduce plaque better than brushing alone.

Suggested regimen

The following plaque control steps are suggested when a permucosal healing abutment is placed into the implant body at the time of implant insertion using a flapless procedure.

- For the first 2 days after implant placement, the implant surfaces should be cleaned using a 0.12% chlorhexidine rinse followed by a microbrush soaked in 0.12% chlorhexidine (Fig 9-19).
- From the third day, the implant surfaces should be cleaned using a sequence of oral rinse with 0.12% chlorhexidine, a microbrush soaked in 0.12% chlorhexidine, and a soft toothbrush soaked in 0.12% chlorhexidine (Fig 9-20).
- From the sixth day, surfaces should be cleaned using the following four methods in sequence (Fig 9-21): an oral

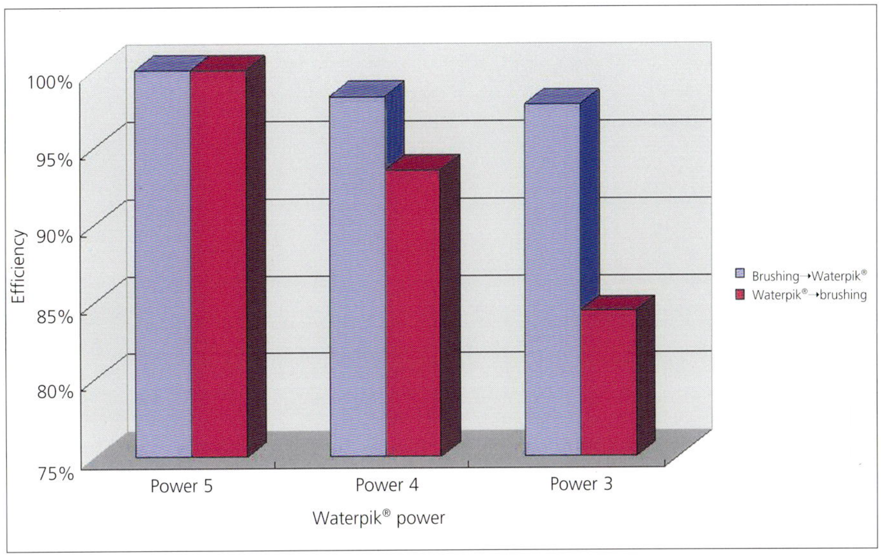

Fig 9-17 Using a toothbrush first is more effective than using an oral irrigator first.

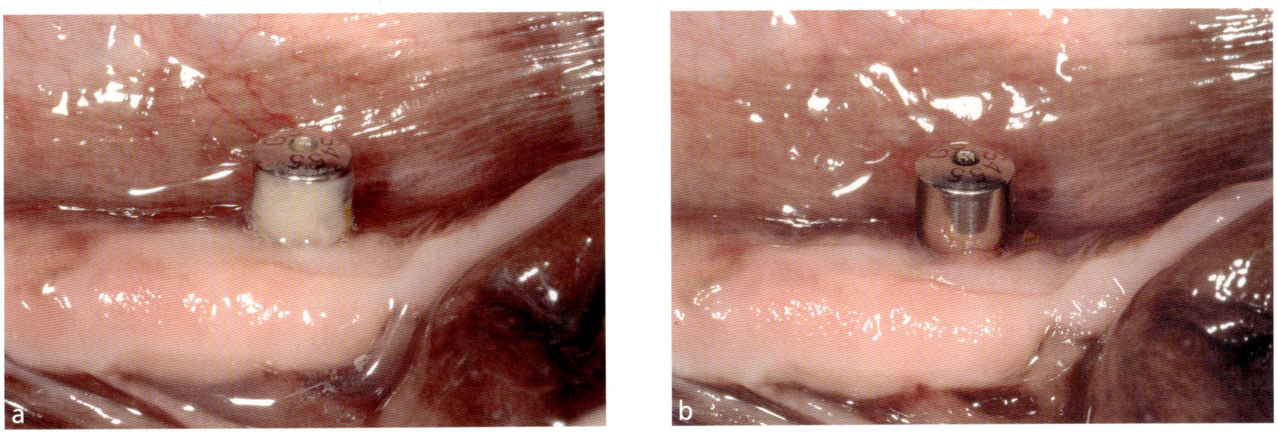

Fig 9-18 Intraoral views (a) before and (b) after the use of a toothbrush combined with oral irrigation.

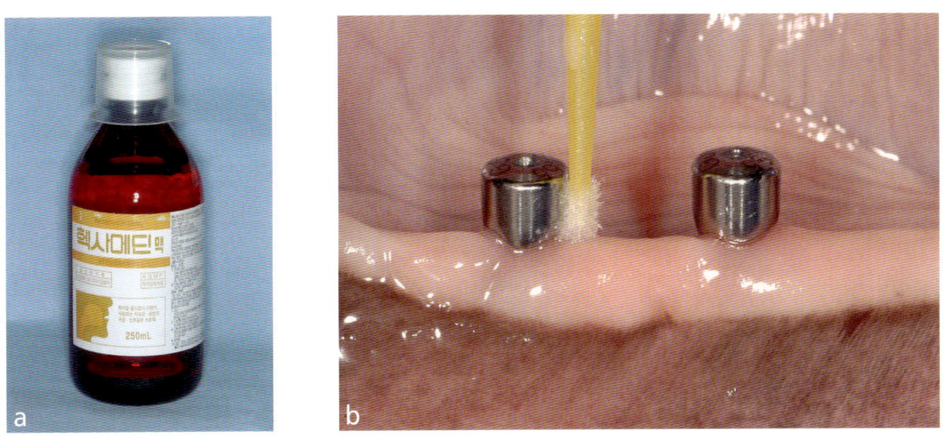

Fig 9-19 For the first two days after flapless implant placement, implant surfaces should be cleaned using two methods in sequence: an oral rinse with 0.12% chlorhexidine and a microbrush soaked in 0.12% chlorhexidine.

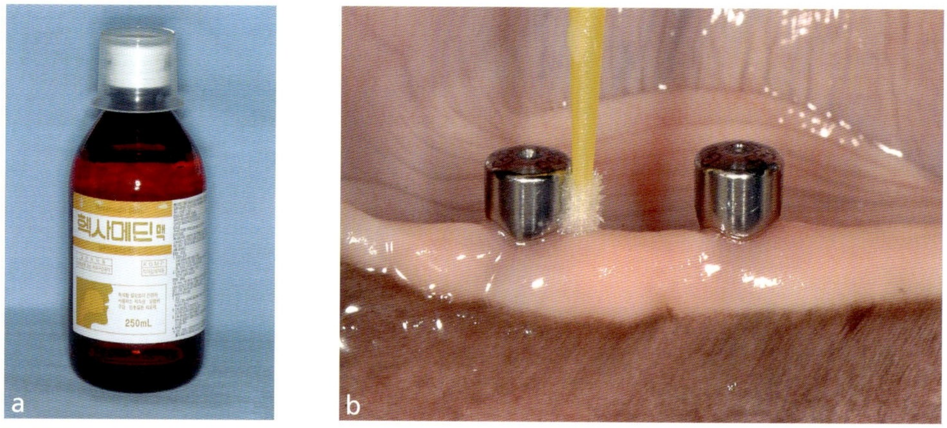

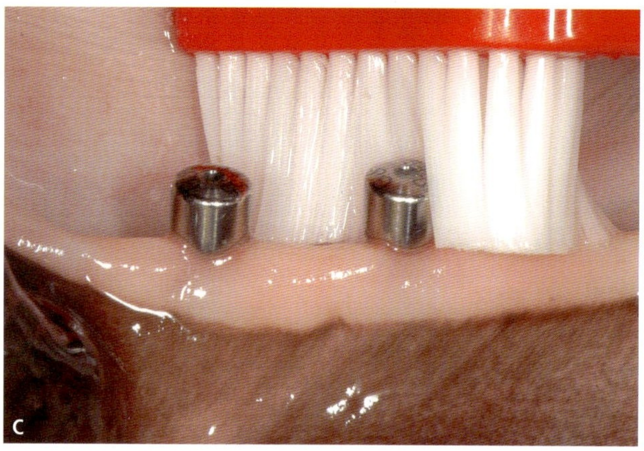

Fig 9-20 From the third day, the implant surfaces should be cleaned using a sequence of three methods: an oral rinse with 0.12% chlorhexidine, a microbrush soaked in 0.12% chlorhexidine, and a soft toothbrush soaked in 0.12% chlorhexidine.

Fig 9-21 *(bottom)* From the sixth day, implant surfaces should be cleaned in sequence using the following four methods: an oral rinse with 0.12% chlorhexidine, a microbrush soaked in 0.12% chlorhexidine, a soft toothbrush soaked in 0.12% chlorhexidine, and an oral irrigator on the lowest setting.

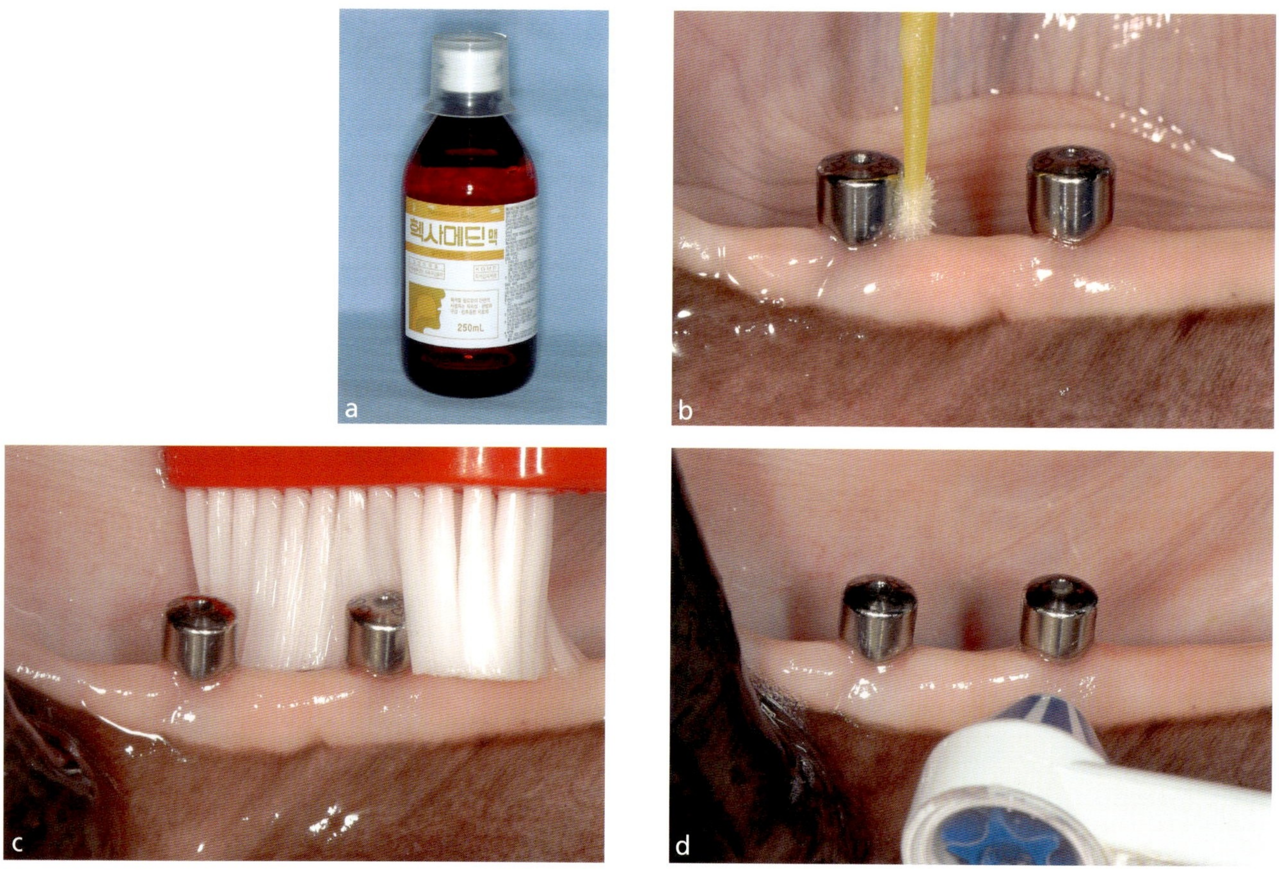

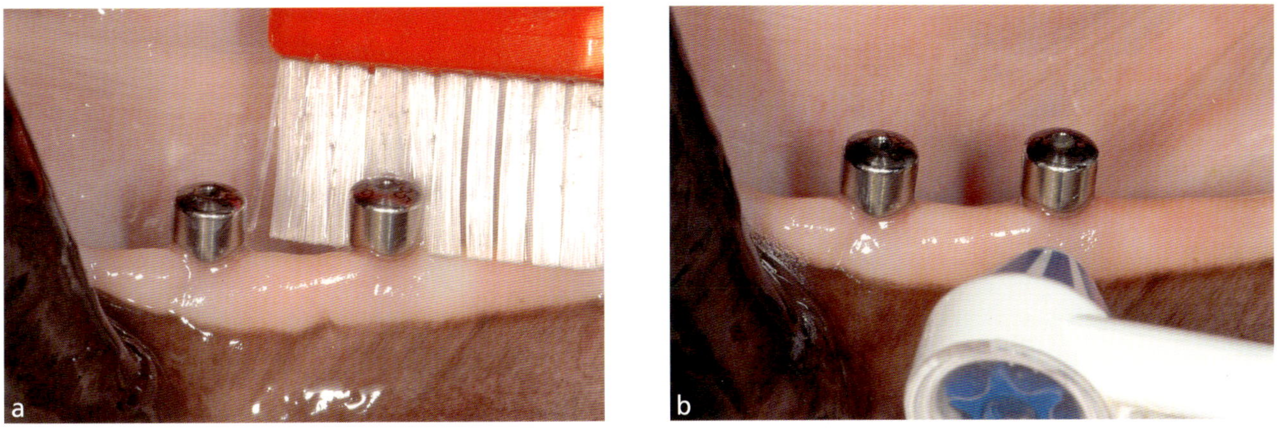

Fig 9-22 (a and b) From the 15th day, the implants should be cleaned with a normal toothbrush and an oral irrigator on higher settings.

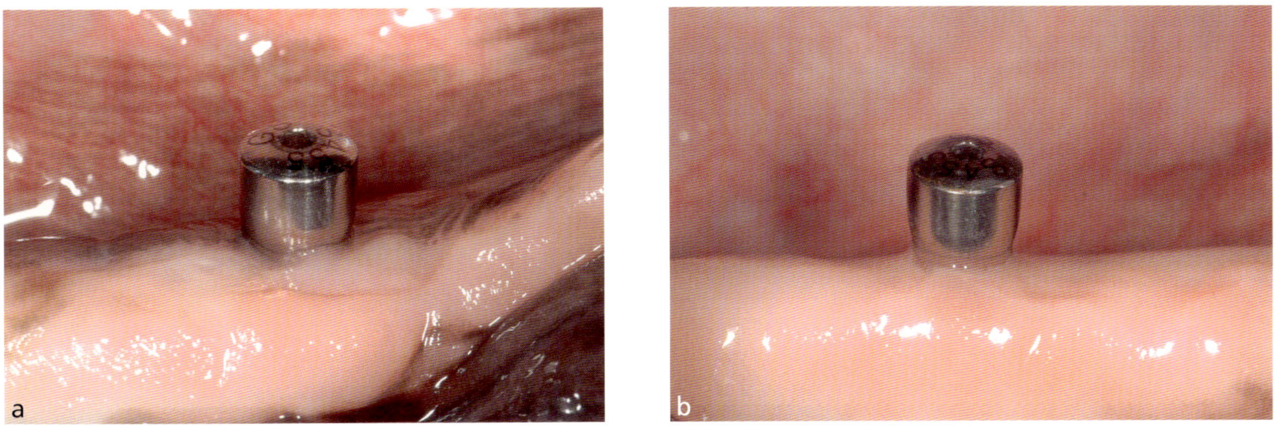

Fig 9-23 Implants that have been cleaned using the suggested methods for 3 months, showing healthy peri-implant mucosa.

rinse with 0.12% chlorhexidine, a microbrush soaked in 0.12% chlorhexidine, a soft toothbrush soaked in 0.12% chlorhexidine, and an oral irrigator (Waterpik®) on the lowest setting.

- From the 15th day, the implants should be cleaned with a normal toothbrush and an oral irrigator (Waterpik®) on higher settings (Figs 9-22 and 9-23).

Results of early plaque control on peri-implant tissues

An animal study was carried out to determine the influence of early, meticulous plaque control on the healing of nonsubmerged implants. Bilateral, edentulated, flat alveolar ridges were created in the mandible of six mongrel dogs. After a 3-month period, two implants were placed on each side using the flapless procedure. After placing the fixture, a permucosal healing abutment was connected to the fixture so that the coronal portion of the abutment remained exposed to the oral cavity (Fig 9-24). The implants on each side were assigned randomly to one of two plaque control programs.

- For the early plaque control group, the regimen was initiated immediately on placing the implant. On the first 2 days the implant surfaces were cleaned using the following in sequence: local irrigation with 0.12% chlorhexidine and a microbrush soaked in 0.12% chlorhexidine. From the third day, the implant surfaces were cleaned using a triple sequence: local irrigation with 0.12% chlorhexidine, a microbrush soaked in 0.12% chlorhexidine, followed by a soft toothbrush soaked in 0.12% chlorhexidine. From the sixth day, the implants were cleaned using a four-stage sequence that involved the addition of an oral irrigator (Waterpik®). From the 15th day, the implants were cleaned with a normal toothbrush and a Waterpik®.
- For the late control group, local irrigation with 0.12% chlorhexidine was performed for the first 2 weeks after implant placement. From the 15th day, the implants were cleaned with a normal toothbrush and a Waterpik®.

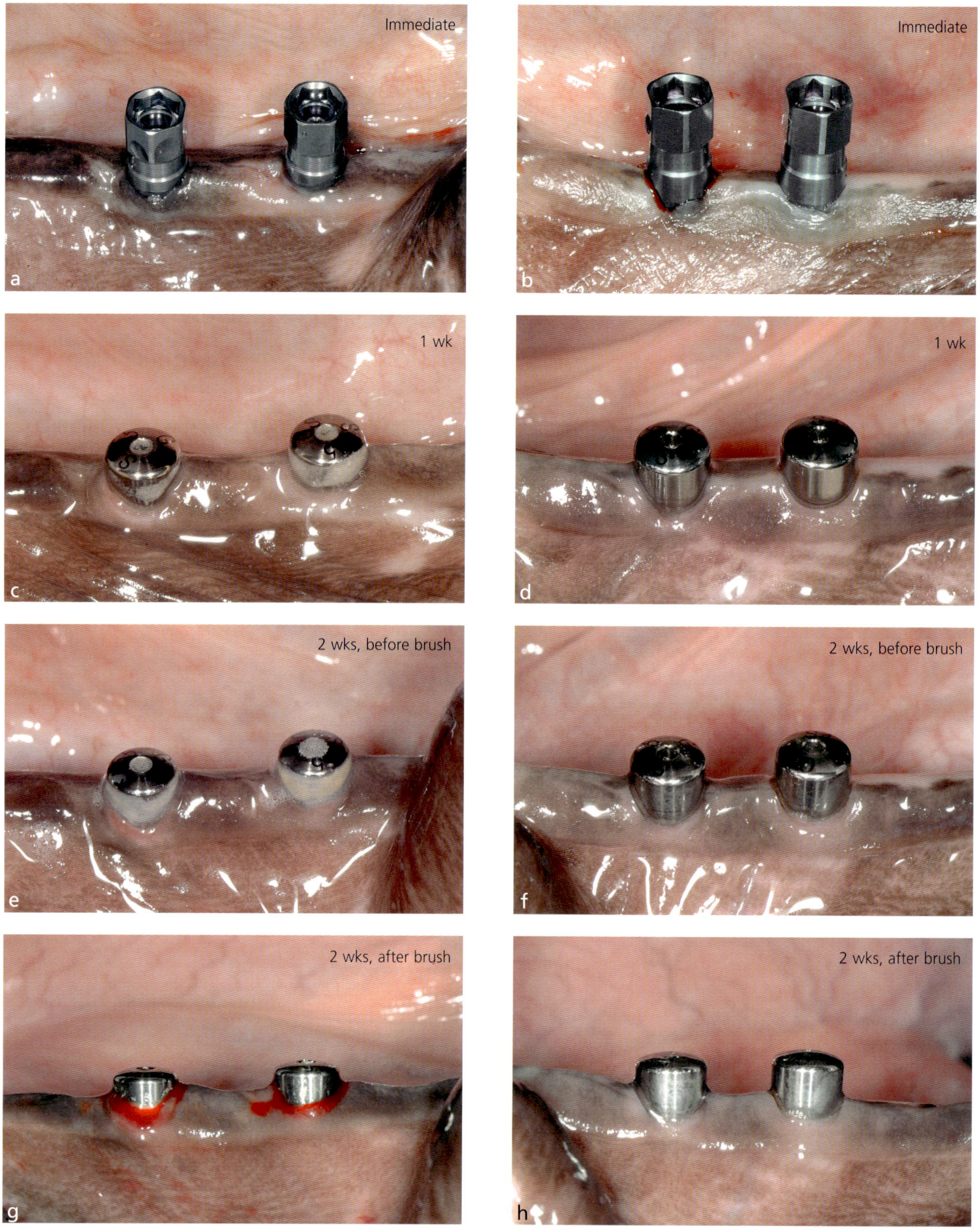

Fig 9-24 Influence of early, meticulous plaque control on the healing of nonsubmerged implants. In six mongrel dogs, the implants on the right side of the mandible (a, c, e, g) were cleaned with local irrigation using 0.12% chlorhexidine for the first 2 weeks after flapless implant placement. The implants on the left side of the mandible (b, d, f, h) were cleaned with the suggested methods immediately after flapless implant placement. Clinical examination performed at 2 weeks showed that the implants cleaned with a chlorhexidine irrigation alone bled with a normal toothbrush. However, the implants cleaned with a microbrush, a soft brush, and Waterpik® did not bleed with a normal toothbrush at 2 weeks.

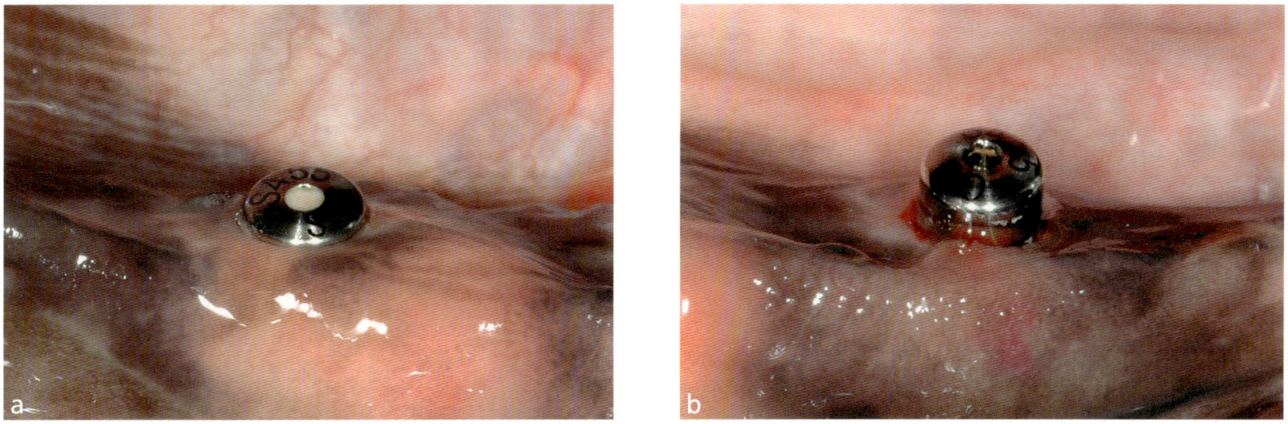

Fig 9-25 (a and b) Clinical features in the late plaque control group 8 weeks after flapless implant placement. Inflammatory lesions were observed in the marginal portion of the peri-implant mucosa.

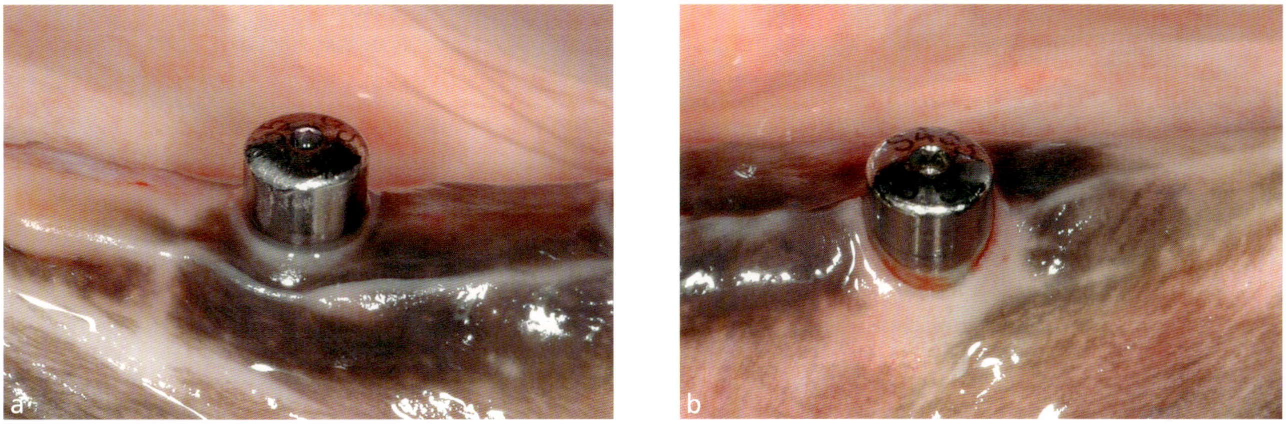

Fig 9-26 The Gingival Index and bleeding on probing were all significantly lower in the implants in the early plaque control group (a) than in the late plaque control group (b).

Clinical examinations performed at 2 weeks revealed gross amounts of plaque on the implants cleaned with chlorhexidine irrigation alone, and the peri-implant mucosa surrounding the implants bled when brushed with a normal toothbrush. However, no plaque accumulation was observed on the implants that had been cleaned with a microbrush, a soft brush, and Waterpik®, and the soft tissue around the implants showed no signs of inflammation nor did they bleed when brushed with a normal toothbrush at 2 weeks. From the 15th day (when a regimen including daily cleaning of the implants with a normal brush and a Waterpik® was initiated in both groups), all implant surfaces were free of visible plaque *in both groups*. However, at 8 weeks, inflammatory lesions in the marginal portion of the peri-implant mucosa were observed in the late control group, whereas there were no visible signs of inflammation around the peri-implant mucosa in the early control group (Figs 9-25 and 9-26). Clinical examinations showed that the Gingival Index, bleeding on probing, and probing depth were all significantly higher in the late control group than in the early control group (Fig 9-27; Table 9-1). Approximately 0.7 mm of crestal bone was lost in the late control group, whereas only 0.2 mm was lost in the early control group (Fig 9-28).

Table 9-1 Gingival Index, bleeding upon probing, and probing depth in the early and late plaque control groups.

	Early plaque control group	Late plaque control group
Gingival Index	0	1.1
Probing depth (mm)	1.3	1.6
Bleeding Index	0	0.8
Marginal bone loss	0.2	0.7

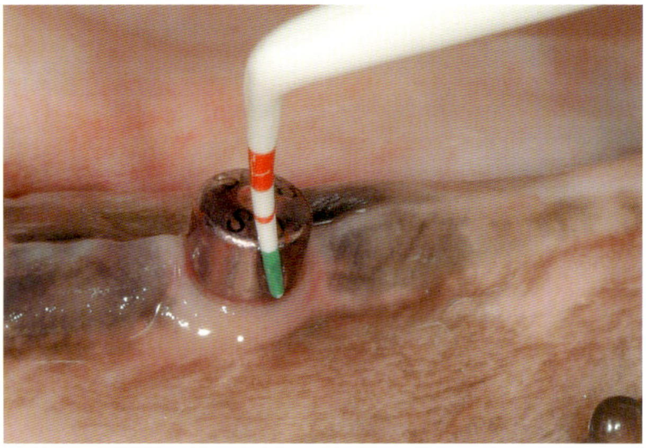

Fig 9-27 The probing depth was significantly greater in the implants in the late plaque control group than in those in the early plaque control group.

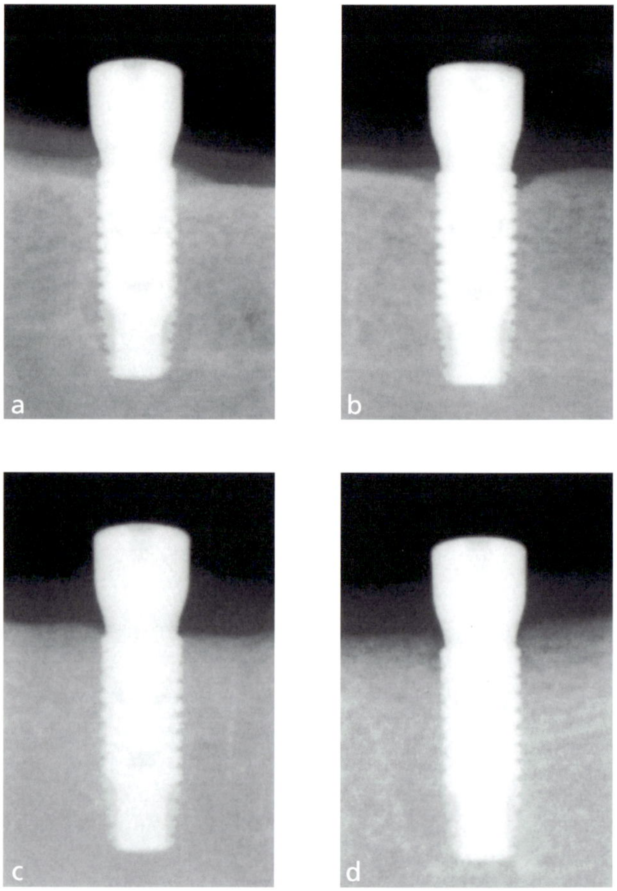

Fig 9-28 The crestal bone loss was less in the early plaque control group (a and c) than in the late plaque control group (b and d).

Further considerations

Early plaque control for mini-incision submerged implants

It is advisable to clean the implant sites using an antibacterial mouthwash alone for the first 2 weeks after surgery (Fig 9-29). The use of a toothbrush and an oral irrigator might lead to wound dehiscence, because irrigation flow and mechanical irritation caused by brushes or hydraulic pressure can damage the sutured wounds.

Early plaque control after stage II surgery

After stage II surgery using the flapless procedure, the implants should be cleaned using the same plaque control methods as those used after stage I surgery using the flapless technique.

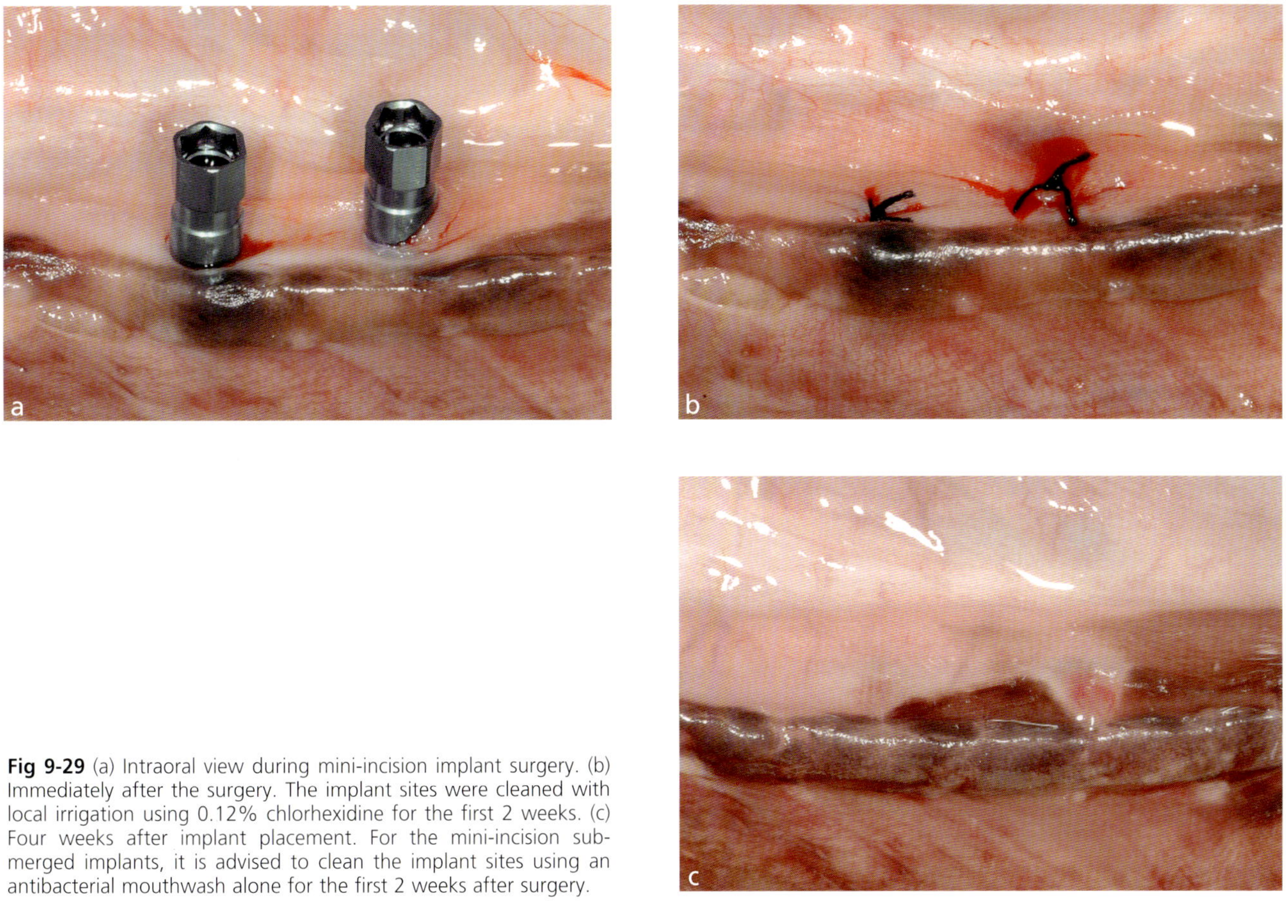

Fig 9-29 (a) Intraoral view during mini-incision implant surgery. (b) Immediately after the surgery. The implant sites were cleaned with local irrigation using 0.12% chlorhexidine for the first 2 weeks. (c) Four weeks after implant placement. For the mini-incision submerged implants, it is advised to clean the implant sites using an antibacterial mouthwash alone for the first 2 weeks after surgery.

Patient oral hygiene after implant prosthetic mounting

The clinician should instruct the patient on the use of toothbrushes, tufted brushes, floss, oral irrigators, and interdental brushes (Fig 9-30). When choosing and recommending oral hygiene tools and practices, the clinician should consider the appropriate oral hygiene measures that will allow access to the implant–gingiva margin and interdental space.[13,14] Daily removal of supragingival plaque using a toothbrush can significantly reduce the amount and composition of subgingival microbiota. This reduction translates to a decreased risk of periodontal disease initiation or recurrence. Further, the decreased prevalence of periodontal pathogens in the supragingival plaque reduces the potential reservoirs of these species.[15] It is important to educate patients about their responsibility to decrease plaque effectively, particularly if they have a history of periodontal disease.

Because patients are likely to have some fear of damaging their implants with oral hygiene tools, detailed education is critical. Frequent recall visits after implant prosthetic mounting will be essential to evaluate and establish good oral hygiene. The recall visit should also be used to detect potential problems and encourage early intervention should a problem arise. A review check-up is needed every 3 months, and an examination of bone loss through periapical radiography will be necessary every 6 months.

Summary

With nonsubmerged implants, early plaque control is very important because peri-implant wounds are vulnerable to bacterial infection for the first 2 weeks. The following plaque control steps are suggested after flapless implant placement. For the first 2 days after implant placement, the implant surfaces should be cleaned with chlorhexidine mouthwash and a microbrush. From the third day, a soft toothbrush should be added to the regimen. From the sixth day, an oral irrigator should be added. From the 15th day, the implants should be cleaned with a normal toothbrush and oral irrigator. Meticulous early plaque control plays a key role in promoting health in the peri-implant mucosa and preventing peri-implant bone loss.

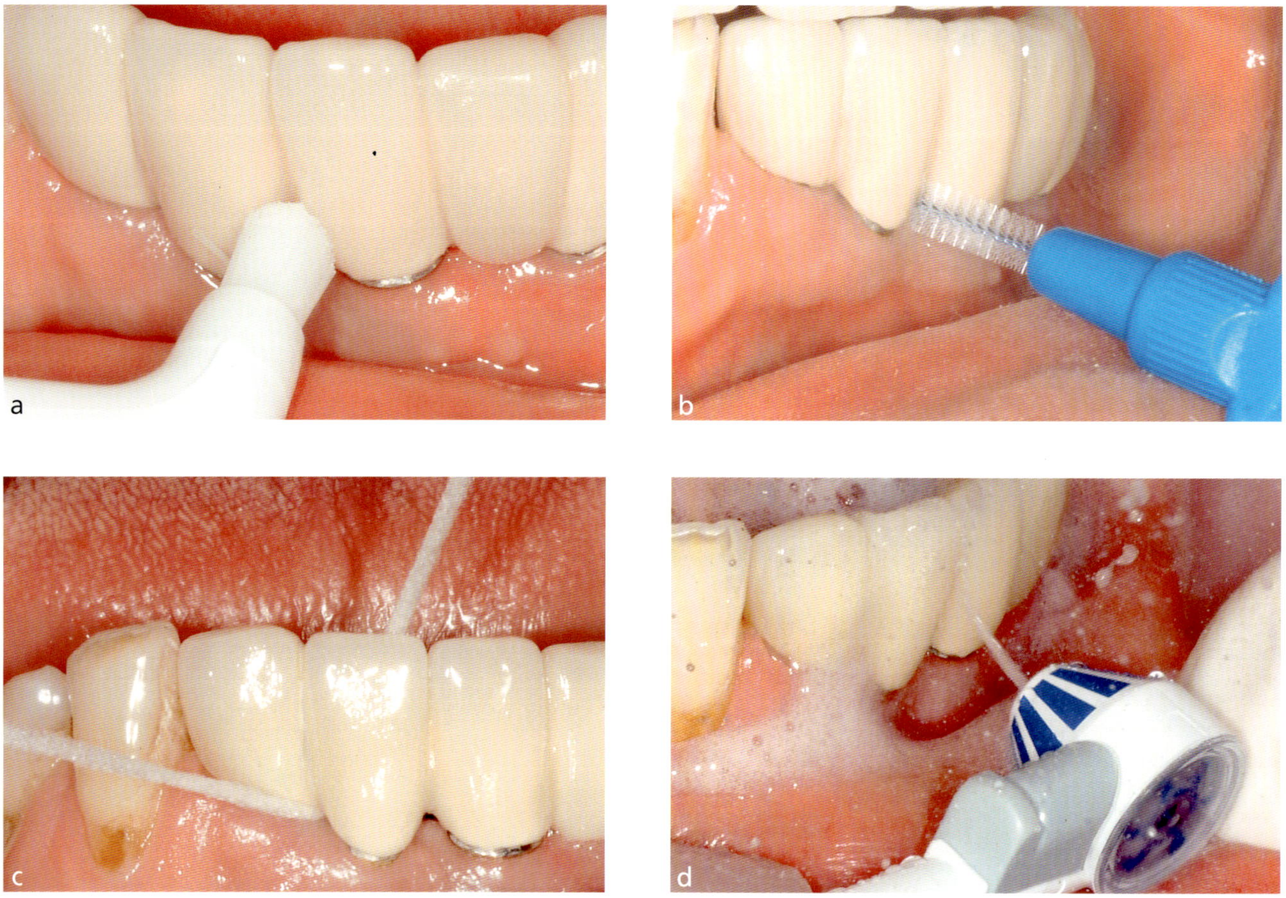

Fig 9-30 The clinician should instruct the patient on the use of (a) a tufted brush, (b) an interdental brush, (c) floss, and (d) an irrigator.

References

1. Van Steinberghe D, Lekholm U, Bolender C et al. The application of osseointegrated oral implants in the rehabilitation of partial edentulism: a prospective multicenter study on 558 fixtures. Int J Oral Maxillofac Implants 1990;5:272–281.
2. Joly C, de Lima AFM, da Silva RC. Clinical and radiographic evaluation of soft and hard tissue changes around implants: a pilot study. J Periodontol 2003;74:1097–1103.
3. Weber HP, Buser D, Donath K. Comparison of healed tissues adjacent to submerged and non-submerged unloaded titanium dental implants: a histomorphometric study in beagle dogs. Clin Oral Implants Res 1996;7:11–19.
4. Berglundh T, Lindhe J, Ericsson I, Marinello CP, Liljenberg B, Thomsen P. The soft tissue barrier at implants and teeth. Clin Oral Implants Res 1991;2:81–90.
5. Berglundh T, Lindhe J, Marinello C, Ericsson I, Liljenberg B. Soft tissue reaction to de-novo plaque formation on implants and teeth: an experimental study in the dog. Clin Oral Implants Res 1992;3:1–8.
6. Berglundh T, Abrahamsson I, Welander M, Lang NP, Lindhe J. Morphogenesis of the peri-implant mucosa: an experimental study in dogs. Clin Oral Implants Res 2007;18:1–8.
7. Ericsson I, Persson LG, Berglundh T, Marinello CP, Lindhe J, Klinge B. Different types of inflammatory reactions in peri-implant soft tissues. J Clin Periodontol 1995;22:255–261.
8. Noma H, Kaneko Y. A Color Atlas of Teeth Extraction in Dental Practice. Tokyo: Ishiyaku, 1991.
9. Briner WW, Grossman E, Buckner RY. Effect of chlorhexidine gluconate mouthrinse on plaque bacteria. J Periodont Res 1986; 16:44–52.
10. Jolkovsky DL, Waki MY, Newman MG. Clinical and microbiological effects of subgingival and gingival marginal irrigation with chlorhexidine gluconate. J Periodontol 1990;61:663–669.
11. Frascella JA. A randomized, clinical evaluation of the safety and efficacy of a novel oral irrigator. Am J Dent 2000;13:55–58.
12. Barnes CM, Russell CM, Reinhardt RA, Payne JB, Lyle DM. Comparison of irrigation to floss as an adjunct to toothbrushing: effect on bleeding, gingivitis, and supragingival plaque. J Clin Dent 2005;16: 71–77.
13. Wilken E. Clinical Practice of the Dental Hygienist, ed 7. Philadelphia, PA: Williams & Wilkins, 1994.
14. English C. Hygiene, maintenance, and prosthodontic concerns for the infirm patient: clinical report and discussion. Implant Dent 1995;4:166–172.
15. Lindhe J, Karring T, Lang N. Clinical Periodontology and Implant Dentistry. Copenhagen: Munksgaard, 2000.

CHAPTER

10

Soft Tissue around Flapless Implants

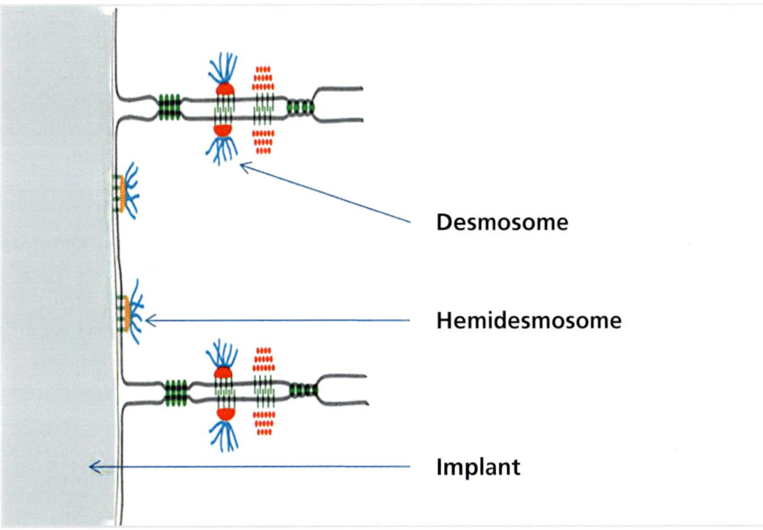

Key point

Healthy peri-implant soft tissue promotes a healthy implant.

Overview

Flapless implant surgery has an important advantage over flap surgery in that it provides a good environment for the healing of soft tissue. This difference leads to the formation of the peri-implant soft tissue structures that are essential for maintaining healthy implants. This chapter addresses the attachment structures of peri-implant soft tissues, the factors influencing formation of the attachment, and the effects of flapless implant surgery on the attachment.

Structural aspects of the interface between titanium implants and peri-implant mucosa

In 1956, Weinmann introduced a theory on the biological seal around implants.[1] James and Kelln were the first to systematically examine the biological seal.[2] Many researchers reported that the biological seal was composed of two portions: a junctional epithelial zone and a connective tissue zone.[3–8] The marginal junctional epithelium is continuous with the zone of connective tissue attachment (Fig 10-1).

Interface between the implant surface and epithelium

Junctional epithelial cells interface with surgically placed titanium implants.[4] The junctional epithelial cells then attach to the implant through hemidesmosome attachment with a lucida and a lamina densa layer, as well as a sublaminal zone and glycoaminoglycan layer (Figs 10-2 to 10-4).[5,9,10] These junctional epithelial cells are morphologically similar to those observed around natural teeth.[11] However, the junctional epithelial zone has less attachment strength to the implant than to the natural teeth.

Interface between the implant surface and connective tissue

Fibroblasts adhere to the implant through focal adhesion contacts (Figs 10-5 and 10-6).[12,13] Proteoglycans and collagen fibers participate in the formation of these focal adhesion contacts. Collagen fibers in the connective tissue attachment around an implant run parallel to the implant surface, not perpendicular, which is observed with natural teeth (Fig 10-7).[5,12–14]

Roles

The attachment of soft tissue acts as a barrier between the oral environment and underlying bone. This attachment protects the underlying bone from destructive, extraneous substances, such as bacteria, toxins, food remnants, and other harmful factors. Breaking the barrier is closely related to peri-implant disease and bone loss. Therefore, the success of a dental implant depends strongly on good attachment of the surrounding tissue to the implant.[10,15]

Differences between tooth-adjacent and peri-implant soft tissues

The implant surface is devoid of root cementum, whereas natural teeth have root cementum.

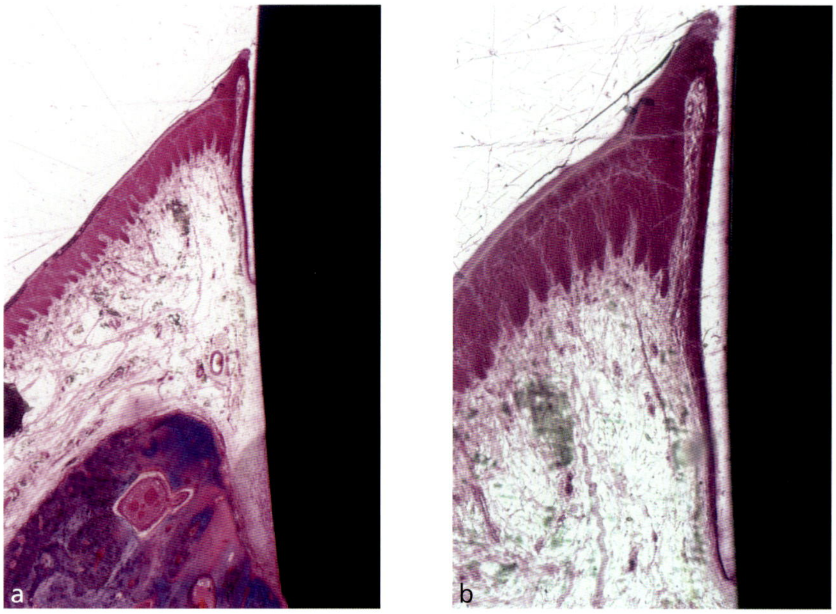

Fig 10-1 (a and b) The interface between the surface of a dental implant and peri-implant mucosa is composed of two portions: a marginal junctional epithelium (a) that is continuous with a zone of connective tissue attachment (b).

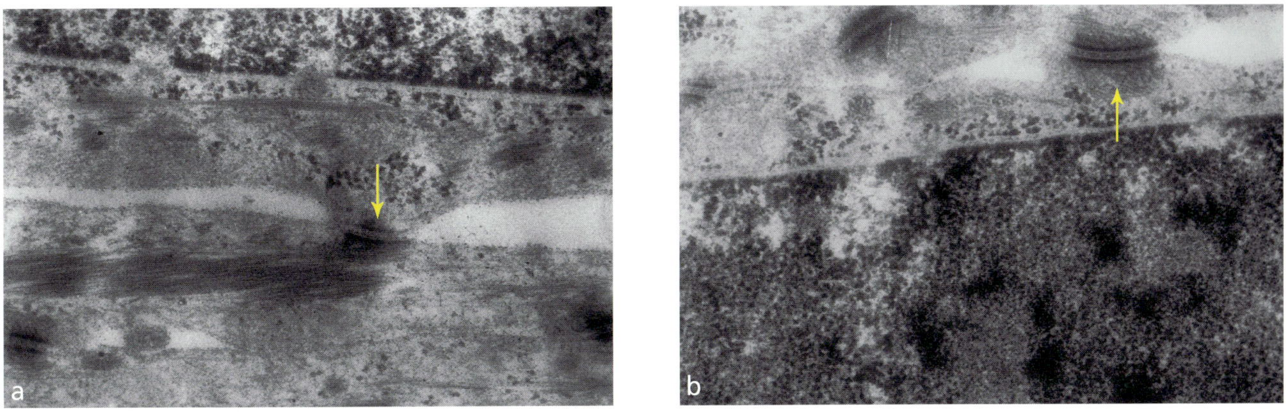

Fig 10-2 (a) The desmosome of a human gingival epithelial cell. (b) The junctional epithelial cells attach to the implant via a hemidesmosome attachment.

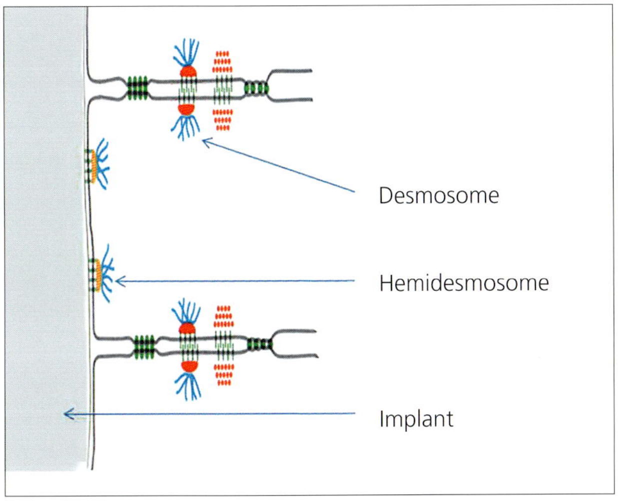

Fig 10-3 Schematic of epithelial cell attachment.

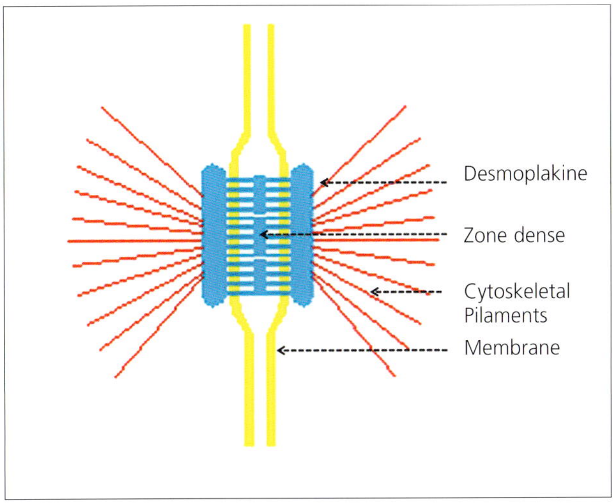

Fig 10-4 Schematic of a desmosome.

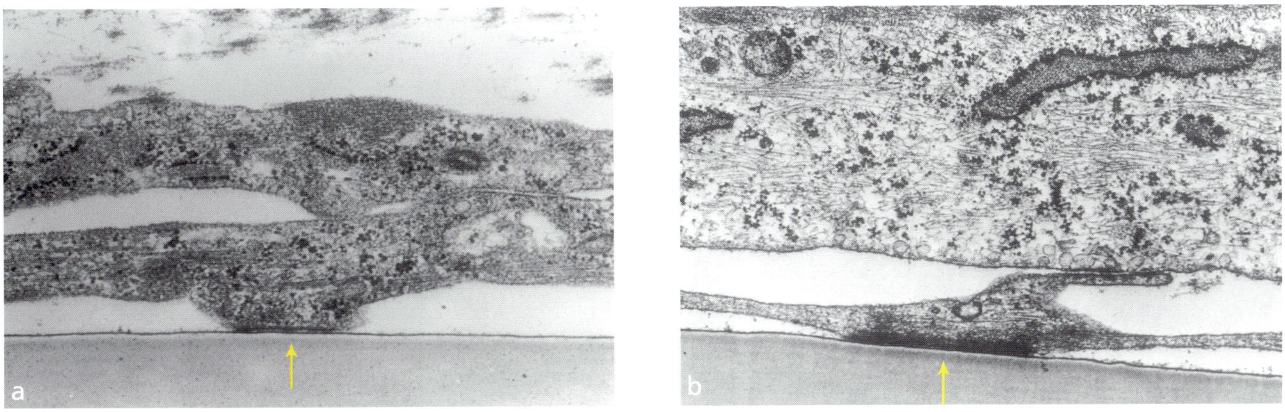

Fig 10-5 (a and b) Focal adhesion contact of a human gingival fibroblast growing on a plastic surface.

The collagen fibers in the supra-alveolar region run a course more or less parallel to the implant surface, whereas collagen fibers attach to the natural teeth perpendicularly. This is partly why inflammation around the implant migrates more easily into the underlying bone than around the natural teeth.[16] The inner zone of connective tissue attachment has more collagen around the implants than around the teeth.

The inner zone of connective tissue attachment has fewer fibroblasts around the implant than around the teeth.

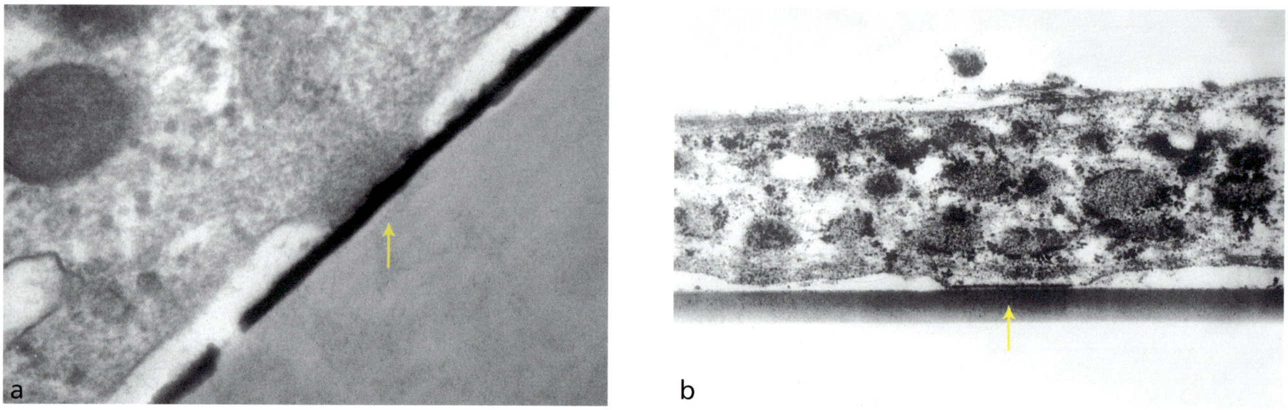

Fig 10-6 (a and b) Focal adhesion contact of a human gingival fibroblast growing on a titanium-coated plastic surface.

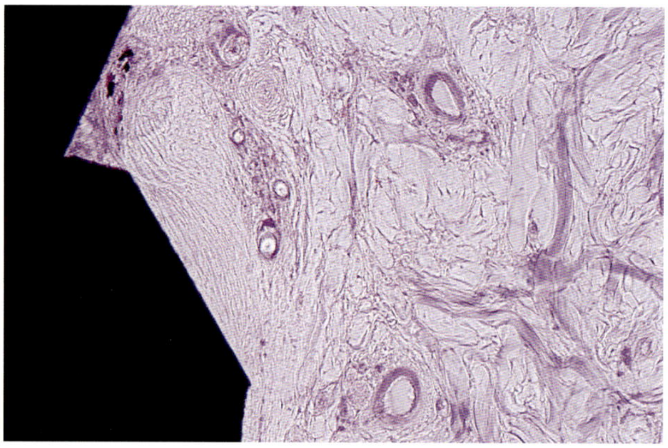

Fig 10-7 Zone of connective tissue attachment around a dental implant.

The infiltration of inflammation into the underlying bone is more likely to occur around an implant than around teeth. This suggests that peri-implant tissue has weaker defense against bacterial attack than teeth.[17] The connective tissue layer around a natural tooth has abundant blood vessels originating from the periodontal ligament, whereas the peri-implant connective layer has few blood vessels. This means that peri-implant tissues have weak defensive ability against inflammation.[16]

Wound repair biology in the peri-implant mucosa after implant placement

Tissue injury initiates a cascade of wound repair processes to restore tissue integrity. After a nonsubmerged implant installation procedure, wound repair consists of inflammatory, proliferative, and remodeling phases.

The inflammatory phase

A coagulum occupies the compartments between the mucosa and implant immediately after surgery. After hemostasis, the local vessels dilate secondary to the effects of coagulation. Reactive and inflammatory edema occurs in the gingival margin. The blood clot is infiltrated by numerous neutrophil granulocytes. The neutrophils scavenge debris, foreign bodies, and bacteria in the wound. This inflammatory phase is present at the wound for 1–6 days after surgery. In wounds containing necrotic tissue, sutures, foreign material, bacterial infection, blood flow problems, or mechanical irritation, there is an increase in neutrophil infiltration and the inflammatory phase is prolonged, which can delay the move to the next phase. When a bacterial infection occurs, bacterial toxins weaken the function of leukocytes and slow fibroblast proliferation, thereby impairing the healing process. The hematoma appearing after flap implant surgery increases the risk of a bacterial infection because a hematoma is a suitable culture medium for bacteria. A blood flow problem in the wound also affects the length and quality of wound healing (Fig 10-8).[18]

The proliferation phase

Fibroblasts proliferate at the wound site. They become the main cell type after 3–5 days in clean and uninfected wounds. Fibroblasts synthesize and secrete collagens. The fibroblasts and collagen begin filling the gap between the mucosa and implant from the bottom and then advance upward. These fibroblasts adhere to the implant surface when they come into contact with it. The marginal basal cells of the epithelium at the wound margin migrate over the wound defect and grow down into the gap.[19] Epithelial cells migrate as a sheet over the wound matrix formed in the gap and adhere to the implant surface. An interface between the implant surface and peri-implant mucosa is

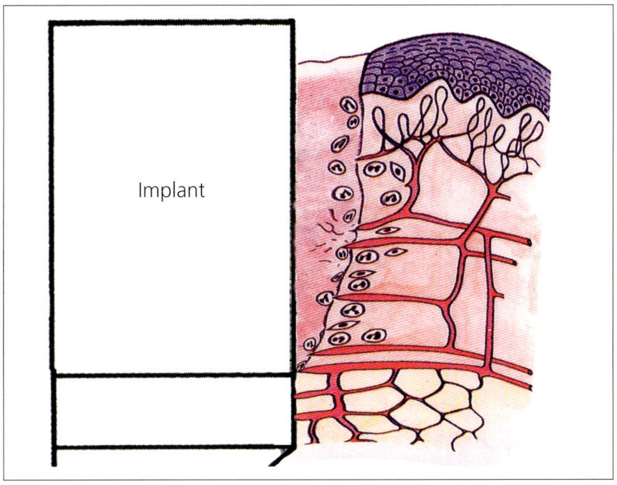

Fig 10-8 Schematic of the inflammatory phase. A coagulum occupies the compartments between the mucosa and implants immediately after surgery. The blood clot is infiltrated by numerous neutrophil granulocytes. The neutrophils scavenge debris, foreign bodies, and bacteria in the wound. This inflammatory phase is present at the wound by 1–6 days after surgery.

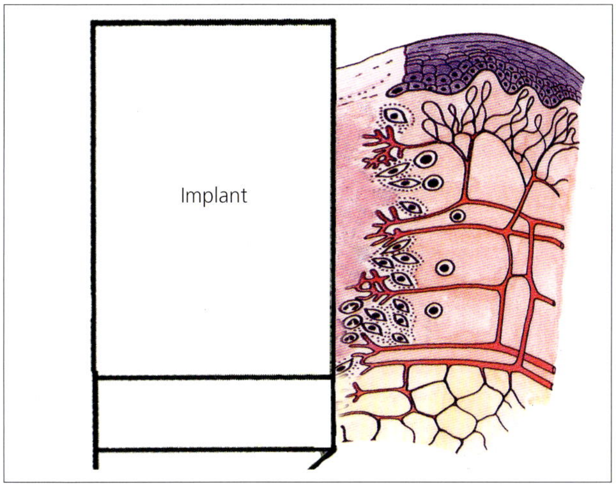

Fig 10-9 Schematic of the early proliferation phase. Fibroblasts proliferate at the wound site. They become the main cell type after 3–5 days in a clean, uninfected wound. Fibroblasts synthesize and secrete collagen.

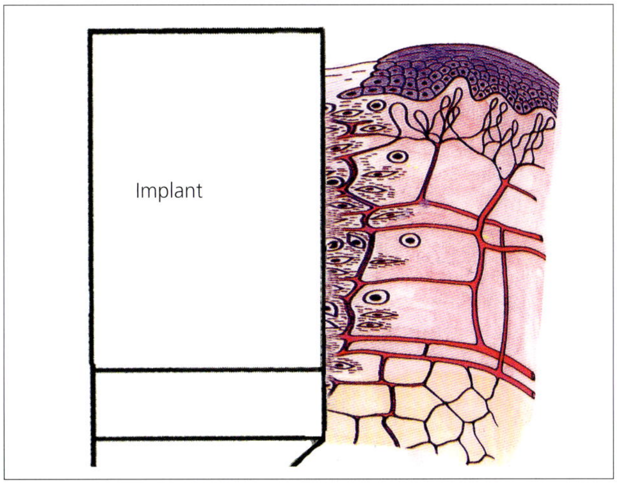

Fig 10-10 Schematic of the late proliferation phase. Fibroblasts and collagen fill the gap between the mucosa and implants from the bottom and then advance upward. The epithelial cells migrate as a sheet over the wound matrix formed in the gap. The formation of a connective tissue layer is complete in 4–6 weeks and that of barrier junctional epithelium in 6–8 weeks.

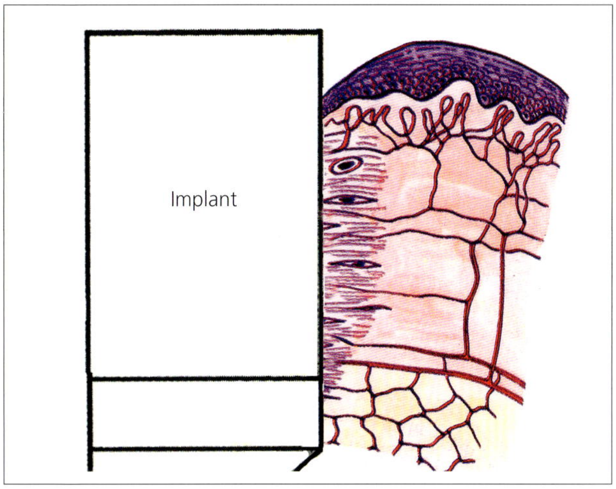

Fig 10-11 Schematic illustrating the remodeling phase. Wound scar remodeling occurs over months to years to form a mature scar.

formed when the fibroblasts and epithelial cells adhere to the implant surface. The formation of this interface is completed at between 6 and 8 weeks. This proliferation phase is prolonged in wounds with inflammation or mechanical irritation (Figs 10-9 and 10-10).[19]

The remodeling phase

When the wound matrix is filled with collagen fibers, fibroblasts will have the form and properties of fibrocytes in the so-called "silent period." Wound scar remodeling occurs during the course of months or years to form a mature scar (Fig 10-11).

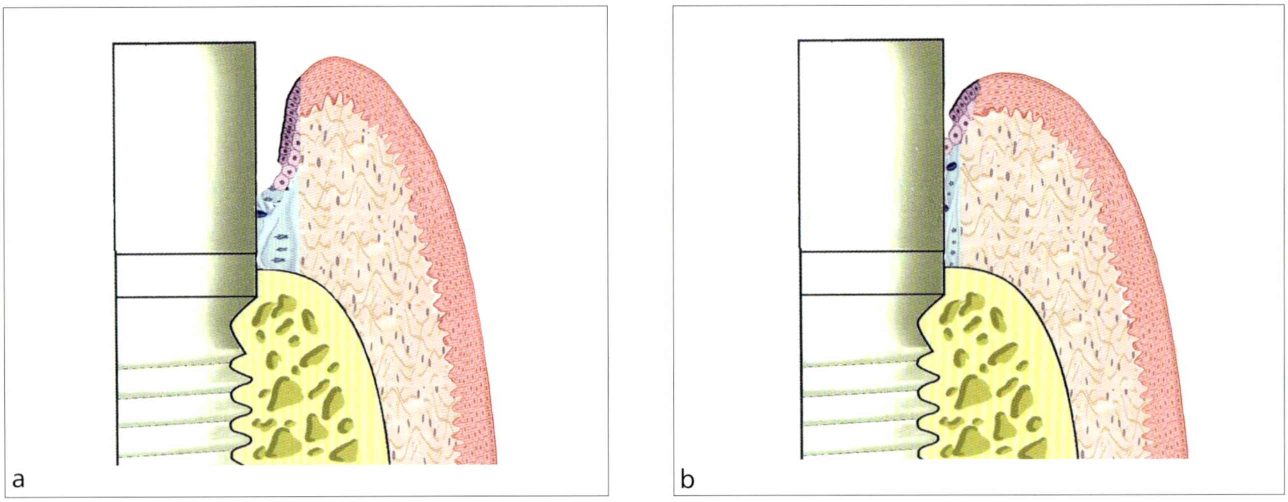

Fig 10-12 (a) With flap implant surgery, a wide gap between the implants and surrounding mucosa is created. Epithelial cells grow even deeper down into the gap and the height of the junctional epithelium is increased. (b) With flapless implant surgery, a small gap between the implant and surrounding mucosa is created, and epithelial cells grow down a lot less and the length of the junctional epithelium is shorter.

Differences in wound healing between flap and flapless surgery

Wound healing after flap implant surgery

A wide gap is created between the implant and surrounding mucosa. More fibroblasts and collagen are necessary to fill the gap. If the proliferative phase is prolonged, epithelial cells grow even deeper down into the gap and the height of the junctional epithelium is increased (Fig 10-12). A large amount of collagen is generated in the wide gap as the mucosa thickens.[20] This type of tissue heals with extensive scar formation, resulting in weakened healing and defensive ability.[16]

Wound healing after flapless implant surgery

Only a small gap is created between the implant and surrounding mucosa. The gap is filled quickly with the wound matrix. Epithelial cells grow down a lot less and the length of the junctional epithelium is shortened (Figs 10-12 and 10-13). Such tissue heals with very little scar formation, resulting in improved healing and defensive ability.

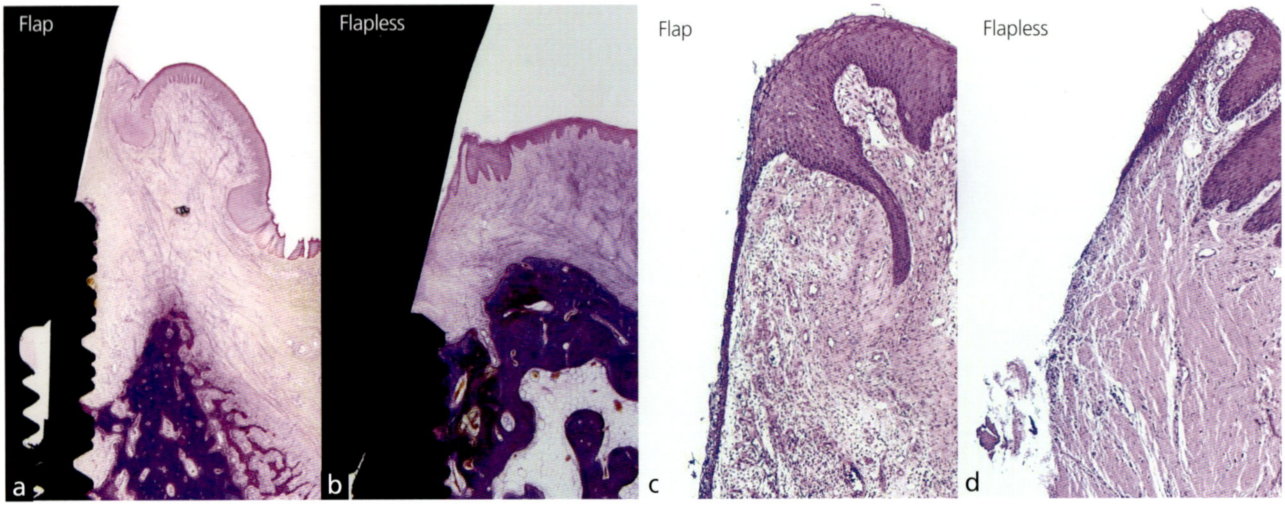

Fig 10-13 Morphogenesis of the peri-implant mucosa: a comparison between (a, c) flap and (b, d) flapless procedures. Histological examinations performed 3 months after the procedures show that the junctional epithelium extends more apically in the flap implants than in the flapless implants.

Table 10-1 Histometric measurements, vessel measurements, and parameters of probing depth, Gingival Index, and bleeding on probing around implants when placed with or without a flap.

	Flap implant	Flapless implant	*P* value
PM–B (mm ± SD)	3.5 ± 0.8	2.2 ± 0.2	< .05
PM–aJE (mm ± SD)	2.2 ± 0.3	1.2 ± 0.3	< .05
aJE–B (mm ± SD)	1.3 ± 0.2	1.0 ± 0.2	< .05
Vessel fraction (% ± SD)	1.2 ± 0.3	1.7 ± 0.7	< .05
Vessel number (± SD)	38.2 ± 8.1	51.4 ± 9.2	< .05
Probing depth (mm)	1.7	1.0	< .05
Gingival Index	0.9	0	< .05
Bleeding on probing	0.7	0	< .05

PM – marginal position of the peri-implant mucosa; aJE – apical termination of the junctional epithelium; B – marginal level of "bone to implant contact".

Comparison of morphogenesis of the peri-implant mucosa

Thickness of the peri-implant mucosa

With flap implants, the junctional epithelium is approximately 2 mm in length and the connective tissue compartment is approximately 1–1.5 mm high.[21-24] When implants are placed without flap elevation, the length of the junctional epithelium is approximately 1.2 mm and the zone of connective tissue integration is 1.0 mm, indicating that the junctional epithelium extends more apically in the flap implants than in the flapless implants (Figs 10-13 and 10-14; Table 10-1).

Blood vessels of the peri-implant mucosa

Abrahamsson et al.[23] examined the attachment zone of the peri-implant mucosa in three different implant systems and stated that the connective tissue in a 300–600 µm wide zone lateral to the implant surface had the composition of a scar; that is, a high density of collagen and a low density of cells and vascular structures. Berglundh et al.[16] studied the attachment zone of the connective tissue in a Brånemark implant system and reported that the supracrestal connective tissue apical to the junctional epithelium was almost devoid of vessels in an approximately 300–500 µm wide zone surrounding the implant surface.

In an animal study, a more detailed analysis of the vessels within the attachment zone was carried out. The findings from morphometric analysis performed using optical microscopy indicated significant differences between the flap and flapless implants. In the flap group, the vessel number and vessel fraction were approximately 38.2 and 1.2%, respectively. In some sections, the surgical zone was almost devoid of vascular structures (Fig 10-15). These results corroborate the previously reported data.[16,23] When

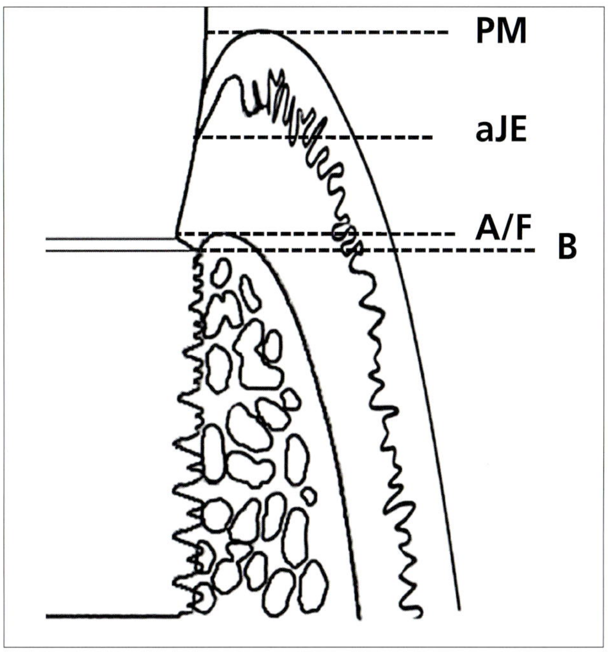

Fig 10-14 Schematic illustrating the landmarks used for histometric measurements. PM – the marginal portion of the peri-implant mucosa; aJE – the level of the apical termination of the junctional epithelium; B – the marginal level of bone to implant contact; A/F – the abutment–fixture borderline

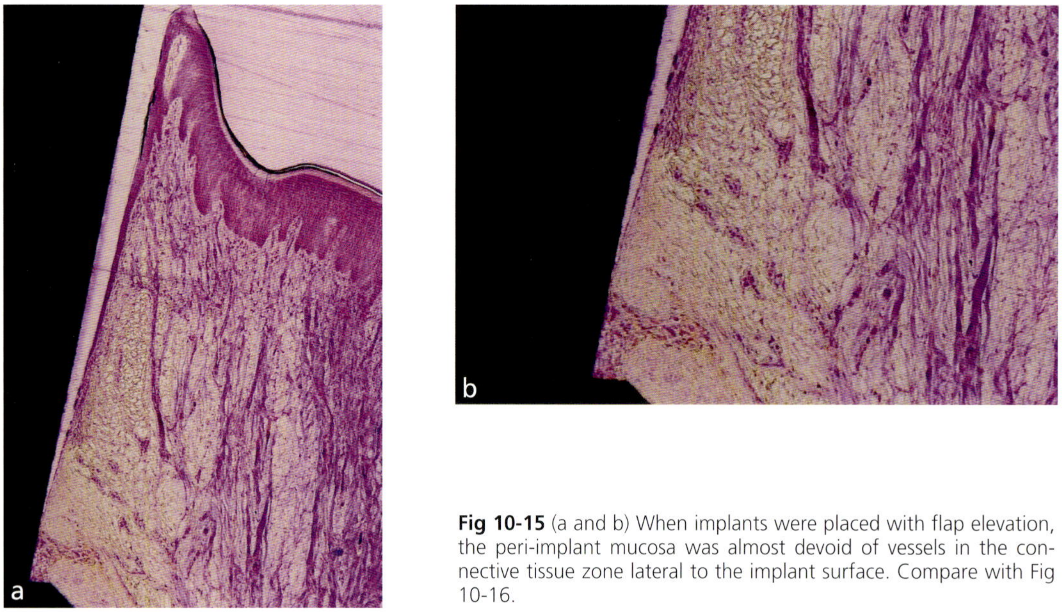

Fig 10-15 (a and b) When implants were placed with flap elevation, the peri-implant mucosa was almost devoid of vessels in the connective tissue zone lateral to the implant surface. Compare with Fig 10-16.

the implants were placed without flap elevation, the vessel number and vessel fraction were approximately 51.4 and 1.7%, respectively (Fig 10-16). This indicates that the peri-implant mucosa was more richly vascularized in the flapless group than in the flap group (see Table 10-1). The more richly vascularized peri-implant mucosa is directly related to an increased blood supply around the implant, which may strengthen the resistance to inflammation. This indicates that the flapless procedure may increase the vascularity of the peri-implant mucosa.

Peri-implant mucosal health

The peri-implant mucosal health of flap and flapless implants was compared using a canine mandible model (Fig 10-17). In six mongrel dogs, bilateral, edentulated, flat alveolar ridges were created in the mandible. After 3 months, two implants were placed in each side using either the flap or flapless procedure. After another healing period of 3 months, the peri-implant mucosa was evaluated using clinical parameters, including the Gingival Index (GI), bleeding on probing, and probing pocket depth. These examinations showed a significantly higher GI, bleeding on probing, and probing depth in the dogs that had undergone the flap procedure than those that had undergone the flapless procedure (see Table 10-1). The more apically positioned junctional epithelium was related directly to an increased probing depth around the implant, which might provide an environment that is conducive to peri-implantitis. There were more cases of peri-implantitis in the flap group than in the flapless group, as confirmed by the higher GI scores. More marginal bone resorption was observed at the flap implant sites than at the flapless implant sites. The results of this study show that the mucosal health of the peri-implant was better in the flapless group than in the flap group.

Soft tissue around flapless implants after prosthesis fabrication

The fabrication of a final prosthesis begins with the replacement of a healing abutment with a permanent abutment (Figs 10-18 and 10-19). This severs the soft tissue attachment. Abrahamsson et al.,[25] in a study using beagle dogs, demonstrated that repeated disconnection and reconnection of implant abutments causes an apical shift in the marginal bone levels as well as soft tissue recession. It was suggested that repeated injury to the mucosal barrier was associated with apical proliferation of the epithelium, and that bone resorption occurs to reestablish the connective tissue attachment of a sufficient dimension. At sites where the abutments were disconnected and reconnected five times over a 6-month period (once a month), the bone level was found to be located 0.7 mm more apical of the abutment–fixture junction than at the control sites at which the abutments were left unchanged.

According to the results of our animal experiment, a single shift from a healing abutment to a permanent abut-

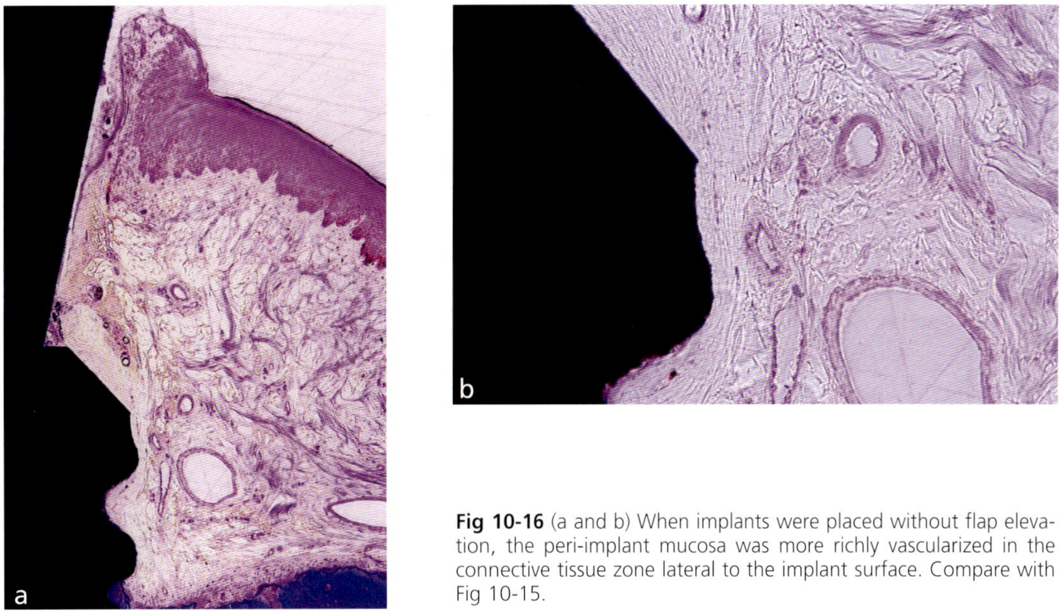

Fig 10-16 (a and b) When implants were placed without flap elevation, the peri-implant mucosa was more richly vascularized in the connective tissue zone lateral to the implant surface. Compare with Fig 10-15.

ment resulted in the reestablishment of transmucosal attachment, the dimension and quality of which were similar to those of the mucosal barrier formed to an abutment left unchanged (Fig 10-20).

It is possible that the change from a healing abutment to a permanent abutment does not compromise the mucosal attachment, and that the soft tissue attachment to the titanium abutment is reestablished after a single abutment shift.

Factors affecting formation of the peri-implant soft tissue attachment

Oral hygiene

The peri-implant attachment between the implant surface and mucosa, which is established early during soft tissue healing after implant surgery, constitutes an effective barrier between the oral environment and peri-implant bone. Plaque formation on the mucosa around implants can cause inflammation of the peri-implant tissue. Plaque-induced inflammation can impede the formation of a biological seal in the initial healing of peri-implant tissue. In addition, the existing peri-implant soft tissue attachment may also be destroyed by plaque-induced inflammation. Therefore, meticulous plaque control after implant placement is required to prevent inflammation in the peri-implant mucosa.

Surgical trauma

Scar tissue is an area different from normal tissue in terms of esthetics, function, and blood supply. Formation of the peri-implant attachment during the initial healing period is closely related to the scar volume. Little scar formation leads to the formation of healthy peri-implant soft tissue structures that are essential for maintaining healthy implants. Therefore, implant surgery should be performed to minimize the surgical trauma.

Soft tissue condition

The condition of the soft tissue is also important for formation of the peri-implant attachment. Implants placed in the attached gingiva have a more stable interface.[26,27] Implants in the mucosa or movable soft tissue have a less stable interface and are likely to experience soft tissue problems, such as infection.

The thickness of the mucosa is also associated with establishment of the peri-implant mucosa. Implants placed in thick mucosa have a greater pocket depth, and thicker junctional epithelium and connective tissue layers. In our animal experiment, at the sites where the vertical dimension of the mucosa was twice as thick, the heights of the junctional epithelium and connective tissue layers were almost double the corresponding dimensions at the normal mucosa sites. The influence of a thick mucosa on peri-implant tissue healing around implants is described in more detail in Chapter 11.

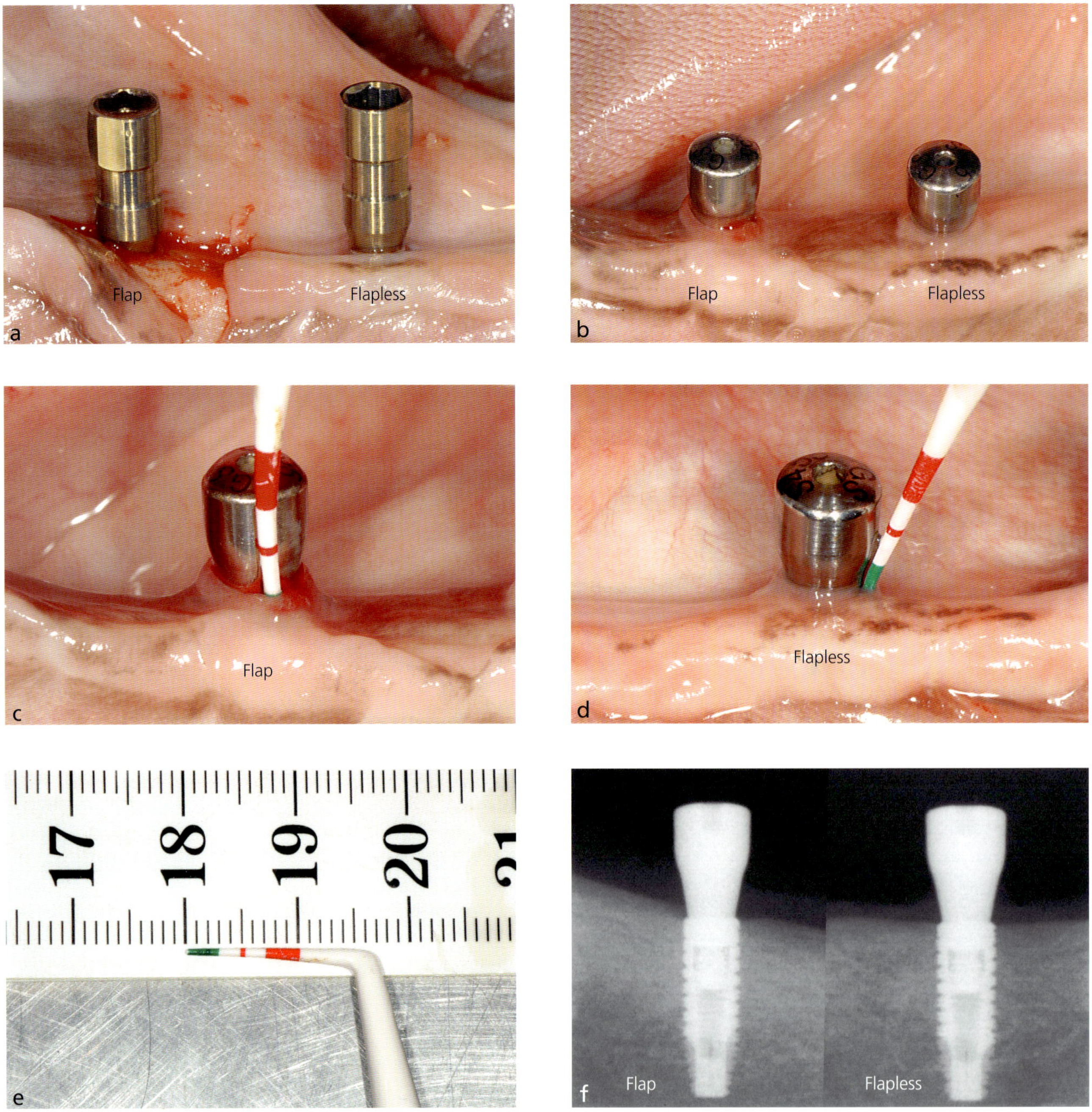

Fig 10-17 Comparison of peri-implant mucosal health between the flap and flapless procedures using a canine mandible model. (a) Two implants were placed using either the flap or the flapless procedure. (b–d) Clinical examinations after a 3-month healing period showed significantly greater Gingival Index, bleeding on probing, and probing depth in the dogs that had undergone the flap procedure. (e) The probe used to measure the probing depth. (f) Radiographs 3 months after implant placement. Note the marginal bone resorption at the flap implant site and no marginal bone resorption at the flapless implant site.

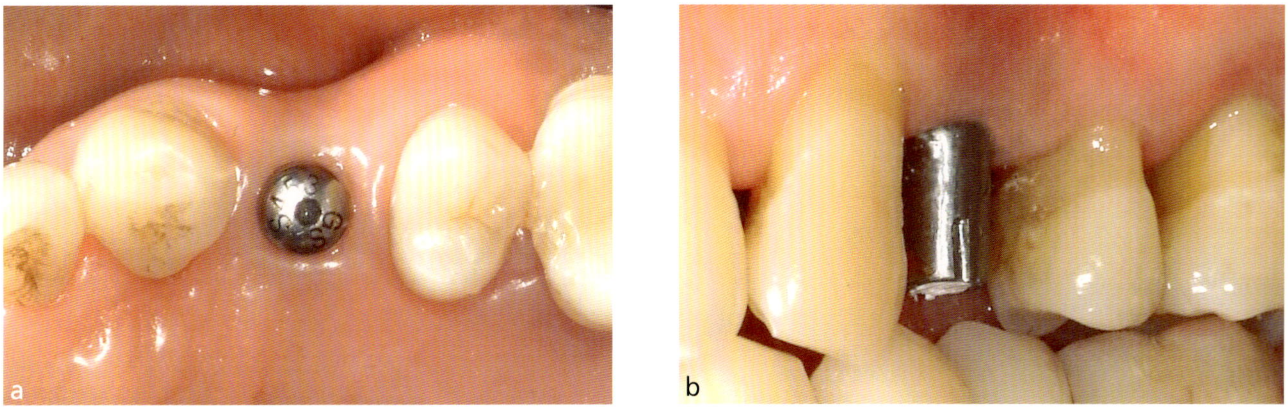

Fig 10-18 (a and b) A healing abutment is changed to a permanent abutment before prosthesis fabrication.

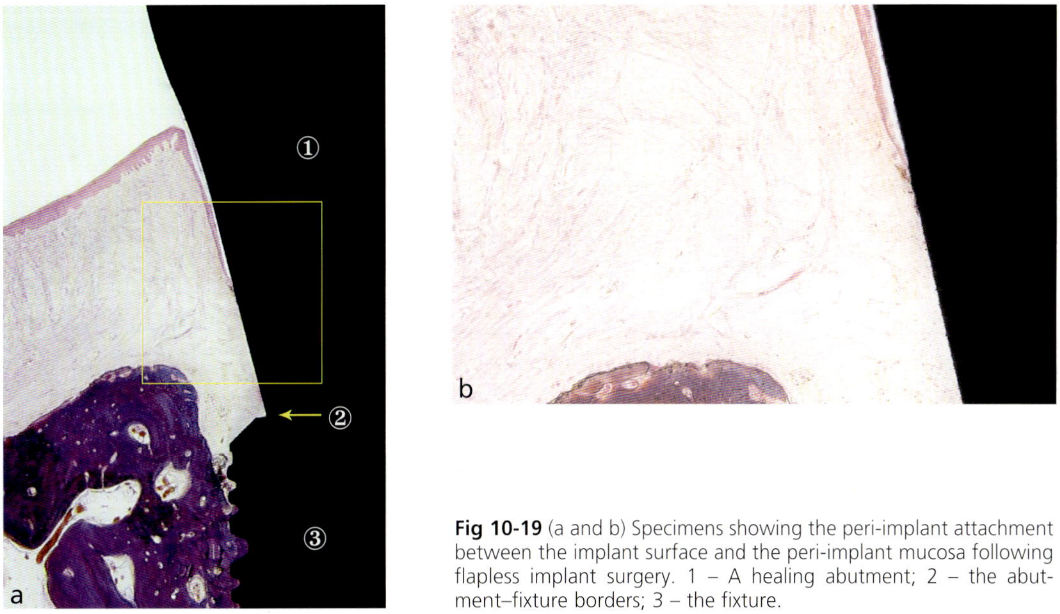

Fig 10-19 (a and b) Specimens showing the peri-implant attachment between the implant surface and the peri-implant mucosa following flapless implant surgery. 1 – A healing abutment; 2 – the abutment–fixture borders; 3 – the fixture.

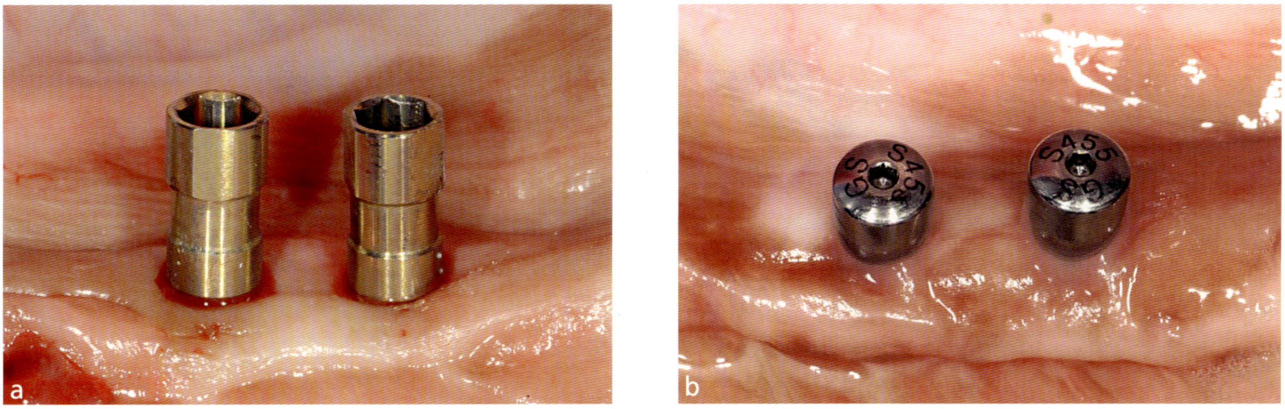

Fig 10-20 (a–h) Soft tissue reactions that occur in the transmucosal attachment after changing the healing abutment to a permanent abutment. (a) Two fixtures were placed within the edentulated ridge on each side of the canine mandible using flapless implant techniques. (b) Implants were nonsubmerged.

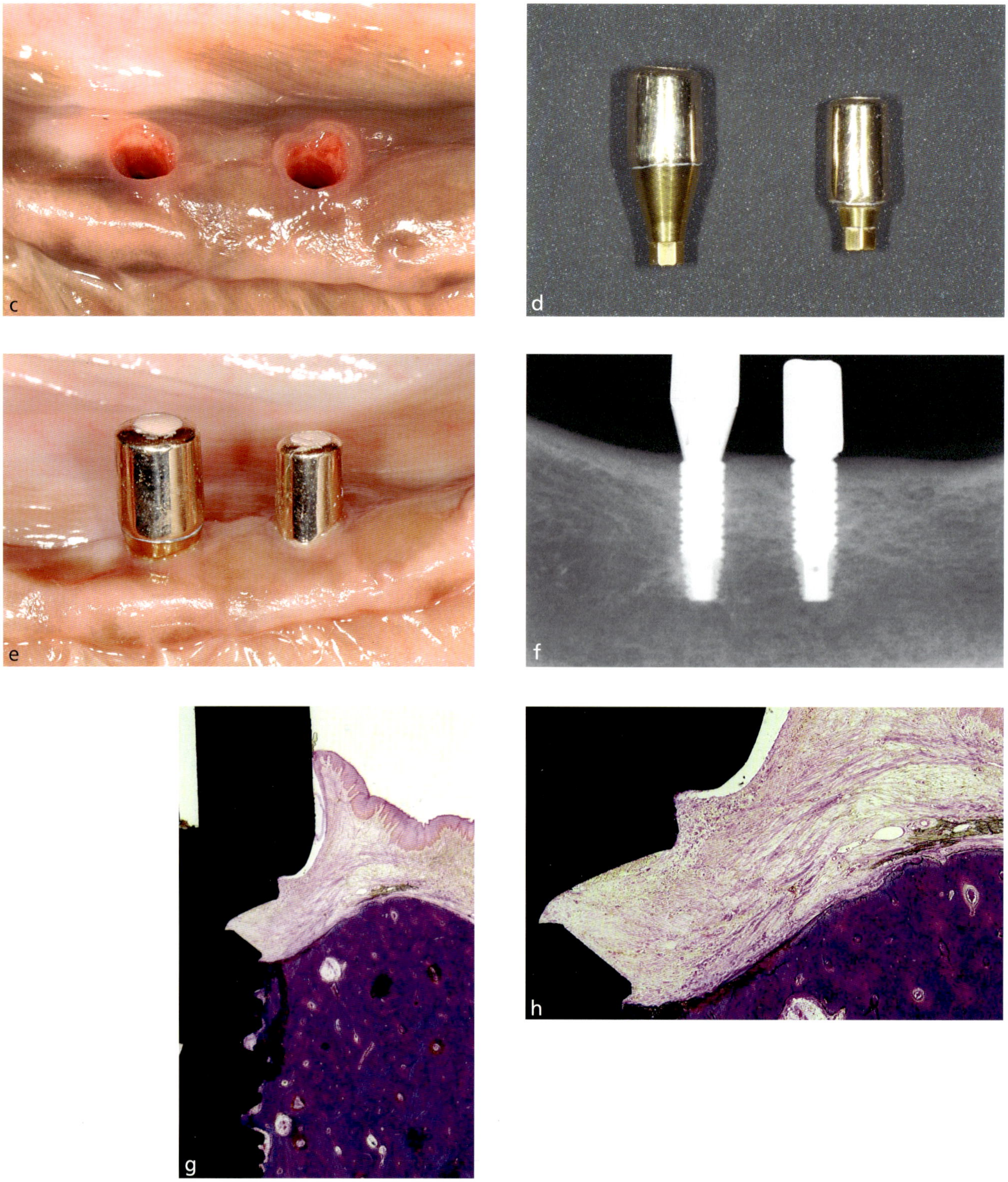

Fig 10-20 (*cont.*) (c and d) After a healing period of 3 months, healing abutments were changed to permanent abutments and the prostheses were fabricated. (e–h) Six months after implant placement: intraoral view, radiograph, and histological specimens. Note that the change from a healing abutment to a permanent abutment does not compromise the mucosal attachment, and the soft tissue attachment to the titanium abutment is reestablished after a single abutment shift.

Abutment material and its surface roughness

The abutment material influences the location and quality of the mucosal attachment that forms after abutment connection. Abrahamsson et al.[28] revealed through experiments on dogs that abutments made from titanium or ceramic allowed mucosal attachment. No proper attachment formed at the abutment level at sites where abutments were made from gold alloy.

In terms of the abutment surface roughness, the difference in the surface roughness of titanium abutments has no impact on the formation of mucosal attachment.[29,30] Abrahamsson's team reported similar attachments between the peri-implant mucosa and titanium abutments with either a smooth or a rough surface, and the lengths of the barrier epithelium and the zone of connective attachment were similar at smooth and rough surfaces. A similar result was obtained after 6 months of observation – daily plaque control was managed after the connection of titanium abutments with different surface roughnesses (machined surface, Ra = 1.5) (Fig 10-21). Although the soft tissue attachment was not influenced by the roughness of the titanium surface,[31–33] choosing abutments with smooth surfaces is advisable because a rough surface tends to accumulate more plaque.[34]

Submerged or nonsubmerged procedures

It has been reported that the attachment that forms between the mucosa and implant is similar regardless of whether implant placement was performed using a submerged or nonsubmerged technique. In addition, the soft tissue dimensions are similar regardless of whether the

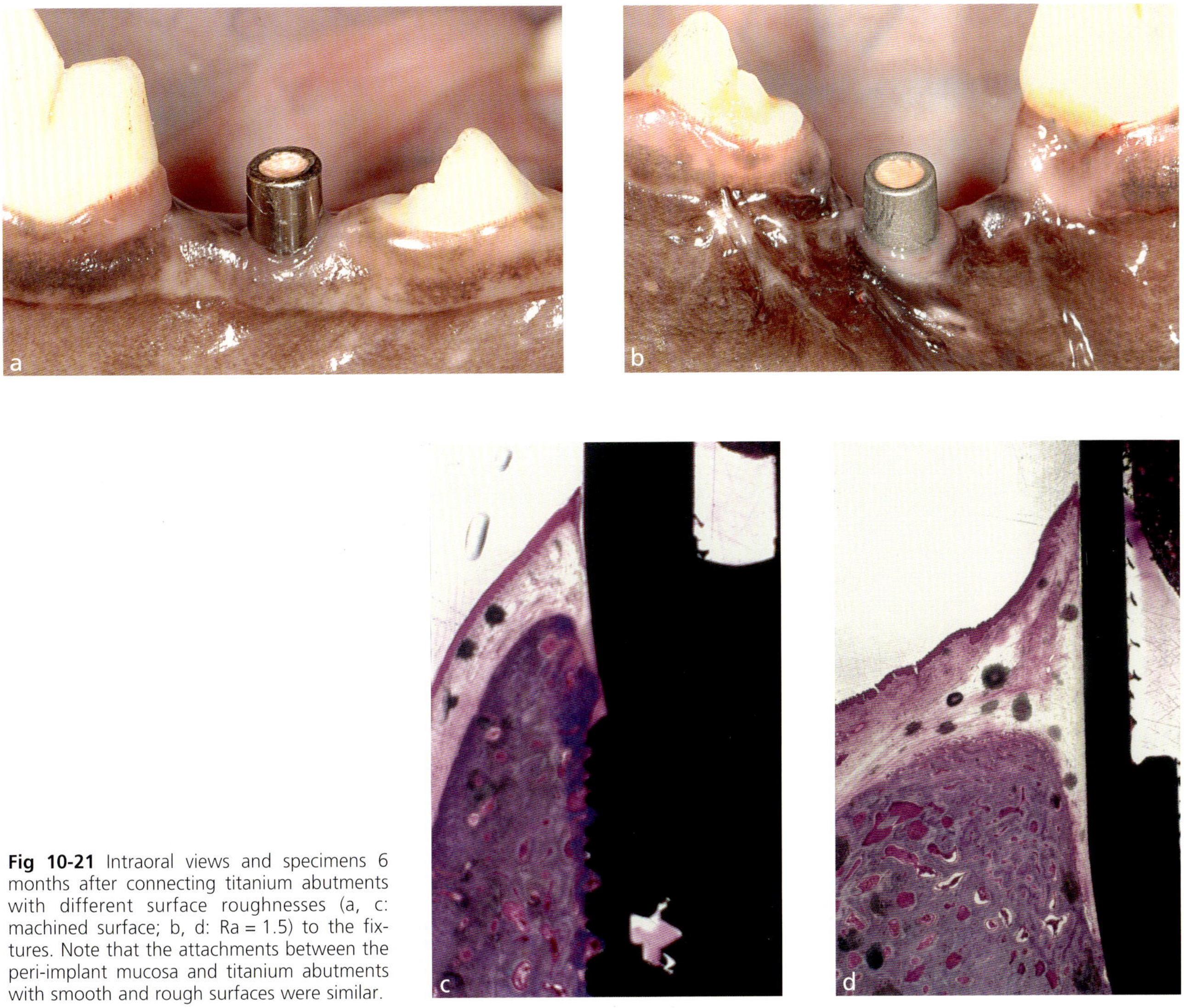

Fig 10-21 Intraoral views and specimens 6 months after connecting titanium abutments with different surface roughnesses (a, c: machined surface; b, d: Ra = 1.5) to the fixtures. Note that the attachments between the peri-implant mucosa and titanium abutments with smooth and rough surfaces were similar.

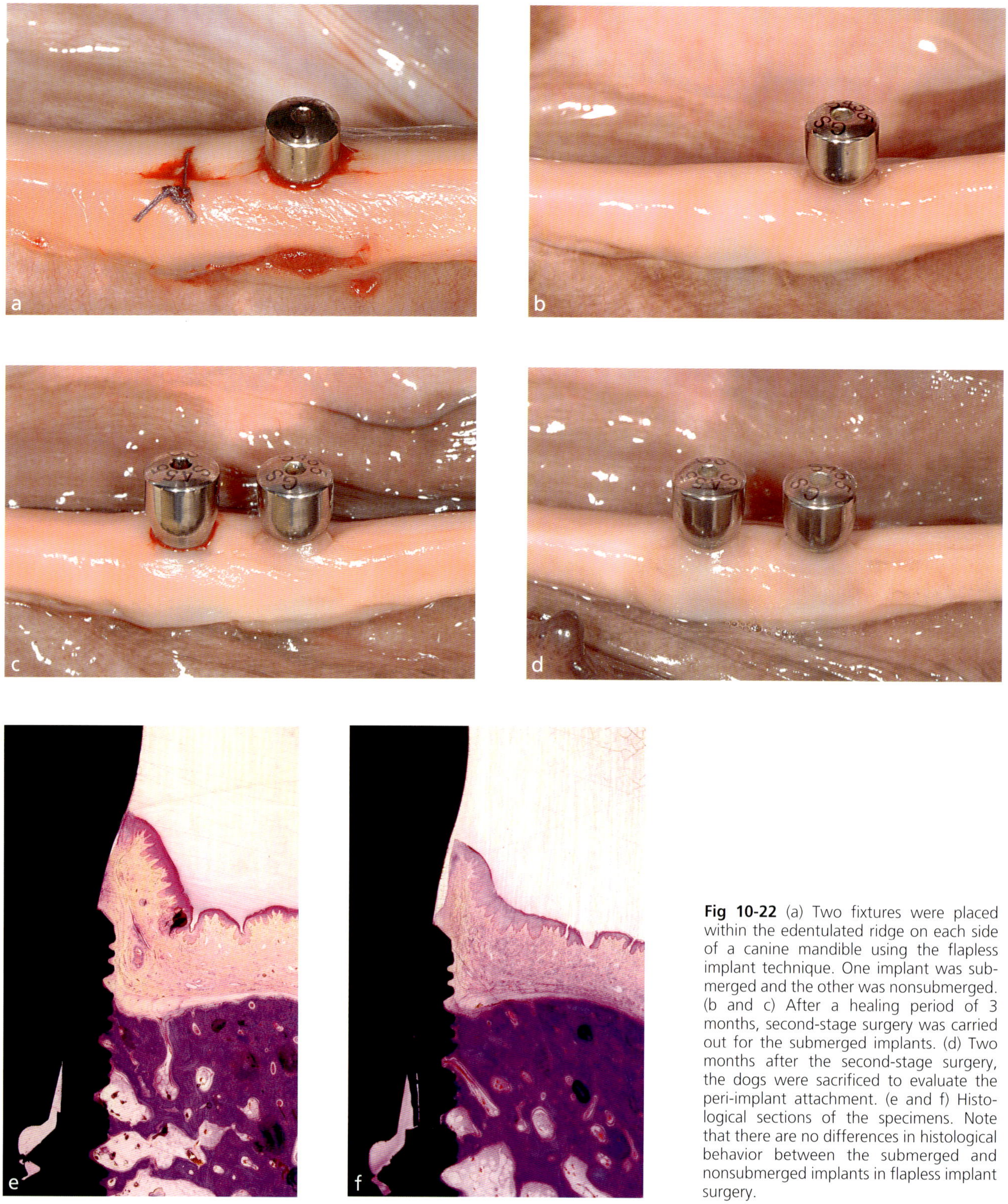

Fig 10-22 (a) Two fixtures were placed within the edentulated ridge on each side of a canine mandible using the flapless implant technique. One implant was submerged and the other was nonsubmerged. (b and c) After a healing period of 3 months, second-stage surgery was carried out for the submerged implants. (d) Two months after the second-stage surgery, the dogs were sacrificed to evaluate the peri-implant attachment. (e and f) Histological sections of the specimens. Note that there are no differences in histological behavior between the submerged and nonsubmerged implants in flapless implant surgery.

implants are initially submerged or nonsubmerged.[23–25] Our animal experiment using flapless implant surgery showed similar results: the mucosal attachment was independent of whether implant placement was performed using a submerged or a nonsubmerged installation technique. There were no differences in histological features between the submerged and nonsubmerged implants in flapless implant surgery (Fig 10-22).

Factors affecting maintenance of the peri-implant attachment

Oral hygiene

The long-term success of a dental implant depends strongly on good attachment of the surrounding soft tissue. This can protect the zone of osseointegration from the factors released from plaque and from the oral cavity. Meticulous plaque control is essential for protecting the biological seal.[35]

Overload

It has been reported that most implant failures occur in the first year after implant placement. Significantly higher rates of crestal bone resorption occur during this period than in any other post-loading periods.[36–38] The crestal bone loss that takes place after prosthesis fabrication can be associated with implant overload. This occurs when the magnitude of the bite forces exceeds the biomechanical capacity of the bone. Micro-fractures of the bone at the implant interface can occur once the biomechanical demand has exceeded the load-bearing ability of the bone. Loading forces are concentrated at the coronal portion of the implant.[39] The continuous application of cyclic loads can cause constant micro-motion at the interface, which can result in the formation of scar tissue. Such fibrous tissue loses its capacity to differentiate into bone. At this stage, down-growth of the junctional epithelium can occur, ultimately damaging the peri-implant attachment.[40]

Summary

For the formation of a good peri-implant soft tissue attachment, it is essential to use flapless implant surgery and perform early plaque control. Maintaining the peri-implant attachment requires meticulous plaque control and avoidance of implant overload (Figs 10-23 and 10-24).

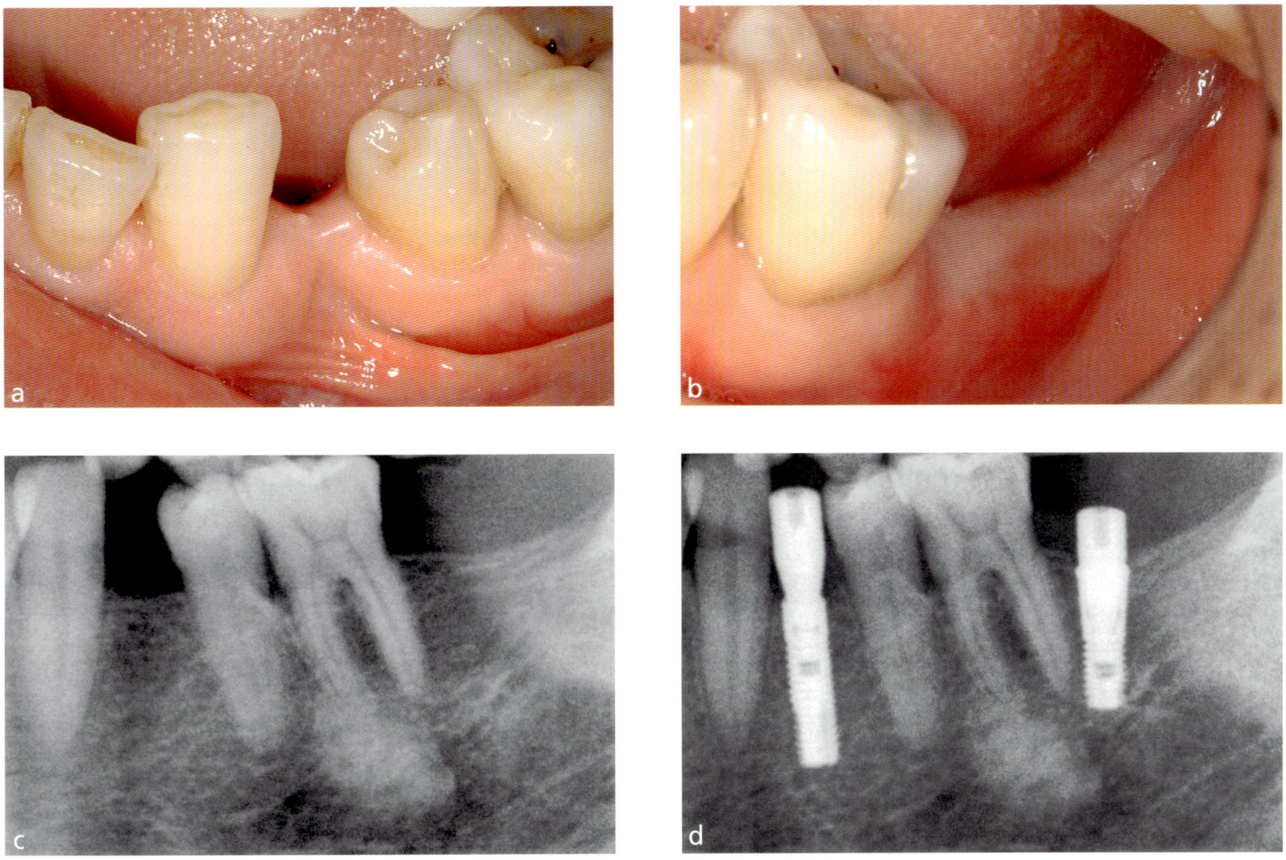

Fig 10-23 (a and b) Intraoral views of a patient with a missing lower first premolar and second molar. (c and d) Radiographs before and immediately after implant placement.

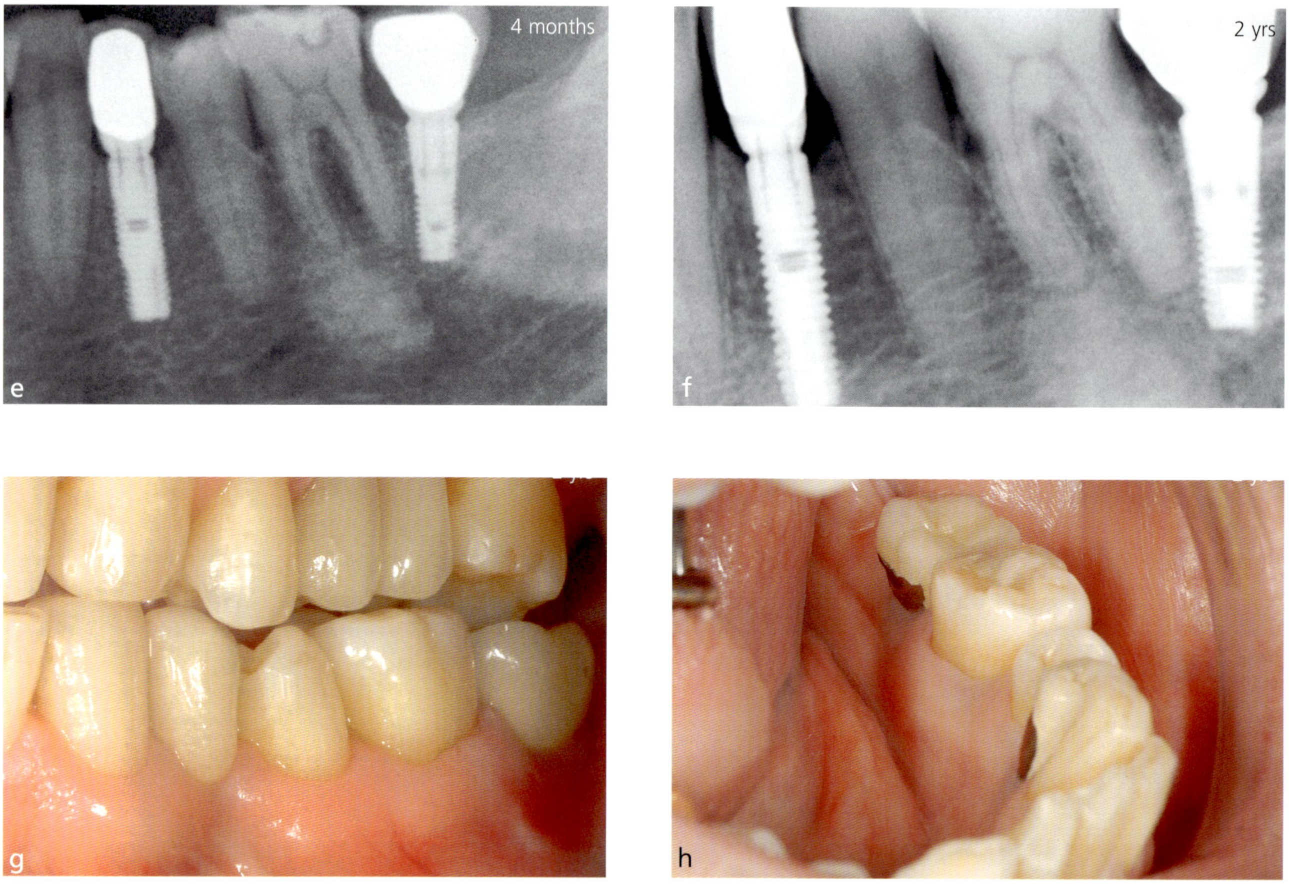

Fig 10-23 (*cont.*) (e and f) Radiographs 4 months and 2 years after placement. (g and h) Intraoral views 2 years after placement. Note the healthy peri-implant mucosa and bone.

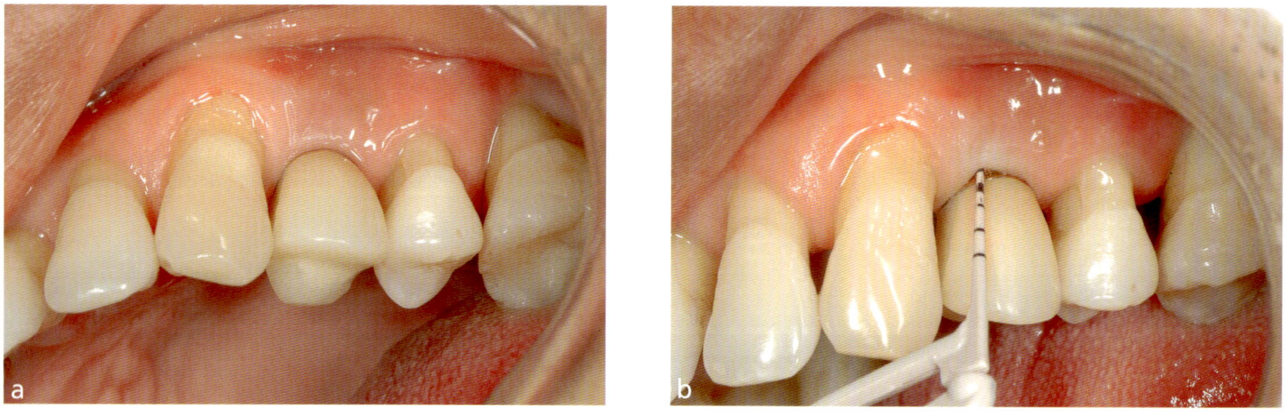

Fig 10-24 (a and b) Intraoral views of the implant prosthesis in the maxillary left first premolar region 1 year after prosthesis fabrication. Note the healthy peri-implant mucosa and shallow pocket depth around the implant.

References

1. Weinmann JP. Biological factors influencing implant denture success. J Implant Dent 1956;2:12–15.
2. James RA, Kelln E. A histopathological report on the nature of the epithelium and underlying connective tissue which surrounds implant posts. J Biomed Mat Res 1974;5:373.
3. McKinney RV, Steflik DE, Koth DL. Ultrastructural surface topography of the single crystal sapphire endosseous dental implant. J Prosthet Dent 1984;51:372–379.
4. McKinney RV Jr, Steflik DE, Koth DL. Evidence for a junctional epithelial attachment to ceramic dental implants: a transmission electron microscopic study. J Periodontol 1985;56:579–591.
5. Hansson HA, Ablrektsson T, Brånemark PI. Structural aspects of the interface between tissue and titanium implants. J Prosth Dent 1983;50:108–113.
6. Gould TR, Brunette DM, Westbury L. The attachment mechanism of epithelial cells to titanium in vitro. J Periodontal Res 1981;16:611–616.
7. Gould TR, Westbury L, Brunette DM. Ultrastructural study of the attachment of human gingiva to titanium in vivo. J Prosth Dent 1984;52:418–420.
8. Hashimoto M. Ultrastructure of the peri-implant junctional epithelium on single-crystal sapphire endosseous dental implant loaded with functional stress. J Oral Rehabil 1989;16:261–270.
9. Campbell JH, Terranova VP. Laminin: molecular organization and biological function. J Oral Pathol 1988;17:309–323.
10. McKinney RV, Steflik DE, Koth DL. The epithelium dental implant interface. J Oral Implants 1988;13:622–641.
11. Moon IS, Berglundh T, Abrahammson I, Lindhe E, Lindhe J. The barrier between the keratinized mucosa and the dental implant: an experimental study in the dog. J Clin Periodontol 1999;26:658–663.
12. Groessner-Schriber B. Focal adhesion contact formation by fibroblasts cultured on surface-modified dental implants: an in vitro study. Clin Oral Implants Res 2006;17:726–745.
13. Listgarten MA, Buser D, Steinemann SG, Donath K, Lang NP, Weber HP. Light and transmission electron microscopy of the interface between non-submerged titanium-coated epoxy resin implants and bone or gingiva. J Dent Res 1992;71:364–371.
14. Berglundh T, Lindhe J, Marinello C, Ericsson I, Liljenberg B. Soft tissue reaction to de-novo plaque formation on implants and teeth: an experimental study in the dog. Clin Oral Implants Res 1992;3:1–8.
15. Akagawa Y, Takata T, Matsumoto T, Nikai H, Tsuru H. Correlation between clinical and histological evaluations of the periimplant gingiva around the signe-crystal sapphire endosseous implant. J Oral Rehabil 1989;16:581–587.
16. Berglund T, Lindhe J, Jonsson K, Ericsson I. The topography of the vascular systems in the periodontal and peri-implant tissues in the dog. J Clin Periodontol 1994;21:189–193.
17. Ericsson I, Berglundh T, Marinello C, Liljenberg B, Lindhe J. Long standing plaque and gingivitis at implants and teeth in the dog. Clin Oral Implants Res 1992;3:99–103.
18. Noma H, Kaneko Y. A Color Atlas of Teeth Extraction in Dental Practice. Tokyo: Ishiyaku, 1991.
19. Berglundh T, Abrahamsson I, Welander M, Lang NP, Lindhe J. Morphogenesis of the peri-implant mucosa: an experimental study in dogs. Clin Oral Implants Res 2007;18:1–8.
20. Cardaropoli G, Lekholm U, Wennström JL. Tissue alterations at implant supported single tooth replacement: a 1-year prospective clinical study. Clin Oral Implants Res 2006;17:165–171.
21. Berglundh T, Lindhe J. Dimension of the peri-implant mucosa: biological width revisited. J Clin Periodontol 1996;23:971–973.
22. Berglundh T, Lindhe J, Ericsson I, Marinella CP, Liljenberg B, Thomsen P. The soft tissue barrier at implants and teeth. Clin Oral Implants Res 1991;2:81–90.
23. Abrahamsson I, Berglundh T, Wennström J, Lindhe J. The peri-implant hard and soft tissues at different implant systems: a comparative study in the dog. Clin Oral Implants Res 1996;7:212–219.
24. Buser D, Weber HP, Donath K, Fiorellini JP, Paquette DW, Williams RC. Soft tissue reactions to non-submerged unloaded titanium implants in beagle dog. J Periodontol 1992;63:226–236.
25. Abrahamsson I, Berglundh T, Lindhe J. The mucosal barrier following abutment dis/reconnection: an experimental study in dogs. J Clin Periodontol 1997;24:568–572.
26. Artzi Z, Tal H, Moses O, Kozlovsky A. Mucosal considerations for osseointegrated implants. J Prosth Dent 1993;70:427–432.
27. Zarb GA, Schmitt A. The longitudinal clinical effectiveness of osseointegrated dental implants (the Toronto study). III: Problems and complications encountered. J Prosth Dent 1990;64:185–194.
28. Abrahamsson I, Berglundh T, Glantz PO, Lindhe J. The mucosal attachment at different abutments: an experimental study in dogs. J Clin Periodontol 1998;25:721–727.
29. Abrahamsson I, Zitzmann NU, Berglundh T, Linder E, Wennerberg A, Lindhe J. The mucosal attachment to titanium implants with different surface characteristics: an experimental study in dogs. J Clin Periodontol 2002;29:448–455.
30. Wennerberg A, Sennerby L, Kultje C, Lekholm U. Some soft tissue characteristics at implant abutments with different surface topography: a study in humans. J Clin Periodontol 2003;30:88–94.
31. Bollen CM, Papaioannou W, Van Eldere J, Schepers E, Quirynen M, van Steenberghe D. The influence of abutment surface roughness on plaque accumulation and peri-implant mucositis. Clin Oral Implants Res 1996;7:201–211.
32. Quirynen M, van Steenberghe D. Bacterial colonization of the internal part of two-stage implants: an in-vitro study. Clin Oral Implant Res 1993;4:158–161.
33. Zitzmann NU, Abrahamsson I, Berglundh T, Lindhe J. Soft tissue reactions to plaque formation at implant abutments with different surface topography: an experimental study in dogs. J Clinical Periodontol 2002;29:456–461.
34. Sawase TWA, Hallgren C, Albrektsson T, Baba K. Chemical and topographical surface analysis of five different implant abutments. Clin Oral Implant Res 2000;11:44–50.
35. Esposito M, Hirsch J-M, Lekholm U, Thomsen P. Biological factors contributing to failures of osseointegrated oral implants. I: Success criteria and epidemiology. Eur J Oral Sci 1998;106:527–551.
36. Jemt T, Linden B, Lekholm U. Failures and complications in 127 consecutively placed fixed partial prostheses supported by Brånemark implants: from prosthetic treatment to first annual checkup. Int J Oral Maxillofac Implants 1992;7:40–44.
37. Misch CE. Early crestal bone loss etiology and its effect on treatment planning for implants. Postgrad Dent 1995;3:3–17.
38. Friberg B, Jemt T, Lekholm U. Early failures in 4641 consecutively placed Brånemark dental implants: a study from stage I surgery to the connection of completed prostheses. Int J Oral Maxillofac Implants 1991;6:142–146.
39. Misch CE. Contemporary Implant Dentistry, ed 2. St Louis, MO: Mosby, 1999:125–142.
40. Lindquist LW, Rockler B, Carlsson GE. Bone resorption around fixtures in edentulous patients treated with fixed tissue integrated prostheses. J Prosth Dent 1988;59:59–63.

CHAPTER 11

The Thick Mucosa

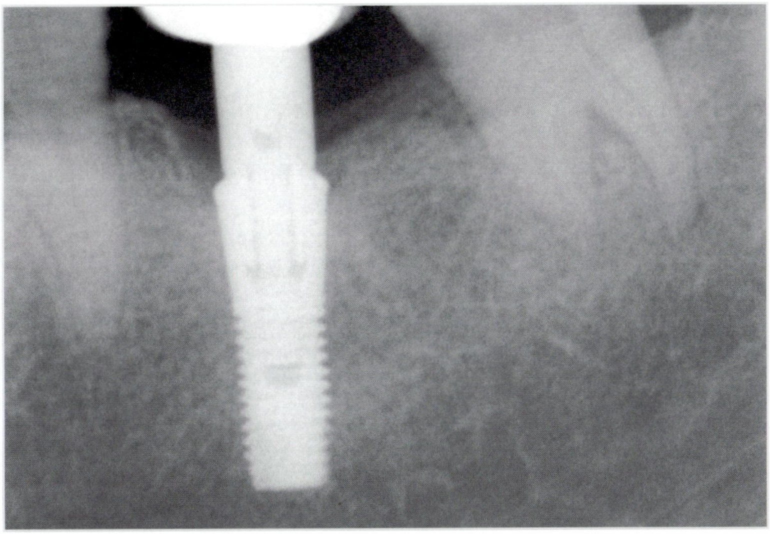

Key point

Flapless implant surgery helps to optimize the health of the peri-implant tissue in areas with thick mucosa.

Overview

The average thickness of the peri-implant mucosa is 3.0–3.5 mm.[1] It has been suggested that soft tissue thicker than 4 mm induces deep pockets, plaque accumulation, and mucositis around implants. However, the present authors have found that thick mucosa around flapless implants does not adversely affect peri-implant health and implant stability. This chapter addresses flapless implant surgery in areas with thick mucosa and the considerations related to surgery as well as its effects on peri-implant tissue healing.

Review of the literature

Studies have shown that the thick mucosa has significantly greater periodontal probing depth than thin mucosa.[2] Misch[3] reported that a mucosa thicker than 4 mm will result in a less-than-ideal pocket depth around the implant. As the sulcus depth increases beyond 4 mm, the incidence of anaerobic bacteria in the sulcus increases. When 75% of the bacteria are anaerobic, an active process places the region at risk of disease.[4–6] Dharmar et al.[7] identified elevated levels of proteolytic enzymes in the sulcus around implants with deep pockets. For this reason, many clinicians expect that the placement of implants in areas with thick mucosa can lead to deep pocket formation, progressive bone resorption, and a loss of the implant.[8–11] These clinicians recommend a correction of soft tissue thicker than 4 mm to achieve an ideal pocket depth around the implant.

However, the relationship between pocket depth and peri-implant tissue health is controversial. The hypothesis that the presence of thick mucosa will always lead to the destruction of the peri-implant tissue has not been proven. Lekholm et al.[12] reported that deep pockets are not always accompanied by accelerated marginal bone loss around the implants or by microflora or histological changes indicative of periodontitis. The suggestion that the presence of periodontitis-associated bacteria will necessarily lead to a destructive process in the peri-implant tissues also has not been proven. Some researchers have reported that deep pockets do not play a decisive etiological role in implant failure.[6,13] A review of the literature showed that no study has addressed this issue directly. For this reason, we performed experiments in animal models to determine the effect of thick mucosa on peri-implant tissue healing around dental implants.

Effect of thick mucosa on peri-implant tissues after flap implant surgery

When implants were placed in dogs in the alveolar ridge with 6–8 mm thick mucosa using a flap implant procedure and meticulous plaque control, the condition of the peri-implant mucosa 6 months later was normal – it showed no signs of inflammation. Histometric measurements showed that, in the alveolar ridge with 6–8 mm thickness of mucosa, the length of the junctional epithelium was 3.1 mm and the zone of connective tissue integration was 4.1 mm long (Table 11-1). Hence the height of the mucosa, the length of the junctional epithelium, and the height of the zone of connective tissue integration were significantly higher in the thick mucosa than in normal mucosa. This suggests that implantation in areas with thick mucosa may provide conditions for mucosa integration with longer zones of both the junctional epithelium and connective tissue. In this study, the junctional epithelium was located coronal to the abutment/fixture border with respect to the apical termination of the junctional epithelium. Although the junctional epithelium was extended more apically into the thick mucosa than in the normal mucosa, neither marginal bone resorption nor signs of inflammation were observed at the thick mucosa sites during a 6-month observation period (Figs 11-1 and 11-2).[14]

Table 11-1 Effect of thick mucosa on peri-implant tissue after flap implant surgery.

	Normal mucosa	Thick mucosa	*P* value
PM–B (mm ± SD)	3.5 ± 0.7	7.2 ± 1.8	< .05
PM–aJE (mm ± SD)	1.5 ± 0.3	3.1 ± 0.6	< .05
aJE–B (mm ± SD)	2.0 ± 0.4	4.1 ± 1.2	< .05
A/F–B (mm ± SD)	0.5 ± 0.3	0.3 ± 0.2	> .05

PM – marginal position of the peri-implant mucosa; aJE – apical termination of the junctional epithelium; B – marginal level of bone to implant contact

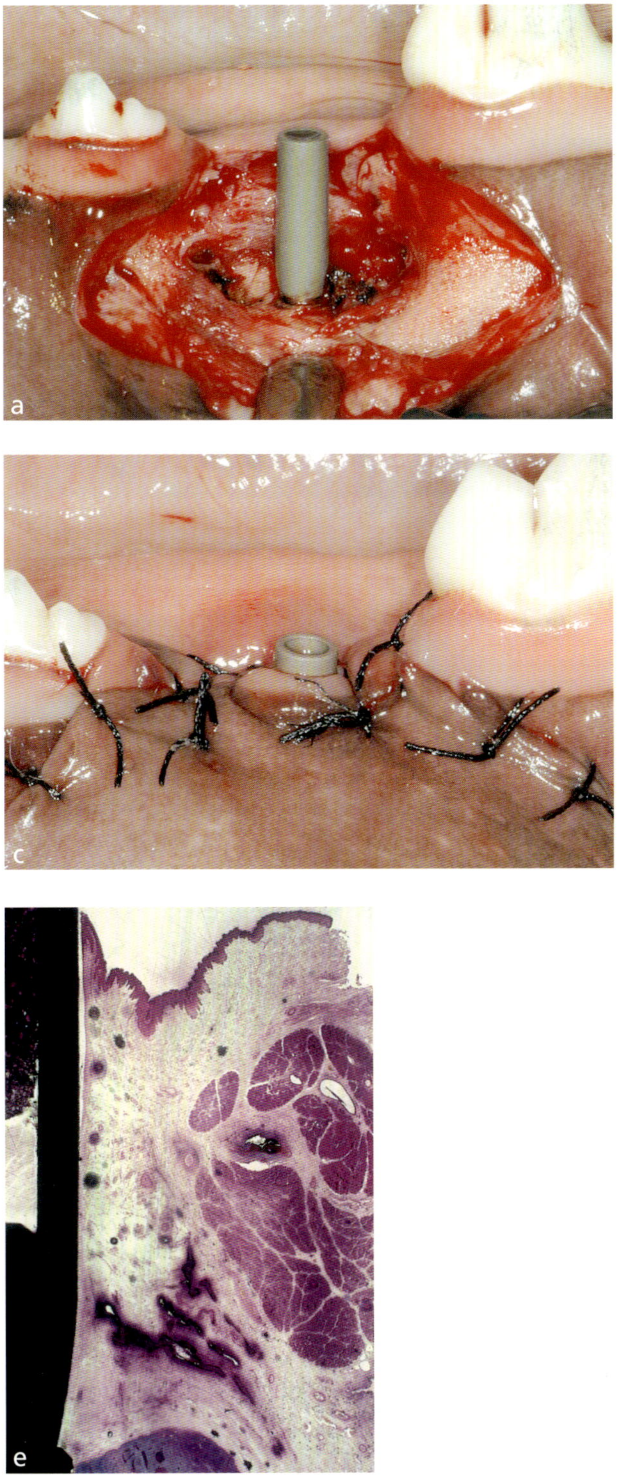

Fig 11-1 Effect of thick mucosa on peri-implant tissues after flap implant surgery in a canine model. (a–c) An implant was placed in the mandibular region with bone defect (8.0 mm in height) using a flap procedure and a long abutment was connected to the fixture. (d) After 6 months of plaque control, the condition of the mucosa at the implant site is normal. (e) Histological sections show that the height of the mucosa, the length of the junctional epithelium, and the height of the zone of connective tissue integration are significantly greater in the thick mucosa than in the normal mucosa. This suggests that the junctional epithelium extends more apically in the thick mucosa than in the normal mucosa.

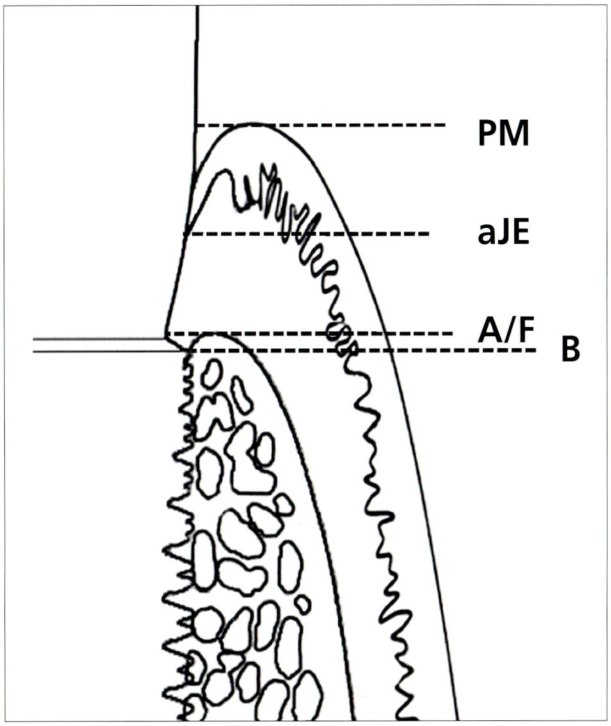

Fig 11-2 Schematic illustrating the landmarks used for histometric measurements. PM – the marginal portion of the peri-implant mucosa; aJE – the level of the apical termination of the junctional epithelium; B – the marginal level of bone to implant contact; A/F – the abutment–fixture borderline

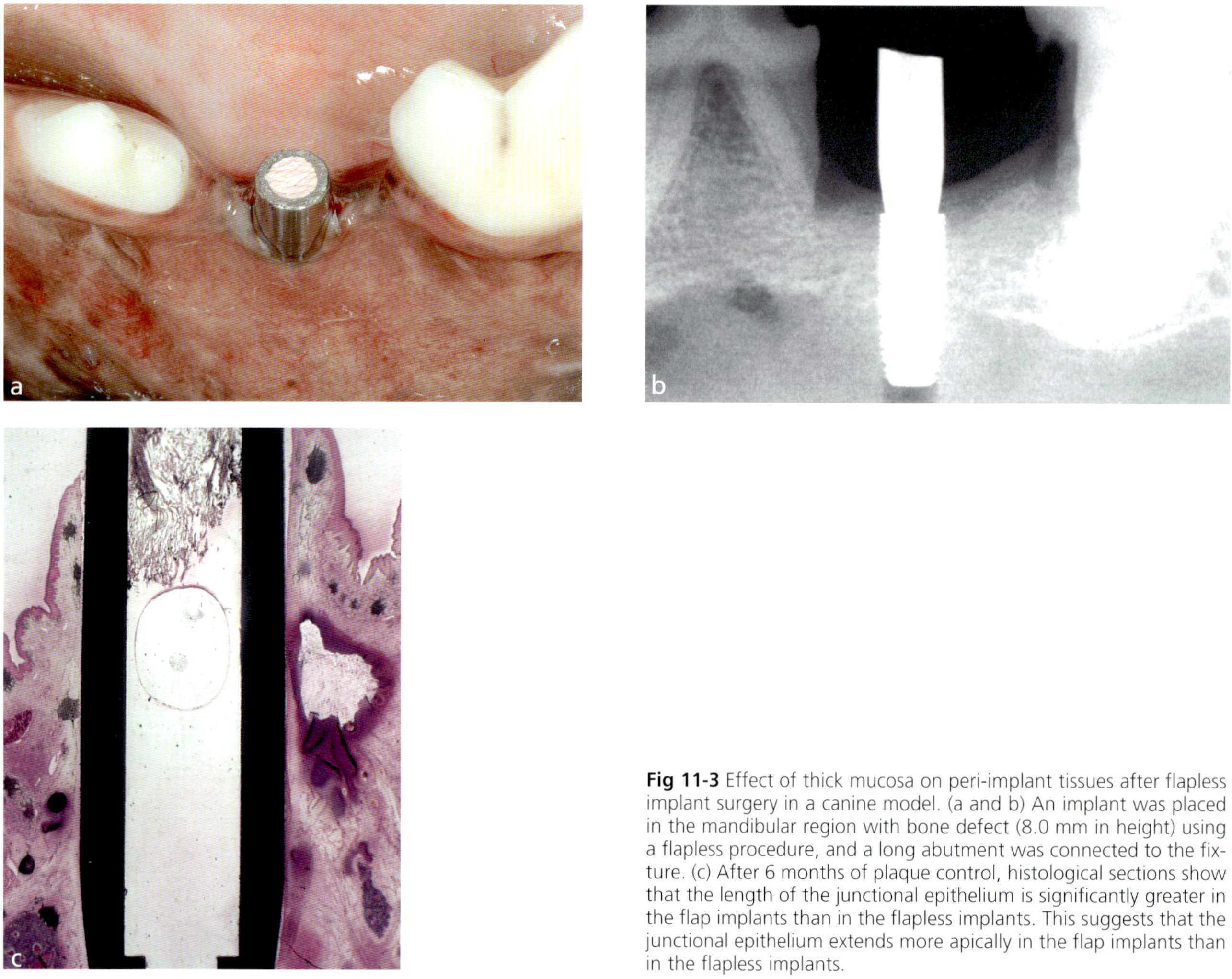

Fig 11-3 Effect of thick mucosa on peri-implant tissues after flapless implant surgery in a canine model. (a and b) An implant was placed in the mandibular region with bone defect (8.0 mm in height) using a flapless procedure, and a long abutment was connected to the fixture. (c) After 6 months of plaque control, histological sections show that the length of the junctional epithelium is significantly greater in the flap implants than in the flapless implants. This suggests that the junctional epithelium extends more apically in the flap implants than in the flapless implants.

These findings support the clinical use of implants in sites with a thick mucosa. The peri-implant sulcus depth increases when implants are placed in alveolar ridges with thick mucosa, but the peri-implant tissue can remain healthy provided meticulous plaque control is performed.

Comparison of flap and flapless procedures on peri-implant tissue healing

A canine study was carried out to compare the effects of flap and flapless surgery on peri-implant tissue healing around the implants placed in areas with thick mucosa (Fig 11-3). When implants were placed in the alveolar ridge with 6–8 mm thickness of mucosa using flap or flapless implant procedures followed by meticulous plaque control, the length of the junctional epithelium was signifi-

Table 11-2 When implants were placed in the alveolar ridge with thick mucosa using flap or flapless implant procedures, the length of the junctional epithelium is significantly greater in the flap implants than in the flapless implants.

	Flap implants	Flapless implants	*P* value
PM–B (mm ± SD)	7.2 ± 1.8	7.0 ± 1.3	> .05
PM–aJE (mm ± SD)	3.1 ± 0.6	2.3 ± 0.4	< .05
aJE–B (mm ± SD)	4.1 ± 1.2	4.5 ± 0.7	> .05
A/F–B (mm ± SD)	0.3 ± 0.2	0.2 ± 0.3	> .05

PM, marginal position of the peri-implant mucosa; aJE, apical termination of the junctional epithelium; B, marginal level of bone to implant contact.

Table 11-3 Description of all implants placed at the thick mucosa sites for the flap group.

Patient no	Mucosal thickness (mm)	Implant location	Implant size (diameter × length)	Observation time (months)	Number of implants
1	ï6	14	4.0 × 13	24	1
2	6, 5, 6	24, 25, 26	4.5 × 13, 4.5 × 13, 4.5 × 11	27	3
3	5, 7	15, 17	4.5 × 11, 4.5 × 9	27	2
4	5	13	4.5 × 13	34	1
5	6	14	4.0 × 13	33	1
6	7	14, 16	4.5 × 13, 4.5 × 9	25	2
7	5	22	4.5 × 13	39	1
8	5	14	4.0 × 13	38	1
9	6	23	4.5 × 15	32	1
10	7	12	3.5 × 15	36	1

Implant location: 16 is the maxillary right first molar. 22 is the maxillary left lateral incisor.

cantly higher in the flap implants than in the flapless implants (Table 11-2). Hence flapless implant surgery is advantageous in terms of reducing the sulcus depth around the implants in the areas with thick mucosa.

To determine whether the results of the animal study are in accordance with clinical findings, a prospective clinical study was carried out in 25 implants placed in areas with thick mucosa using either flap or flapless implant procedures. The inclusion criteria were a mucosa thickness of at least 5 mm at the time of implant placement and a more than 2-year follow-up period after the treatment.

- *Flap implant group.* This consisted of ten patients (seven females) ranging in age from 21 to 65 years (mean 41.5 years). A total of 14 Astra dental implants (Astra Tech Implant System™, Mölndal, Sweden) of various lengths were used (Table 11-3). Implant placement was performed with flap elevation. The mucosal flaps were closed with sutures, and the implants were fully submerged. In the second-stage procedure, the submerged fixtures were uncovered using the same flap procedure (Figs 11-4 and 11-5).
- *Flapless implant group.* This consisted of eight patients (five females) ranging in age from 37 to 68 years (mean

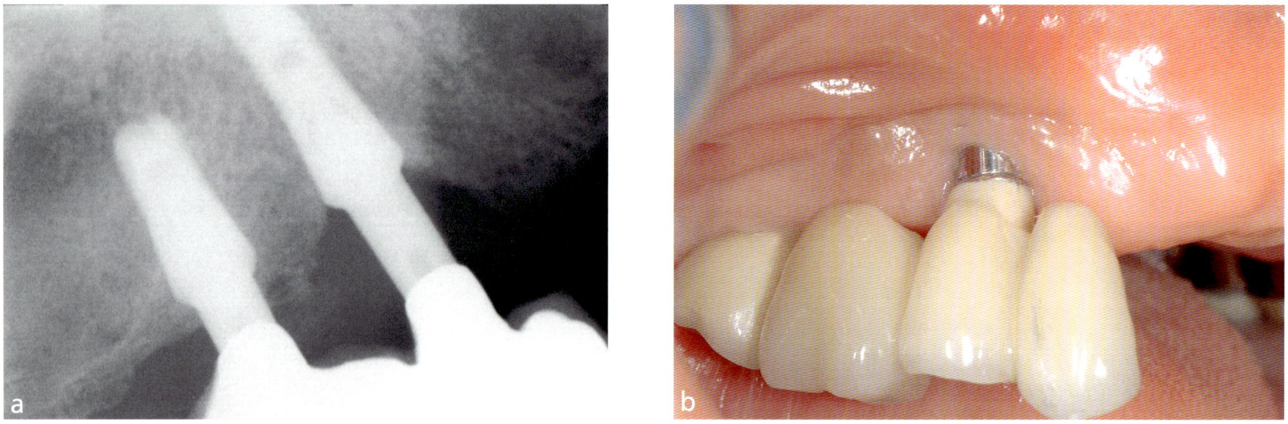

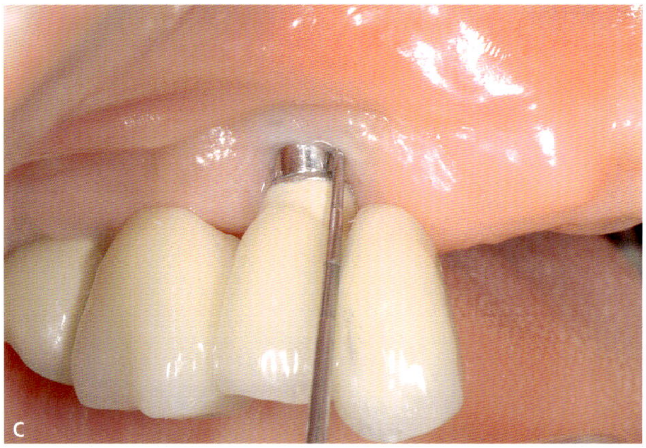

Fig 11-4 (a–c) Implant placement was performed with flap elevation in a patient with an alveolar ridge with 7 mm thickness of mucosa. Over a 2-year follow-up, the probing depths increased up to 5.7 mm in areas with thick mucosa, but the patient had no marginal bone loss or inflammation during this period.

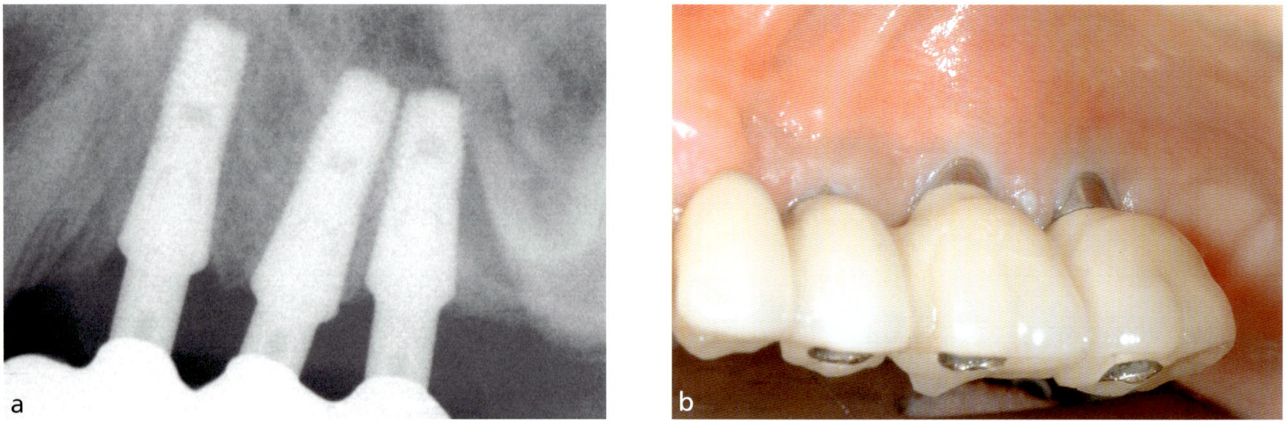

Fig 11-5 (a and b) Implant placement was performed with flap elevation in a patient with a 5–6 mm thickness of mucosa in the alveolar ridge. Over a 2-year follow-up, the probing depths increased up to 4.3 mm in the areas with thick mucosa, but the patient had no marginal bone loss or inflammation during this period.

51.4 years). A total of seven Astra dental implants (Astra Tech Implant System™) of various lengths were used in addition to four Osstem implants (Osstem Implant Co., Seoul, Korea) (Table 11-4). The implants were placed without flap elevation and fully submerged. In the second-stage procedure, the submerged fixtures were uncovered using the same flapless procedure (Figs 11-6 and 11-7).

The implants that had been in function for 2 years at the follow-up examination were evaluated using clinical and radiological parameters, including the Plaque Index, Gingival Index, presence of bleeding on probing, probing pocket depth, degree of mobility, and amount of marginal bone loss (Table 11-5).

There was no marginal bone resorption in either the flap or flapless groups. The pocket probing depth was

Table 11-4 Description of all implants at the thick musoca sites for the flapless group.

Patient no	Mucosal thickness (mm)	Implant location	Implant size (diameter × length)	Observation time (months)	Number of implants
1	7, 6	14, 16	4.0 × 13, 4.5 × 11	25	2
2	6	36	4.5 × 13	27	1
3	5	13	4.0 × 15	29	1
4	6	25	4.5 × 13	25	1
5	7	15	4.5 × 11	24	1
6	5, 6	24, 26	4.0 × 13, 4.0 × 9	26	2
7	5, 6	15, 27	3.5 × 13, 4.0 × 11	24	2
8	5	14	4.5 × 13	28	1

Implant location: 16 is the maxillary right first molar; 22 is the maxillary left lateral incisor.

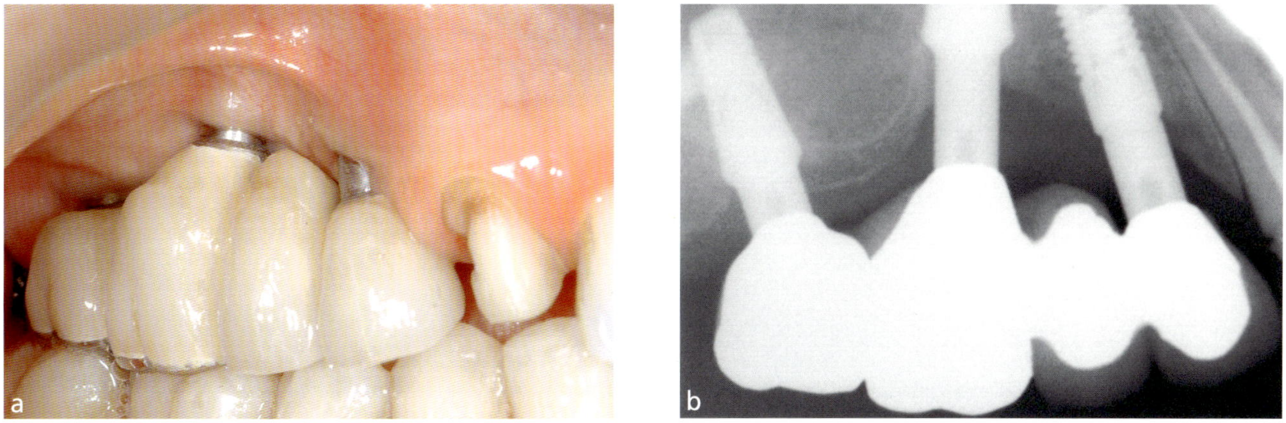

Fig 11-6 (a and b) Implant placement was performed without flap elevation in a patient with a 6–7 mm thickness of mucosa in the alveolar ridge. The average probing depth over a 2-year follow-up was 3.1 mm in areas with thick mucosa. The patient showed no marginal bone loss or inflammation during this period.

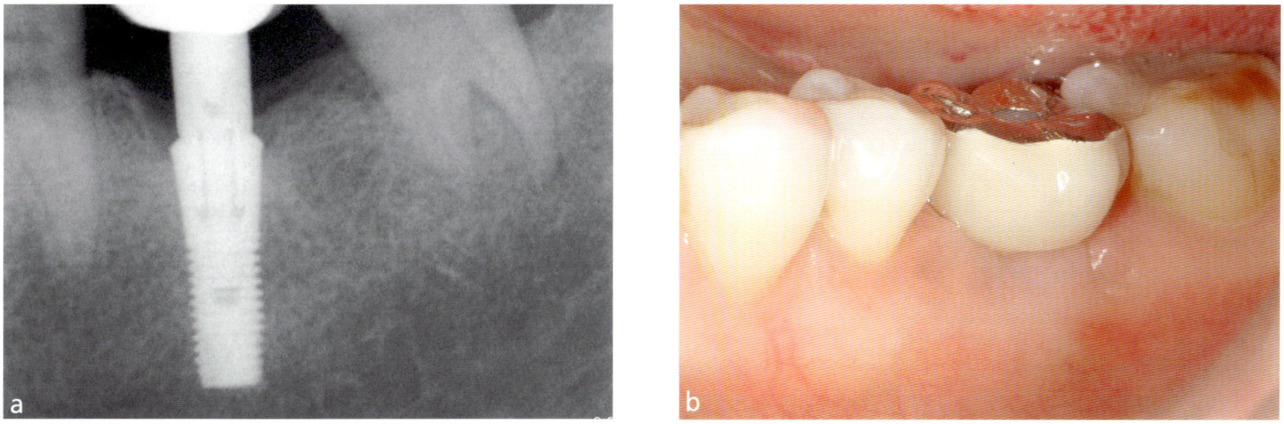

Fig 11-7 (a and b) Implant placement was performed without flap elevation in a patient with a 6 mm thickness of mucosa in the alveolar ridge. Over a 2-year follow-up, the probing depth was 3.1 mm in the area with thick mucosa. The site had no marginal bone loss or inflammation during this period.

Table 11-5 Average measures of the probing pocket depth (PPD), marginal bone loss, Modified Plaque Index (mPI), Gingival Index (GI) assessments, and the presence of bleeding on probing (BOP) for the flap and flapless implants placed at the thick mucosa sites.

	Flap group	Flapless group	*P* value
PPD (mean ± SD)	5.5 ± 0.9 mm	3.3 ± 0.8 mm	< .05
Marginal bone loss	0.0 ± 0.0 mm	0.0 ± 0.0 mm	> .05
Perio-test value (± SD)	–(4.0 ± 3.4)	–(4.6 ± 2.9)	> .05
Percentage of sites with:			
mPI > 0	30.1	34.3	> .05
GI > 0	59.3	30.1	< .05
BOP = 1	49.1	37.1	< .05

significantly higher in the flap group. The average pocket probing depths were 5.5 ± 0.9 mm and 3.3 ± 0.8 mm in the flap and flapless groups, respectively ($P < .05$). With respect to the status of the peri-implant mucosal health or inflammation, 59.3% and 30.1% of the sites were labeled with a Gingival Index greater than zero in the flap and flapless groups, respectively; this difference was statistically significant ($P < .05$). The majority of sites corresponded to a Gingival Index of 1. Bleeding on probing was detected in 49.1% and 37.1% of the sites in the flap and flapless groups, respectively, mostly in the form of a discrete blood point at the place where the periodontal probe had been applied. The study described above showed that, although the probing depths increased up to 5.5 mm (range 4.2–6.8) in the areas with thick mucosa, no marginal bone loss was observed at 2-year follow-up; that is, the probing depth itself does not appear to affect the marginal bone loss. Interestingly, other implants placed in the areas with normal mucosa showed even higher resorption values than the sites with thick mucosa. The reason for this is unclear. One explanation might be that the tissue thickness acts as a cushion over the implant, protecting the zone of osseointegration from the factors released from plaque and the oral cavity. Another interpretation might be that oral hygiene was acceptable in all patients during the follow-up years, which may have had a positive influence on the results. In patients with the appropriate oral hygiene, a thick mucosa around the implants does not appear to adversely affect the peri-implant health and stability. One interesting finding was that the probing depth in the flap group was greater than the corresponding value in the flapless group. It appears that when no flaps are reflected, the preservation of the soft tissue around the implants may help to optimize the healing of the peri-implant tissue and reduce the pocket depth. Flapless implant procedures should be considered in areas with thick mucosa because they have the advantage of reducing probing depths in a thick mucosa.

Considerations related to implant placement in thick mucosal sites

Vertical bone resorption before implant placement may result in increased soft tissue height in the edentulous sites. In these cases, the geometry of the soft tissue is an important factor to take into account when considering ridge augmentation. The soft tissue is evaluated to assess the height, width, and crown height space. The soft tissue volume is the most important dimension for esthetic results because the increased height and thin width of the soft tissue in implant sites increases the risk of gingival shrinkage after implant placement (Fig 11-8).

If there is inadequate soft tissue volume, surgical techniques – such as ridge augmentation or soft tissue grafting – are indicated to prevent gingival recession. The peri-implant mucosa usually requires more than 2 mm of soft tissue thickness to ensure a sufficient soft tissue blood supply around the implant for predictable survival. Therefore, a flapless implant procedure without a ridge augmentation procedure should be considered when implants are placed in regions with a relatively thick bulk of soft tissue.

The crown height space measured from the crest of the bone to the occlusal plane increases owing to vertical bone resorption in the thick mucosal sites (Fig 11-9). Two options should be considered in the case of excessive crown height space.[15-20] The first is the surgical method to increase the bone height. Surgical augmentation of the residual ridge height will reduce the crown height space and improve implant biomechanics (Fig 11-10).[15-17] The second option is a stress reduction method for the prosthesis.[18,19] If prosthesis stress reduction methods cannot compensate for the increase in force to the implants and the patient demands an esthetic prosthesis, an augmentation procedure may be required before surgical placement of the implants.

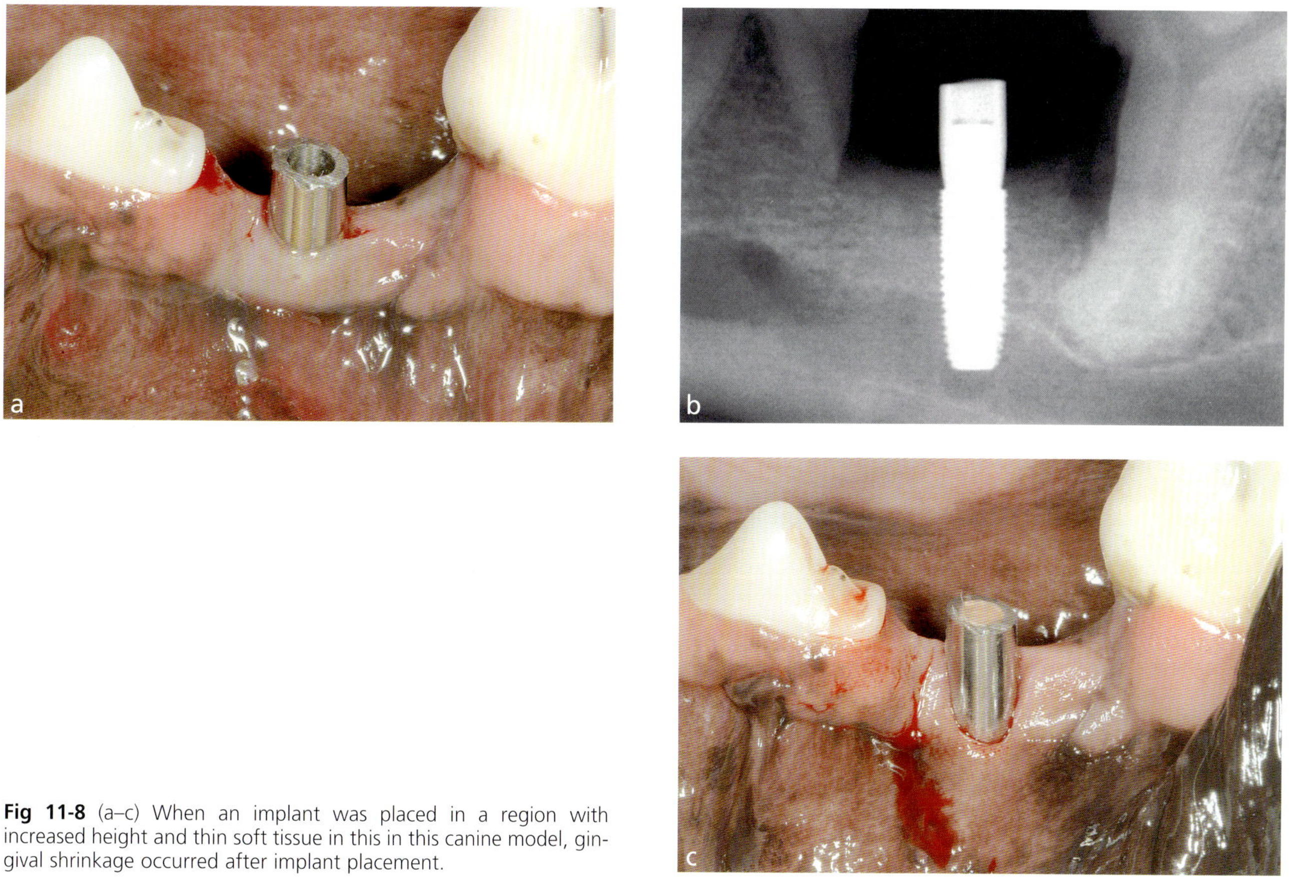

Fig 11-8 (a–c) When an implant was placed in a region with increased height and thin soft tissue in this in this canine model, gingival shrinkage occurred after implant placement.

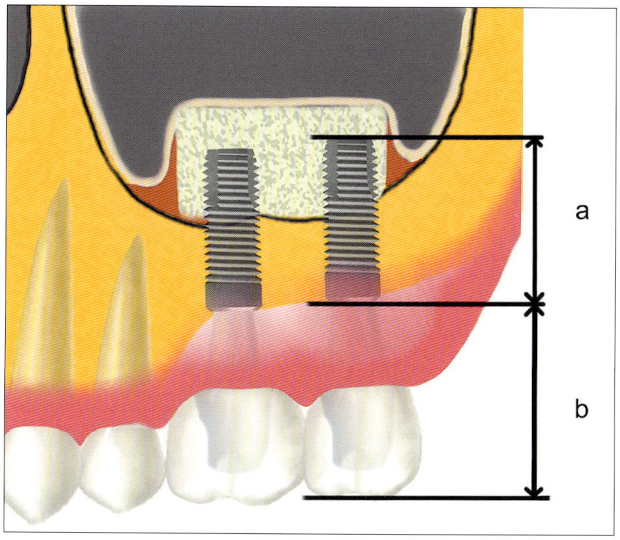

Fig 11-9 Crown height space measured from the crest of the bone to the occlusal plane increases owing to vertical bone resorption in the thick mucosal sites. The force applied to the implants increases with increasing height of the space.

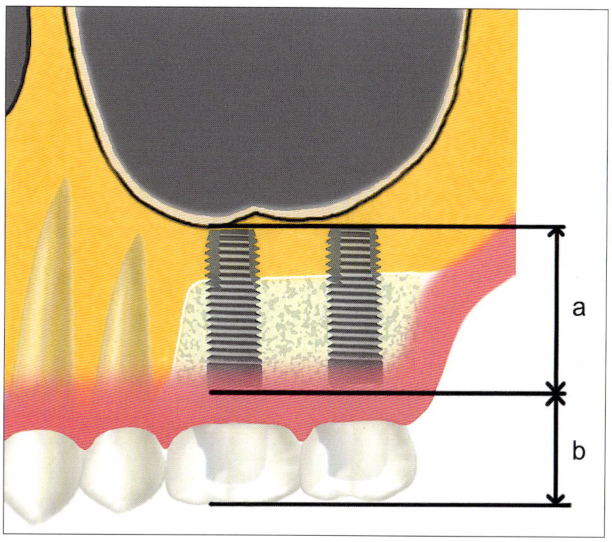

Fig 11-10 Bone augmentation should be performed to increase bone height if the crown height to bone height ratio is significantly large owing to a decreased alveolar bone height.

Arguments against the necessity for thick mucosa correction

Misch[3] recommended correction of soft tissue thicker than 4 mm to ensure an ideal pocket depth around the implant. However, the necessity of correcting the thick mucosa as a precondition for implant success appears to be questionable for the following reasons.

- Complications associated with gingivoplasty to reduce the tissue thickness must be considered. Gingivoplasty performed at the initial implant surgery can cause complications, such as wound dehiscence, infection, bone loss, or implant failure. The procedure performed at stage II uncovering after initial bone healing can also cause bone loss or implant failure.
- The integrity and vascularity of the mucosa must be considered when handling the mucosa. Surgery to thin the soft tissue may damage the blood vessels of the periosteum. The bone regeneration capability of the periosteum can also be damaged by surgical trauma. The surgical process can cause extensive scar formation around the implants, with the loss of blood vessels. A decrease in blood vessels will result in diminished healing and defensive ability.[21]
- As the surgery to reduce tissue thickness is delicate and sensitive to the technique, occasional poor clinical outcomes occur in association with the surgical procedure.
- Flapless implant surgery without a correction of the thick mucosa in regions with a thick bulk of soft tissue is effective in developing inflammation resistance of soft tissue surrounding the implants. The soft tissue adjacent to the implant has blood vessels after flapless surgery, which may increase its resistance to inflammation. Maintaining a good environment for the health of the tissue adjacent to the implant will ensure the success of the implant.
- The flapless implant procedure has the advantage of reducing the peri-implant sulcus depth.
- Thick soft tissue can act as a cushion over the implant, protecting the zone of osseointegration.
- A thick mucosa is more resistant to trauma and inflammation than a thin mucosa.
- There is no correlation between the peri-implant mucosa thickness and peri-implant tissue health.[22]

Considering all these points, flapless implant placement should be considered without the need to correct the thick mucosa in regions with thick soft tissue.

Flapless implant procedure in a thick mucosa

A comprehensive evaluation of the surgical site is essential for surgical planning. This evaluation includes the soft and hard tissue topography and esthetic concerns. The height of the soft and hard tissues is evaluated using radiographs (Fig 11-11).

Preparation and antisepsis

Preparation of the surgical site is important for reducing contamination by the patient's own normal flora. Intraoral preparation of the surgical site should be performed using a 0.12% chlorhexidine gluconate scrub and rinse. Extraoral presurgical scrubbing of the skin should also be carried out with chlorhexidine antiseptics. Adequate infiltration anesthesia can be obtained at the implant site.

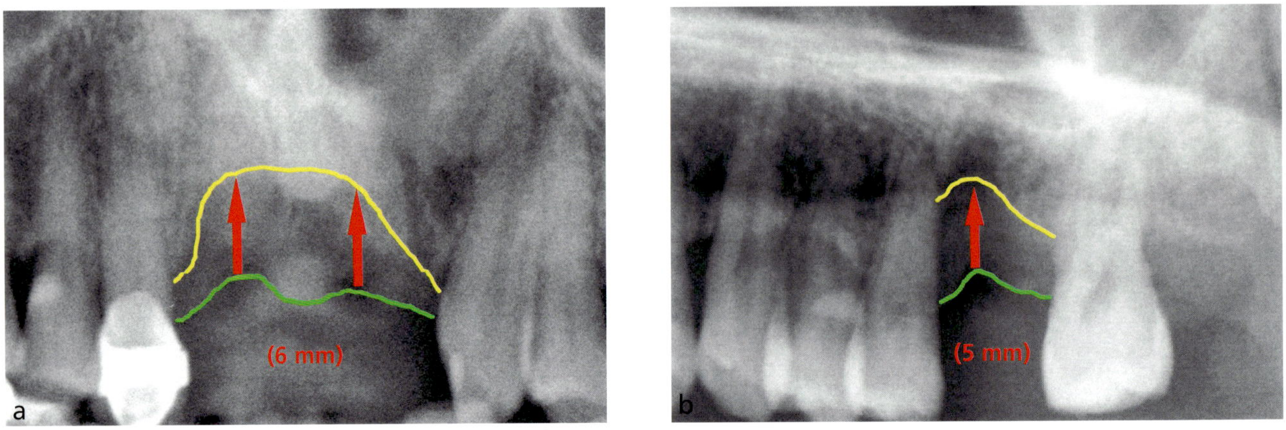

Fig 11-11 (a and b) The height of soft and hard tissues is evaluated using radiographs.

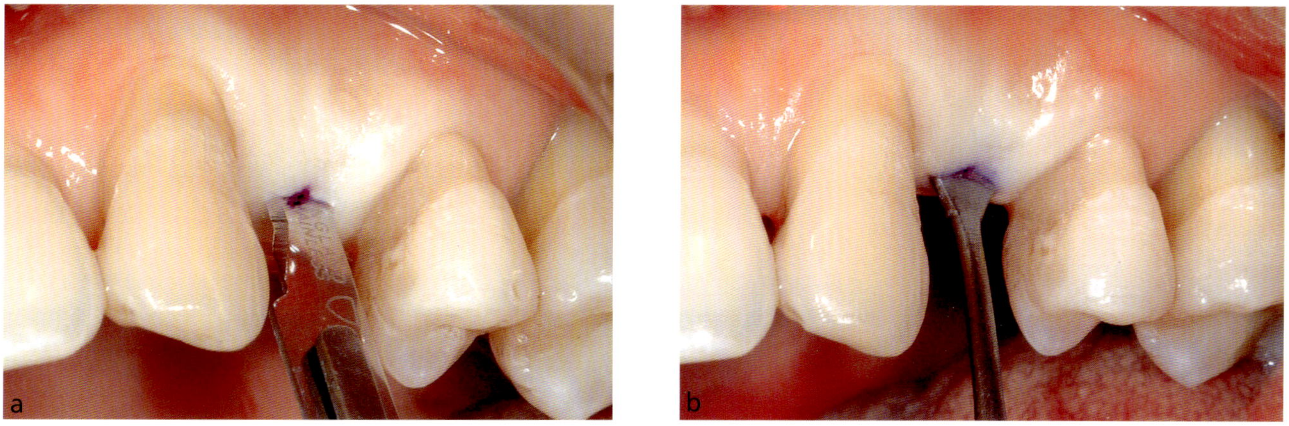

Fig 11-12 (a and b) For implant placement in areas with thick mucosa, a crestal mini-incision approximately 5 mm horizontally with the alveolar crest is made at the center of the implant site, and then local undermining of the gingiva is performed. The amount of undermining should not exceed 5 mm and should fall within the range of a large-diameter implant.

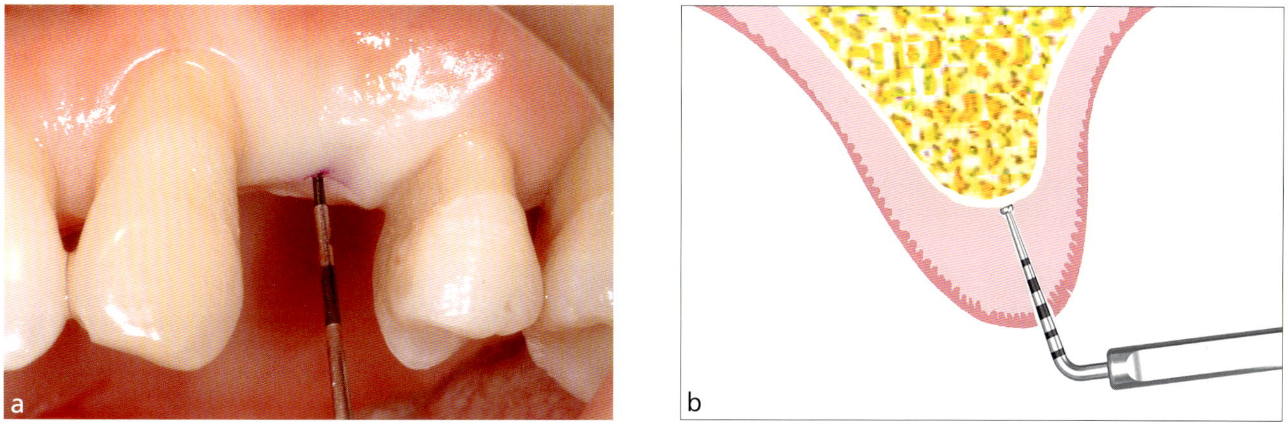

Fig 11-13 (a and b) Prior to drilling, the mucosal thickness is measured using a periodontal probe or a depth gauge to control the depth of drilling above the mucosa.

The incision

For mini-incision implant placement, a crestal mini-incision approximately 5 mm horizontally with the alveolar crest is made at the center of the implant site, followed by local undermining of the gingiva. The amount of undermining at the implant site should not exceed 5 mm and must fall within the range of a large-diameter implant (Fig 11-12).

Intraoperative measurement of mucosal thickness

To control the depth of drilling, the mucosal thickness is measured using a periodontal probe or a depth gauge prior to drilling (Fig 11-13). The sum of the length of the implant and the thickness of the mucosa is marked on the drills.

Drilling

To minimize damage to the mucosa while preparing the implant site, the drills should be used at low speed to prepare the implant site because the cutting surface of the drill contacts the mucosa (Figs 11-14 and 11-15). Soft tissue is likely to be cut while drilling through a small opening. As a result, the use of drills with a cutting surface on the tip and a rounded surface on the other parts is advisable. Osteotomes may be used to prepare the osteotomy site in the maxilla instead of drills because they can protect the soft tissue. The surgical sites are rinsed thoroughly and suctioned to remove any debris or contaminants before inserting the implant.

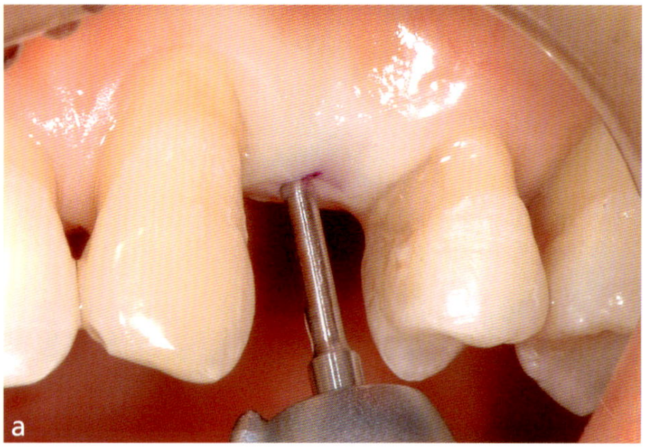
a

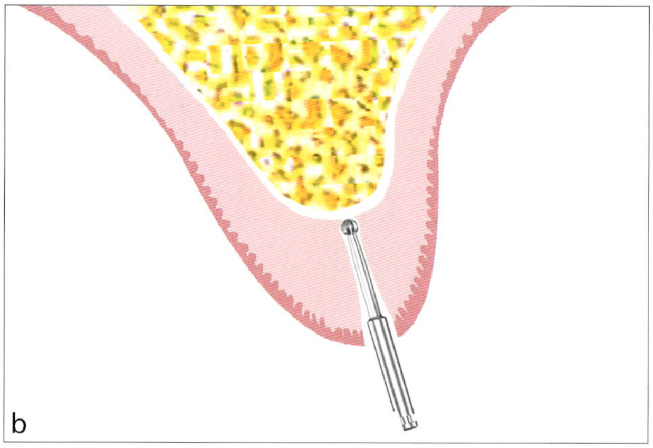
b

Fig 11-14 (a and b) A pilot hole for the implant osteotomy is made with a round or pilot bur.

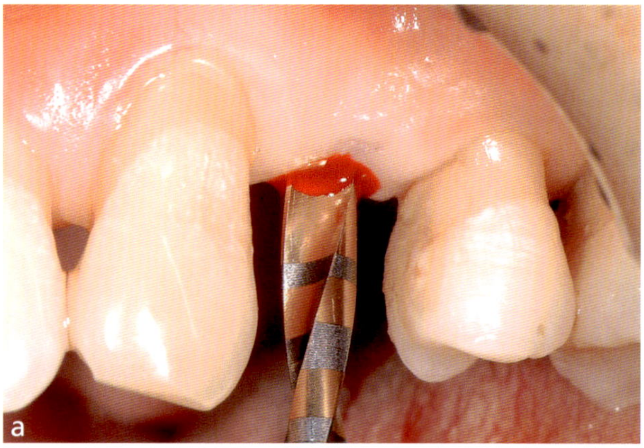
a

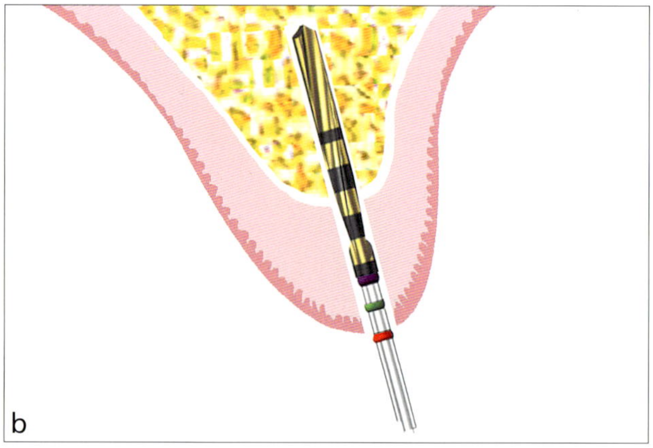
b

Fig 11-15 (a and b) Drilling at the areas with thick mucosa is likely to damage the adjacent mucosa, because the cutting surface of the drill contacts the mucosa. Drills should be used to prepare an implant site at a low speed to minimize such damage. The use of flapless implant drills with cutting surfaces on their tips and rounded surfaces on their other parts is advisable.

Implant placement

The depth of implant insertion above the mucosa is controlled by the depth line corresponding to the sum of the implant length and mucosa thickness. The implant crest module is located at the level of the bone crest (Fig 11-16). The cover screw is inserted (Fig 11-17), and then the implant is submerged for a two-stage approach or a permucosal healing abutment is inserted for a one-stage approach. A two-stage approach is used when the implant is threaded into position with 20 Ncm or less (Fig 11-18). A one-stage surgical approach is used when the implant is threaded into position with more than 20 Ncm (Fig 11-19). This one-stage approach eliminates the second-stage surgery and allows the tissue to mature at the time of prosthetic fabrication.

After inserting the healing abutments, the peri-implant mucosa is evaluated for any irregular edges. These should be cut and removed because the final soft tissue contour is dependent on the early form of the soft tissue.

For nonsubmerged implants in areas with thick mucosa, caution is needed to prevent an excessive load on the implants. When a lateral force is applied to the abutment, the forces are magnified in proportion to the abutment height. The abutment height is a force magnifier. The force applied to the implants increases with increasing height of the healing abutment to the crest of the bone. Implant failure can occur as a result of overload. Crestal bone loss can also be related to excessive load to the implants.

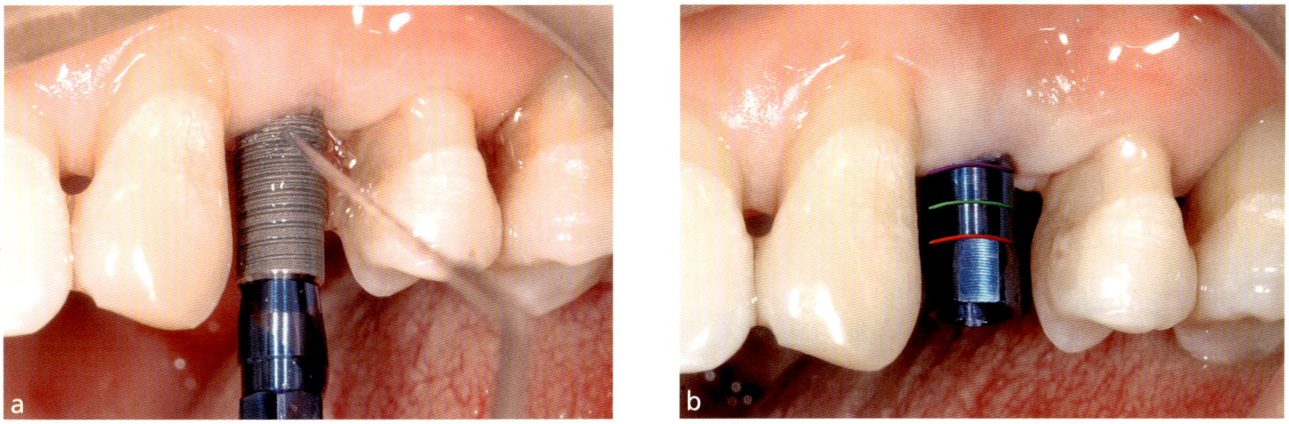

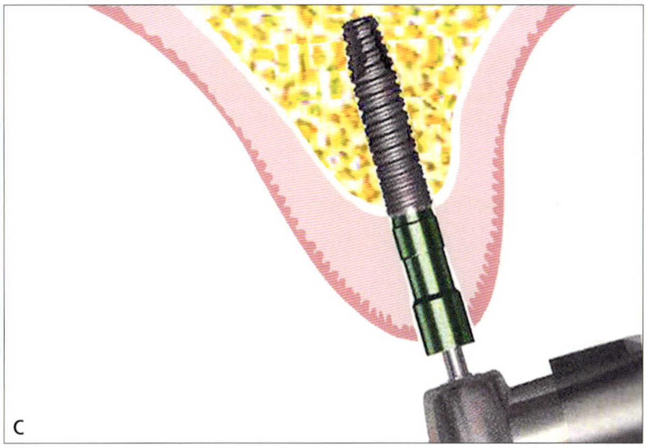

Fig 11-16 (a–c) The depth of implant insertion is controlled above the mucosa by a depth line corresponding to the sum of the length of the implant and the thickness of the mucosa. The implant crest module is located in the level of the bone crest.

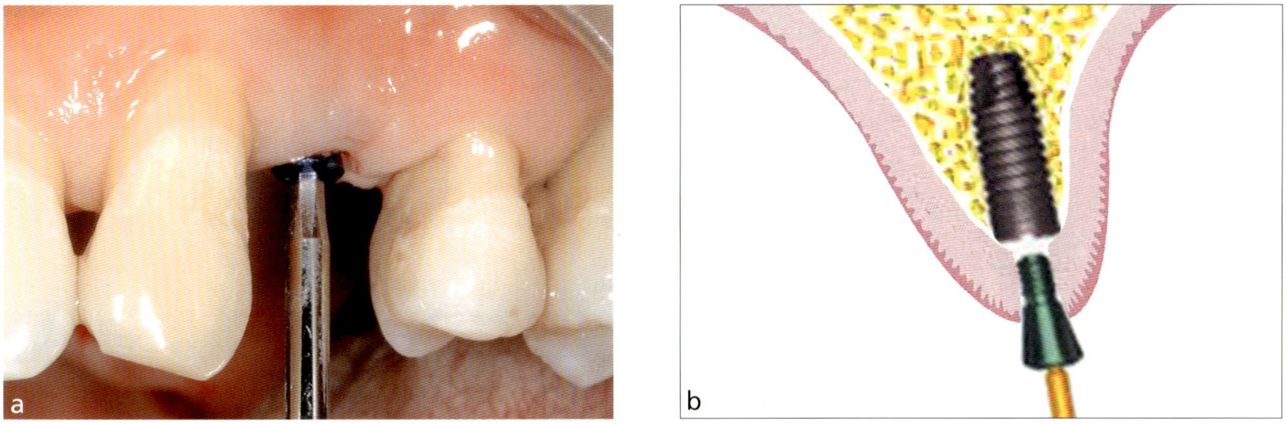

Fig 11-17 (a and b) Cover screw insertion.

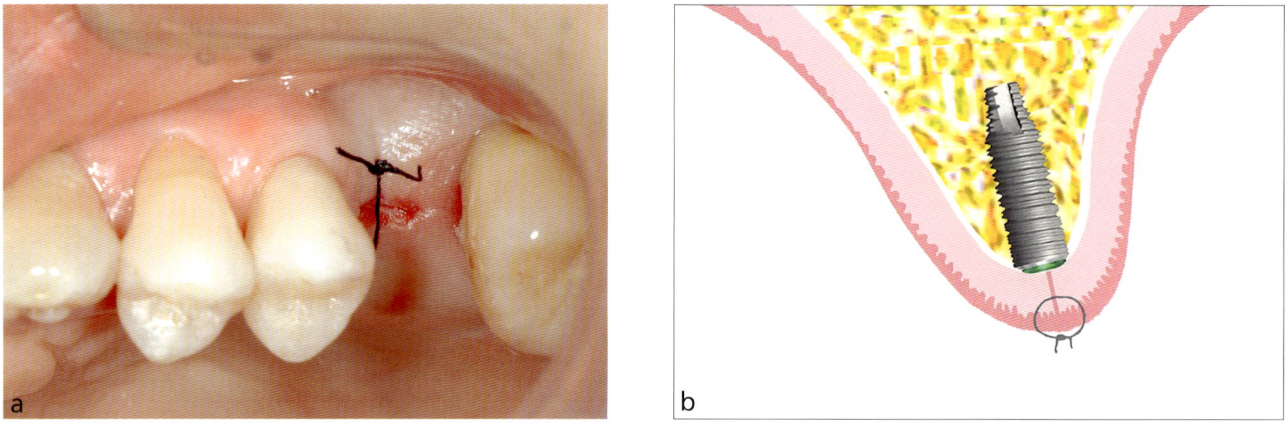

Fig 11-18 (a and b) The implant is submerged after being threaded into position with a maximum torque of 20 Ncm.

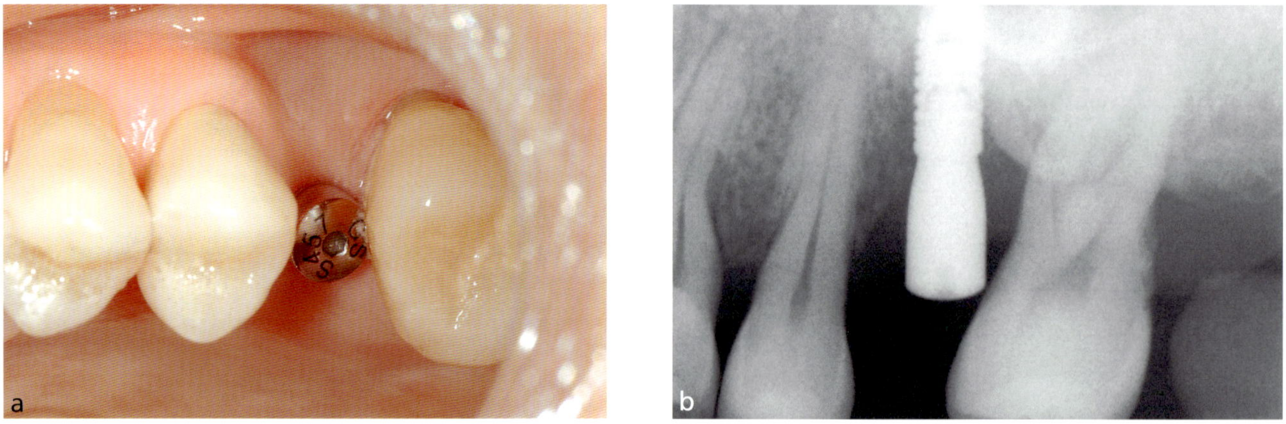

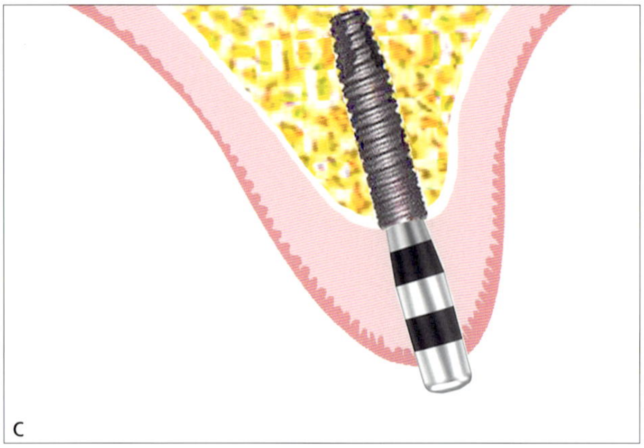

Fig 11-19 (a–c) A permucosal healing abutment is inserted and not submerged when the implant is threaded into position with more than 20 Ncm torque.

Uncovering procedure

Implants covered with soft tissue after placement require second-stage surgery to uncover them. The surgery is performed 4 months later in the maxilla and 3 months later in the mandible. It is performed in a manner similar to the original stage I procedure. Once the cover screws are identified by probing into the screws with an explorer, a crestal mini-incision approximately 3 mm is made horizontally with the alveolar crest at the center of the implant site, and the cover screws are then located using a surgical curette. After removing the screws, a guide pin is connected to the implant fixture. Along the guide pin, the mucosa is punched using 3.0–3.5 mm tissue punches. A permucosal healing abutment that is 1.0–1.5 mm wider than the tissue punch is then connected to the implant fixture. This procedure allows the peri-implant mucosa to be in tight contact with implants after the uncovering procedure (Fig 11-20).

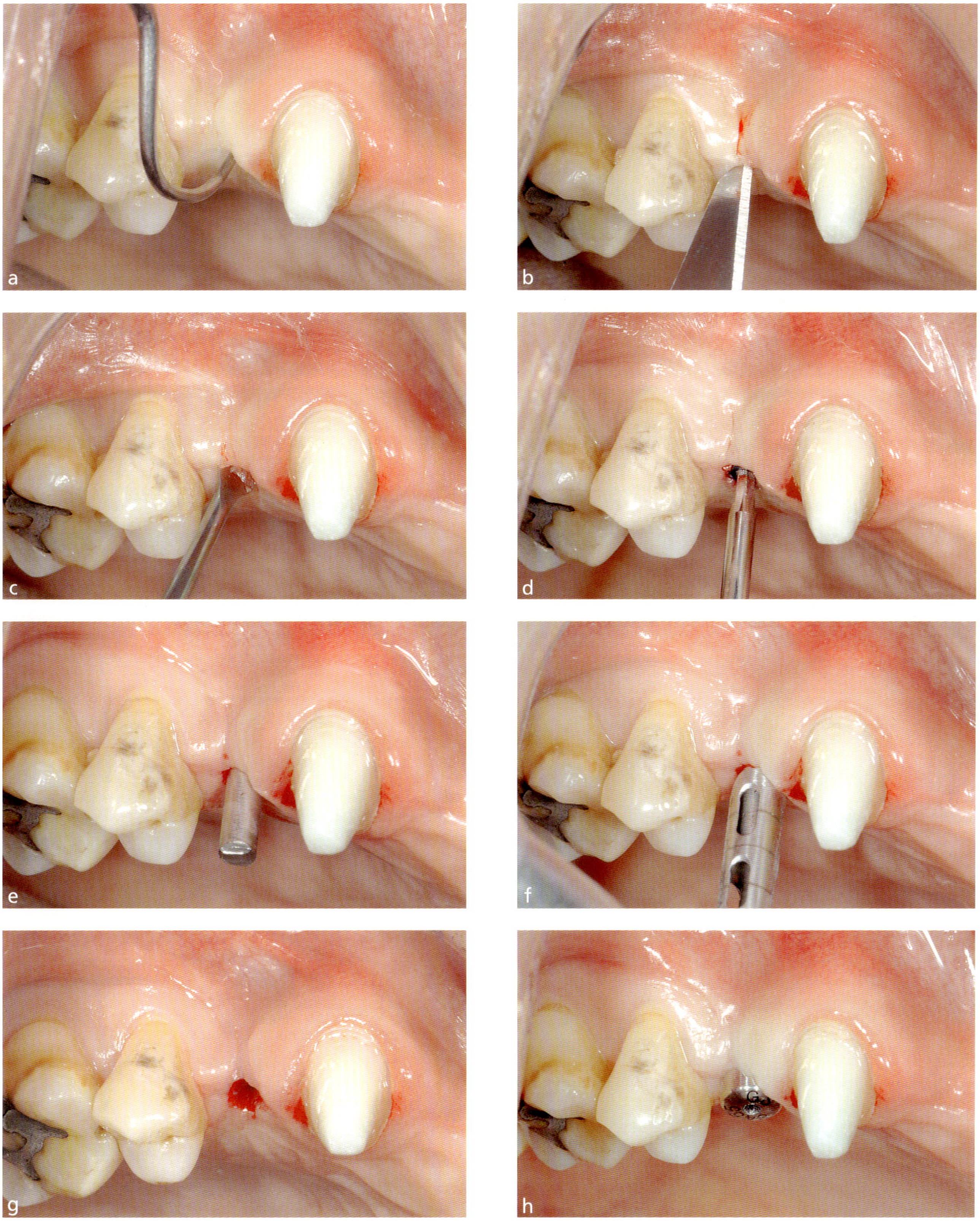

Fig 11-20 Uncovering procedure. (a) The cover screws are identified by probing with an explorer. (b) A crestal mini-incision approximately 3 mm horizontal to the alveolar crest is made at the center of the implant site. (c) The cover screws are located using a surgical curette. (d and e) After removal of the screws, a guide pin is connected to the implant fixture. (f and g) Along the guide pin, the mucosa is punched with 3.0–3. 5 mm tissue punches. (h) A permucosal healing abutment that is 1.0–1.5 mm wider than the tissue punch is then connected to the implant fixture. This procedure allows the peri-implant mucosa to be in tight contact with the implant after the uncovering procedure.

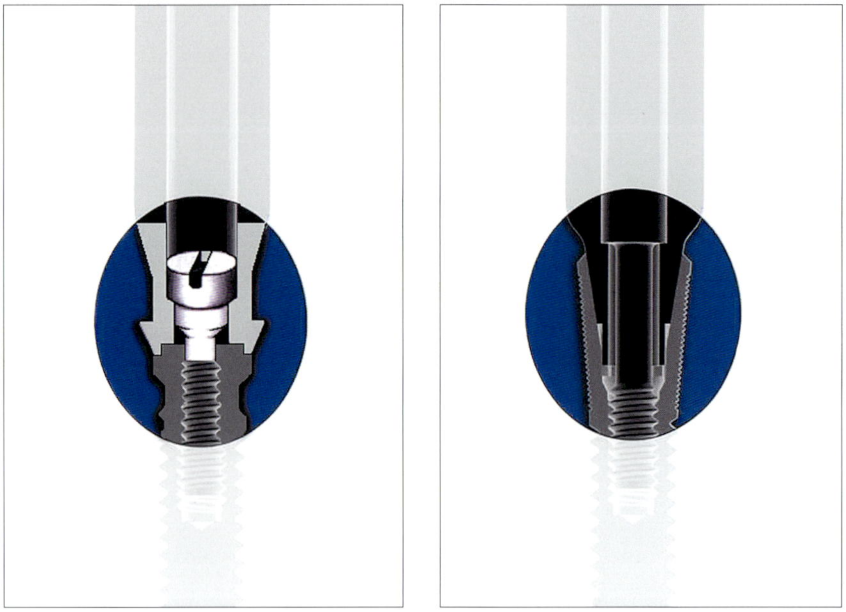

Fig 11-21 Comparison of (a) Brånemark and (b) Astra Tech implants. The latter has a conical fixture–abutment interface, which decreases micro-movement of the abutment.

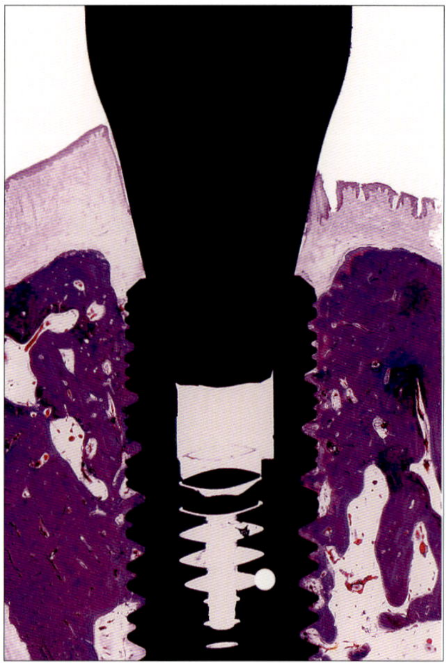

Fig 11-22 The apical extension of the epithelium is located at or above the fixture–abutment border at the Astra Tech implant site.

The soft tissue thickness sometimes obstructs location of the cover screws in the flapless procedure. A mucoperiosteal flap is reflected to expose the screws if the soft tissue is too thick to allow location of the cover screws.

Considerations related to prosthetic attachments in thick mucosa

Implant system

The use of an implant system that reduces the peri-implant sulcus depth in a thick mucosa is crucial. Brånemark implants with external hex attachments have a gap between the fixture and abutment part (Fig 11-21). The apical extension of the epithelium is always located below the fixture–abutment gap because of the subtle movement caused by the gap or the risk of bacterial contamination inside the gap.[23] It was previously reported that, after the abutment connection, the bacteria from the oral cavity can contaminate the inner region (including the microgap) of the system.[24]

Recent publications are reporting radiographs and marginal bone levels over time suggest that there is less bone loss with a conical, inward-shifted connection compared with the butt-joint connections with external hex attachments. For this reason, the use of implants without a fixture–abutment gap or with a conical fixture–abutment interface is advisable (see Fig 11-21). The cone-screw abutment has been shown to decrease micro-movement and provide a seal against invasion by microorganisms. Our animal experiments showed that apical termination of the junctional epithelium is located coronal to the abutment–fixture border using an implant system with the conical connection (Fig 11-22).

Abutments

In the thick mucosa, long abutments are connected to the fixture (Figs 11-23 and 11-24). Care should be taken to minimize the mechanical trauma to the peri-implant soft tissue attachment while removing a healing abutment and placing the prosthetic abutment. To prevent the intracrevicular position of the restoration margin from causing injury to the mucosal barrier, the crown margin should not be submerged too deeply in the gingiva. In the non-esthetic posterior region, the margin of the crowns is placed at the gingival level.

The material used in the abutment portion of the implant affects the location and quality of the soft tissue attachment that develops between the peri-implant mucosa and the implant. Abutments made from titanium or ceramic allow the formation of mucosal attachment and help to anchor the attachment in place.[25] However, no proper attachment forms at the abutment level at sites where abutments made from gold alloy are used. Therefore, the use of long titanium abutments is advisable at sites with thick mucosa (Fig 11-25).

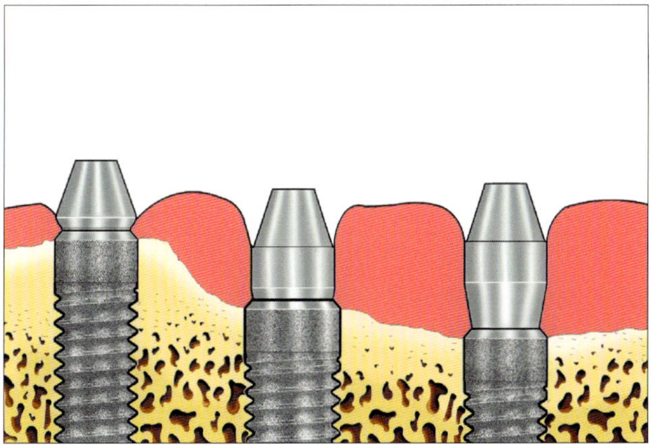

Fig 11-23 In thick mucosa, long abutments are connected to the fixture.

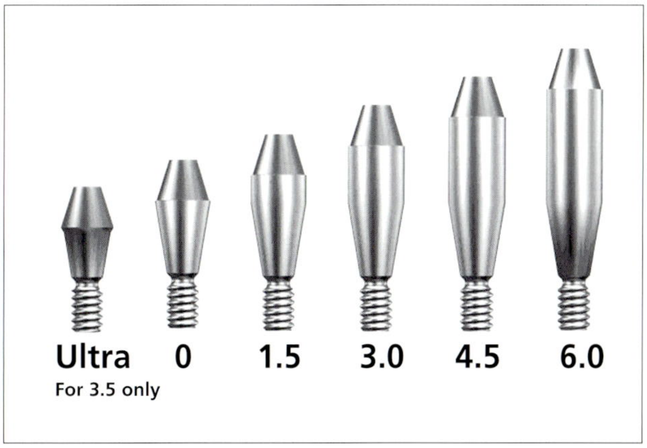

Fig 11-24 Titanium abutments with various heights.

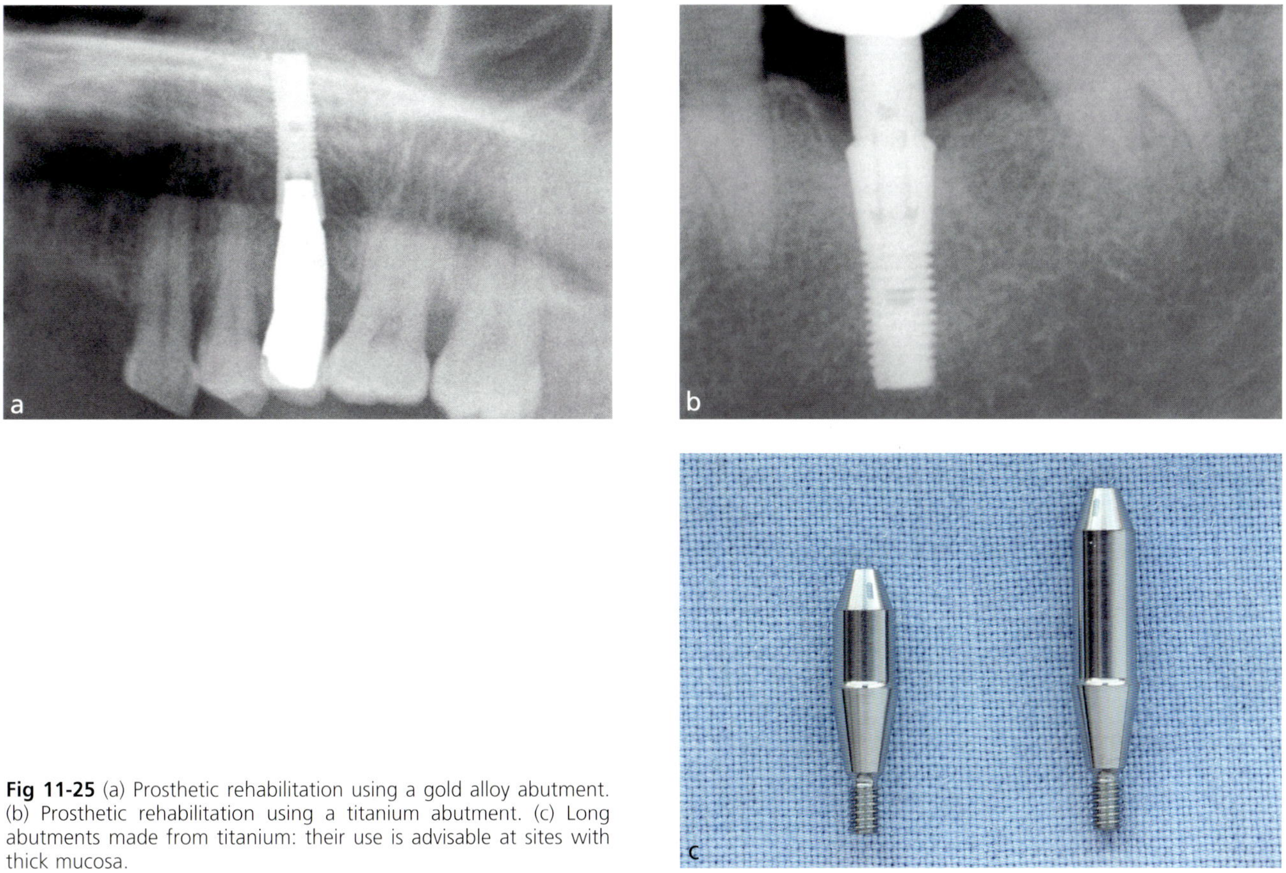

Fig 11-25 (a) Prosthetic rehabilitation using a gold alloy abutment. (b) Prosthetic rehabilitation using a titanium abutment. (c) Long abutments made from titanium: their use is advisable at sites with thick mucosa.

Plaque control at thick mucosal sites

The peri-implant sulcus depth increases when implants are placed in areas with thick mucosa. As a result, the health of peri-implant tissue placed in alveolar ridges with thick mucosa is strongly dependent on plaque control. Daily removal of supragingival plaque using a toothbrush can significantly reduce the amount and composition of subgingival microbiota. This reduction should translate to a decreased risk of periodontal disease initiation or recurrence. Furthermore, the decreased prevalence of periodontal pathogens in supragingival plaque reduces the potential reservoirs of these species.[26] The clinician should instruct the patient in the proper use of toothbrushes, tufted brushes, floss, oral irrigators, and interdental brushes. The use of a Pik Pocket® subgingival irrigation tip connected to a Waterpik® enables more effective control of subgingival plaque (Fig 11-26).

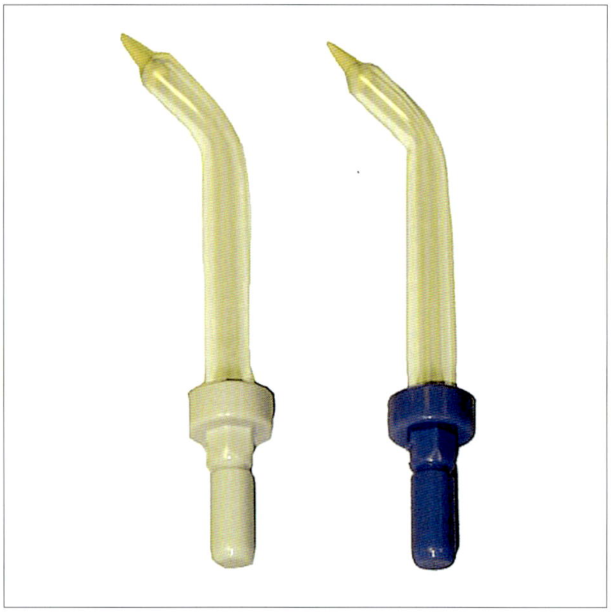

Fig 11-26 Pik Pocket® subgingival irrigation tips.

Summary

The peri-implant sulcus depth increases when implants are placed in the alveolar ridges with thick mucosa, but the peri-implant tissue can remain healthy with meticulous plaque control. The use of the flapless implant procedure in areas with thick mucosa can reduce the peri-implant sulcus depth and increase the resistance to inflammation. In view of these points and the complications associated with gingivoplasty to reduce tissue thickness, flapless implant placement should be considered in regions with a thick bulk of soft tissue without correction of the thick mucosa.

References

1. Berglundh T, Lindhe J, Ericsson I. The soft tissue barrier at implants and teeth. Clin Oral Implants Res 1991;2:81–90.
2. Cardaropoli G, Lekholm U, Wennström JL. Tissue alterations at implant-supported single-tooth replacements: a 1-year prospective clinical study. Clin Oral Implants Res 2006;17:165–171.
3. Misch CE. Contemporary Implant Dentistry, ed 2. St Louis, MO: Mosby, 1999:397–407.
4. Newman MG, Flemming TF. Periodontal considerations of implants and implant associated microbiota. J Dent Educ 1988;52:737–744.
5. Lekholm U, Adell R, Lindhe J. Marginal tissue reactions at osseointegrated titanium fixtures. II: A cross sectional retrospective study. Int J Oral Maxillofac Surg 1986;15:53–61.
6. Papaioannou W, Quirynen M, Nys M, van Steenberghe D. The effect of periodontal parameters on the subgingival microbiota around implants. Clin Oral Implants Res 1995;6:197–204.
7. Dharmar S, Yoshida K, Adachi Y. Subgingival microbial flora associated with Brånemark implants. Int J Oral Maxillofac Implants 1994;9:314–318.
8. Kirsch A, Mentag P. The IMZ endosseous two-phase implant system: a complete oral rehabilitation treatment concept. J Oral Implants 1986;12:576–589.
9. Steflik DE, Koth DC, McKinney RV. Human clinical trials with the single crystal sapphire endosteal implant. J Oral Implants 1986;13:39–53.
10. Yukna RA. Periodontal considerations for dental implants. In: Block MS, Kent JN (eds). Endosseouos Implants for Maxillofacial Reconstruction. Philadelphia, PA: WB Saunders, 1995:587–590.
11. Misch CE. The maxillary anterior single tooth implant aesthetic-health compromise. Int J Dent Symp 1995;3:4–9.
12. Lekholm U, Adell R, Lindhe J et al. Marginal tissue reactions at osseointegrated titanium fixtures. II: A cross-sectional retrospective study. Int J Oral Maxillofac Surg 1986;15:53–61.
13. Leonhardt A, Adolfsson B, Lekholm U, Wirkström M, Dahlen G. A longtitudinal microbiological study on osseointegrated titanium implants in partially edentulous patients. Clin Oral Implants Res 1993;4:113–120.
14. Jeong SM, Choi BH, Li J, Xuan F. The effect of thick mucosa on peri-implant tissues: an experimental study in dogs. J Periodontol 2008; 79:2151–2155.
15. Papavasiliou G, Tripodakis AP, Kamposiora P, Strub JR, Bayne SC. Finite element analysis of ceramic abutment–restoration combinations for osseointegrated implants. Int J Prosthodont 1996;9:254–260.
16. Lin S, Shi S, LeGeros RZ, LeGeros JP. Three-dimensional finite element analyses of four designs of a high-strength silicon nitride implant. Implant Dent 2000;9:53–60.
17. Penny RE, Kraal JH. Crown to root ratio: its significance in restorative dentistry. J Prosth Dent 1979;42:34–38.
18. Misch CE, Goodacre CJ, Finley JM. Consensus conference panel report: crown-height space guidelines for implant dentistry – part 1. Implant Dent 2005;14:312–318.
19. Misch CE, Goodacre CJ, Finley JM. Consensus conference panel report: crown-height space guidelines for implant dentistry – part 2. Implant Dent 2006;15:113–121.
20. Jensen OT, Cockrell R, Kuheke L. Anterior maxillary alveolar distraction osteogenesis: a prospective 5-year clinical study. Int J Oral Maxillofac Implants 2002;17:507–516.

Further reading

Berglundh T, Lindhe J, Jonsson K. The topography of the vascular systems in the periodontal and peri-implant tissues in the dog. J Clin Periodontol 1994;21:189–193.

Kan JYK, Rungcharassaeng K, Umezu K, Kois JC. Dimensions of peri-implant mucosa: an evaluation of maxillary anterior single implants in humans. J Periodontol 2003;74:557–565.

Fiorellini JP, Martuscelli G, Weber HP. Longitudinal studies of implant systems. Periodontology 2000;17:125–131.

Ericsson I, Persson LG, Berglundh T, Marinello CP, Lindhe J, Klinge B. Different types of inflammatory reactions in peri-implant soft tissues. J Clin Periodontol 1995;22:255–261.

Abrahamsson I, Berglundh T, Glantz PO, Lindhe J. The mucosal attachment at different abutments: an experimental study in dogs. J Clin Periodontol 1998;25:721–727.

Lindhe J, Karring T, Lang N. Clinical Periodontology and Implant Dentistry. Copenhagen: Munksgaard, 2000.

CHAPTER

12

The Deficient Alveolar Ridge

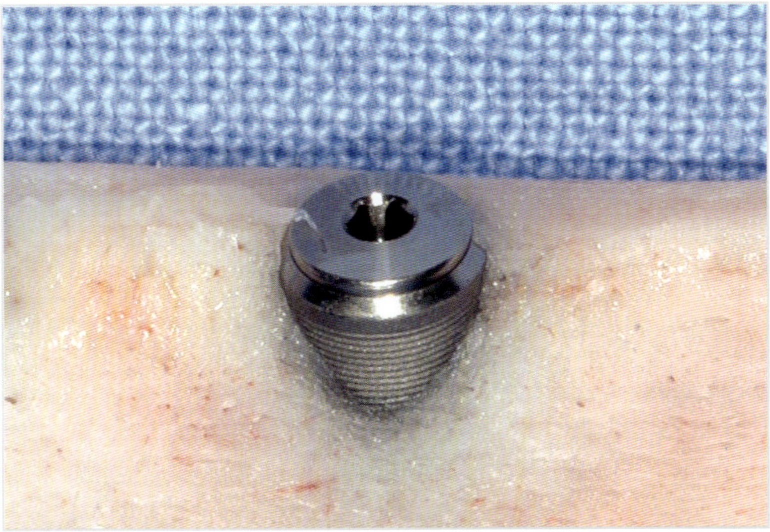

Key point

Flapless implant surgery is possible in an alveolar ridge with insufficient bone width.

Overview

Most of the conditions that lead to tooth loss result in the loss of some bone in the region of the missing tooth. In addition, a decrease in width and height of the bone occurs after tooth loss. The resorption pattern occurs first in width and then in height. The loss of bone width occurs primarily from the facial region because the labial plate is much thinner than the palatal plate.[1,2] The height of available bone decreases as the resorption process continues. As a result, the alveolar ridge has inadequate bone available for proper-size implants. Because flapless implant surgery does not allow direct visualization or access to the bone, there is some concern that this procedure might not be suitable for placing implants in a deficient alveolar ridge. This chapter addresses how to deal with a deficient alveolar ridge and how to use the flapless implant procedure in challenging cases.

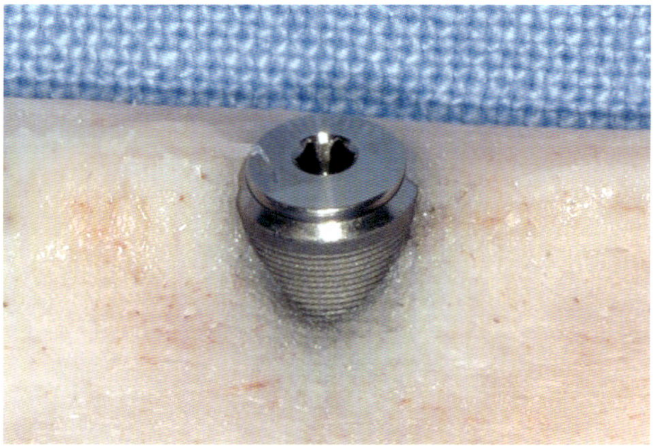

Fig 12-1 Implant threads are exposed on the buccal side of the implant after placing the implant in a sloping ridge.

Effect of exposed implant threads on the adjacent tissue

Placement of implants using flapless implant surgery in alveolar ridges with insufficient bone width might result in incomplete bone coverage on the labial or buccal side (Fig 12-1). There is some concern that threads exposed owing to incomplete bone coverage can irritate the adjacent peri-implant soft tissues, and, in a worst-case scenario, lead to gingival recession, progressive bone resorption, and loss of the implant. However, the necessity for complete bone coverage of the implant surface as a precondition for implant success appears to be questionable from a clinical and biomechanical point of view.[3–5] There is very little risk associated with exposed implant threads when abundant soft tissue is present. Lekholm et al.[3] reported that one to five exposed threads at implant surgery did not result in any measurable increase in the incidence of complications over a 5-year period compared with fully bone-covered control implants.

The results of the present authors' animal study are in accordance with that (Fig 12-2). Sloping alveolar ridges were created in the mandibles of five mongrel dogs. After 3 months, one implant was placed on each side of the mandible using a flapless procedure. The oblique alveolar bone defects resulted in exposure of the implant threads for approximately 5 mm on the buccal aspects of the implants. Clinical examinations after 6 months of plaque control showed a normal condition of the mucosa at all

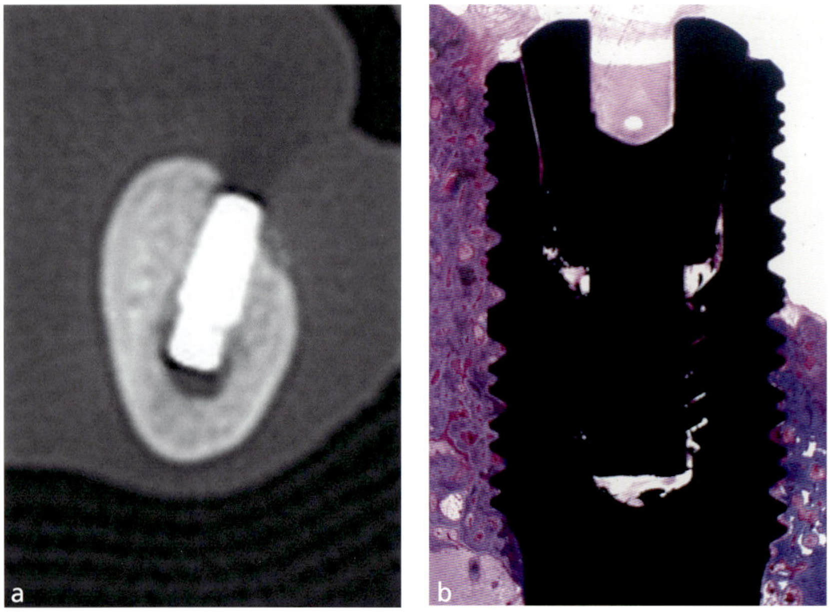

Fig 12-2 (a and b) Sloping alveolar ridges were created in the mandibles of five mongrel dogs. After 3 months of healing, one implant was placed on either side of the mandible using a flapless procedure. The oblique alveolar bone defects resulted in exposure of the implant threads, approximately 5 mm on the buccal aspects of the implants. Clinical and histological examinations were carried out after 6 months of plaque control.

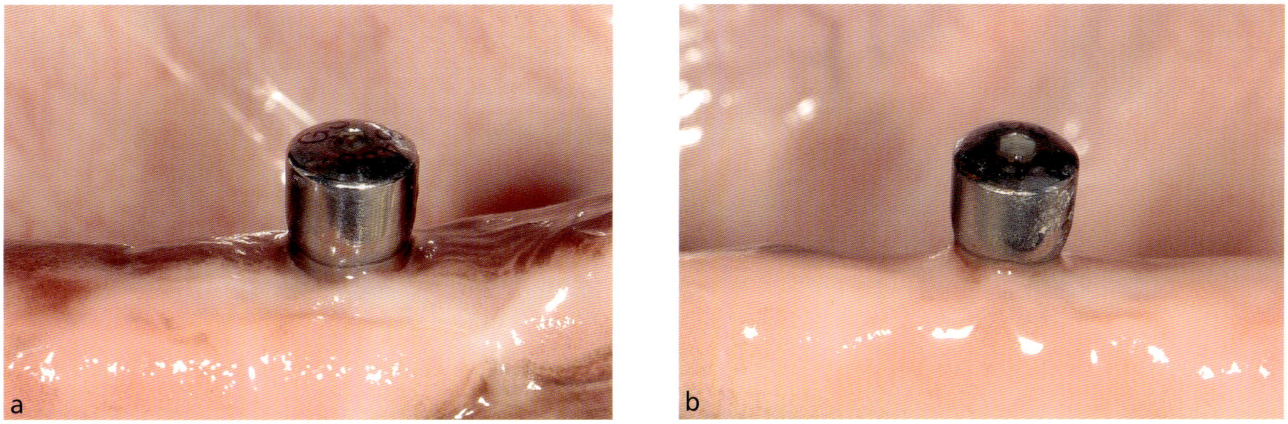

Fig 12-3 Clinical examinations after 6 months of plaque control showed that the condition of the mucosa at all implant sites was normal – the mucosa showed no signs of inflammation or gingival shrinkage.

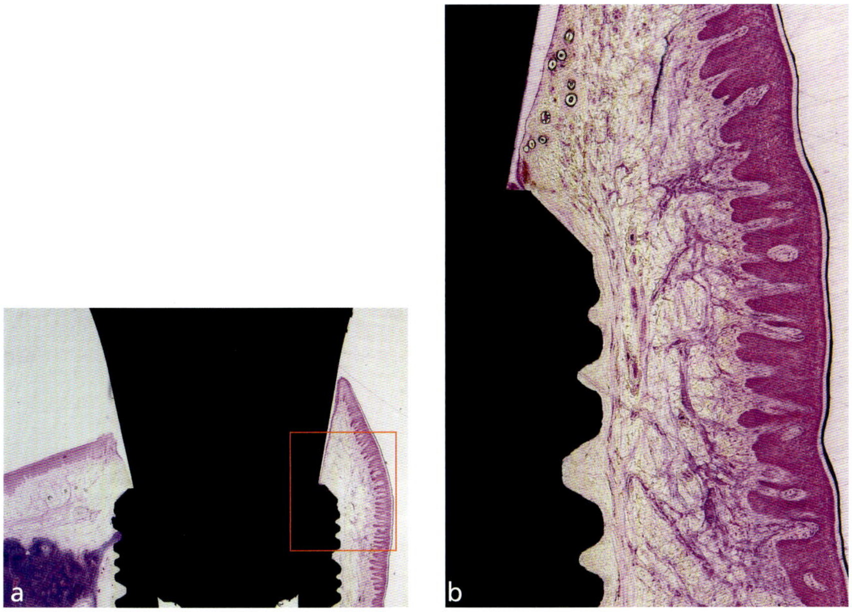

Fig 12-4 Results of the histological evaluation showing that the junctional epithelium contacts were at the abutment connection and did not extend beyond the abutment–fixture borderline of the implants. The implant surface apical to the junctional epithelium appeared to be in direct contact with the connective tissue.

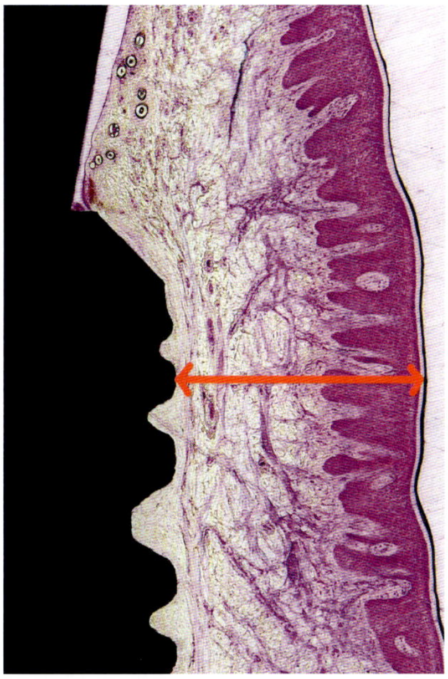

Fig 12-5 The thickness of the overlying mucosa (arrow) is an important factor to consider when gingival recession occurs in cases of exposed implant threads.

implant sites – there were no signs of inflammation or crestal bone loss (Fig 12-3). A histological evaluation showed that the junctional epithelial contacts were at the abutment connection and did not extend beyond the abutment–fixture borderline of the implants (Fig 12-4). The implant surface apical to the junctional epithelium appeared to be in direct contact with the connective tissue. This suggests that the exposed threads themselves cause no peri-implantitis. In addition, gingival recession does not occur when abundant soft tissue is present, even though threads are exposed outside the bone.

The thickness of the overlying mucosa is an important factor with regard to gingival recession in the cases of exposed implant threads (Fig 12-5). The implant threads can be exposed outside the mucosa, and gingival recession can occur if the threads are exposed outside the bone and covered with relatively thin overlying mucosa (Figs 12-6 to 12-8). Gingival recession will result in poor esthetics in some patients, particularly at the facial aspects with thin mucosa (Fig 12-9). In contrast, gingival recession does not occur if the overlying mucosa is thick. Hence, bone grafting to cover the exposed threads is indicated if the over-

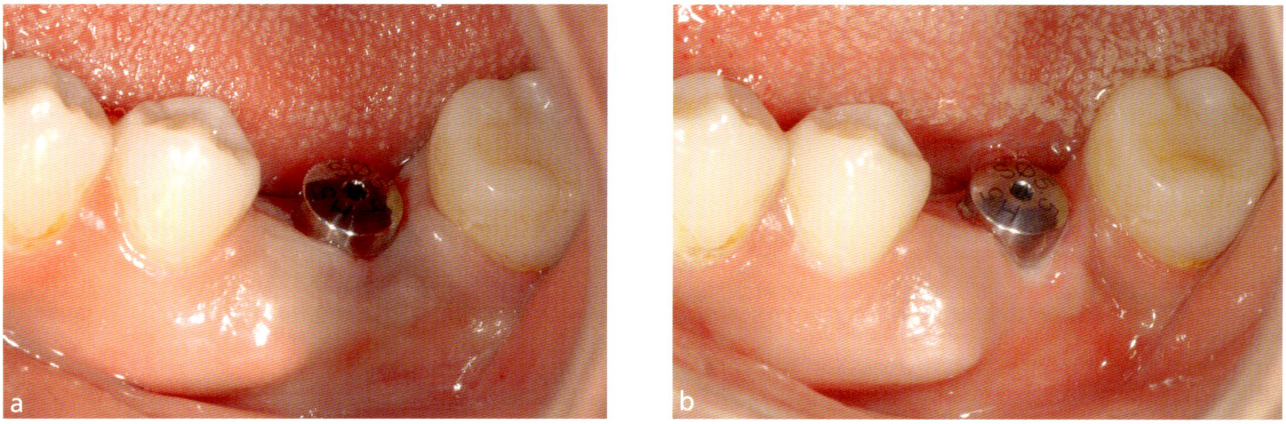

Fig 12-6 (a and b) Gingival recession occurs in patients with a thin mucosa when the implant surface is exposed outside the bone and covered with the thin mucosa. See also Fig 12-7.

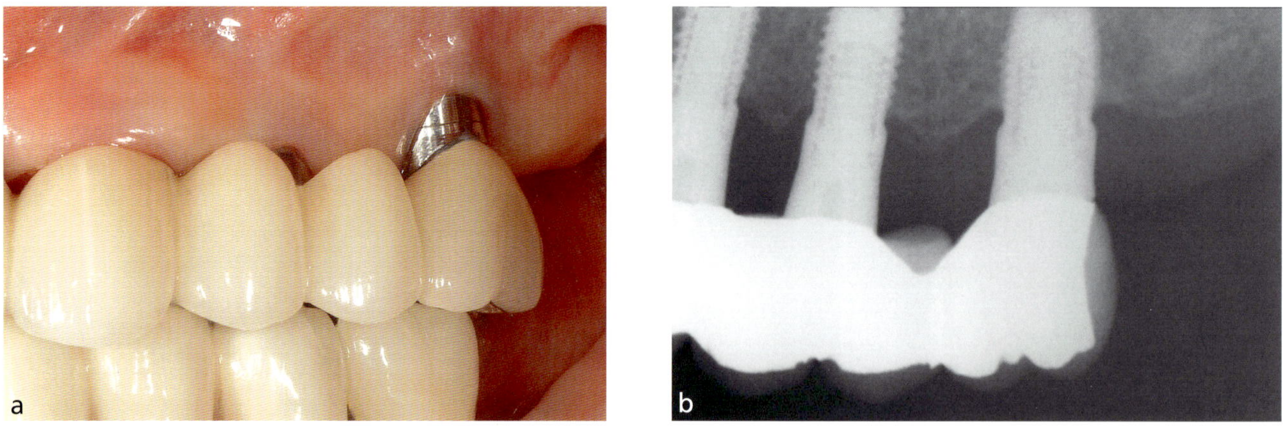

Fig 12-7 (a and b) Gingival recession occurs in patients with a thin mucosa when the implant surface is exposed outside the bone and covered with the thin mucosa. See also Fig 12-6.

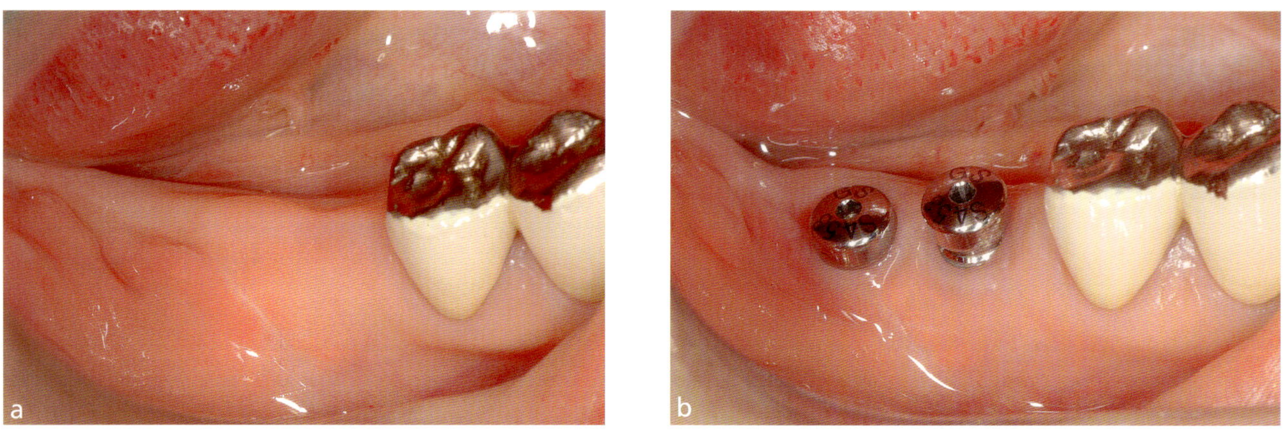

Fig 12-8 (a and b) Gingival recession commonly occurs when the implant threads on the buccal side of the alveolar bone are exposed outside the bone and covered with thin mucosa, and the threads are exposed to the oral cavity.

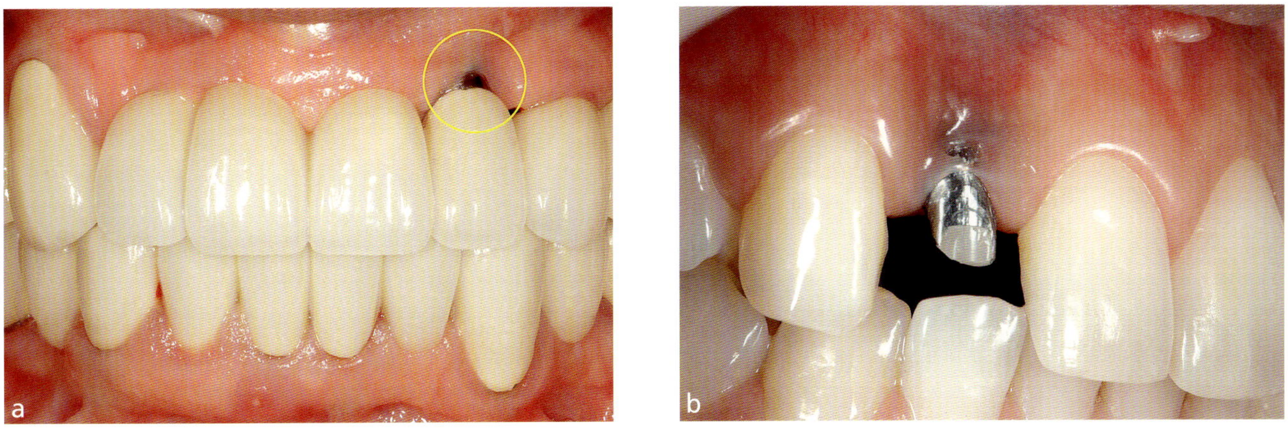

Fig 12-9 (a and b) Soft tissue shrinkage and poor esthetics will result if the exposed implant threads are covered with a thin mucosa.

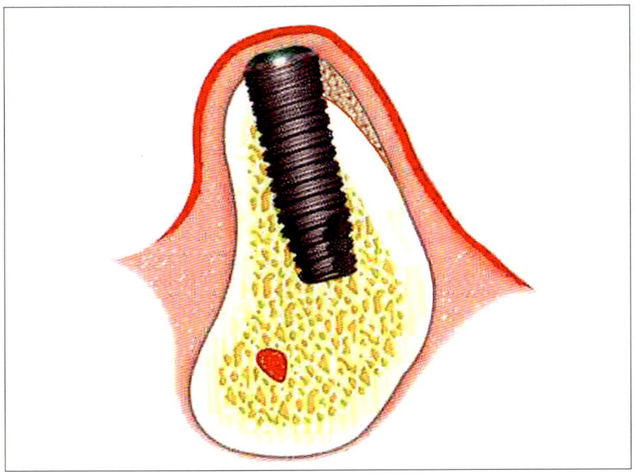

Fig 12-10 Bone grafting to cover the exposed threads is indicated in the esthetic zone if the overlying mucosa is thin.

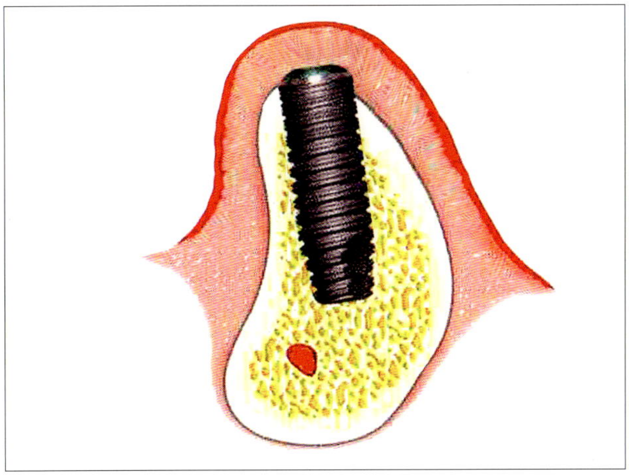

Fig 12-11 There is no need to cover the exposed threads of the implant with grafting material if implant threads are exposed outside the bone after flapless implant placement in the non-esthetic zone with thick mucosa, provided the primary stability of the implant is secured.

lying mucosa is thin (Fig 12-10). The bone foundation sets the tone for the soft tissue drape.

Bone augmentation is often an important aspect of the treatment when ideal soft tissue is desired or a reconstruction of labial alveolar bone contour is demanded to improve the esthetics. There is no need to cover the exposed threads of the implant with grafting material if implant threads are exposed outside the bone after flapless implant placement in the zone with thick mucosa, provided the primary stability of the implants is secured (Figs 12-11 and 12-12).

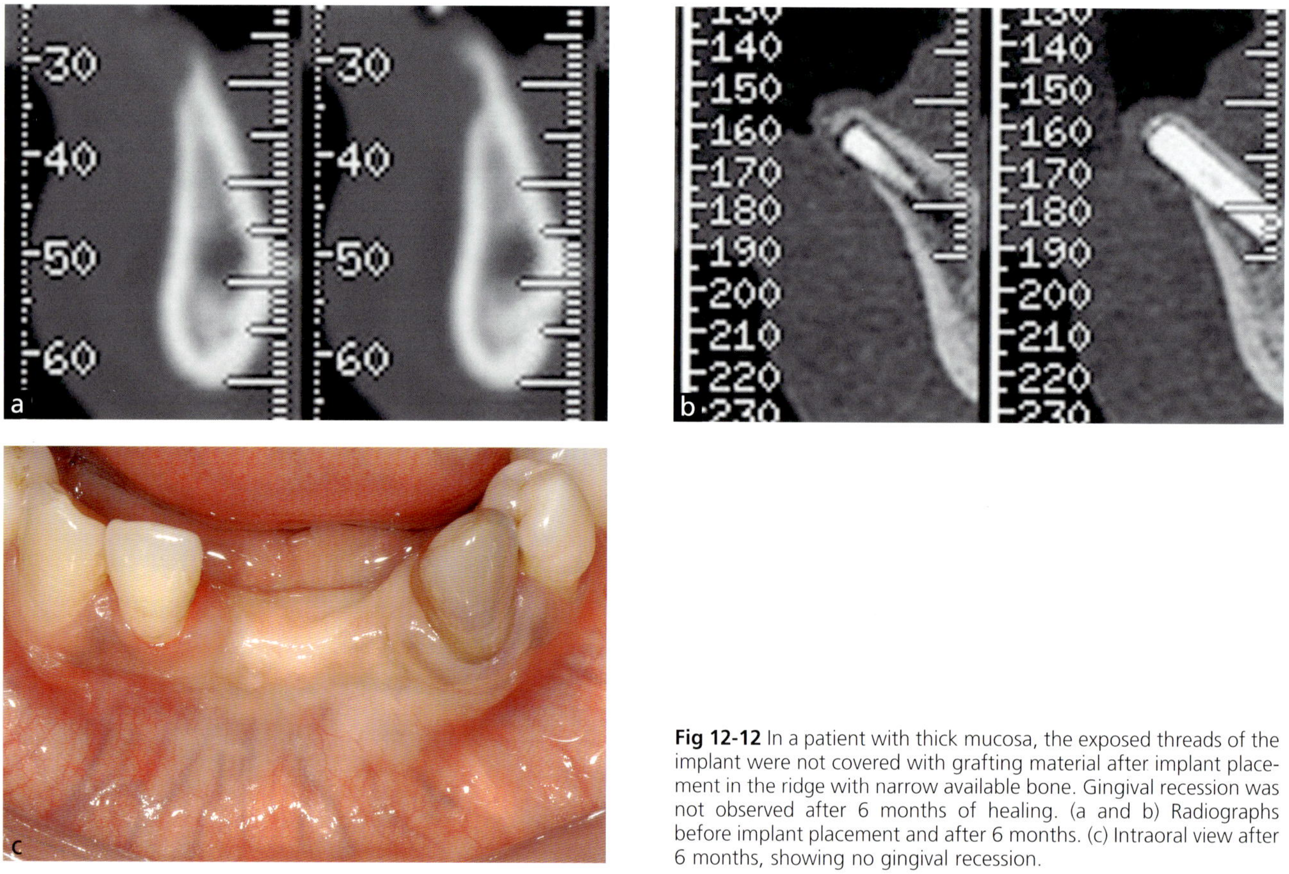

Fig 12-12 In a patient with thick mucosa, the exposed threads of the implant were not covered with grafting material after implant placement in the ridge with narrow available bone. Gingival recession was not observed after 6 months of healing. (a and b) Radiographs before implant placement and after 6 months. (c) Intraoral view after 6 months, showing no gingival recession.

Bone graft materials or barrier membranes for bone regeneration

Autogenous bone particles alone

It is possible to avoid problems with the procurement of autogenous bone by recovering the autogenous bone particles from the drilling procedure of the alveolar bone while preparing the implant site. Some authors have reported that marrow stem cells are present in these bone particles,[6] and others have been able to cultivate osteoblast-like cells from this material.[7] This material is commonly used to cover the exposed threads of the implants. Based on our animal experiments, the autogenous bone particles alone have little or no effect on bone regeneration (Fig 12-13). The major reason for the lack of bone regeneration might be that the particles are dispersed and lost owing to the pressure of the overlying soft tissue. Therefore, the use of autogenous bone particles derived from bone preparation during implant placement for the repair of alveolar bone defects appears to be unreliable.

Autogenous bone particles and resorbable membranes

The use of autogenous bone particles and resorbable membranes to restore the alveolar bone contour has little (or only a small) enhancing effect on bone regeneration (Fig 12-14). These results are consistent with a previous report showing that there is only a small increase in bone regeneration in defects augmented with autogenous bone particles with resorbable membrane coverage.[8] The major reason for the lack of a general increase in bone formation might be that the space available for bone regeneration was collapsed by the pressure of the overlying soft tissue during the healing period of soft tissue. Hence, augmentation using autogenous bone particles with resorbable membranes appears to be unreliable.

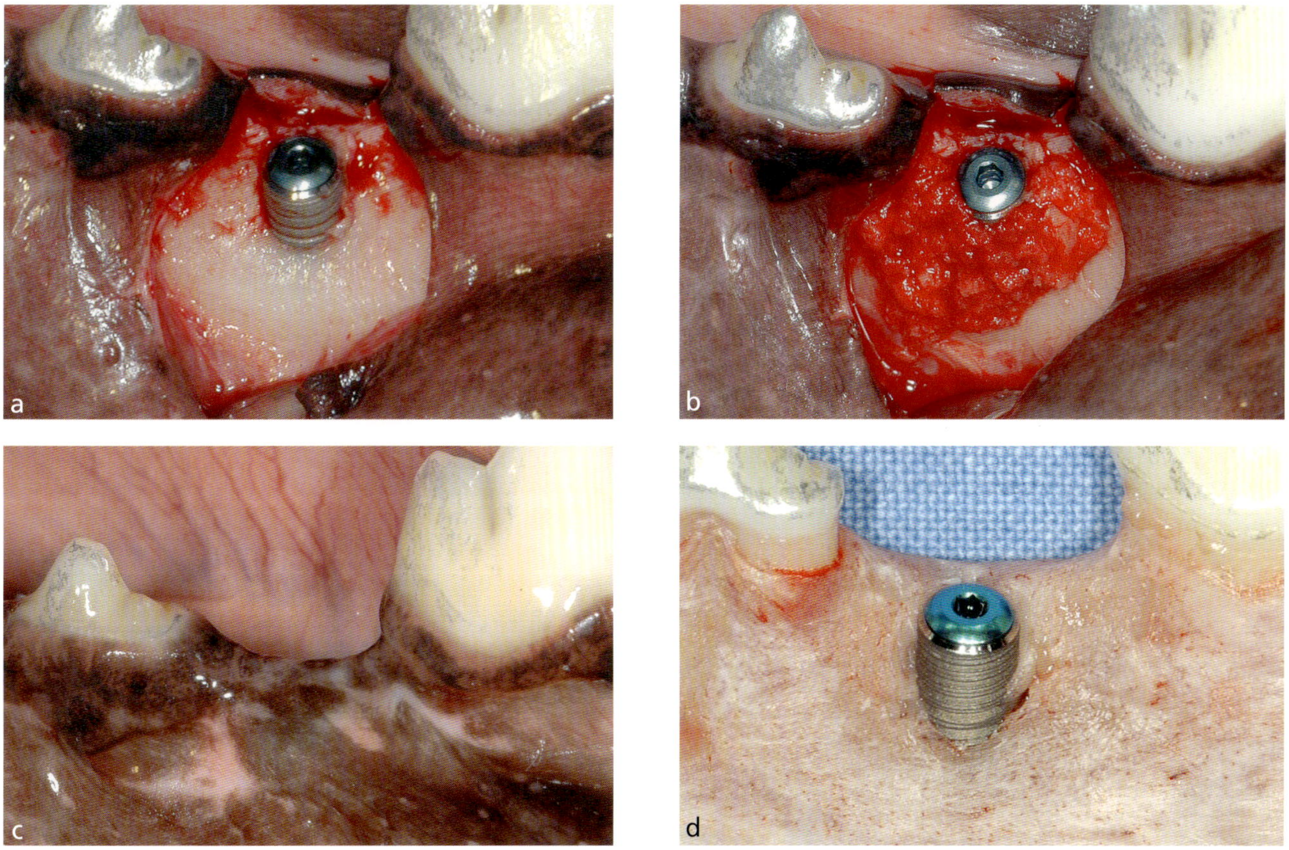

Fig 12-13 (a and b) Autogenous bone particles derived from the bone preparation during implant placement were used to cover the exposed implant threads. (c) A view of the overlying mucosa showing that healing is uneventful. (d) A view of the implant showing no bone regeneration in the peri-implant defect. The autogenous bone particles had little or no effect on the outcome of the bone regeneration procedures around the exposed implant threads.

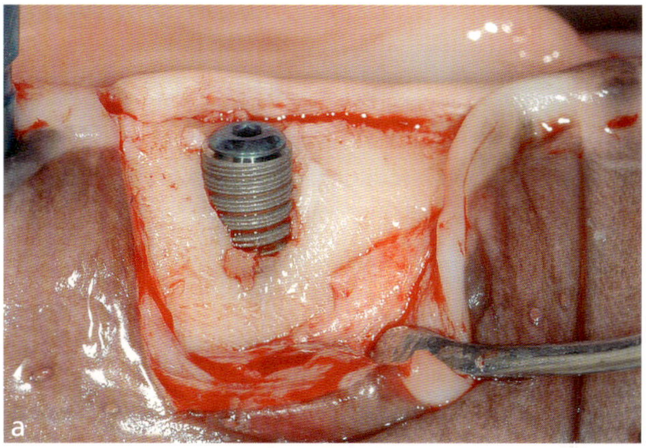

Fig 12-14 The use of resorbable membranes and autogenous bone particles for restoration of the alveolar bone contour has only a small enhancing effect on the results of the reconstruction. (a) Implant threads are exposed to the buccal aspects after placement in a deficient alveolar ridge. (b) Resorbable collagen membranes and autogenous bone particles are used to cover the exposed threads. (c) Three months after surgery.

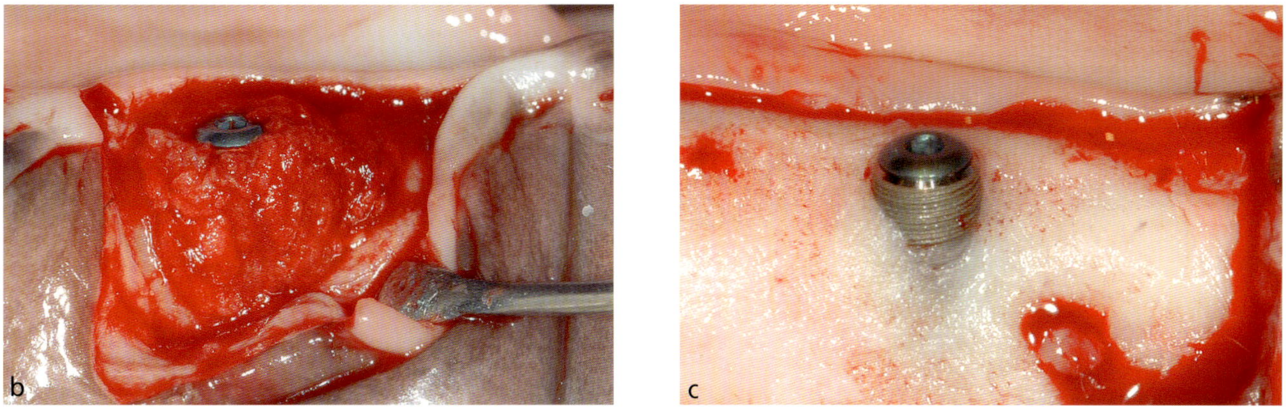

Bio-Oss® (Geistlich, Wolhusen, Switzerland)

Bio-Oss® is deproteinized bovine cancellous bone with a similar structure to human bone and with osteoconductive properties. The material is available in either particulate or block forms (Fig 12-15). One of the main advantages of the block-type material is that it can be shaped to fit in the anatomical structure of a recipient site.

Bio-Oss® is chemically and physically identical to human bone and is highly osteoconductive.[9] It provides an ideal scaffold for new bone formation.[9-12] Bio-Oss® contributes to the osteoconductive effect of bone formation because new bone forms by resorption or apposition from the surrounding bone, a process known as creeping substitution[13] (Fig 12-16). When a mixture of Bio-Oss® particles and autogenous bone particles are used, the autogenous bone provides bone cells and osteogenic growth factors.

The resorption rate of Bio-Oss® depends on the remodeling ability of the surrounding cells or tissue. When placed in a poor remodeling condition, the material remains unchanged without new bone formation even 1 year after grafting (Fig 12-17). However, when placed in a good remodeling condition, new bone forms on its surface with the concomitant resorption of the material. Six months later, the newly formed bone can contribute to implant stability, even though the material is not completely substituted for bone (Fig 12-18).

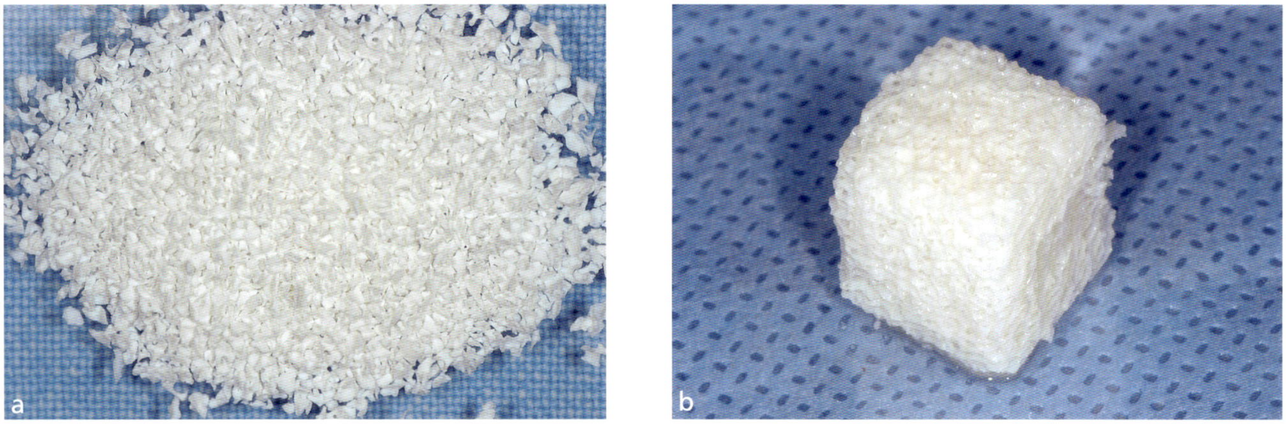

Fig 12-15 Bio-Oss® in particulate (a) and block (b) forms.

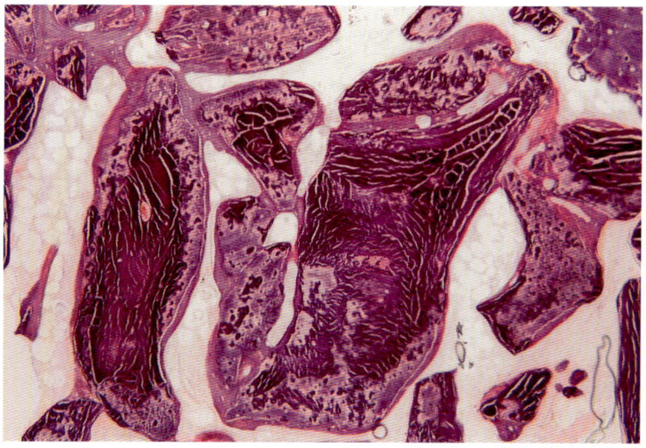

Fig 12-16 Three months after grafting, new bone had formed through the resorption of Bio-Oss® particles and the apposition of bone on the surface of the particles.

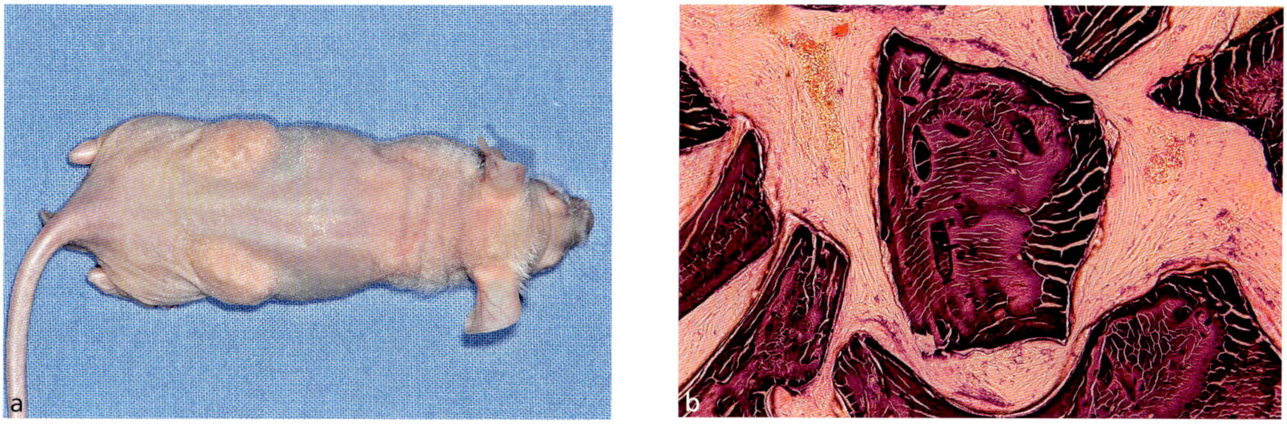

Fig 12-17 (a and b) Bio-Oss® particles did not grow bone when the material was placed into subcutaneous tissues of a nude mouse. The material remained unchanged even 1 year after grafting.

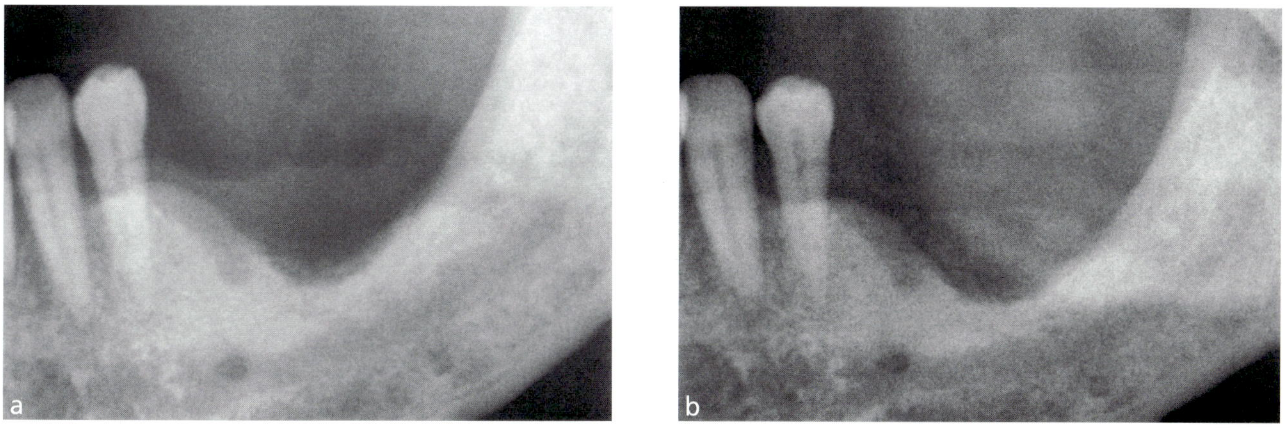

Fig 12-18 (a and b) Radiographs of the mandible before and immediately after surgery. Bio-Oss® block was placed in the mandible.

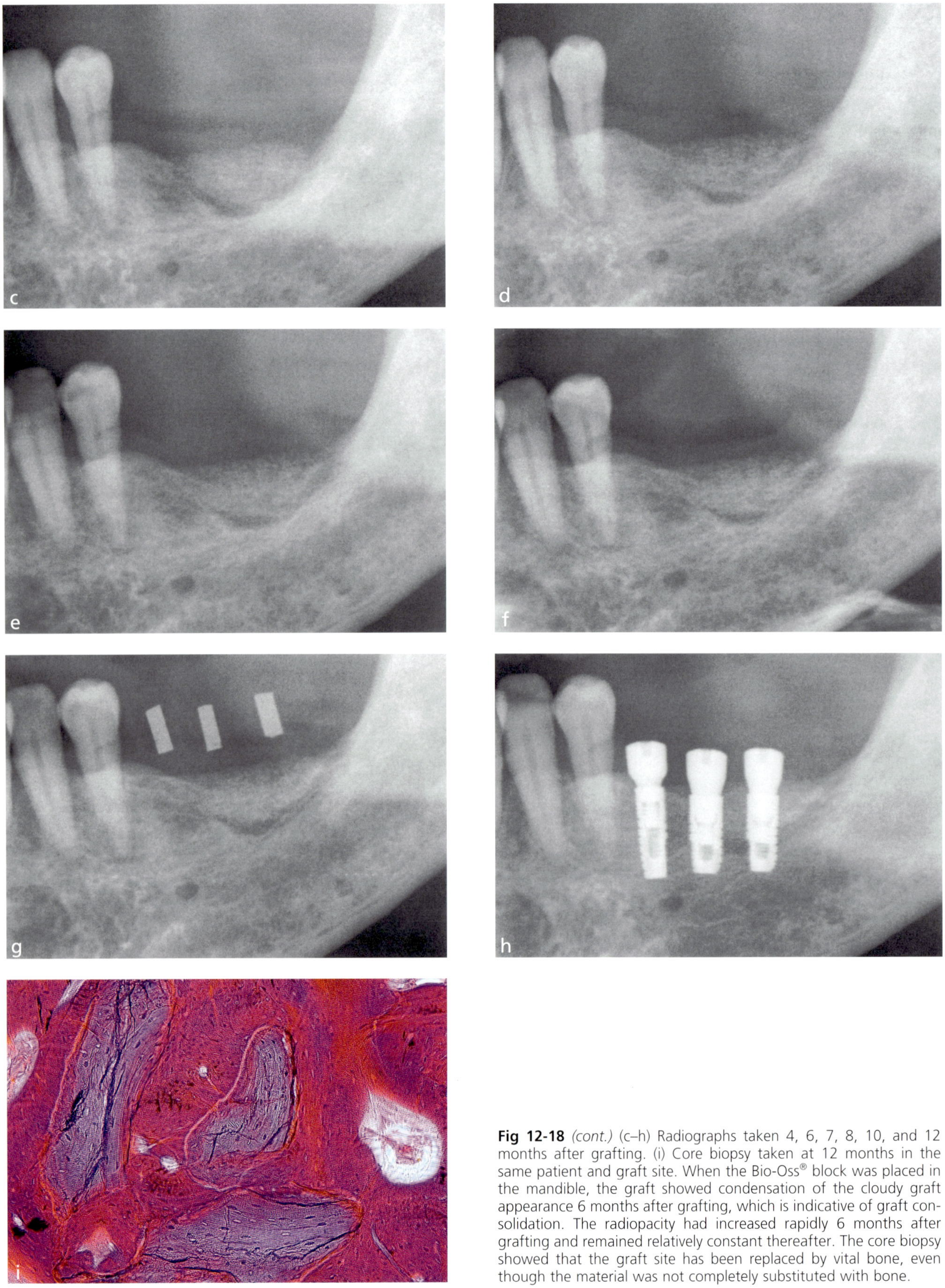

Fig 12-18 *(cont.)* (c–h) Radiographs taken 4, 6, 7, 8, 10, and 12 months after grafting. (i) Core biopsy taken at 12 months in the same patient and graft site. When the Bio-Oss® block was placed in the mandible, the graft showed condensation of the cloudy graft appearance 6 months after grafting, which is indicative of graft consolidation. The radiopacity had increased rapidly 6 months after grafting and remained relatively constant thereafter. The core biopsy showed that the graft site has been replaced by vital bone, even though the material was not completely substituted with bone.

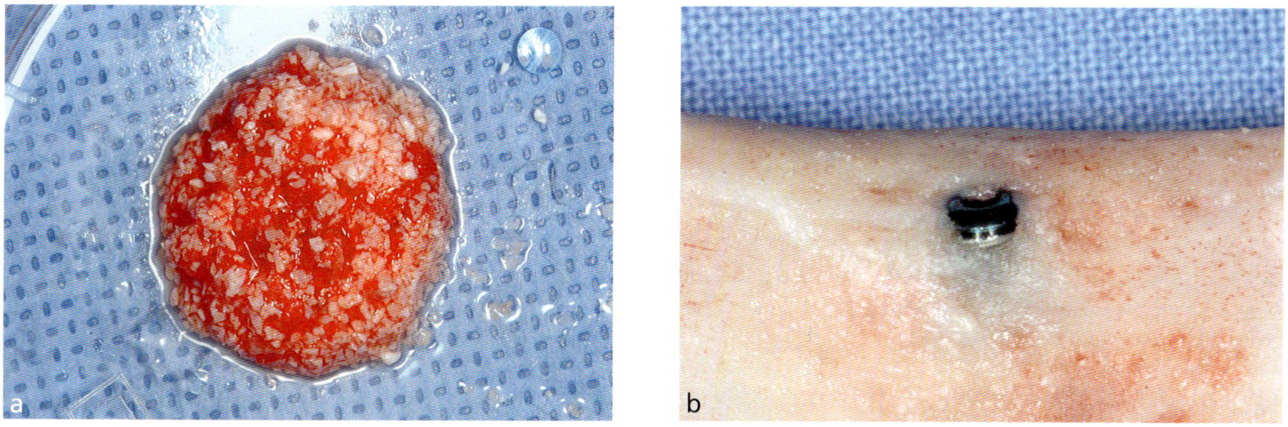

Fig 12-19 (a) Bone particles recovered from the alveolar ridge during bone preparation were mixed with Bio-Oss® particles in a 1:1 ratio. The mixture was then used to cover the exposed implant threads. (b) After 3 months, the peri-implant defect is covered with bone and the graft is well incorporated in the grafted area.

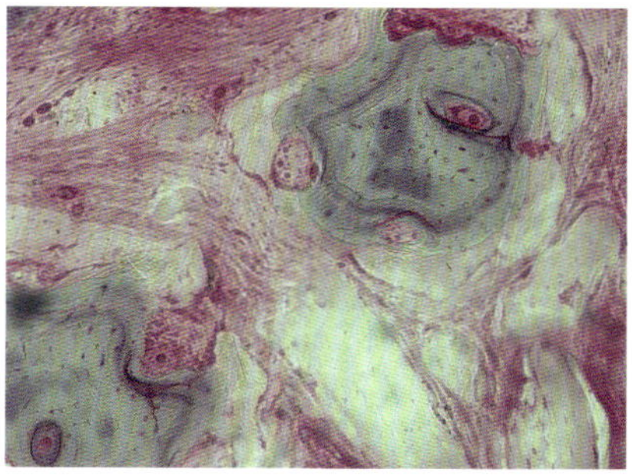

Fig 12-20 A buccal–lingual ground section of Fig 12-19b specimen. New bone had formed on the surface of the Bio-Oss® particles. A zone of dense connective tissue is interposed between the particles.

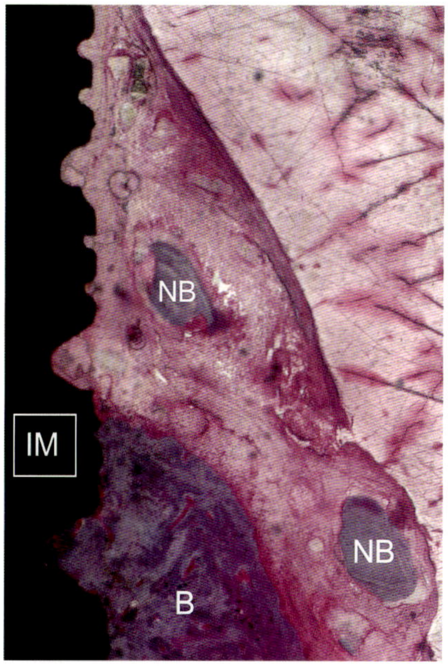

Fig 12-21 The new bone (NB) is not in direct contact with the implant (IM), and connective tissue is interposed between the implant surface and host bone (B).

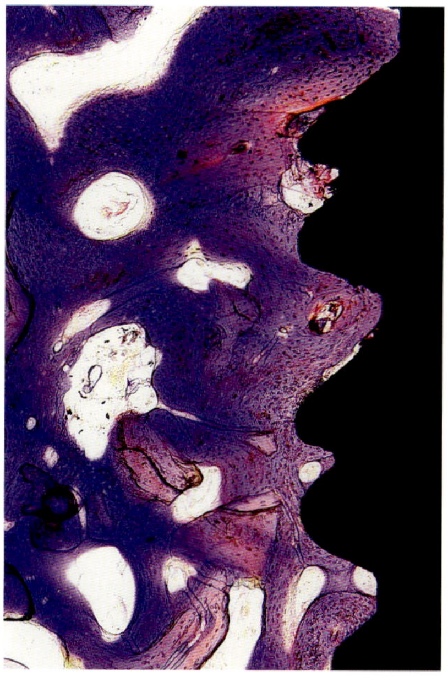

Fig 12-22 The bone–implant contact area was increased significantly when the implant was placed 6 months after Bio-Oss® graft.

The sequence of augmentation and implant placement procedures is an important factor for enhancing osseointegration. When Bio-Oss® is used to cover peri-implant defects after implant placement, the new bone is generally not in direct contact with the implants, and connective tissue is interposed between the implant surface and bone (Figs 12-19 to 12-21).[14] When peri-implant defects are covered with Bio-Oss®, the newly formed bone does not contribute to the increase of the bone–implant contact. This finding is in accordance with earlier published reports,[4,5] showing that the newly formed bone does not contribute to implant stability when the exposed implant surface is treated using a barrier membrane technique to provide for bone augmentation. However, the bone–implant contact area is increased significantly when implant placement is delayed for secondary surgery after the graft has healed (Fig 12-22). For this reason, in order to enhance the bone–implant contact, an augmentation procedure is advisable before placing the implant in the posterior region of the mouth.

Barrier membrane

The most common complication of guided bone regeneration using a barrier membrane is exposure of the membrane and subsequent inflammation. The incidence of membrane exposure is approximately 16–53%.[15–17] Pretorius et al.[18] revealed that complications associated with barrier membranes occur even if the procedure is performed by a proficient practitioner. Therefore, the use of barrier membranes always carries the risk of membrane exposure and subsequent infection.

The simultaneous use of a barrier membrane and implant placement increases the risk of membrane exposure. Gotfredsen et al.[19] reported that the incidence of soft tissue dehiscence was 61% when bone defects around implants were covered with a polytetrafluoroethylene membrane.

Another common complication is membrane collapse caused by pressure from the overlying soft tissue on the membrane during the healing period.[20,21] Araújo et al.[22] reported that when a soft collagen membrane (Bio-Gide®, Geistlich Pharma AG) was used for lateral ridge augmentation, 30% of the height and 50% of the length had been resorbed 6 months later. When a strong membrane is used, stiffness renders clinical management difficult and increases the risk of membrane exposure.[23,24] Pretorius et al.[18] reported that the periosteum can replace the covering membrane provided the grafting material retains space for bone formation.

Considering these points, we advocate treating bone defects using slowly resorbable Bio-Oss® without a barrier membrane.

Available bone and dental implant treatment plans

The available bone, which is the amount of bone in the edentulous area considered for implantation, is particularly important in implant dentistry. It is measured in width, height, and length. The existing bone volume is the primary factor used to develop a treatment plan. A panoramic radiograph is the most common method for making a preliminary determination of the available bone height. The height of available bone is measured from the crest of the edentulous ridge to the opposing landmark.

When there is adequate height available, the next most important dimension is the width of available bone. The mesiodistal length is the third determinant for available bone. As a rule, the implant should be at least 1.5 mm from an adjacent tooth and 3 mm from an adjacent implant.

Classfication of residual bone was developed based on the width and height of available bone.

- Misch[25] established four divisions of available bone for implant dentistry in the edentulous maxilla and mandible: division A (abundant bone), division B (barely sufficient bone), division C (compromised bone), and division D (deficient bone).
- Engelke[26] developed a bone mapping system based on a multiple cube concept. The implant sites are represented as a column of cubes with 5 mm sides.
- Vertical and horizontal bone mappings of the available bone have been presented: vertical bone dimension (abundant [>20 mm], sufficient [>15 mm], critical [>10 mm], insufficient [<10 mm]) and horizontal bone dimension (sufficient [>5 mm], insufficient [<5 mm]).
- Implant treatment plans are developed based on the divisions of available bone.

Treatment of ridges with "abundant" bone

Flapless implant surgery is optimal in abundant bone where the bone width is >6 mm and the bone height is >12 mm (division A in the Misch classification). A width >6 mm is predicated on an implant diameter of 4 mm at the crest module. Implants with a crestal diameter of 4 mm usually require more than 6 mm of bone width to ensure adequate bone thickness and blood supply around the implant. These dimensions provide more than 1 mm of bone on each side of the implant at the crest.

Treatment of ridges with "insufficient" bone

Implant placement using flapless implant surgery in alveolar ridges with insufficient bone width requires greater experience, caution, and training than in cases with sufficient bone. However, excellent results can be achieved. An evaluation of the existing bone volume is the primary factor for developing a treatment plan in the ridges. To assess the amount of labiolingual bone, CT should be integrated into the pretreatment imaging (Fig 12-23). The following treatment options are available for flapless implant surgery if there is inadequate bone width available for proper-size implants.

Barely sufficient bone

Four treatment options are available if the ridge offers sufficient available bone height but the available bone width is 2.5–6 mm (division B in the Misch classification).

The first treatment option is to countersink the implant below the bone surface to ensure that the entire area of threads is inside the bone (Figs 12-24 to 12-26). The crest of the edentulous ridge is most often supported by a wider base of bone. In most cases, countersinking provides greater bone width because of this triangular-shaped

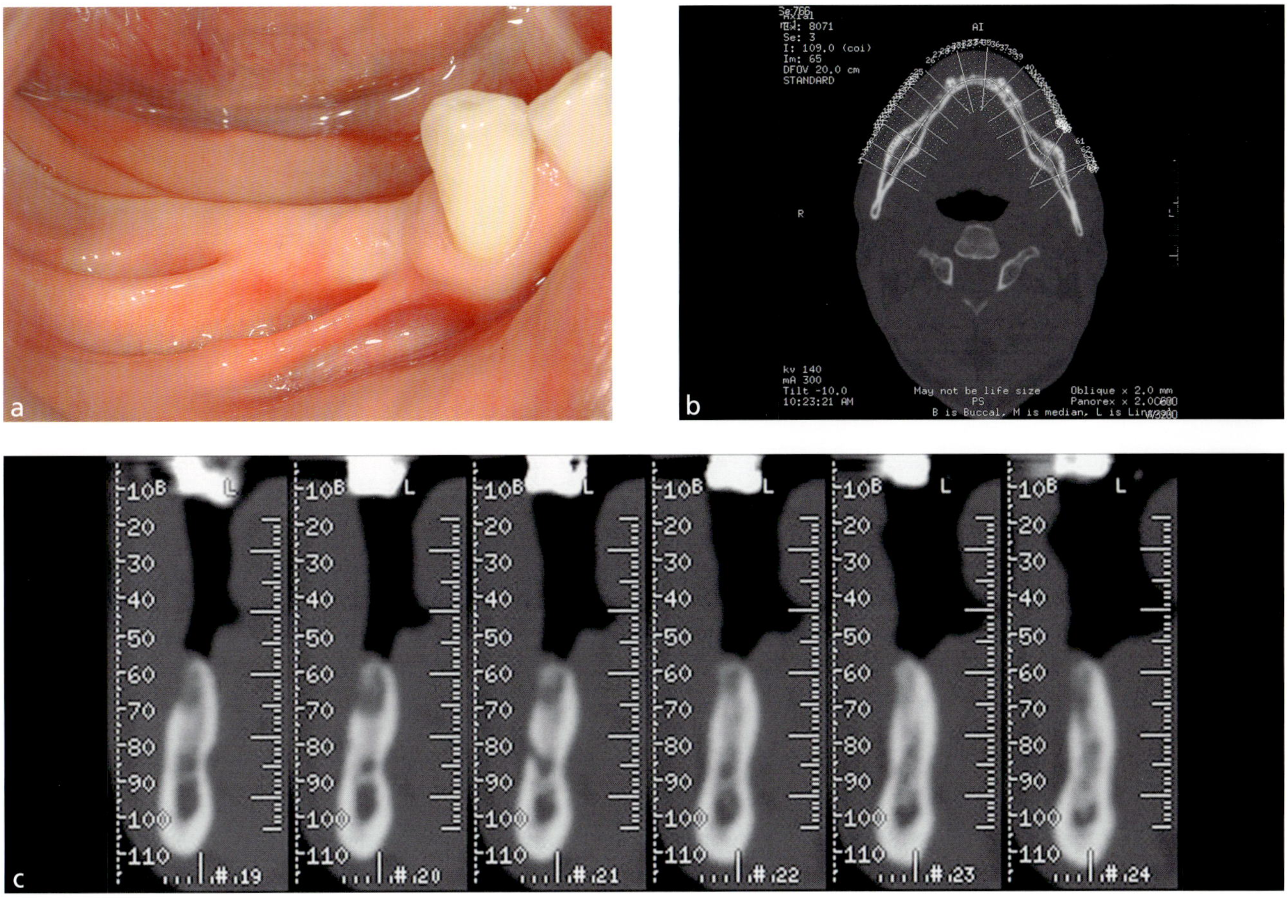

Fig 12-23 (a–c) Computerized tomography should be integrated into the pretreatment imaging process in complex cases or when accurate representation of the buccolingual amount of bone is needed.

cross-section, even though there is reduced height. This option is more likely the treatment of choice in the posterior region where adequate crown height space is created.

The second treatment option is to increase the width of bone by grafting the edentulous ridge with an autogenous or Bio-Oss® graft with or without guided bone regeneration. Bone grafting is performed using a subperiosteal tunneling procedure. The subperiosteal tunnel ensures a favorable condition for the healing of a soft tissue adjacent to the flapless implant, promotes bone generation, and reduces the incidence of membrane exposure. After augmenting the ridge, flapless implant placement can be performed. When using fixation screws or unresorbable barrier membranes for guided bone regeneration, a separate incision is made away from the flapless implant site to remove screws or membranes at the time of implant placement (Fig 12-27).

The third treatment option is simultaneous flapless implant placement and peri-implant defect correction. The treatment may be influenced by the amount of

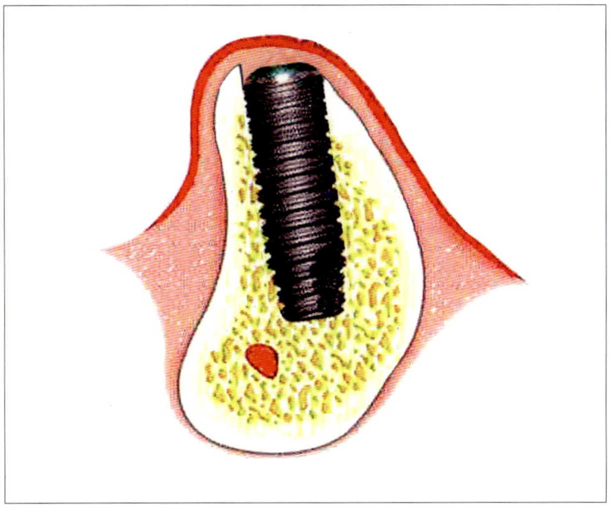

Fig 12-24 One treatment option for narrow available bone is to countersink the implant below the bone surface so that the entire area of threads is inside the bone. This option is more likely the treatment of choice in the posterior region where adequate crown height space is created.

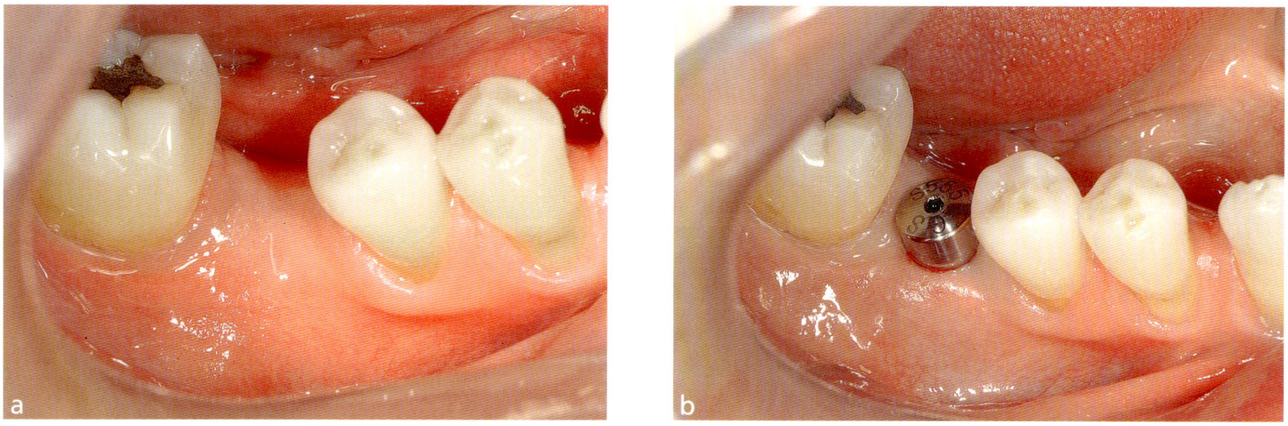

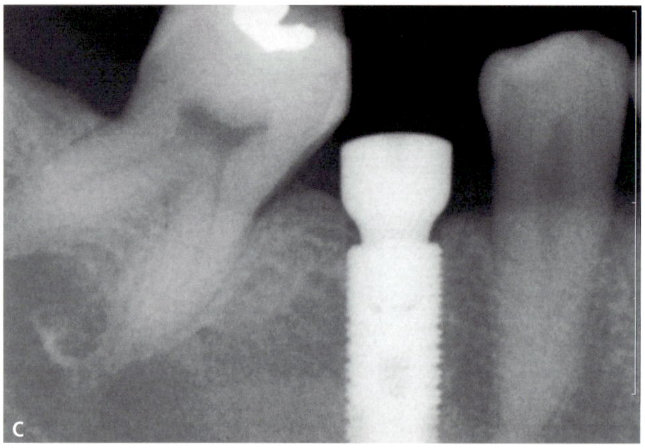

Fig 12-25 (a–c) In the case of a sloping alveolar ridge in the posterior region, this implant was countersunk below the bone surface to place the entire area of the threads inside the bone. See also Fig 12-26.

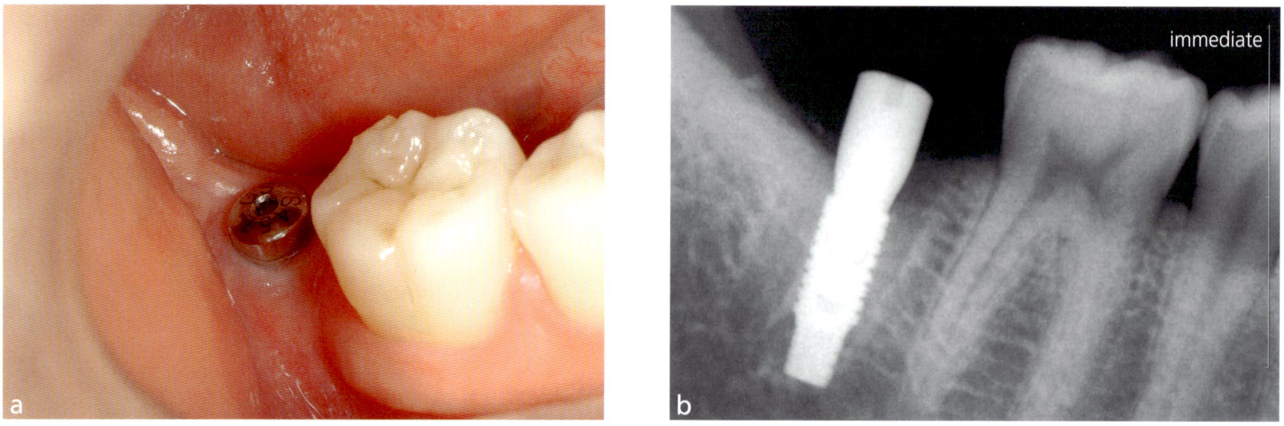

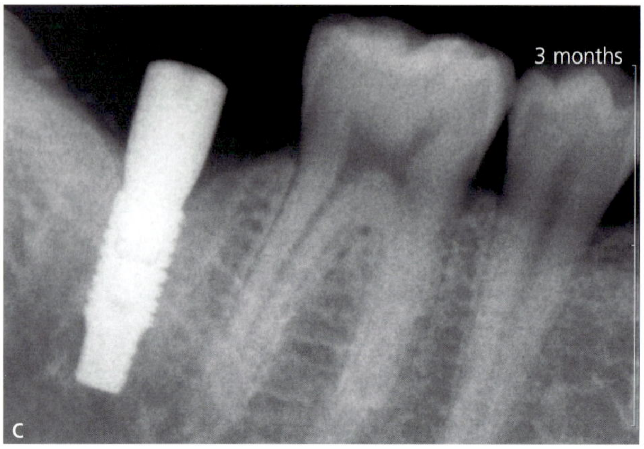

Fig 12-26 (a) Another case of a sloping alveolar ridge in the posterior region. The implant was countersunk below the bone surface to place the entire area of the threads inside the bone. (b and c) Radiographs immediately after implant placement and at 3 months.

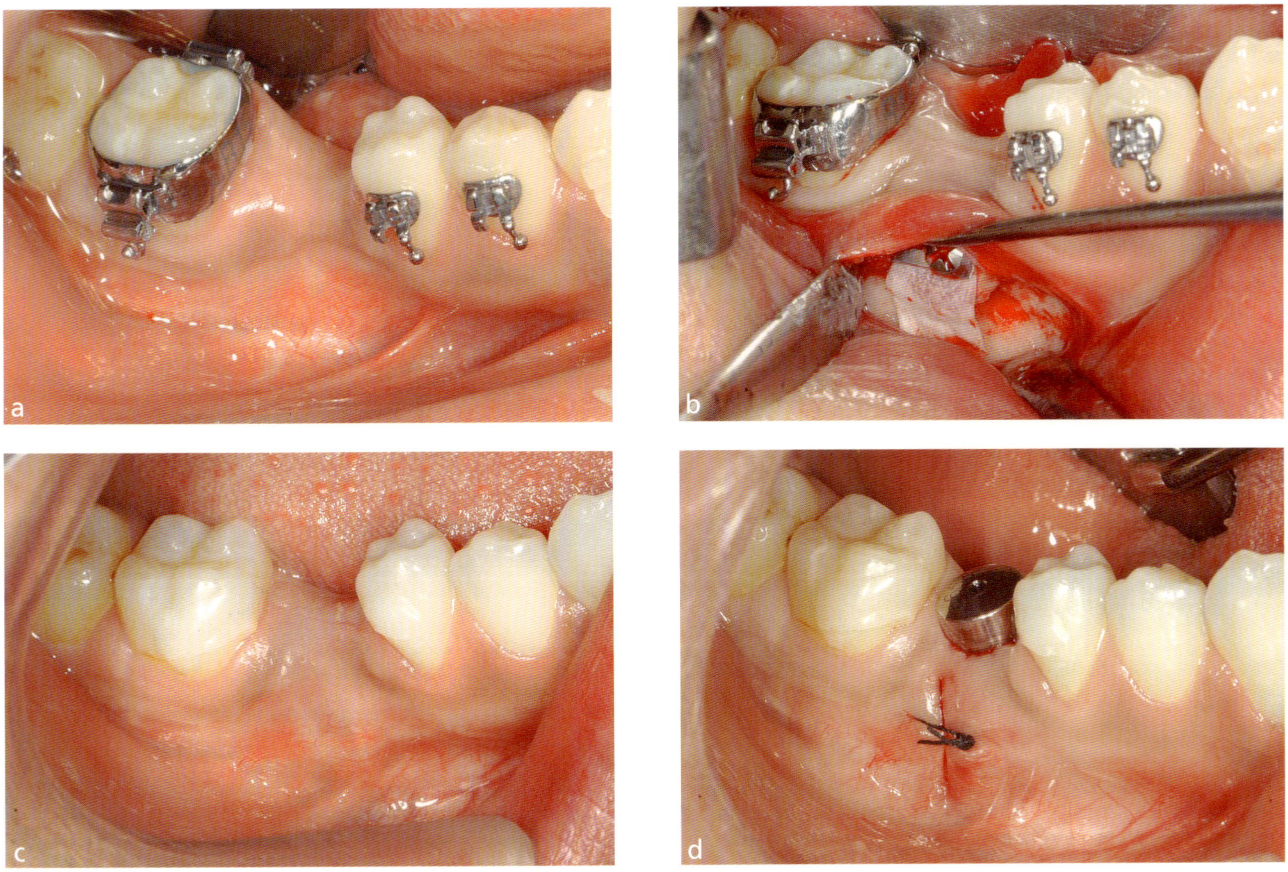

Fig 12-27 (a) Intraoral view before surgery showing the narrow available bone. (b) A block graft was positioned in the key implant region and a barrier membrane was placed over the bone graft. Both the block graft and membrane were fixed with a screw. These procedures were performed using a subperiosteal tunnel. (c) Healing after 6 months. (d) Flapless implant placement was performed. A separate incision was made away from the flapless implant site to remove the screw and membrane at the time of flapless implant placement.

exposed threads and the thickness of the overlying mucosa. Bone grafts to cover the exposed threads using a subperiosteal tunneling procedure are indicated if implant threads <5 mm are exposed outside the bone and covered with relatively thin overlying mucosa after mini-incision implant placement (see Chapter 3). In contrast, if the overlying mucosa is thick, there is no need to cover the exposed threads of the implant with grafting material provided that the primary stability of the implants is secured. If implant threads >5 mm are exposed on the buccal or labial aspects of the implants after flapless implant placement, they should be covered with a graft material using a subperiosteal tunneling procedure. Bio-Oss® in either particulate or block form is used to cover the bone defects (Figs 12-28 and 12-29). If the primary stability of the implant cannot be secured, implant placement should be delayed for secondary surgery.

The fourth treatment option is bone spreading. A narrow osteotomy can be performed between the bony plates, and bone spreaders can be tapped into the edentulous site to expand the ridge. Both bone spreading and implant placement can be performed simultaneously using the flapless method.

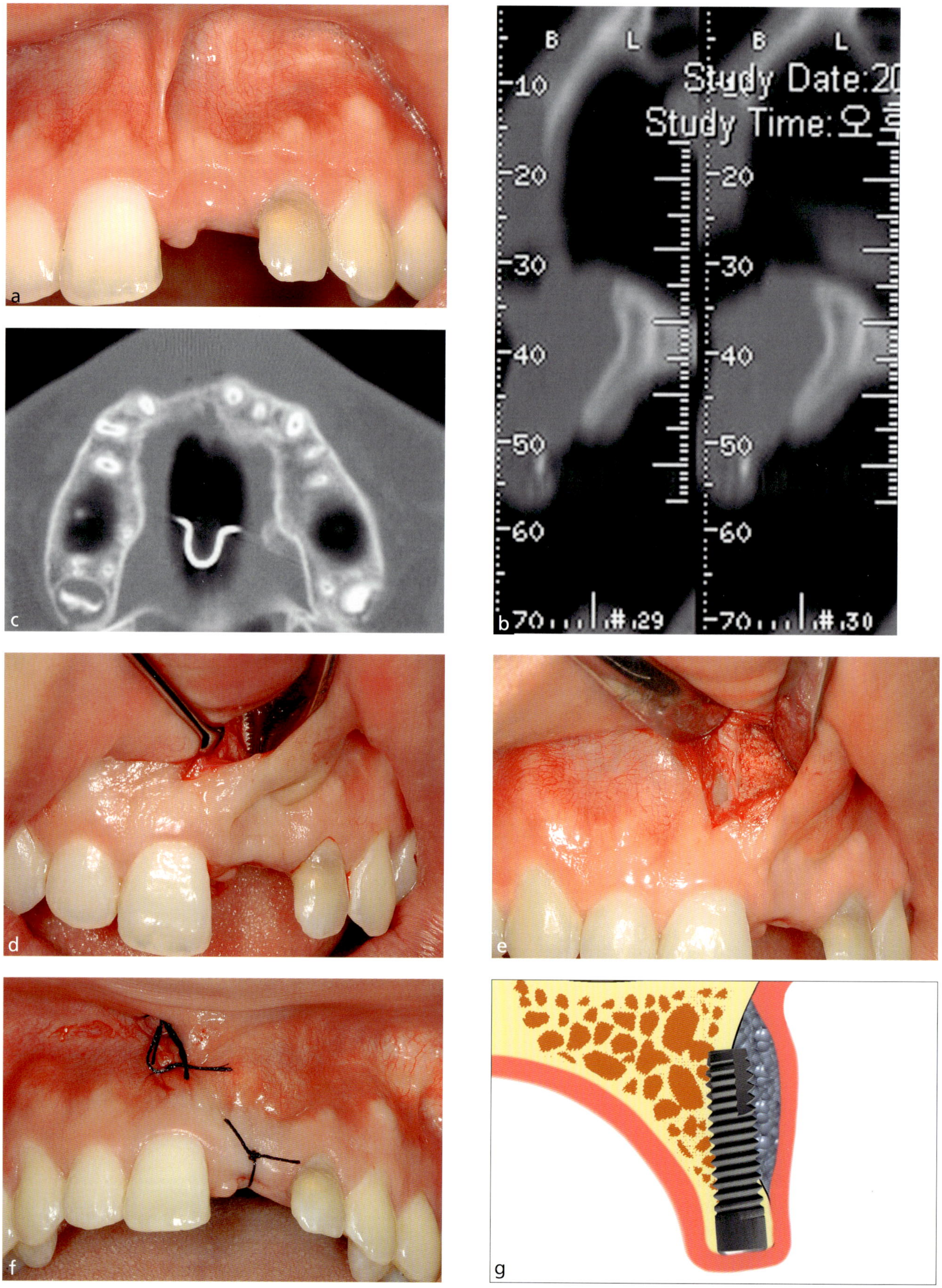
a
B
L
Study Date:20
Study Time:오
10
20
30
40
50
60
70
#29
#30
b
c
d
e
f
g

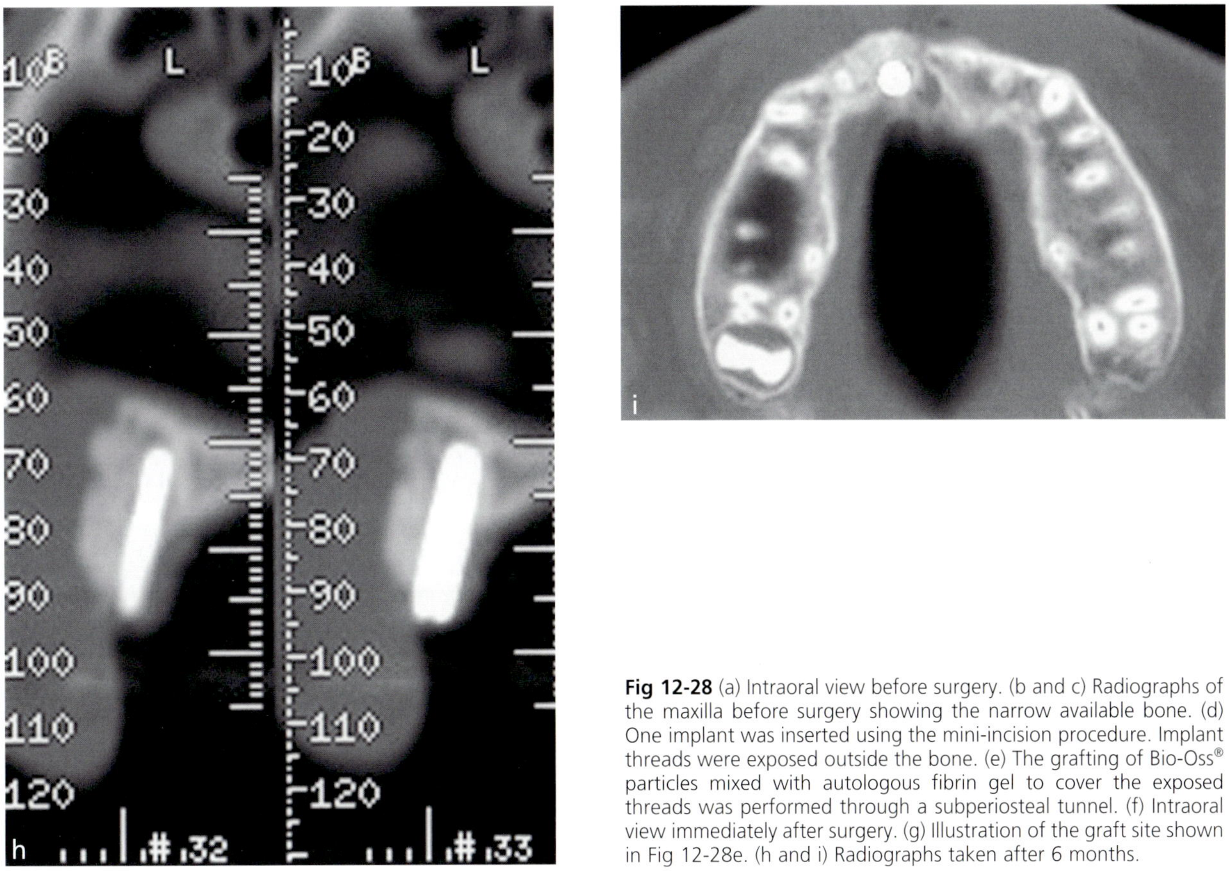

Fig 12-28 (a) Intraoral view before surgery. (b and c) Radiographs of the maxilla before surgery showing the narrow available bone. (d) One implant was inserted using the mini-incision procedure. Implant threads were exposed outside the bone. (e) The grafting of Bio-Oss® particles mixed with autologous fibrin gel to cover the exposed threads was performed through a subperiosteal tunnel. (f) Intraoral view immediately after surgery. (g) Illustration of the graft site shown in Fig 12-28e. (h and i) Radiographs taken after 6 months.

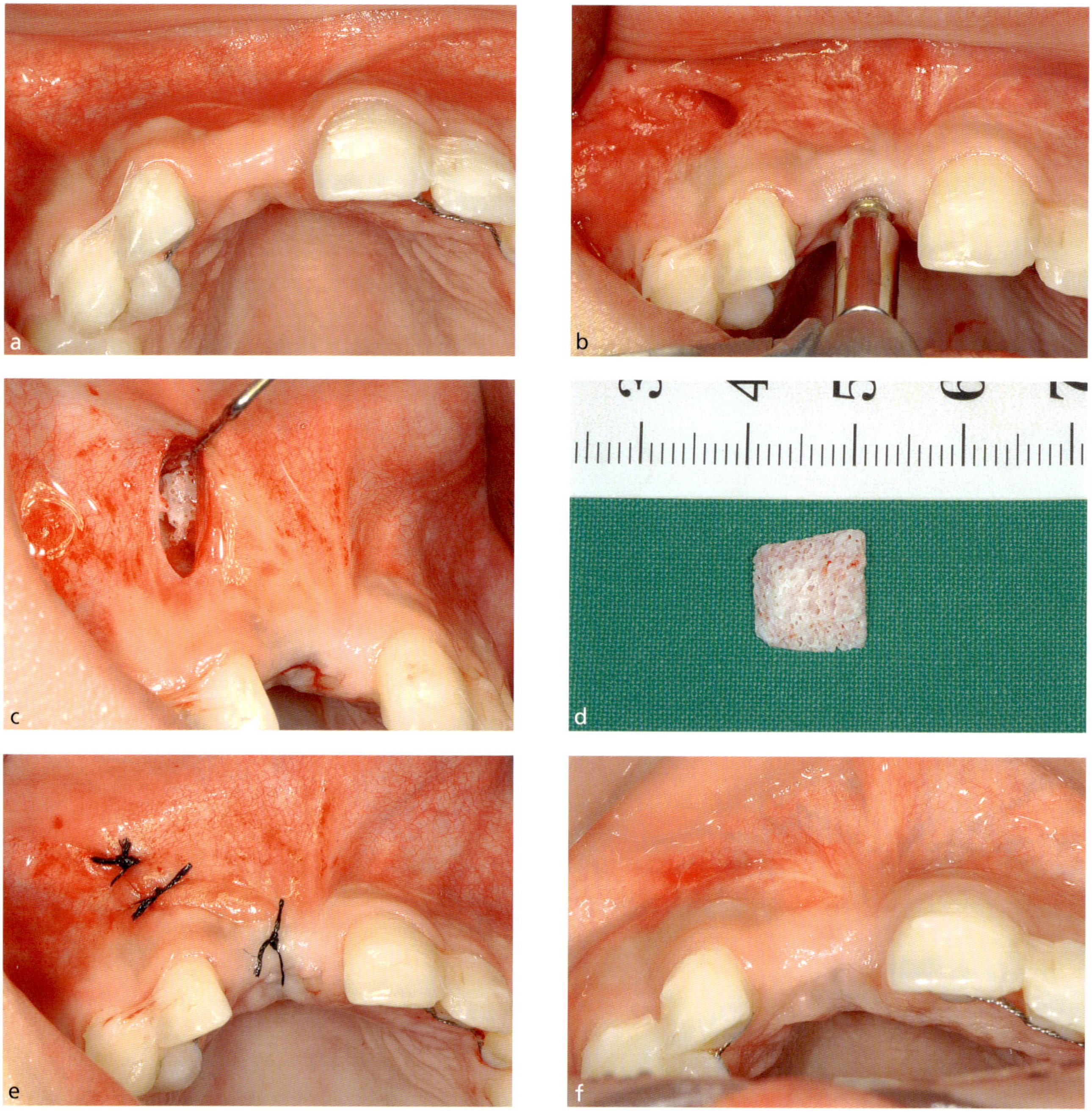

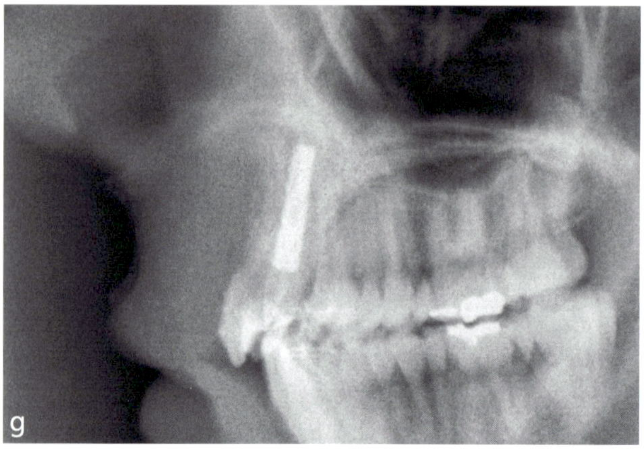

Fig 12-29 (a) Intraoral view before surgery. (b) One implant was inserted using the mini-incision procedure. (c) A layer of Bio-Oss® block was placed on the labial surface of the recipient site through a subperiosteal tunnel. (d) The Bio-Oss® block should be shaped to conform to the recipient site contours. (e and f) Intraoral views immediately after surgery and at 3 months. (g) Radiograph taken after 3 months.

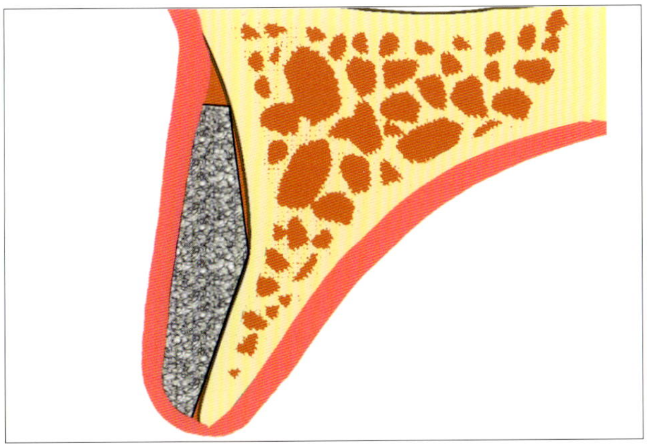

Fig 12-30 If the available bone width is <2.5 mm, bone augmentation was performed before implant placement by grafting the edentulous ridge with a block graft, which was fixed with a screw. The grafting was performed using a subperiosteal tunneling procedure. Flapless implant surgery was performed after augmenting the ridge.

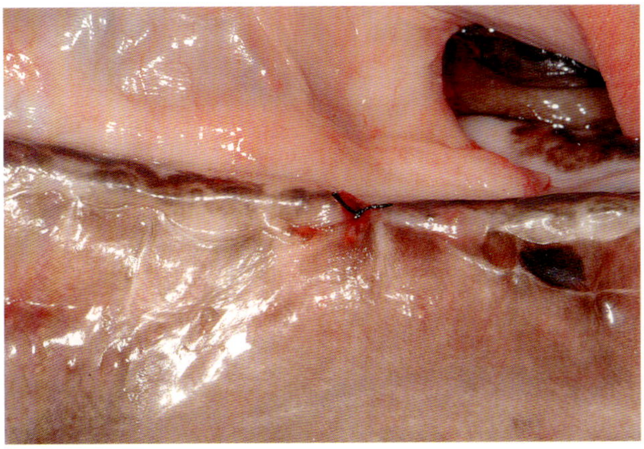

Fig 12-31 An implant was inserted in a narrow alveolar ridge using a mini-incision flapless technique.

Compromised bone

If the ridge offers sufficient available bone height but the available bone width is <2.5 mm (division C-w in the Misch classification), bone augmentation is performed before implant placement by grafting the edentulous ridge with either an autogenous or a Bio-Oss® graft with or without guided bone regeneration (Fig 12-30). Bone grafting is performed using a subperiosteal tunneling procedure. Flapless implant surgery is performed after the ridge is augmented.

Simultaneous flapless implant placement and peri-implant defect correction

Mini-incision implant placement

Implant placement using a flapless procedure is performed prior to bone grafting. The mini-incision technique is selected to submerge the implant body below the soft tissue. For mini-incision implant placement, a crestal mini-incision and local undermining is performed in the gingiva at the center of the implant site. The amount of undermining at the implant site does not exceed 5 mm. After preparing the implant site, the implants are inserted into the bone. The implants should be rigid after implant placement. If the primary stability of the implant cannot be secured, placement should be delayed to allow secondary surgery. After fixture placement, a cover screw is connected and the incised gingiva is sutured to submerge the fixture (Fig 12-31).

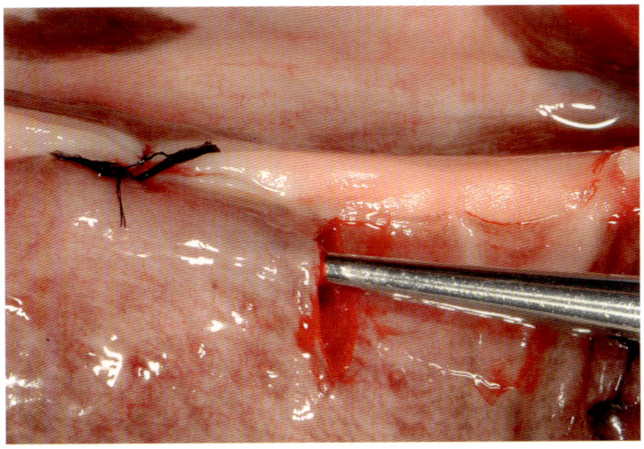

Fig 12-32 A vertical incision was made approximately 8 mm away from the implant and a subperiosteal tunnel was established to the peri-implant defect.

Subperiosteal tunneling

A separate incision is made for a subperiosteal tunnel. A vertical incision is made approximately 8 mm away from the implant on the buccal side of the alveolar ridge. A subperiosteal tunnel to the peri-implant defect is established. Tunneling is performed by lifting the periosteum using an elevator without any releasing incision on the periosteum (Fig 12-32). In the mandible, care must be taken not to damage the mental nerve while detaching the periosteum. Bio-Oss® in either particulate or block form can be used to cover the bone defects (Fig 12-33).

- When using Bio-Oss® particles, autologous fibrin gel made from autologous blood is mixed with the particles (Fig 12-34). The addition of this gel can enhance the hardening of the granular grafting material. The

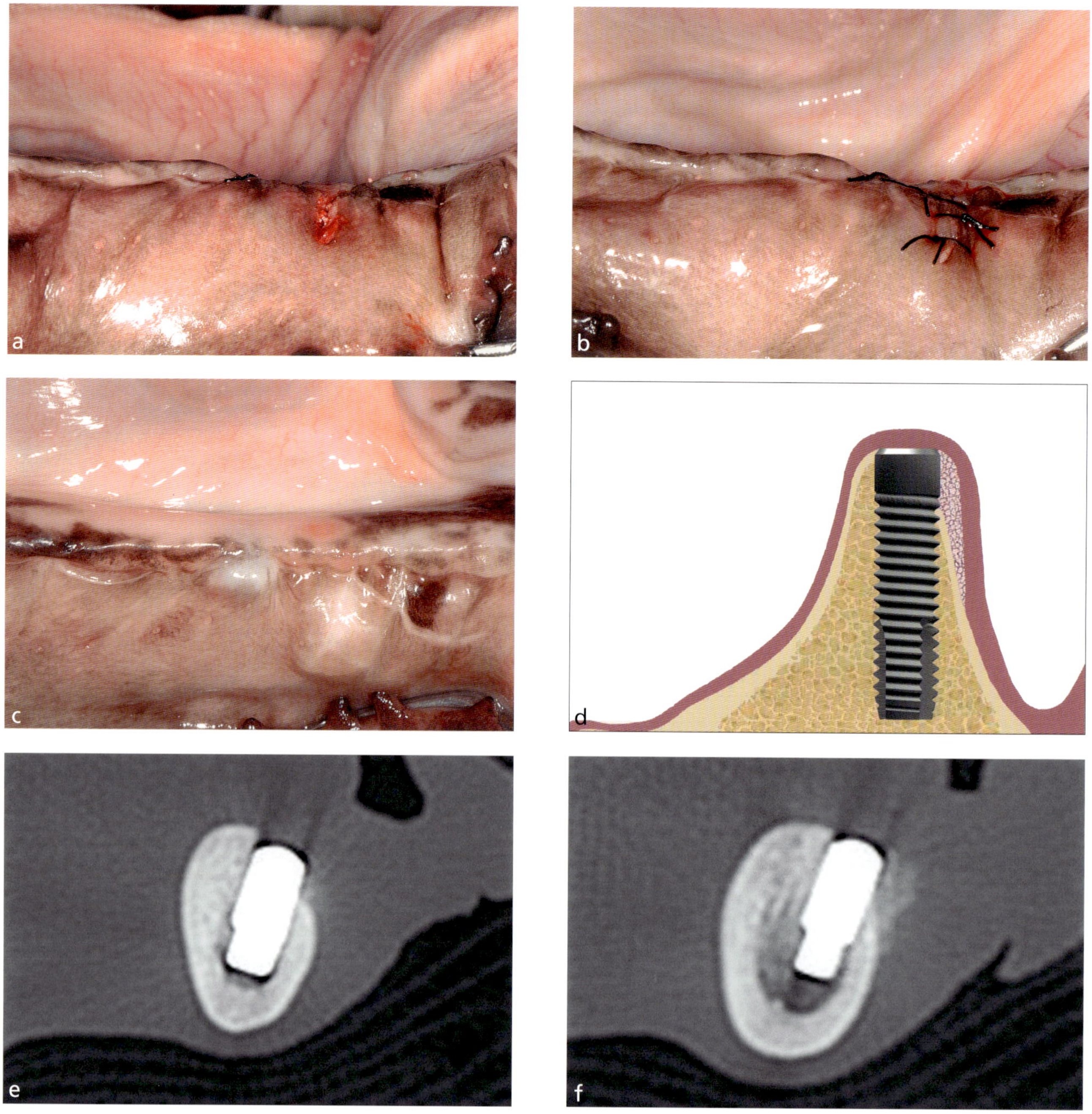

Fig 12-33 (a) View immediately after introducing the graft material to the peri-implant defects through the subperiosteal tunnel. (b) View immediately after closing the vertical incision. (c) Four months after surgery. (d) Illustration of the graft site shown in Fig 12-33b. (e) Computerized tomography scan taken before surgery. (f) Scan taken immediately after the peri-implant defect correction, showing augmentation on the buccal side of the implant.

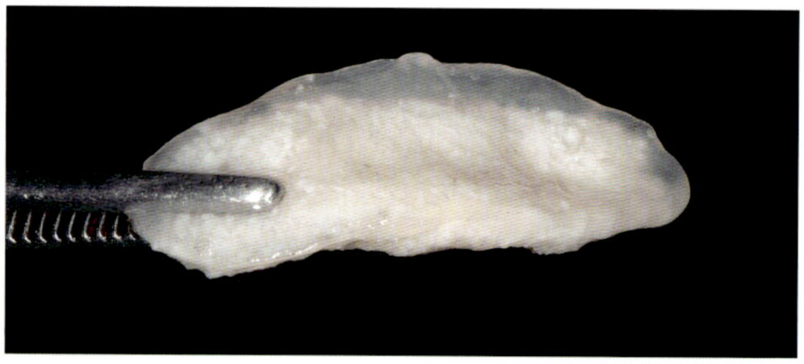

Fig 12-34 Autologous fibrin gel made using autologous blood was mixed with Bio-Oss® particles.

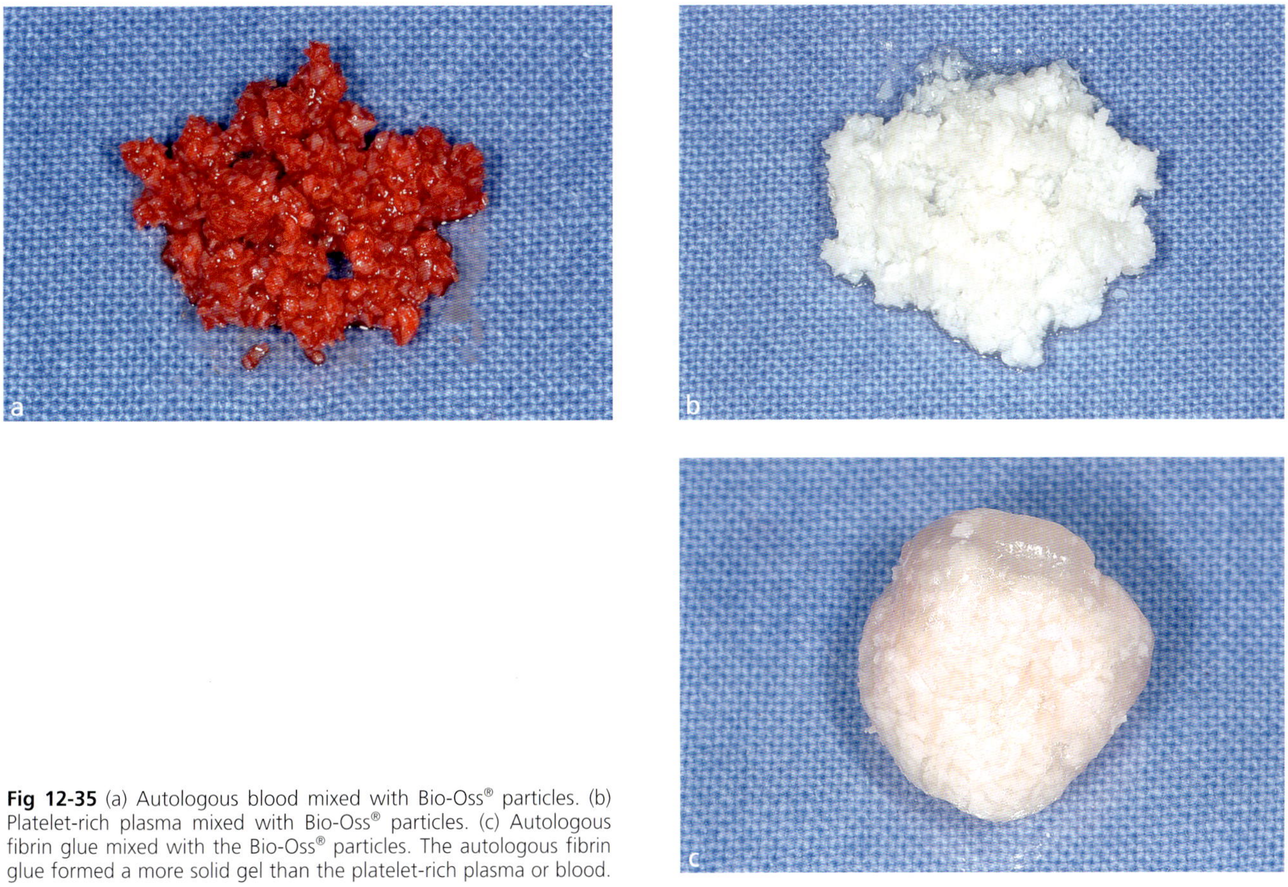

Fig 12-35 (a) Autologous blood mixed with Bio-Oss® particles. (b) Platelet-rich plasma mixed with Bio-Oss® particles. (c) Autologous fibrin glue mixed with the Bio-Oss® particles. The autologous fibrin glue formed a more solid gel than the platelet-rich plasma or blood.

mixture is introduced to the peri-implant defects through the subperiosteal tunnel. The mixture is then molded into the desired contour. After grafting, the vertical incision is closed with interrupted silk sutures (Fig 12-33b). Autologous fibrin forms a more solid gel than platelet-rich plasma or blood (Fig 12-35).

- When using Bio-Oss® blocks, the block graft shaped to fit in the anatomical structure of a recipient site is used without a barrier membrane.

Healing

Bio-Oss® particles are integrated in the host tissues 6–9 months after grafting.[27] Based on our animal experiment using five mongrel dogs,[14] the graft was well incorporated in the grafted area after a healing period of 6 months (Fig 12-36). The peri-implant defects were covered with tissue resembling bone in all cases. There was fairly extensive bone formation, where larger portions of bone particles had been introduced (Fig 12-37). A histological examination showed that, in the graft area, small amounts (spots) of new bone were in direct contact with the trabeculae of the residual Bio-Oss® particles. However, the new bone is not generally in direct contact with the implants. In all cases, a zone of dense connective tissue was interposed between the implant surface and new bone (Fig 12-38).

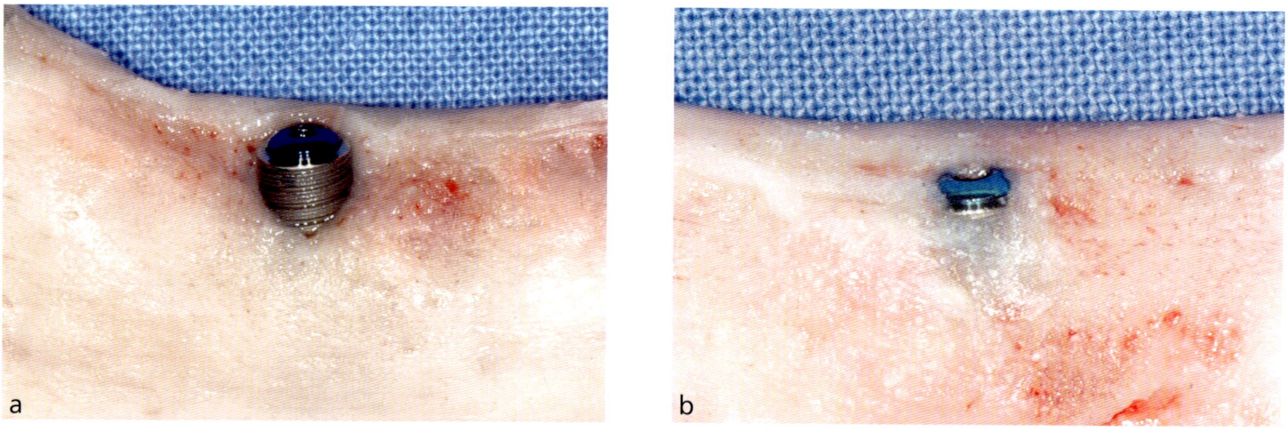

Fig 12-36 (a) In the control site where no graft was used, there is no new bone coverage on the exposed threads. (b) In the test site where the peri-implant defect correction using a subperiosteal tunneling procedure was performed, the peri-implant defect is covered with tissue resembling bone and the graft appears well incorporated in the grafted area.

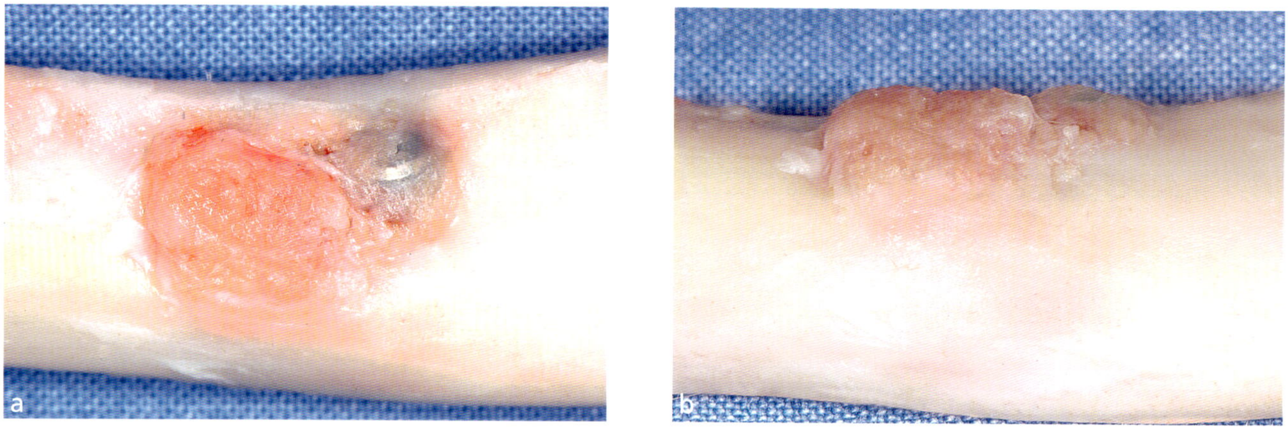

Fig 12-37 (a and b) There is fairly extensive bone formation in the cases where larger portions of Bio-Oss® particles and autologous fibrin gel composites had been introduced.

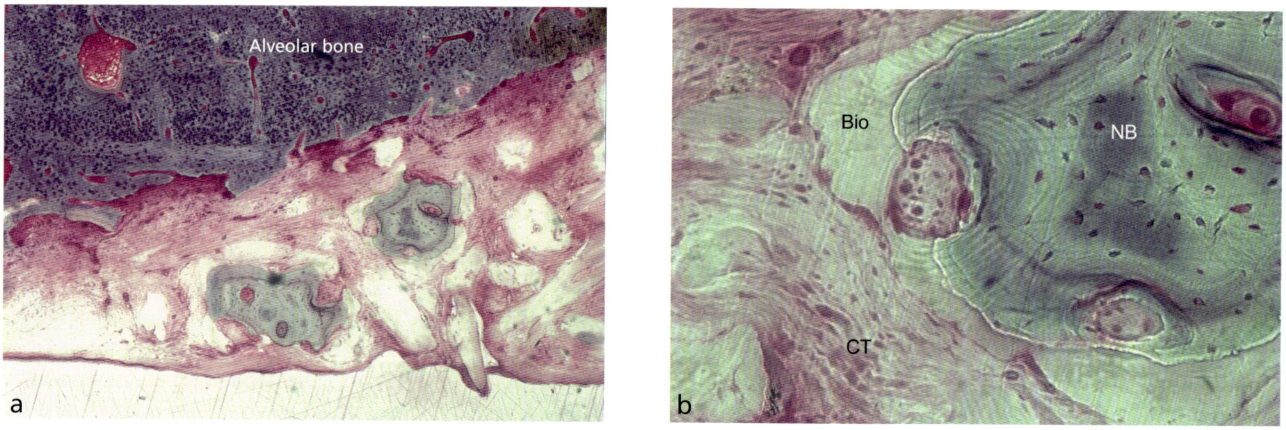

Fig 12-38 (a and b) A zone of dense connective tissue is interposed between the host bone surface and new bone, and newly formed bone is in contact with the trabeculae of the residual Bio-Oss® particles. NB – newly formed bone; Bio – Bio-Oss® particles; CT – connective tissue

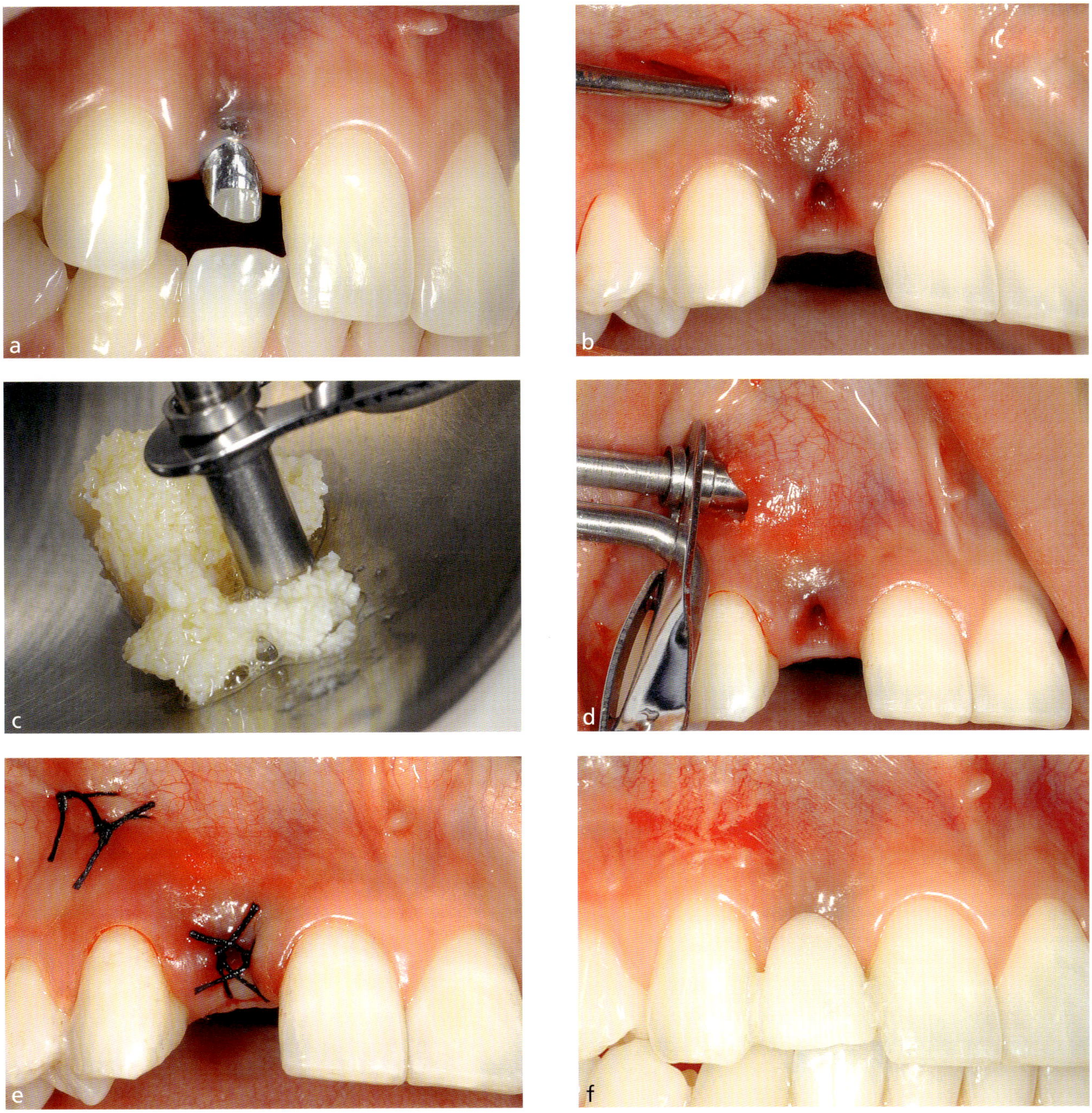

Fig 12-39 (a) Owing to the thin labial plate, bone loss occurred on the labial side of the implant after implant placement. The subsequent recession of the thin mucosa resulted in aesthetic compromise. (b) A vertical incision was made approximately 8 mm away from the implant on the labial side of the alveolar ridge. Tunneling was performed by lifting the periosteum with the periosteal elevator. (c) An amalgam carrier was used to place a Bio-Oss® particle and autologous fibrin gel composite. (d) The graft material was introduced on the labial side of the implant through the subperiosteal tunnel. (e and f) Intraoral views immediately after surgery and 6 months later.

Case report

A 20-year-old female requested treatment of an implant with an exposed metal surface. The implant had been placed in the maxillary right lateral tooth site 2 years earlier at a private dental clinic (Fig 12-39).

Radiography revealed no bone loss on the mesial and distal sides of the implant. Owing to the thin labial plate, bone loss occurred on the labial side of the implant after implant placement, and the very thin mucosa shrank, resulting in esthetic compromise. The treatment plan was to cover the exposed implant surface with a composite of Bio-Oss® particles and autologous fibrin gel using a subperiosteal tunneling procedure.

Before surgery, 20 mL of blood was withdrawn from the patient to make autologous fibrin gel. During surgery, the prosthetic abutment was removed to submerge the implant body below the soft tissue after grafting. Bio-Oss® particles mixed with autologous fibrin gel were grafted on the labial side of the implant through the subperiosteal tunnel. The particles were densely condensed at the graft site. Figure 12-39b–e show the surgical procedure. Figure 12-39f shows the intraoral view 6 months after surgery. Both the labial alveolar bone contour and the esthetics were improved.

Advantages and disadvantages of the flapless approach

- Compared with the flap procedure, in which the most common complication is graft dehiscence and incision line opening, there is little or no risk of complications because the incision line for bone augmentation is made away from the bone grafting site and the periosteum over the graft material is intact.
- The vertical incision helps to prevent impairments of the circulation to the grafted site.
- Lateral ridge augmentation can be performed simultaneously with flapless implant placement.
- The minimally invasive technique offers the advantages of a more conservative surgical entry and less postoperative morbidity, which reduces the surgery time, and minimizes postoperative pain, edema, and infection.
- Flapless implant surgery reduces the peri-implant bone loss, thus contributing to a decreased risk of gingival recession over the implant caused by bone loss.
- Bone regeneration on the exposed implant threads can occur even in the absence of a barrier membrane, thereby preventing the complications associated with a membrane.
- Patient morbidity associated with graft procurement is eliminated.
- The newly formed bone makes little contribution to the support of the implant because new bone is not generally in direct contact with the implants, and connective tissue is interposed between the implant surface and bone.
- Additive surgery is performed to gain additional height if the gingival contour after grafting Bio-Oss® particles is insufficient for a good esthetic result.

Comments on the tunneling technique

To promote the retention of Bio-Oss® particles at the graft site without dispersion, the particles should be densely condensed and contained securely. An amalgam condenser and autologous fibrin gel can help to prevent the particles from dispersing. A benefit of autologous fibrin gel is its ability to form a biological gel, which can provide graft containment and clot stability, and function as an adhesive. The ability to contain the graft material has been

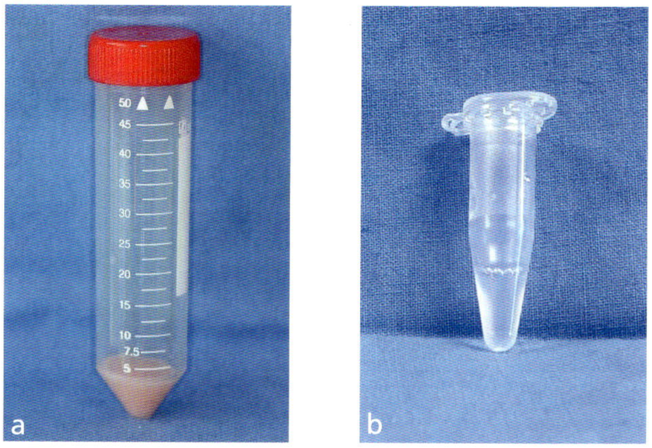

Fig 12-40 (a) Autologous fibrinogen and (b) thrombin prepared using 20 mL of blood.

demonstrated to be important for bone regeneration on the alveolar ridge. Autologous fibrin forms a more solid gel than platelet-rich plasma (Figs 12-40 and 12-41).[28–31] In terms of structural rigidity, Bio-Oss® block grafts offer benefits over Bio-Oss® particulate grafts. They are strong and can be shaped to match the host site.

Treatment of ridges with vertical bone resorption

The available bone is reduced in height as the resorption process continues. The crown height space increases as a result of vertical bone resorption. The crown height space should be measured from the crest of the bone to the occlusal plane if there is inadequate bone height available for proper-length implants.

The crown height space affects the force factors. The force applied to the implants increases with increasing height of the space.[32–34] A crown height space over 15 mm is excessive. Under these conditions, a greater lever action is applied to the implant, which can cause prosthesis failure and bone loss around the implants.

Two options should be considered in these cases. The first is the type of surgical method used to increase the bone height. The second is the type of stress reduction method used with the prosthesis.

The effect of the crown height cannot be reduced by increasing the length of the implant because most forces applied to the osseointegrated implant body are concentrated in the crestal 7–9 mm of the bone. In the case of excessive crown height space, surgical augmentation of the residual ridge may be preferred over prosthetic replacement. Bone augmentation will reduce the crown height space and improve the implant biomechanics. The crown height space also affects the esthetics. As a result, augmentation is selected most often in the area where esthetics is a

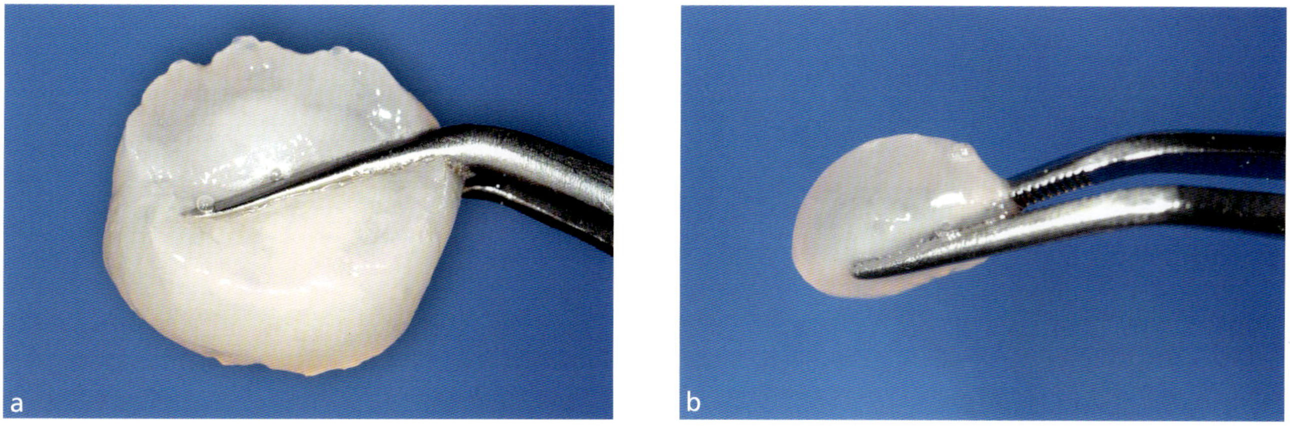

Fig 12-41 Comparison of the gels formed from (a) the autologous fibrin and (b) the platelet-rich plasma. The autologous fibrin formed a more solid gel than the platelet-rich plasma.

primary factor. The augmentation will allow an esthetic prosthesis.

Several surgical techniques have been used to increase the bone height, including block bone grafts, particulate bone grafts with a titanium mesh or barrier membranes, interpositional bone grafts, and distraction osteogenesis. We advocate performing a subperiosteal tunneling procedure with Bio-Oss® block onlay grafting (Fig 12-42). This procedure has several advantages over other bone grafting techniques for vertical bone growth. There is no donor site morbidity, little risk of graft dehiscence and incision line opening, and less postoperative morbidity. Flapless implant surgery is used after the ridge has been augmented (Fig 12-43). Although prosthetics is the most commonly used option to address the excessive crown height space, it should be the last choice. Several prosthetic methods can be used to decrease the level of stress to the implant restoration, including increasing the number of implants, reducing the cantilever lengths, or reducing the angled forces on the prosthesis. These methods will not allow an esthetic prosthesis.

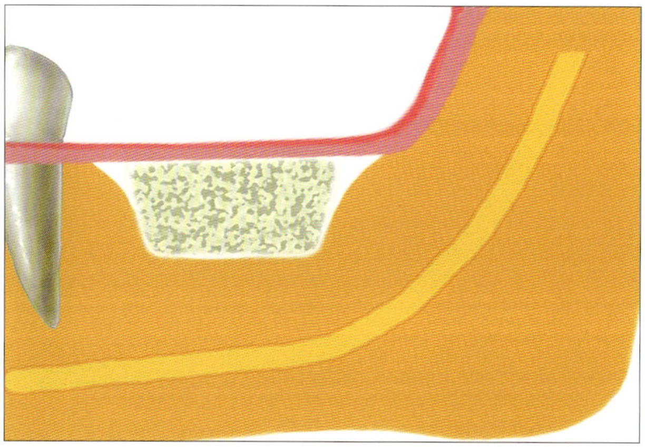

Fig 12-42 Illustration of Bio-Oss® block onlay grafting in the case of excessive vertical bone resorption.

Surgical keys to bone grafting

For successful bone grafting, soft tissue closure and space maintenance are critical factors.[35] Other important factors include graft immobilization and host bone vascularization.

Soft tissue closure

The most common postoperative complication in intraoral bone grafting is incision line opening during initial healing. The consequences of incision line opening are delayed healing, leaking of the graft into the oral cavity, and increased risk of infection.[23] Studies have reported that the rate of occurrence of incision line opening after bone grafting was up to 40%.[20,21] As a result, care should be taken to choose the appropriate surgical method to prevent incision line opening. The subperiosteal tunneling technique is quite advantageous in avoiding this complication.

Space maintenance

Ridge augmentation using guided bone regeneration is frequently compromised by a collapse of the barrier membrane caused by pressure from the overlying soft tissue. The material used for augmentation must provide sufficient stability to resist the soft tissue pressure. If the grafting material is composed of particles, they will be dispersed by the pressure. The particles should therefore be contained securely. Space maintenance in the area of the bone graft is paramount to the bone formation process.[36,37] Space loss means a loss of space for bone to be generated. Therefore, space must exist long enough for the bone to fill the desired region. Accordingly, space maintenance should be ensured, either through the use of a grafting material that does not resorb too rapidly or the use of a barrier membrane that does not lead to the collapse of space under the membrane.

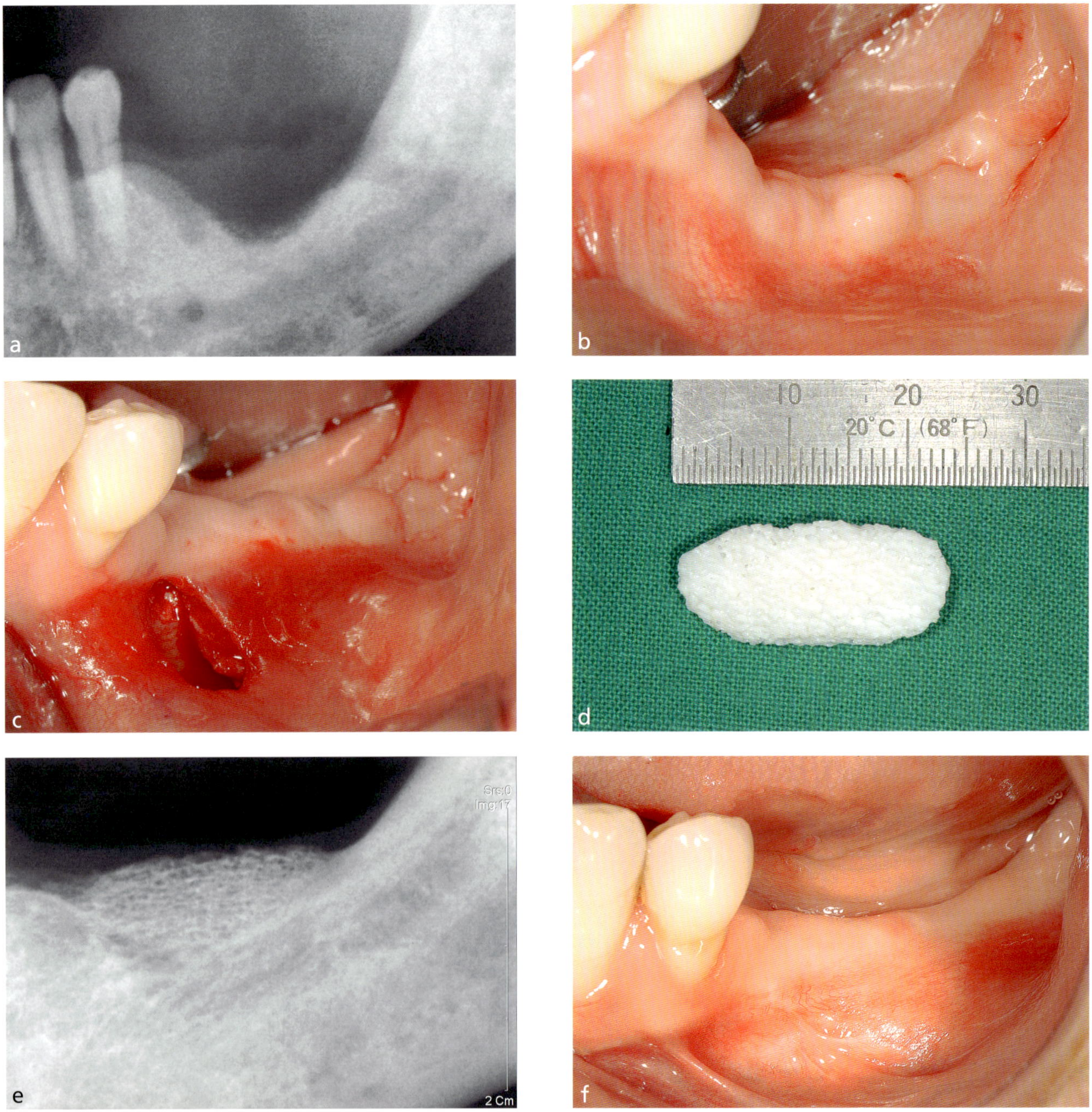

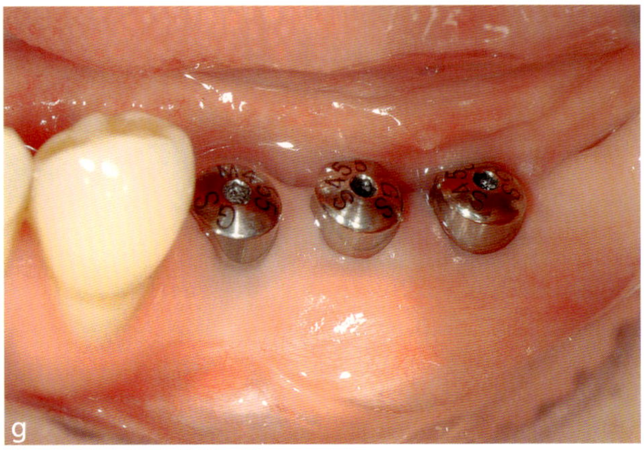

Fig 12-43 (a) Radiograph of the mandible before surgery. (b) Intraoral view before surgery. (c) Intraoral view during surgery. A Bio-Oss® block was placed in a defect area of the mandible through a subperiosteal tunnel. (d) The Bio-Oss® block was shaped to conform to the recipient site contours. (e) Radiograph taken after 12 months. (f) Intraoral view after 12 months. (g) Three implants were inserted using a flapless implant procedure. (h and i) *(facing page)* Radiographs taken immediately after placing the implant and at 24 months.

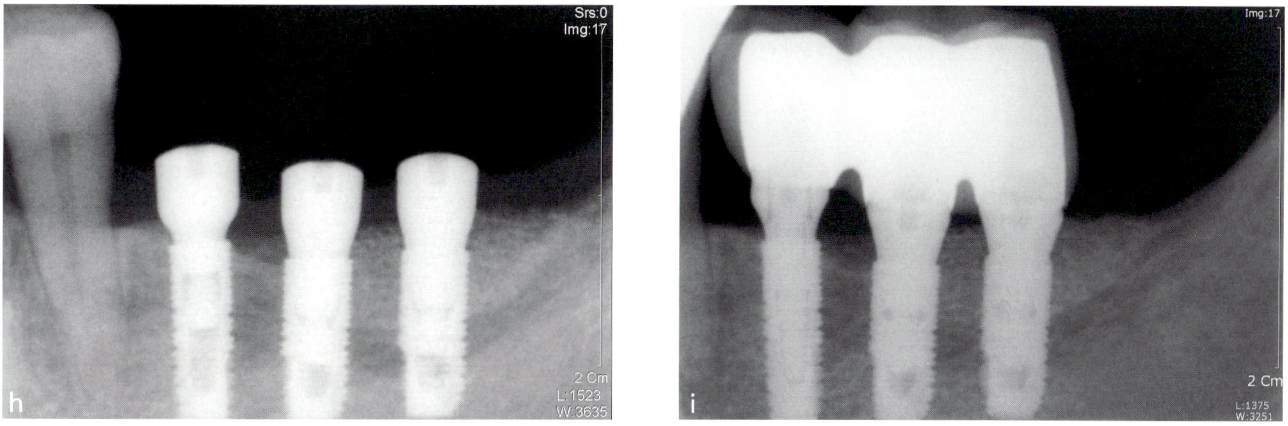

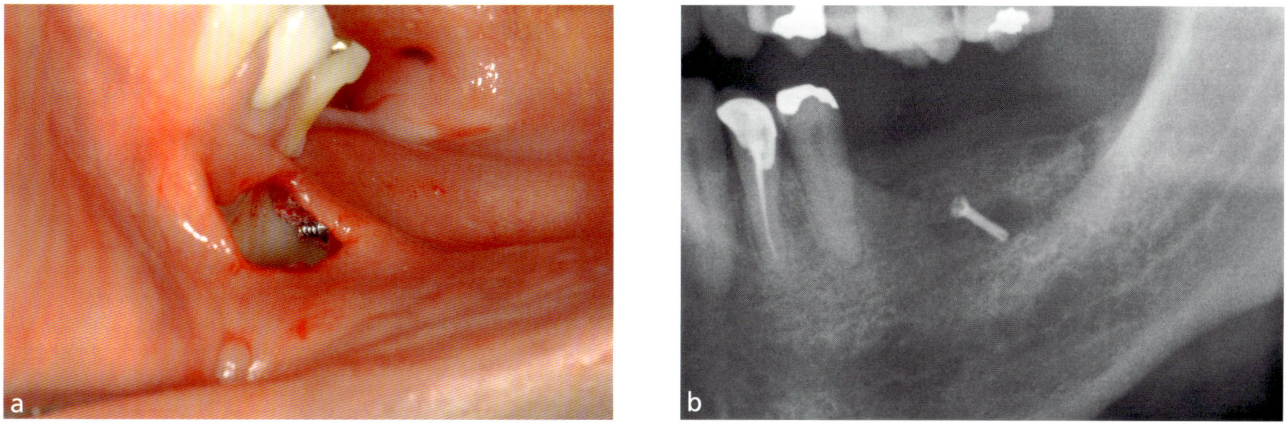

Fig 12-44 When performing a subperiosteal tunneling procedure with a Bio-Oss® block graft, it is essential to fix the block to the recipient site with screws if it is not stable under the periosteum. (a) Intraoral view after fixing the Bio-Oss® block with a screw. (b) Radiograph showing the block and screw.

Graft immobilization

Graft stabilization is essential for achieving predictable bone augmentation.[38,39] If pieces of a particulate graft material or block bone grafts are mobile, they cannot develop a blood supply for new bone formation. Instead, the graft becomes encapsulated in fibrous tissue and often sequestrates. The membrane or graft material should be fixed in order for the barrier membranes and particulate or block graft materials to work most effectively.[40] When performing a subperiosteal tunneling procedure with a Bio-Oss® block graft, it is essential to fix the block to the recipient site with screws if it is not stable under the periosteum (Fig 12-44).

Host bone vascularization

The blood vessels that grow into a bone graft are of primary importance for successful bone augmentation. Not only are the vessels needed to help to maintain the autograft vitality, but they are also required to repopulate the area with osteoblasts to grow new bone. The vessels arise from two primary sources: the host bone and the mucoperiosteum. Care should be taken to cause minimal surgical damage to the mucoperiosteum because it plays a key role in bone regeneration.[21,23] When performing a subperiosteal tunneling procedure, tunneling should be performed without a releasing incision on the periosteum.

Summary

If there is inadequate bone width or height available for proper-size implants, the treatment option is chosen based on the amount of insufficient bone width, the amount of exposed threads, primary stability of the implant, thickness of the overlying mucosa, and crown height space. Implant placement using a flapless procedure is performed prior to bone grafting or simultaneously with grafting. If bone grafting is indicated, the graft can be performed using a subperiosteal tunneling procedure. Bio-Oss® in either particulate or block form can be used to augment the bone defects.

A Bio-Oss® in block can be selected when an augmentation for height is required. When using Bio-Oss® particles, an autologous fibrin gel can be mixed with the particles to promote retention of the particles at the graft site.

References

1. Carlsson GE, Thilander H, Hedegard B. Histologic changes in the upper alveolar process after extractions with or without insertion of an immediate full denture. Acta Odontol Scand 1967;25:21–43.
2. Pietrokovski J, Massler M. Alveolar ridge resorption following tooth extraction. J Prosthet Dent 1967;17:21–27.
3. Lekholm U, Sennerby L, Roos J, Becker W. Soft tissue and marginal bone conditions of osseointegrated implants that have exposed threads: a 5-year retrospective study. Int J Oral Maxillofac Implants 1996;11:599–604.
4. Rasmusson L, Sennerby L, Lundgren D, Nyman S. Morphometrical and dimensional changes after barrier removal in bone formed beyond the skeletal borders at titanium implants: a kinetic study in the rabbit tibia. Clin Oral Implants Res 1996;8:316–322.
5. Rasmusson L, Meredith N, Sennerby L. Measurements of stability changes of titanium implants with exposed threads subjected to barrier membrane-induced bone augmentation. Clin Oral Implants Res 1997;8:316–322.
6. Lauer G, Schilli W. Collected implant cavity borings used as peri-implant osseous augmentation material. Int J Oral Maxillofac Implants 1994;9:437–444.
7. Mailhot JM, Borke JL. An isolation and in-vitro culturing method for human intraoral bone cells derived from dental implant preparation sites. Clin Oral Implants Res 1998;9:43–50.
8. Schliephake H, Dard M, Planck H, Hierlemann H, Stern U. Alveolar ridge repair using resorbable membranes and autogenous bone particles with simultaneous placement of implants: an experimental pilot study in dogs. Int J Oral Maxillofac Implants 2000;15:364–373.
9. Klinge B, Alberius P, Isaksson S, Jonsson J. Osseous response to implanted natural bone mineral and synthetic hydroxyapatite ceramic in the repair of experimental skull bone defects. J Oral Maxillofac Surg 1992;50:241–249.
10. Skoglund A, Hising P, Young C. A clinical and histologic examination in humans of the osseous response to implanted natural bone mineral. Int J Oral Maxillofac Implants 1997;12:194–199.
11. Pinholt EM, Bang G, Haanaes HR. Alveolar ridge augmentation in rats by Bio-Oss®. Scand J Dent Res 1991;99:154–161.
12. Young C, Sandstedt P, Skoglund A. A comparative study of anorganic xenogenic bone and autogenous bone implants for bone regeneration in rabbits. Int J Oral Maxillofac Implants 1999;14:72–76.
13. Araújo MG, Carmagnola D, Berglundh T, Thilander B, Lindhe J. Orthodontic movement in bone defects augmented with Bio-Oss®. An experimental study in dogs. J Clin Periodontol 2001;28:73–80.
14. Jeong SM, Choi BH, Li J, Xuan F. Simultaneous flapless implant placement and peri-implant defect correction: an experimental pilot study in dogs. J Periodontol 2008;79:876–880.
15. Jovanovic SA, Spiekermann H, Richter EJ. Bone regeneration around titanium dental implants in dehisced defect sites: a clinical study. Int J Oral Maxillofac Implants 1992;7:233–245.
16. Becker W, Dahlin C, Becker BE et al. The use of e-PTFE barrier membranes for bone promotion around titanium implants placed into extraction sockets: a prospective multicenter study. Int J Oral Maxillofac Implants 1994;9:31–40.
17. Mellonig JT, Triplett G. Guided tissue regeneration and endosseous dental implants. Int J Periodont Rest Dent 1993;13:109–119.
18. Pretorius JA, Melsen B, Nel JC, Germishuys PJ. A histomorphometric evaluation of factors influencing the healing of bony defects surrounding implants. Int J Oral Maxillofac Implants 2005;20:387–398.
19. Gotfredsen K, Warrer K, Hjørting-Hansen, Karring T. Effect of membranes and porous hydroxyapatite on healing in bone defects around titanium dental implants: an experimental study in monkeys. Clin Oral Implants Res 1991;2:172–178.
20. Buser D, Brägger U, Lang NP. Regeneration and enlargement of jaw bone using guided tissue regeneration. Clin Oral Implants Res 1990;1:22–32.
21. Buser D, Dula K, Belser U. Localized ridge augmentation using guided bone regeneration. I: Surgical procedure in the maxilla. Int J Periodont Prost Dent 1993;13:29–45.
22. Araújo MG, Sonohara M, Hayacibara R, Cardaropoli G, Lindhe J. Lateral ridge augmentation by the use of grafts comprised of autologous bone or a biomaterial: an experiment in the dog. J Clin Periodontol 2002;29:1122–1131.
23. Simion M, Baldoni M, Rossi P. A comparative study of the effectiveness of e-PTFE membranes with and without early exposure during the healing period. Int J Perio Rest Dent 1994;14:167–180.
24. Jensen OT, Greer RO, Johnson L, Dassebaum D. Vertical guided bone-graft augmentation in a new canine mandibular model. Int J Oral Maxillofac Implants 1995;10:335–344.
25. Misch CE. Divisions of available bone in implant dentistry. Int J Oral Implant 1990;7:9–17.
26. Engelke W. Surgical implantation treatment concept for atrophic upper and lower jaw. Niedersachs Zahnarztbl 1991;26:404–409.
27. Buser D, Dula K, Hirt HP. Lateral ridge augmentation using autografts and barrier membranes: a clinical study with 40 partially edentulous patients. J Oral Maxillofac Surg 1996;54:420–432.
28. You TM, Choi BH, Zhu SJ et al. Platelet-enriched fibrin glue and platelet-rich plasma in the repair of bone defects adjacent to titanium dental implants. J Oral Maxillofac Implants 2007;22:417–422.
29. Zhu SJ, Choi BH, Jung JH et al. Comparative histological analysis of tissue-engineered bone using platelet-rich plasma and platelet-enriched fibrin glue. Oral Surg Oral Med Oral Pathol Oral Radiol Endod 2006;102:175–179.
30. You TM, Choi BH, Zhu SJ et al. Treatment of experimental peri-implantitis using autogenous bone grafts and platelet-enriched fibrin glue in dogs. Oral Surg Oral Med Oral Pathol Oral Radiol Endod 2007;103:34–37.
31. Lee HJ, Choi BH, Jung JH et al. Maxillary sinus floor augmentation using autogenous bone grafts and platelet-enriched fibrin glue with simultaneous implant placement. Oral Surg Oral Med Oral Pathol Oral Radiol Endod 2007;103:329–333.
32. Papavasiliou G, Tripodakis AP, Kamposiora P, Strub JR, Bayne SC. Finite element analysis of ceramic abutment-restoration combinations for osseointegrated implants. Int J Prosthodont 1996;9:254–260.
33. Lin S, Shi S, LeGeros RZ, LeGeros JP. Three-dimensional finite element analyses of four designs of a high-strength silicon nitride implant. Implant Dent 2000;9:53–60.
34. Penny RE, Kraal JH. Crown to root ratio: its significance in restorative dentistry. J Prosthet Dent 1979;42:34–38.
35. Misch CE. Contemporary Implant Dentistry, ed 2. St Louis, MO: Mosby, 1999:397–407.
36. Von Arx T, Hardt N, Walikamm B. The TIME technique: a new method for localized alveolar ridge augmentation prior to placement of dental implants. Int J Oral Maxillofac Implants 1996;11:387–394.
37. Widmark G, Andersson B, Ivanoff CJ. Mandibular bone graft in the anterior maxilla for single-tooth implants: presentation of a single method. Int J Oral Maxillofac Surg 1997;26:106–109.
38. Lin KY, Bartlett SP, Yaremchuk M. The effect of rigid fixation on the survival of onlay bone grafts: an experimental study. Plast Reconstr Surg 1990;86:449–456.
39. LaTrenta GS, McCarthy JG, Breitbart AS. The role of rigid skeletal fixation in bone graft augmentation of the craniofacial skeleton. Plast Reconstr Surg 1989;84:578–588.
40. Melcher AH, Accurs GE. Osteogenic capacity of periosteal and osteoperiosteal flaps elevated from the parietal bone of the rat. Arch Oral Biol 1971;16:573–580.

CHAPTER 13

Simultaneous Socket Lift Procedure

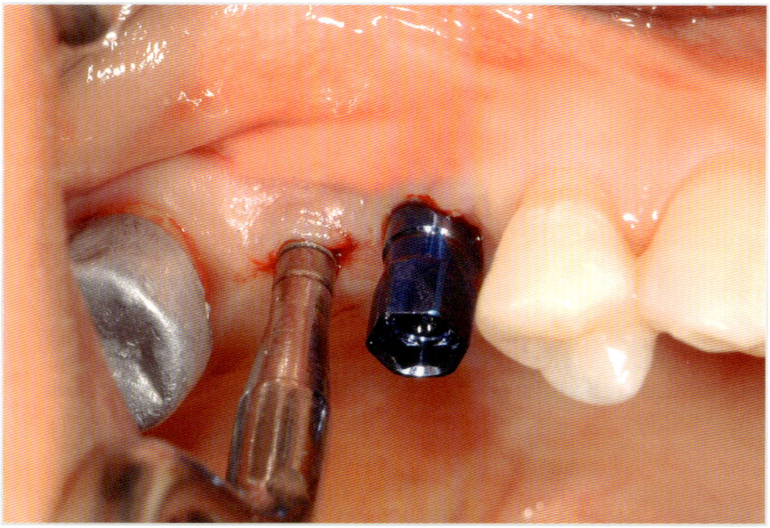

Key point

Socket lift and implant placement can be performed simultaneously using a flapless method.

Overview

The socket lift procedure is used to obtain small, localized elevation of the sinus floor. This technique involves a greenstick-type fracture in the antral floor achieved by compressing the bone below the antrum. Osteotomes are employed with a surgical mallet to compress the sinus floor. This chapter addresses the method of socket lift and immediate flapless implant placement.

Review of the literature

The socket lift procedure can be classified into three types. The first is the alveolar crest-based Summer's osteotome technique.[1] The depth of the implant osteotomy is made approximately 1–2 mm short of the floor of the antrum, and a flat-ended or cupped osteotome with the same diameter as the final osteotomy is then inserted into the osteotomy site and tapped in an attempt to create a greenstick fracture of the antral floor, causing slow elevation of the sinus floor. Summers reported a 96% success rate using the osteotome technique in 46 patients. Horowitz[2] reported a 97% success rate in 18 patients.

The second technique is bone-added osteotome sinus-floor elevation.[3] This involves inserting graft material in the osteotomy and elevating the sinus floor with the graft material.

The third technique is a trephine bone core sinus elevation graft that employs a trephine followed by an osteotome to push the core into the sinus cavity.[4–6] The core is intruded to allow one half to one third of the bone core to remain in contact with the alveolar bone.

Types of osteotome

There are two types of osteotome, depending on the shape of the handle: straight and angled. The straight osteotome is quite efficacious in the pre-maxilla but it is difficult to use to deal with the posterior maxilla. Depending on the end shape, the osteotome can also be classified into convex, flat-ended, or cupped (Fig 13-1). The osteotome with a convex tip may both compress the bone trabeculae and expand the osteotomy site. It is not used to elevate the sinus floor because it cannot push the bone upward. A flat-ended or cupped osteotome is used to elevate the sinus floor. The flat-ended or cupped osteotomes are further subdivided into tapered and cylindrical types. Tapered and flat-ended osteotomes push the bone upward while expanding the osteotomy site, whereas cylindrical and flat-ended osteotomes only push the bone upward.

A tapered flat-ended osteotome is recommended to compress the bone below the antrum and simultaneously expand the osteotomy site. Osteotomes with angled handles are more desirable than straight ones because they are mainly used in the posterior maxilla.

Problems related to the socket lift procedure

There are reports of successful bone formation with socket lift and simultaneous implant placement, which involves reflecting the mucoperiosteum. The mean endosinus bone gain is 2.2 mm.[7] However, there have been problems with implant placement. A common difficulty encountered is crestal peri-implant bone loss after flap implant surgery. The mean crestal bone loss is 1.2 mm, which is 50% of the bone gained from the socket lift (Fig 13-2).[7] It is advisable to use flapless implant placement to prevent or minimize peri-implant bone loss after the procedure. The results of the present authors' study demonstrated that flapless implant surgery, performed simultaneously with socket lift, results in good healing of the peri-implant bone (Fig 13-3).

Socket lift within the implant osteotomy and simultaneous flapless implant placement

This technique is indicated when there is 10–12 mm of vertical bone present, and only 2 mm of bone augmentation in the maxillary sinus is needed to place the implants.

The incision

A crestal mini-incision, approximately 5 mm, is made horizontally with the alveolar crest at the center of the implant site (Fig 13-4), and local undermining of the gingiva is then performed. The amount of undermining at the implant site does not exceed 6 mm and falls within the range of a large-diameter implant.

Drilling

The osteotomy is prepared using drills. Prior to drilling, the mucosal thickness is measured using a periodontal probe or a depth gauge to control the drilling depth to above the mucosa. The distance between the mucosal surface and antral floor is marked on the drills. The depth of the implant osteotomy should be approximately 1–2 mm short of the floor of the antrum (Fig 13-5). In the case of poor bone quality, a 2 mm pilot drill can be used to

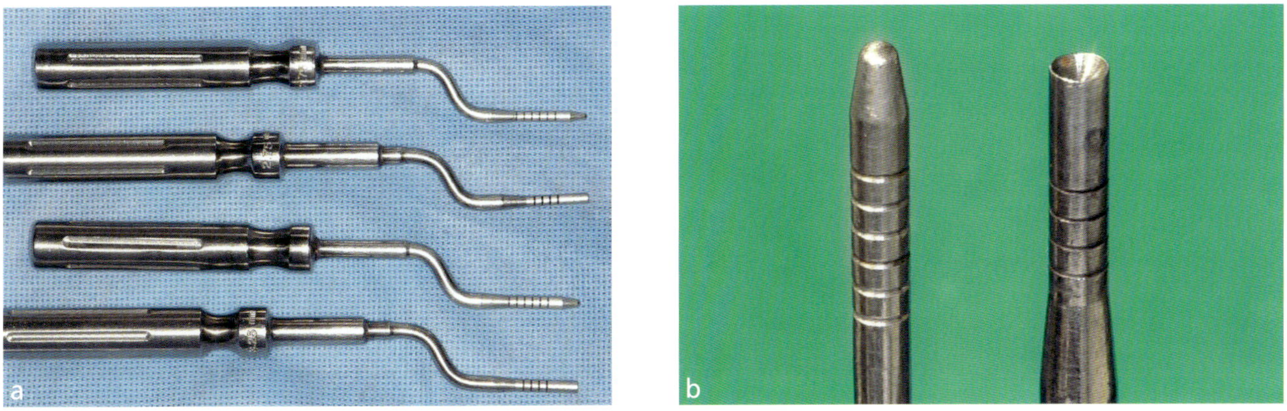

Fig 13-1 (a) Angled osteotomes. (b) The end shape of the osteotome.

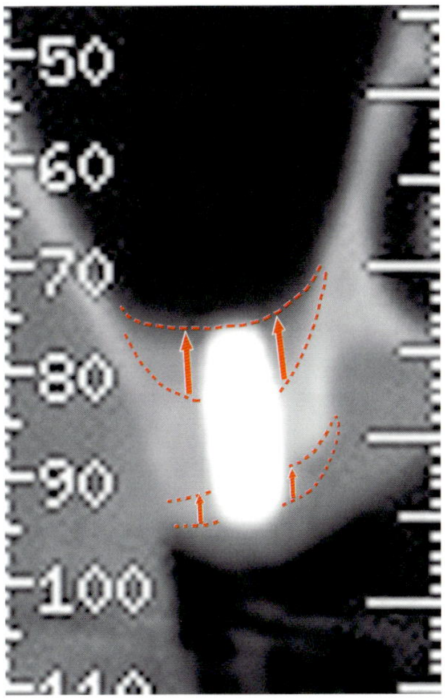

Fig 13-2 Crestal peri-implant bone loss after flap implant surgery is a common problem encountered using the socket lift procedure. The mean crestal bone loss is 1.2 mm, which is 50% of the bone gained from the socket lift.

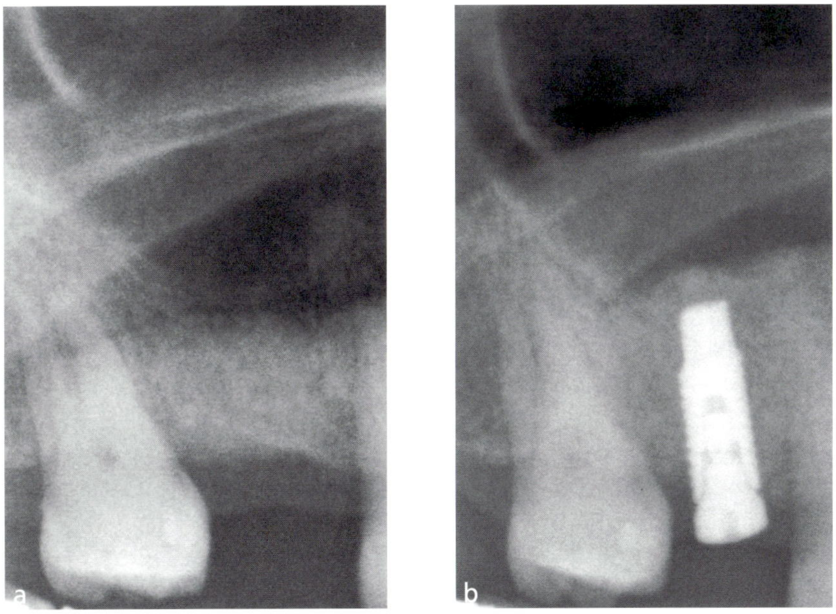

Fig 13-3 Radiographs of a patient with socket lift within the implant osteotomy and immediate flapless implant placement. (a) The proposed implant site. (b) Radiograph taken 4 months after implant placement. Endosinus bone gain is seen at the apical implant surface. There is no crestal peri-implant bone loss.

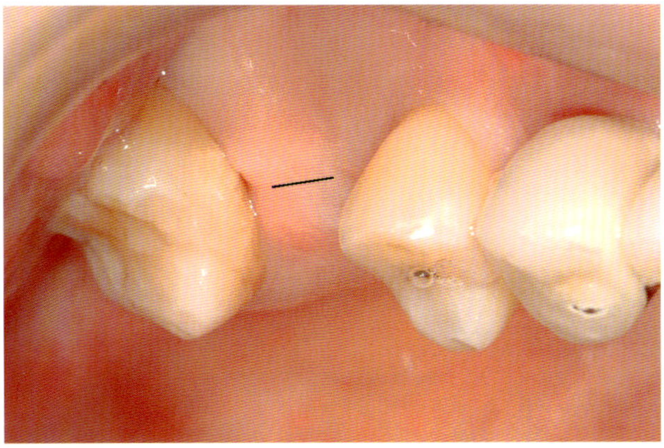

Fig 13-4 A crestal mini-incision, approximately 5 mm, is made horizontally with the alveolar crest at the center of the implant site for a socket lift and immediate flapless implant placement.

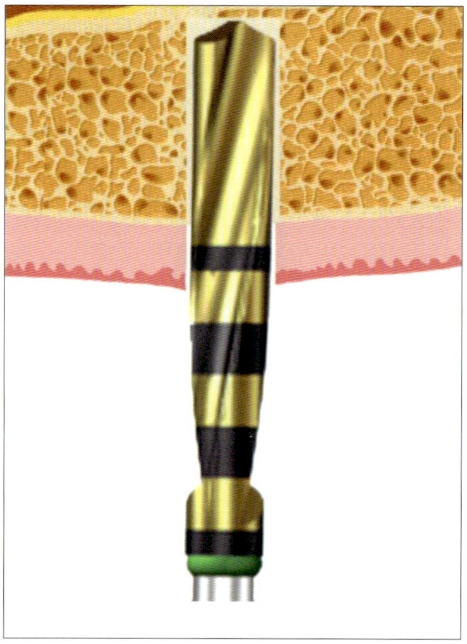

Fig 13-5 The implant osteotomy is prepared using drills. The depth of the osteotomy is approximately 1–2 mm short of the floor of the antrum.

prepare the initial osteotomy, and an osteotome should be used to prepare the osteotomy.

Sinus lift

When the implant osteotomy is prepared to the appropriate final diameter, a flat-ended or cupped osteotome with the same diameter as the final osteotomy is selected. The osteotome is inserted and tapped in 0.5–1.0 mm increments beyond the osteotomy until reaching its final vertical position. The osteotome is tapped up to 2 mm above the floor of the sinus (Fig 13-6). This surgical approach compresses the bone below the antrum, causing a greenstick-type fracture in the antral floor, and slowly elevating the unprepared bone and sinus membrane over the broad-based osteotome. The fracture in the antral floor causes no healing problems because the fractured fragments have a close attachment with the maxillary sinus mucosa.

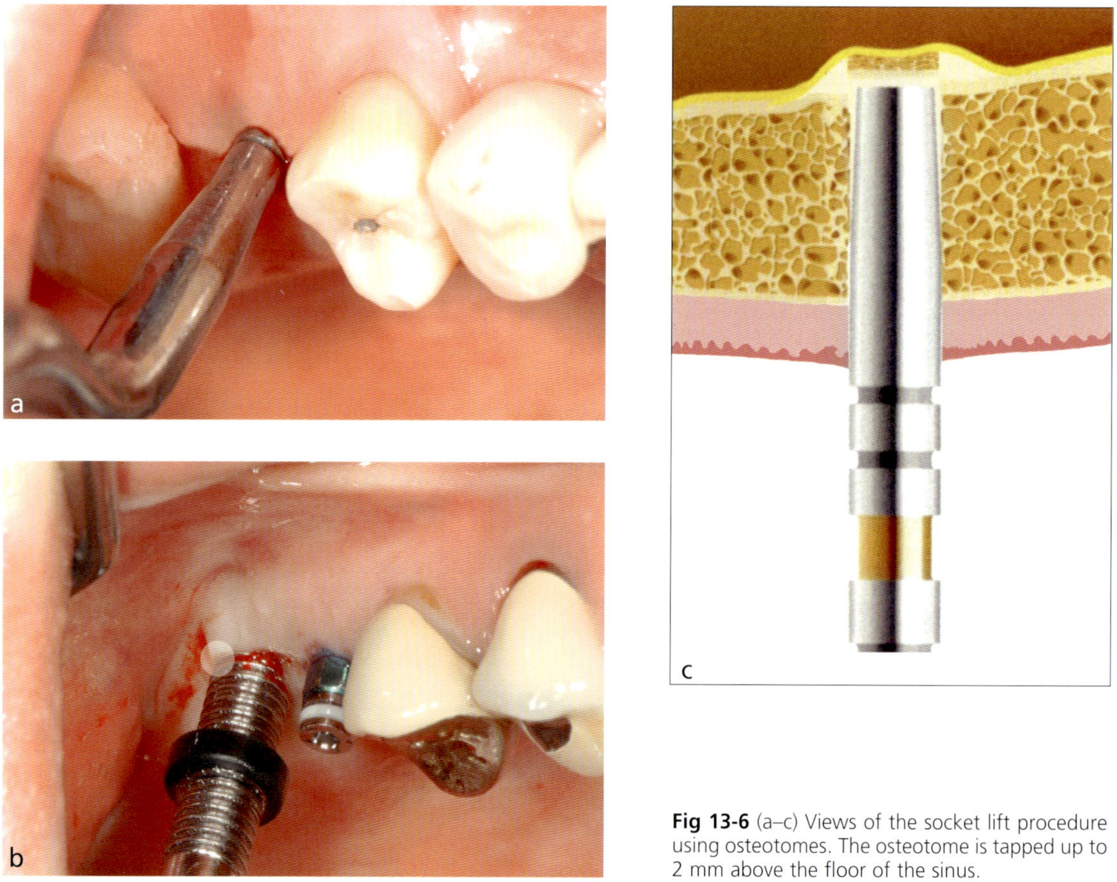

Fig 13-6 (a–c) Views of the socket lift procedure using osteotomes. The osteotome is tapped up to 2 mm above the floor of the sinus.

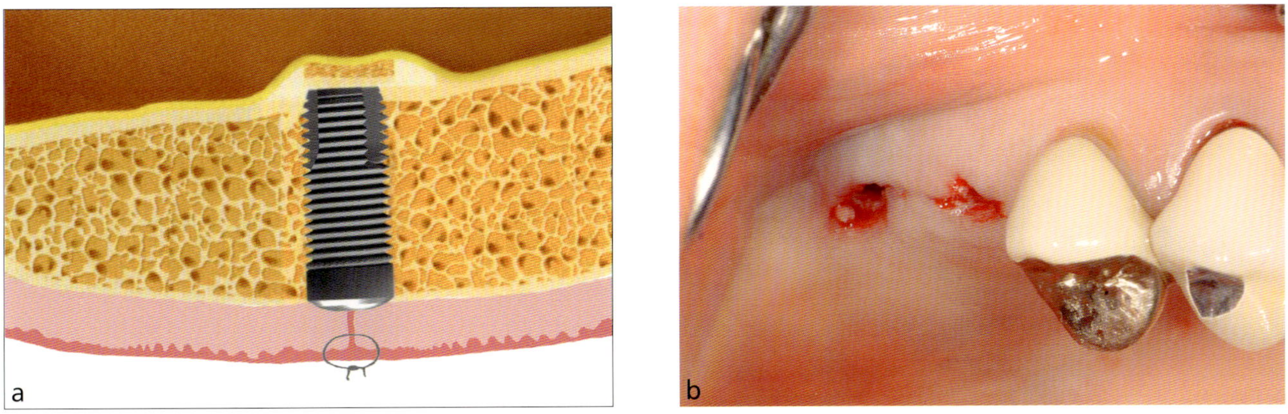

Fig 13-7 (a and b) Views after the socket lift and simultaneous flapless implant placement.

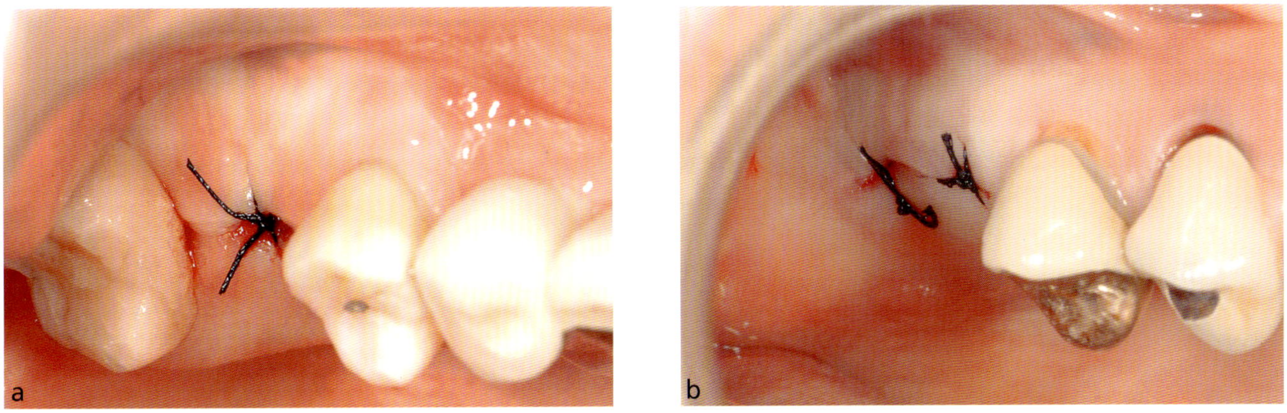

Fig 13-8 (a and b) After connection of a cover screw, the crestal mini-incision is sutured to submerge the fixture.

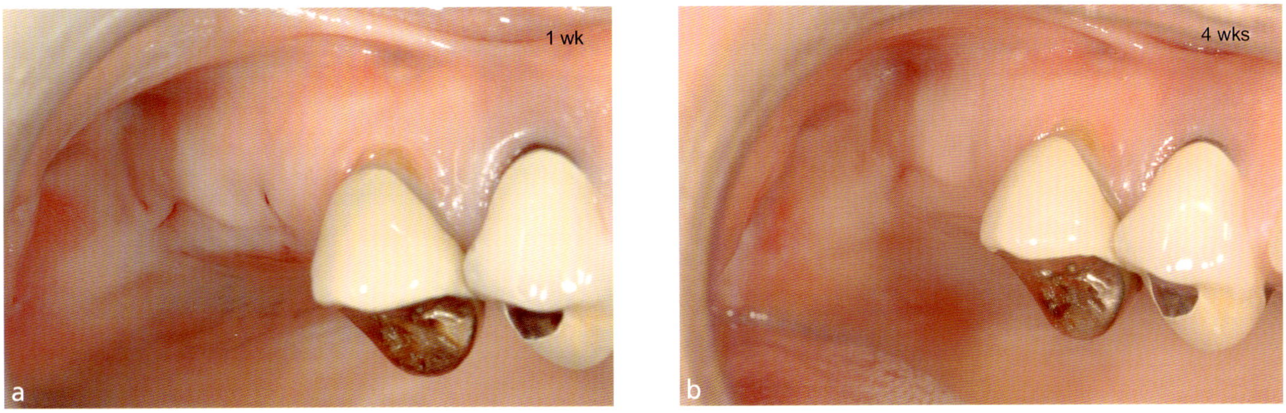

Fig 13-9 Intraoral views (a) 1 week and (b) 4 weeks after socket lift and simultaneous flapless implant placement.

Implant placement

Once the site has been prepared, the implant should be threaded into the osteotomy and extended up to 2 mm above the floor of the sinus (Fig 13-7). The implant is threaded slowly into position so that the membrane is less likely to tear when it is elevated. The upper border of the fixture and the crest of the bone are probed using a periodontal probe to determine whether the fixture top is placed at the same height as the crest. After a cover screw is connected, the crestal mini-incision is sutured to submerge the fixture (Figs 13-8 and 13-9).

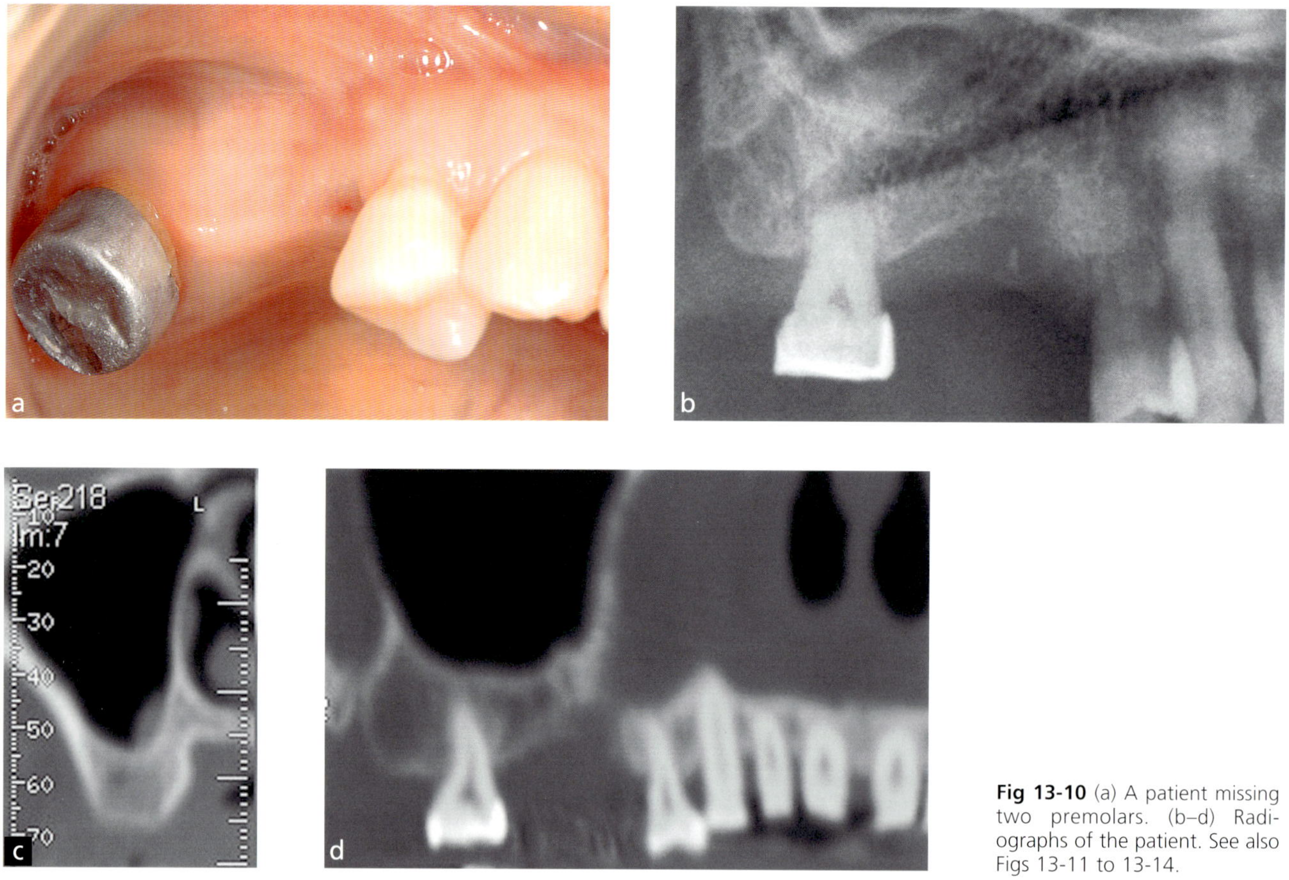

Fig 13-10 (a) A patient missing two premolars. (b–d) Radiographs of the patient. See also Figs 13-11 to 13-14.

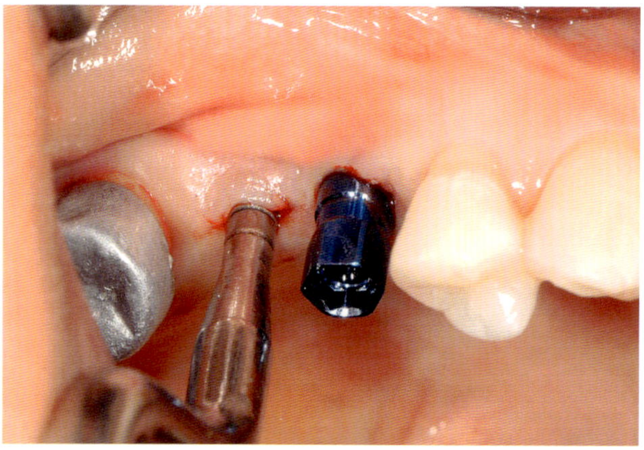

Fig 13-11 Patient as in Fig 13-10: socket lift and simultaneous flapless implant placement.

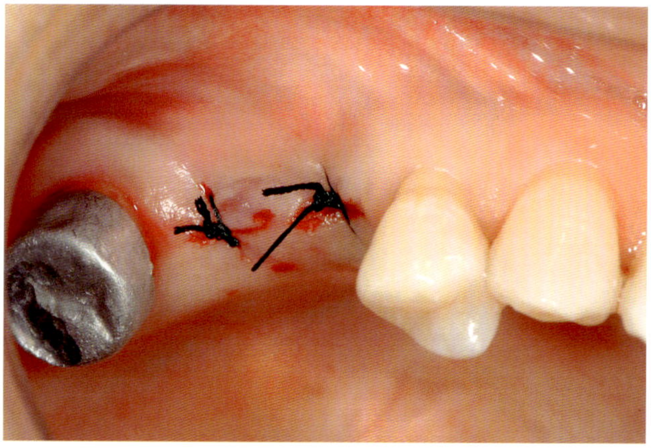

Fig 13-12 Patient as in Fig 13-10: immediately after socket lift and simultaneous flapless implant placement.

Case report

A middle-aged, female patient needed replacement of missing premolars. Figure 13-10 shows an intraoral view and radiographs. A preoperative X-ray study demonstrated deficient alveolar bone height between the crestal bone and the floor of the sinus in the upper right missing area. The bone height from the alveolar crest to the antral floor was measured at approximately 8 mm, and sufficient alveolar bone width was present. Two millimeters of bone augmentation in the maxillary sinus was required to obtain the 10 mm of vertical bone necessary for 10 mm long implants. Socket lift within the implant osteotomy and simultaneous flapless implant placement procedures were used. Two implants, 4.0 mm and 4.5 mm in diameter, were threaded into position (Fig 13-11 and 13-12). Postopera-

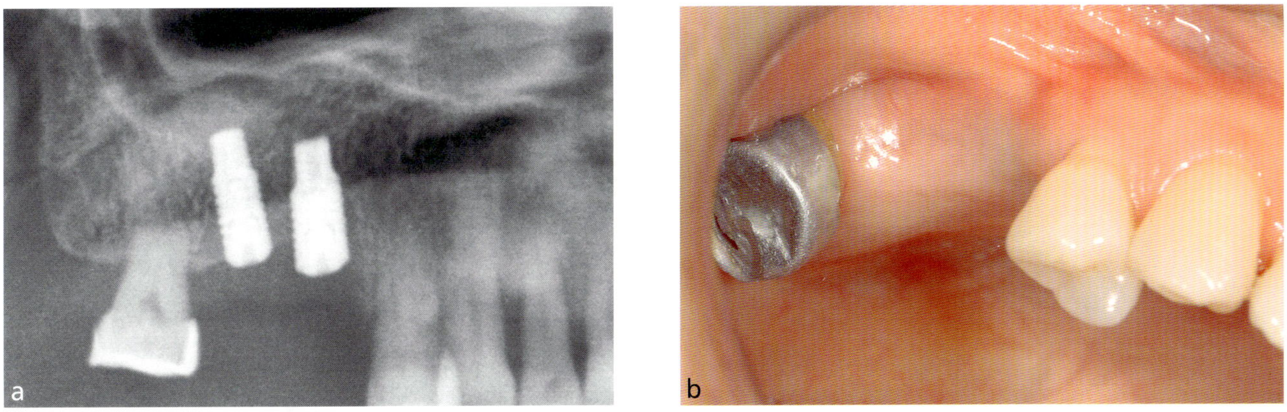

Fig 13-13 Patient as in Fig 13-10: (a) radiograph and (b) intraoral view 4 months after surgery.

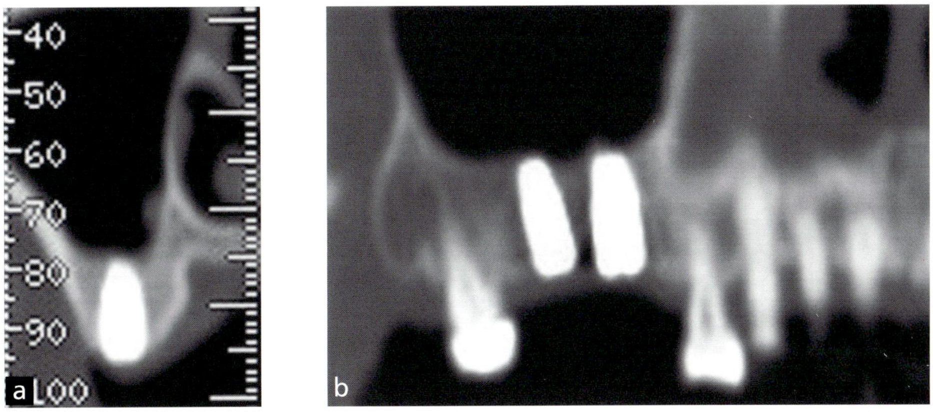

Fig 13-14 Patient as in Fig 13-10: radiographs taken after 4 months indicate that bone formed over the apex of the implant and the maxillary sinus is healthy.

tive radiographs taken after 4 months indicated that bone had formed over the apex of the implant and the maxillary sinus was healthy (Figs 13-13 and 13-14).

Success rates and attainable bone height

The socket lift procedure is quite predictable when the primary stability of the implants is reached. Ferrigno et al.[8] evaluated the outcome of 323 patients with 588 implants placed using the socket lift procedure. The success rate over 12 years was 90.8%. Nedir et al.[7] placed 25 implants in 17 patients using the socket lift procedure and reported a 100% implant success rate after 1 year.

The present authors examined the height of new bone formation in the maxillary sinus after socket lift and simultaneous flapless implant placement by evaluating the endosinus bone gain and crestal peri-implant bone loss 3–4 months after the procedure using CT and dental X-ray studies for 20 implants in 10 patients. Postoperative healing was uneventful in all cases. All implants were clinically stable at the time of stage II surgery (4 months after implant placement). The CT images showed that implants did not have adverse effects on the sinus cavity, such as sinus mucosal thickening. In all 10 patients there was radiographic evidence of ossification around the implants. Bone tissue was observed at the apical implant surface. The mean endosinus bone gain was 2.2 mm. The mean crestal peri-implant bone loss was 0.2 mm. This study demonstrates that flapless implant surgery performed simultaneously with the socket lift procedure produces quite predictable results when 2 mm of bone augmentation in the maxillary sinus is necessary to place the implants.

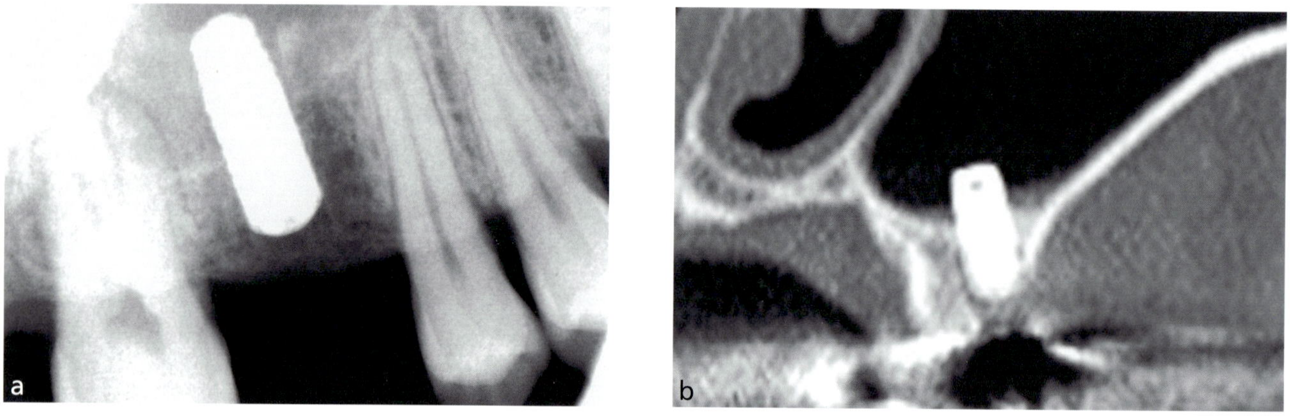

Fig 13-15 (a and b) Increased bone height is unlikely if sinus membrane perforation occurs during the socket lift procedure.

Advantages and disadvantages

Advantages

- Flapless implant surgery reduces the bone loss of the crest during the initial healing period and contributes to enhanced implant stability.
- Among the methods for placing implants simultaneously with elevation of the sinus floor, the socket lift and simultaneous flapless implant placement procedure is the least invasive, thereby shortening surgery time and minimizing postoperative pain, edema, and infection.
- New bone formation over the implant apex is predictable after the socket lift procedure without introducing a graft material because autologous bone is present above the apical portion of the implant and the sinus membrane has an intense vascular network.
- Because 1–2 mm of compressed bone with sinus mucosa covers the implant apex, there is little or no risk of displacing the implant into the sinus.
- The use of a mini-incision implant procedure protects the implants during the early period because the implants are submerged.

Disadvantages

- Only 2 mm of additional bone height can be attempted using this technique.
- The technique is not indicated when the available bone height from the crest of the ridge to the antral floor is very low.
- Sinus membrane perforation can occur during the procedure.

Considerations related to surgery

- The socket lift should raise both the bone and sinus membrane over the osteotome. Sinus membrane perforation is likely to occur if the sinus membrane alone is lifted using the osteotome. Increased bone height is unlikely if sinus membrane perforation occurs during the procedure (Fig 13-15). This is the primary reason why only 2 mm of additional bone height is attempted using this technique.
- Although it has been reported that osteotome sinus floor elevation procedures allow for 2–5 mm of localized sinus floor elevation with simultaneous implant placement, an attempt at only 1–2 mm elevation is safe.
- When the crest of the ridge to the antral floor is up to 6 mm in height, a lateral access opening to the antrum with direct vision and access to elevate the sinus mucosa on the floor is suggested.
- Immediately after socket lift, the implant site is evaluated for perforation of the sinus membrane using the Valsalva maneuver (nose blowing test) – holding the patient's nose and letting him/her blow.
- In a case of sinus mucosa perforation, there is a high risk of displacing the implant into the sinus cavity if the initial stability of the implant is not assured, (Fig 13-16).
- When the primary stability of the implant is not guaranteed the implant is likely to be pushed into the sinus cavity in the case of sinus membrane perforation, and it is prudent to delay implant insertion (Fig 13-17).
- When the primary stability of the implant is ensured in the case of exposing the dental implant to the sinus cavity, care should be taken not to penetrate the bone of the sinus floor more than 2 mm.
- The osteotome should be used with great care. The bone site can be distorted easily, resulting in less initial stability of the implant. The osteotome should be removed from the osteotomy site using a rotating movement instead of shaking it.

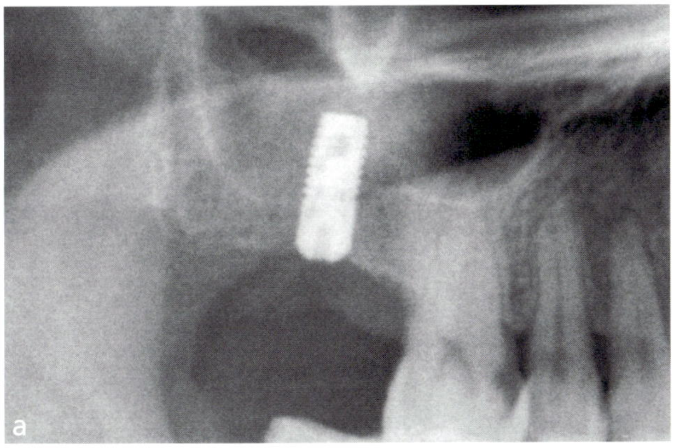

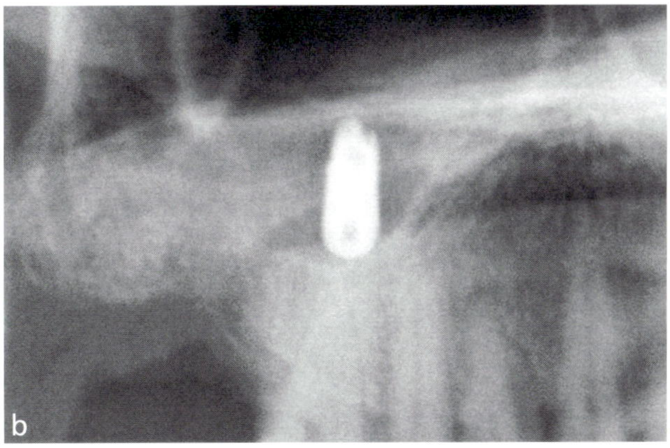

Fig 13-16 (a and b) Radiographs of a patient with a socket lift within the implant osteotomy and immediate implant insertion. The implant is displaced into the sinus during the stage II uncovering procedure. In the case of sinus mucosa perforation, there is a high risk of displacing the implant into the sinus cavity if the initial stability of the implant is not guaranteed.

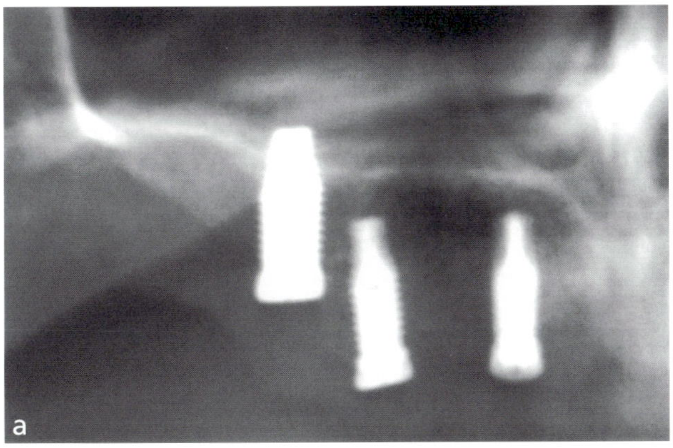

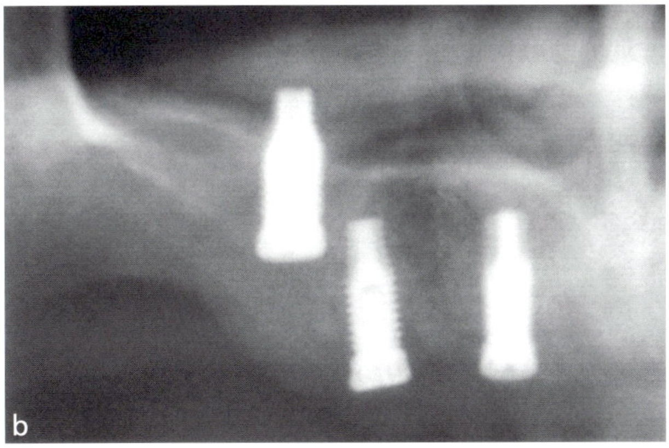

Fig 13-17 (a and b) Radiographs of a patient with a socket lift within the implant osteotomy and immediate implant insertion. An implant exposed to the sinus cavity with uncertain initial stability can be pushed spontaneously into the sinus cavity.

Exposure of implants to the maxillary sinus

The edentulous posterior maxilla generally provides a limited amount of bone volume owing to atrophy of the alveolar ridge and pneumatization of the maxillary sinus.[9] Hence, implant placement in the posterior maxilla is complicated. Such implants are usually inserted marginally to the floor of the maxillary sinus, which carries a high risk of exposing the implant to the maxillary sinus. In general, it has been reported that extension of the implant into the sinus does not play a significant role in the implant outcome.[10,11] The literature focuses primarily on revealing osseointegration, but few report on the effects of exposing dental implants to the sinus cavity in relation to sinus complications. Raghoebar et al.[12] reported a case of maxillary sinusitis.

Therefore, animal and clinical studies were carried out to investigate any complications of exposing dental implants to the maxillary sinus cavity (Fig 13-18).

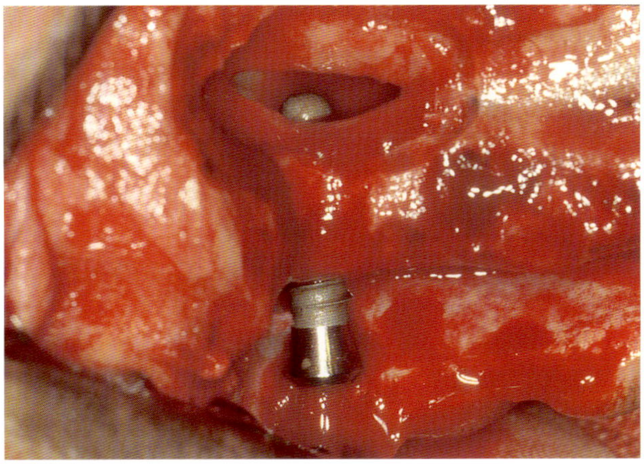

Fig 13-18 To determine whether dental implant exposure to the maxillary sinus cavity increases the risk of maxillary sinus complications, an implant was placed bilaterally in the maxillary sinus of eight adult female mongrel dogs in such a manner that they penetrated the bone and mucous membrane of the maxillary sinus floor to the extent of 2, 4, or 8 mm. The implants were left in place for 6 months. See also Figs 13-19 to 13-22.

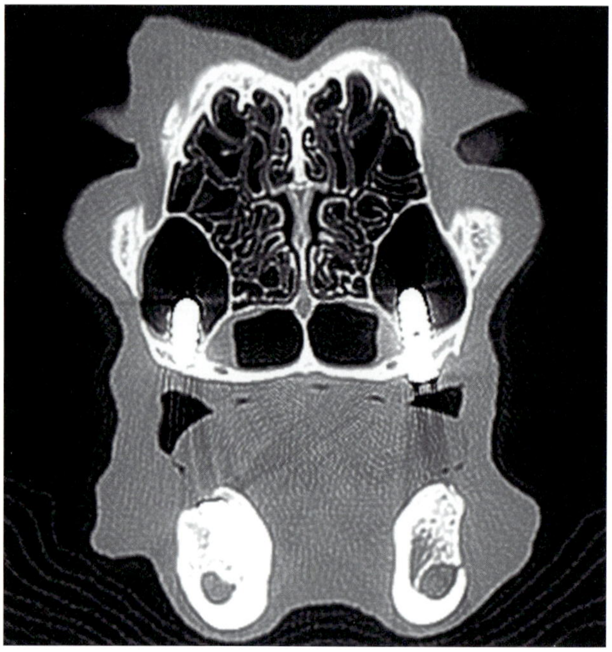

Fig 13-19 Computerized tomography shows implants penetrating the bone and mucous membrane of the maxillary sinus floor to the extent of 4 mm or 8 mm.

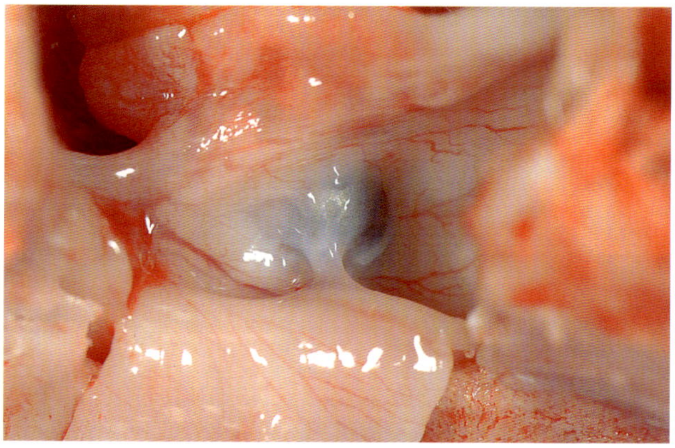

Fig 13-20 Where implants penetrated the cavity by 2 mm, the parts of the implants that were introduced into the sinus cavity were covered with a newly formed membrane. Compare with Fig 13-21.

The animal study

An implant was placed in the maxillary sinus of eight adult dogs in a manner that penetrated the bone and mucous membrane of the maxillary sinus floor to the extent of 2, 4, and 8 mm (Fig 13-19).[13] The implants were left in place for 6 months.

Different results were obtained depending on the height of the implant penetrating into the sinus cavity. On the side with implants penetrating 2 mm, the parts of the implants that had been introduced into the sinus cavity were covered with a new membrane (Fig 13-20). The membrane formed a functional barrier to the sinus cavity. However, on the sides where implants penetrated 4 and 8 mm, the parts of the implants that had been introduced into the sinus cavity were not fully covered with a sinus membrane. Debris had accumulated on the surface of the apical parts of the implants exposed to the sinus cavity (Fig. 13-21). No pathological findings were observed in any of the maxillary sinus cavities with 4 or 8 mm sinus-penetrating implants during the 6 month period. This suggests that implant exposure to the sinus cavity is not related to the development of sinus complications. Regarding the parts that were not covered with the antral membrane, one might expect an increase in debris accumulation over time. After a longer period, accumulating debris can become a source of inflammation. Therefore, care should be taken not to penetrate the bone of the sinus floor to more than 2 mm.

A histological examination revealed that the sinus-penetrating implants were all integrated into the jaw bone without fibrous tissue formation in the interface, and the antral mucosa had no discernible inflammatory reactions in any of the maxillary sinus cavities (Fig 13-22). On the side with 4 or 8 mm penetrating implants, growth of the antral membrane was observed only at the implant base, and the membrane showed direct attachment to the titanium. This attachment forms a barrier to the sinus cavity, which protects the osseointegration of the implants.

The clinical study

Nine patients had 23 implants inserted into the maxillary sinus in such a manner that they penetrated the sinus floor by more than 4 mm (mean 5 mm; range 4–7 mm) without lifting the sinus mucous membranes.[14] All were evaluated for sinus complications 6–10 months after implant insertion, using a questionnaire and CT. The results were slightly different from those of the animal study noted above.

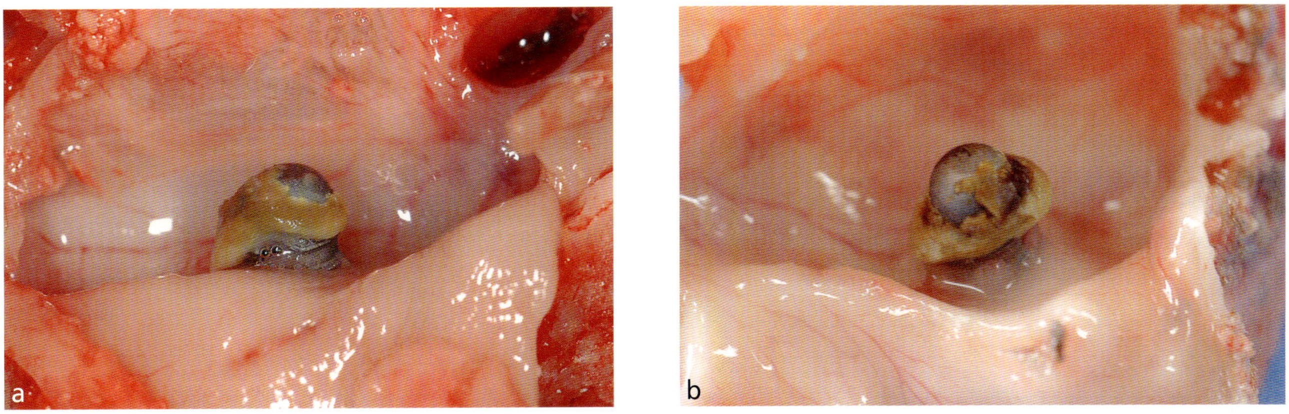

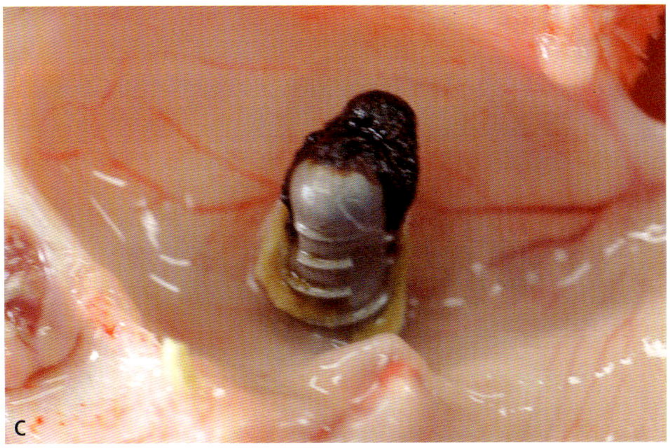

Fig 13-21 (a–c) Where implants penetrated the cavity by 4 and 8 mm, the parts of the implants that were introduced into the sinus cavity were not fully covered with the sinus membrane. Debris accumulates on the surface of the apical parts of the implant exposed to the sinus cavity.

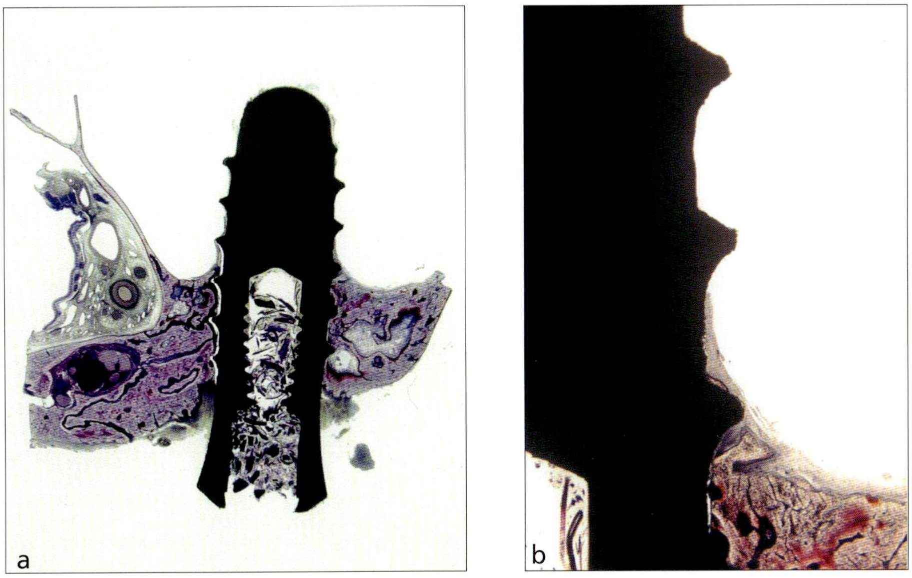

Fig 13-22 (a and b) Histological examination shows that the implants are all integrated into the jaw bone without fibrous tissue formation in the interface, and the antral mucosa has no discernible inflammatory reactions in any of the maxillary sinus cavities. On the sides with 4 and 8 mm penetrating implants, growth of the antral membrane was observed only at the implant base, and the membrane shows direct attachment to the titanium.

Mucosa thickening was observed around the implants in 14 of the 23 implants (61%) (Fig 13-23). The resultant swelling of the mucosal lining was limited to the floor of the sinus and did not affect the ostiomeatal complex (Fig 13-24). In the remaining nine implants there were no indications of adverse mucosal reactions. All penetrating implants remained integrated, and there were no radiographic signs of pathological bone reactions or abnormal loss of anchoring bone (Fig 13-25).

Overall, implant exposure to the maxillary sinus cavity does not affect the bone–implant contact but it can cause sinus mucous thickening around the implants.

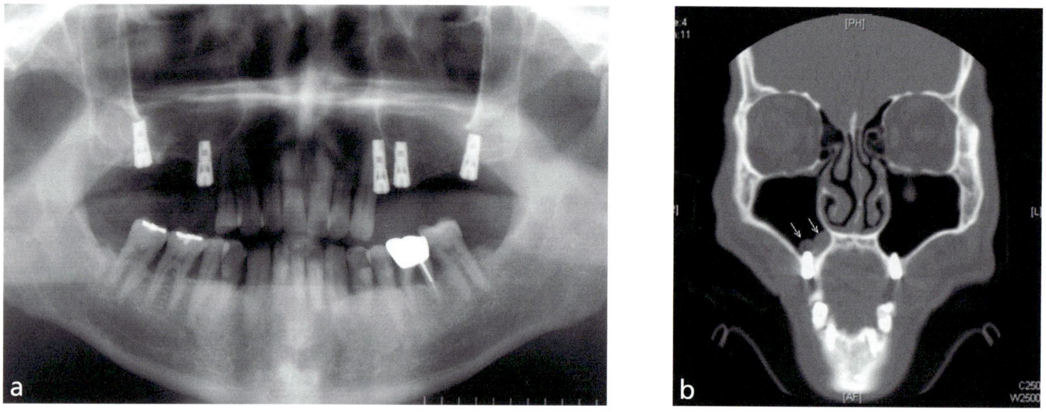

Fig 13-23 Study 7 months after implant insertion of a patient who had implants that extended into the sinus cavity. (a) A panoramic radiograph shows the two implants perforating the sinus floor on both sides. (b) A CT image shows thickening of the sinus mucosa surrounding the implants (arrows).

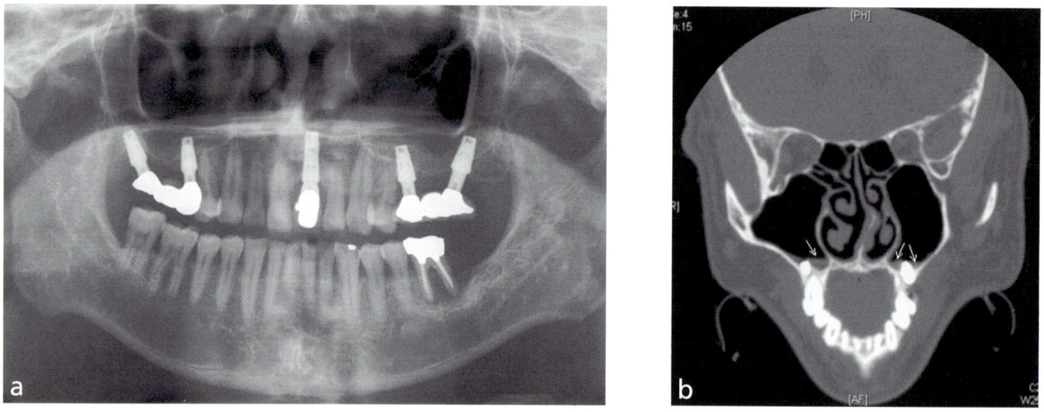

Fig 13-24 Study of a patient 10 months after implant insertion. (a) A panoramic radiograph shows three implants perforating the sinus floor. (b) A CT image shows thickening of the sinus mucosa surrounding the implants (arrows).

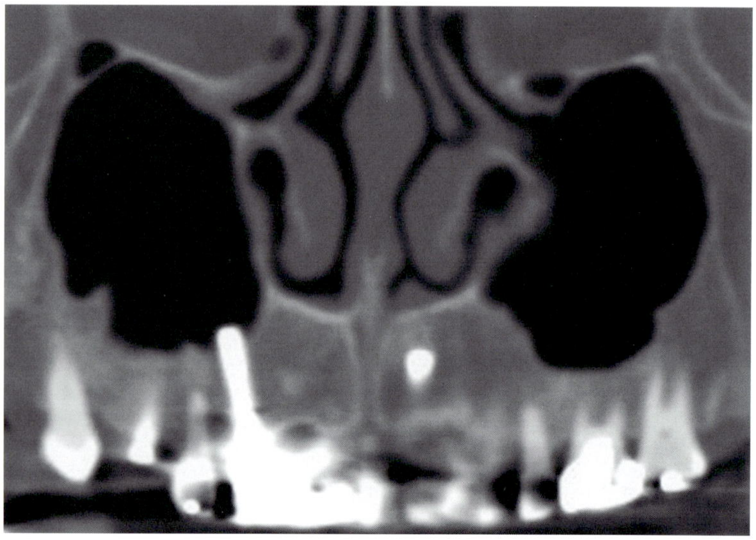

Fig 13-25 An implant was placed in the maxillary sinus in such a manner that it would penetrate further into the sinus floor. The clinical follow-up showed no clinical signs of sinusitis. The penetrating implant remained integrated, and there were no radiographic signs of pathological bone reactions or abnormal loss of anchoring bone.

Summary

Socket lift and simultaneous flapless implant placement is indicated when 10–12 mm of vertical bone is present, and only 2 mm of bone augmentation in the maxillary sinus is needed to place the implants. Flapless implant surgery reduces the bone loss of the crest during the initial healing period, which contributes to enhanced implant stability. In the case of sinus mucosa perforation during osteotome sinus floor elevation procedures, it is advisable to place the implants in such a manner that they do not protrude more than 2 mm into the maxillary sinus once the primary stability of the implant is guaranteed.

References

1. Summers RB. A new concept in maxillary implant surgery: the osteotome technique. Compendium 1994;15:152, 154–156, 158.
2. Horowitz RA. The use of osteotomes for sinus augmentation at the time of implant placement. Compend Contin Educ Dent 1997; 18:441–447, 450–452.
3. Lazzara RJ. The sinus elevation procedure in endosseous implant therapy. Curr Opin Periodontol 1996;3:178–183.
4. Fugazzotto PA. The modified trephine/osteotome sinus augmentation technique: technical considerations and discussion of indications. Implant Dent 2001;10:259–264.
5. Fugazzotto PA. Immediate implant placement following a modified trephine/osteotome approach: success rates of 116 implants to 4 years in function. Int J Oral Maxillofac Implants 2002;17:113–120.
6. Soltan M, Smiler DG. Trephine bone core sinus elevation graft. Implant Dent 2004;13:148–152.
7. Nedir R, Bischof M, Vazquez L, Szmukler-Moncler S, Bernard JP. Osteotome sinus floor elevation without grafting material: a 1-year prospective pilot study with ITI implants. Clin Oral Implants Res 2006;17:679–686.
8. Ferrigno N, Laureti M, Fanali S. Dental implants placement in conjunction with osteotome sinus floor elevation: a 12-year life-table analysis from a prospective study on 588 ITI implants. Clin Oral Implants Res 2006;17:194–205.
9. Zinner ID, Small SA. Sinus lift graft: using the maxillary sinuses to support implants. J Am Dent Assoc 1996;127:51–57.
10. Boyne PJ. Analysis of performance of root-form endosseous implants placed in the maxillary sinus. J Long Term Eff Med Implants 1993;3:143–159.
11. Brånemark PI, Adell R, Albrektsson T, Lekholm U, Lindstrom J, Rockler A. An experimental and clinical study of osseointegrated implants penetrating the nasal cavity and maxillary sinus. J Oral Maxillofac Surg 1984;42:497–505.
12. Raghoebar GM, Weissenbruch R, Vissink A. Rhino-sinusitis related to endosseous implants extending into the nasal cavity: a case report. Int J Oral Maxillofac Surg 2004;33:312–314.
13. Jung JH, Choi BH, Zhu SJ et al. The effects of exposing dental implants to the maxillary sinus cavity on sinus complications. Oral Surg Oral Med Oral Pathol Oral Radiol Endod 2006;102:602–605.
14. Jung JH, Choi BH, Jeong SM, Li J, Lee SH, Lee HJ. A retrospective study of the effects of exposing dental implants to the maxillary sinus cavity on sinus complications. Oral Surg Oral Med Oral Pathol Oral Radiol Endod 2007;103:623–625.

CHAPTER

14

Simultaneous Maxillary Sinus Membrane Elevation

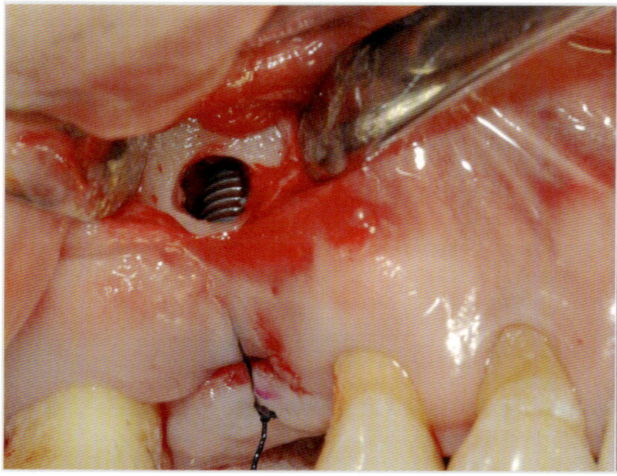

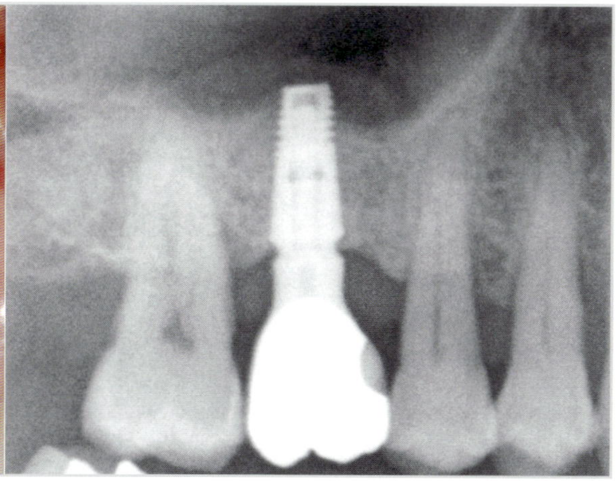

Key point

It is possible to elevate the maxillary sinus mucosa using a small bone window and simultaneously place the implants in the maxillary sinus using flapless implant surgery.

Overview

There are reports of successful bone formation in the sinus floor by simply elevating the maxillary sinus membrane and simultaneously inserting dental implants without the use of a graft material. There are no animal studies that have substantiated the effect of sinus membrane elevation on the endosinus bone gain. This chapter reports a method of sinus membrane elevation performed simultaneously with flapless implant surgery as well as its effect on bone formation around the implants in the maxillary sinus cavity.

Review of the literature

Recently, there has been some controversy regarding the relevance of placing a grafting material in sinus elevation procedures.[1–4] It has been suggested that sinus membrane elevation alone may be enough to obtain new bone formation in the newly created space.

Lundgren et al.[2] treated 10 patients with an average residual bone height of 7 mm. They placed 19 implants that protruded into the sinus after sinus membrane elevation without introducing a grafting material. All their implants gained endosinus bone. Hatano et al.[4] treated six patients who required maxillary sinus floor augmentation. They placed 14 implants in the residual bone penetrating into the sinus cavity after elevating the sinus membrane and filling the sinus cavity below the lifted sinus membrane with peripheral venous blood. They reported that new bone was generated successfully in all implant sites after a minimum 6-month healing period.

The maxillary sinus's potential for bone formation

The environment of the sinus cavity below the lifted sinus membrane after elevation is quite beneficial for bone formation.[5–7] This is in part because the cavity is surrounded by bone, and the primary source of revascularization of the graft originates from the adjacent bony walls. In addition, the sinus membrane has an intensely vascular network (Fig 14-1) and contains mesenchymal progenitor cells and the cells committed to the osteogenic lineage.[7] The periosteum of the lifted sinus membrane is another source of bone-forming cells. Accordingly, bone formation in the newly created space can be induced by elevating the sinus membrane alone, provided that the space is well maintained. Sinus membrane elevation has the advantage of enhancing implant primary stability because implants are placed deeper by going through the cortical bone on the sinus floor.

Mucosal elevation of the maxillary sinus and simultaneous flapless implant surgery

The incision

A vertical incision about 8 mm long is made on the buccal cortical plate approximately 8 mm away from the alveolar crest, and a mucoperiosteal flap is reflected in order to expose the sinus wall (Fig 14-2).

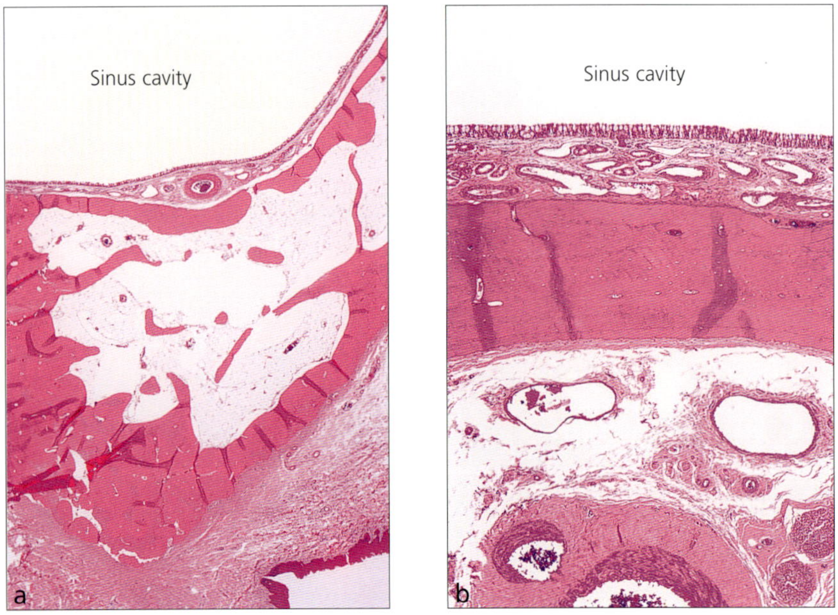

Fig 14-1 (a and b) Histological sections of the maxillary sinus mucosa and the sinus floor. The sinus membrane has an intensely vascular network and the antral floor has cortical bone.

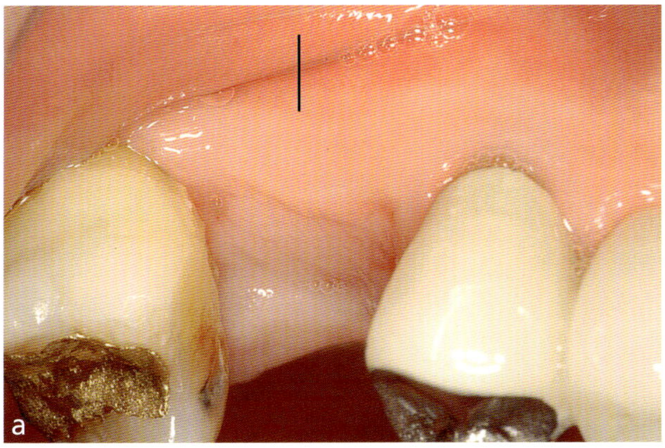
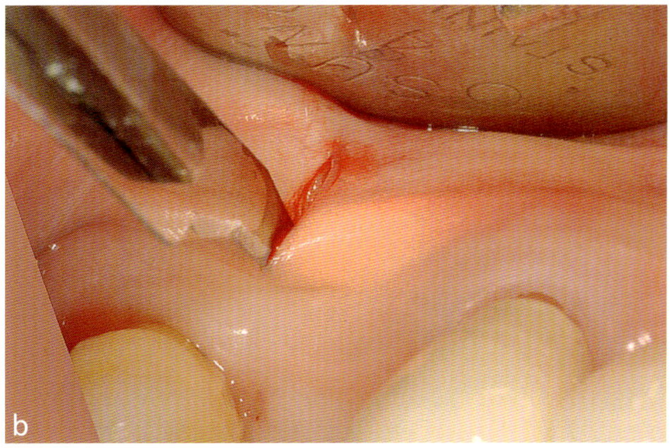

Fig 14-2 (a and b) To access the maxillary sinus, a vertical incision approximately 8 mm in length is made on the buccal cortical plate about 8 mm away from the alveolar crest.

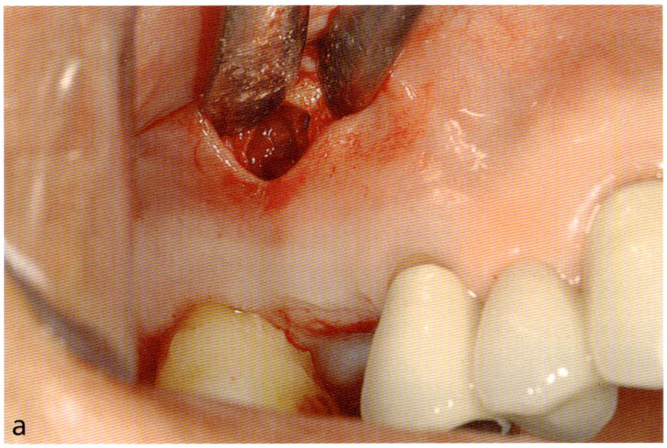
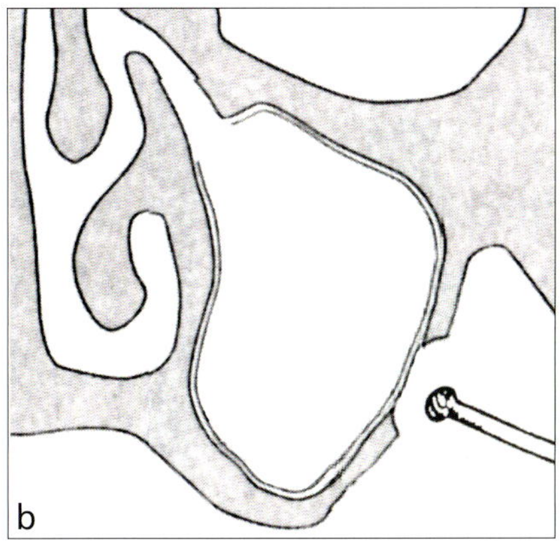

Fig 14-3 (a and b) A 5 mm diameter hole has been made in the lateral sinus wall with a round bur, taking care to avoid perforating the sinus membrane. The hole is placed 2–5 mm above the level of the antral floor.

Access window

A 5 mm diameter hole is made in the lateral sinus wall using a round bur, taking care to avoid perforating the sinus membrane (Fig 14-3). The hole is placed approximately 2–5 mm above the level of the antral floor. Care should be taken not to damage the roots of the adjacent teeth. The sinus membrane is then elevated above the maxillary sinus floor using small curettes. Specially designed and shaped curettes are available to facilitate this maneuver (Fig 14-4). The sinus membrane may be elevated easily from the antral walls because it has few elastic fibers and is not attached to the cortical wall. After elevating the sinus membrane, a rubber dam is cut and placed into the space between the lifted sinus mucosa and sinus floor through the hole. The rubber dam protects the sinus mucosa during drilling (Fig 14-5).

Implant placement

After elevation of the sinus membrane, the implants are placed using a mini-incision procedure. A crestal mini-incision, approximately 5 mm horizontally to the alveolar crest, is made at the center of the implant site, and local undermining of the gingiva is then performed (Fig 14-6). The amount of undermining at the implant site does not exceed 5 mm and falls within the range of a large-diameter implant. The implant osteotomy is prepared to the appropriate final diameter beyond the antral floor (Fig 14-7). In a case of poor bone quality, a 2 mm pilot drill is used to prepare the initial osteotomy, and the osteotome is then used to prepare the osteotomy.

After preparation of the implant site, the implant is threaded into the osteotomy and extends up to 3 mm above the floor of the sinus (Fig 14-8). The incision for

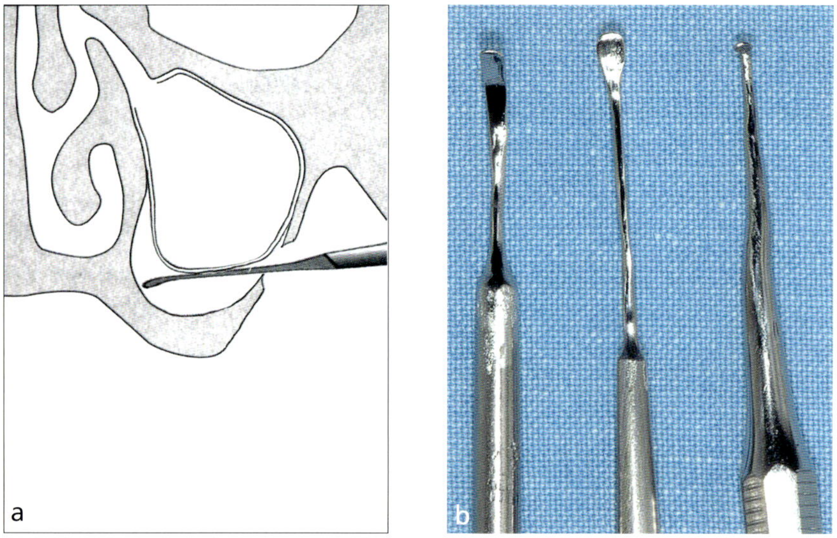

Fig 14-4 (a and b) Specially designed and shaped curettes are available to elevate the sinus membrane above the maxillary sinus floor.

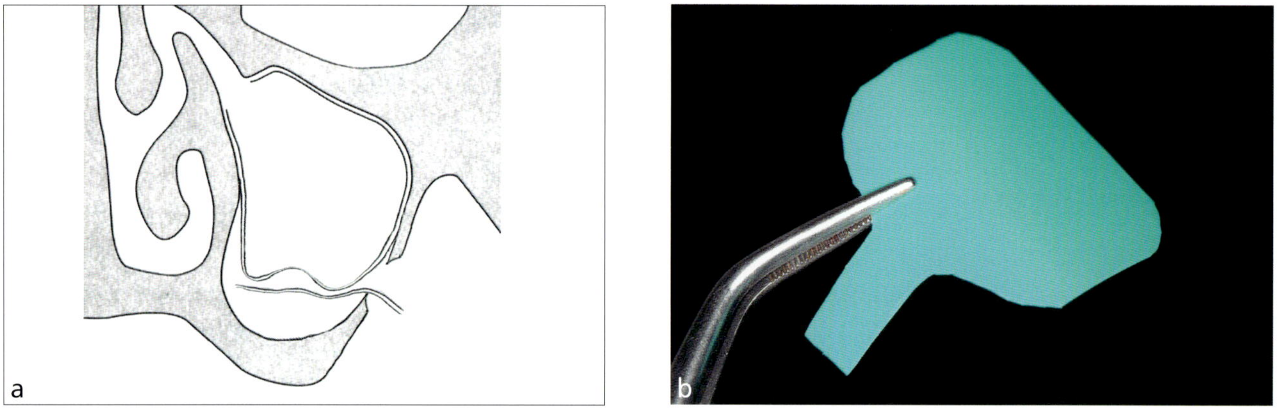

Fig 14-5 (a and b) After elevation of the sinus membrane, a rubber dam is cut and placed into the space between the lifted sinus mucosa and sinus floor through the hole, to protect the sinus mucosa during drilling.

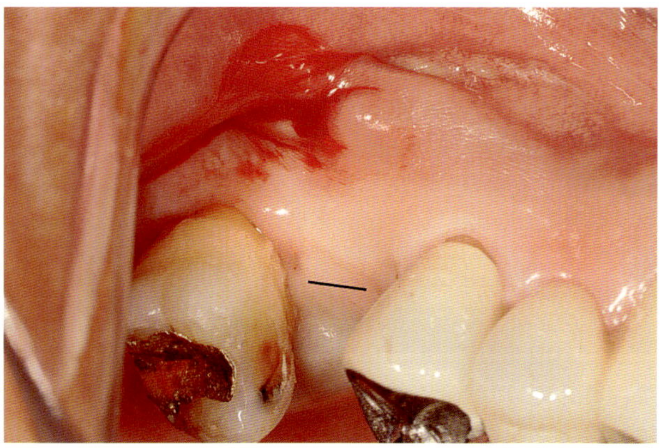

Fig 14-6 A crestal incision for mini-incision implant surgery.

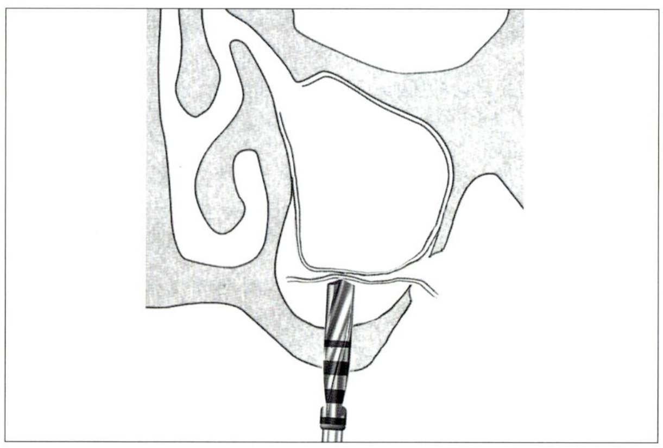

Fig 14-7 An implant osteotomy beyond the antral floor is prepared using a drill.

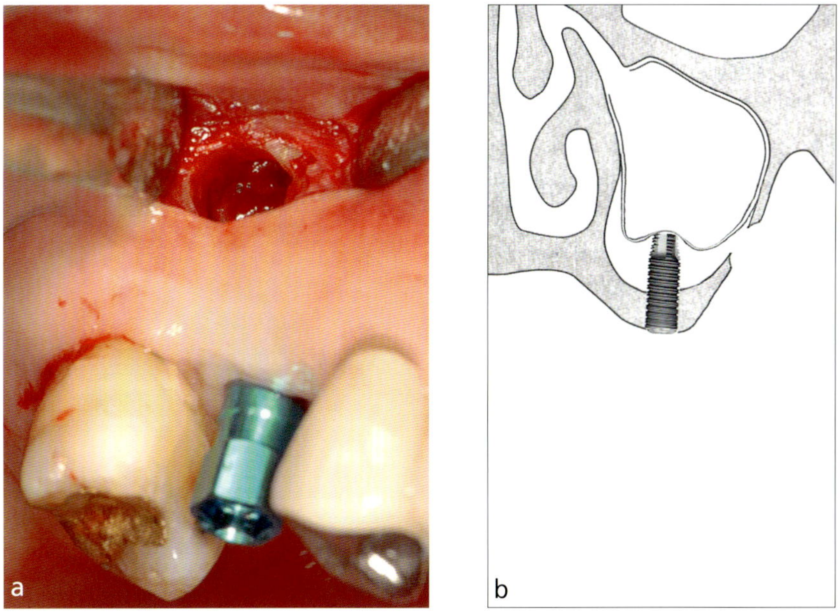

Fig 14-8 (a and b) After preparation of the site, the implant is threaded into the osteotomy and extends up to 3–4 mm above the floor of the sinus.

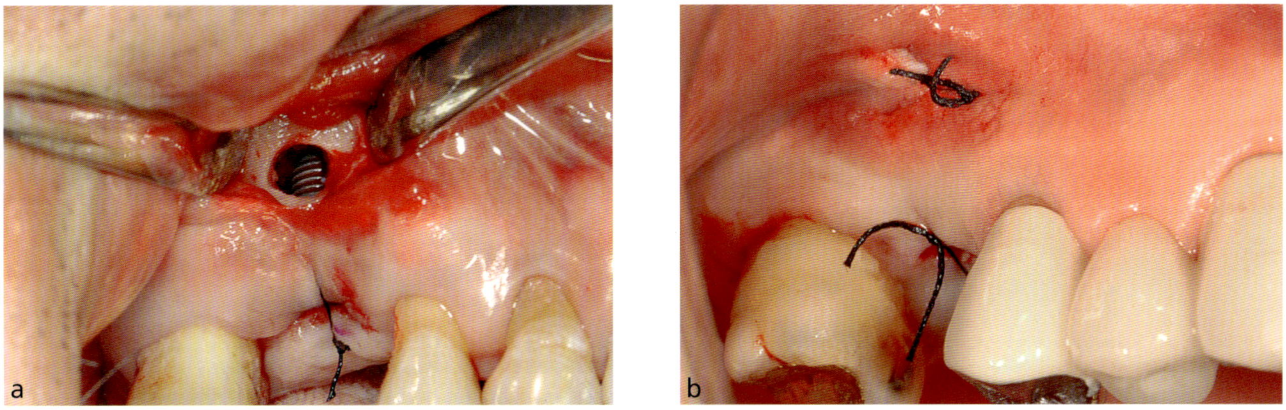

Fig 14-9 (a and b) View of an implant immediately after placement in the maxillary sinus, showing sinus membrane elevation and the inserted implant protruding into the sinus cavity. Once coagulum is observed underneath the elevated sinus membrane, the mucoperiosteal flap is replaced and sutured.

accessing the maxillary sinus is sutured (Fig 14-9). After a cover screw is connected, the crestal mini-incision is sutured to submerge the fixture. A post-insertion radiograph is then made to identify the implant depth (Fig 14-10).

Placement of multiple implants

When patients receive more than two implants within the unilateral maxillary sinus using a method of sinus membrane elevation, two access bone windows on the lateral wall of the sinus are recommended to avoid perforation of the antral membrane (Fig 14-11).

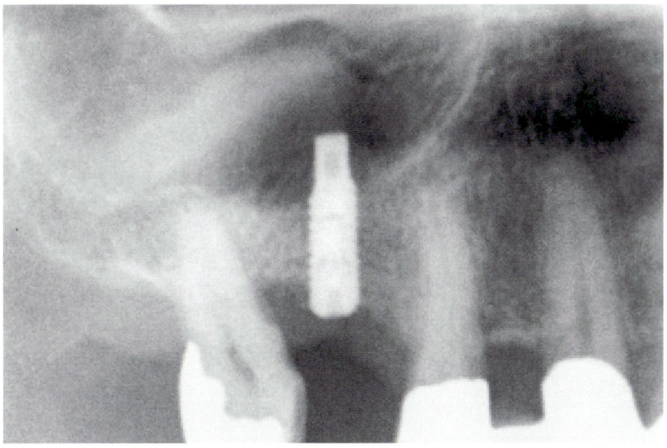

Fig 14-10 Radiograph after sinus membrane elevation and simultaneous flapless implant surgery.

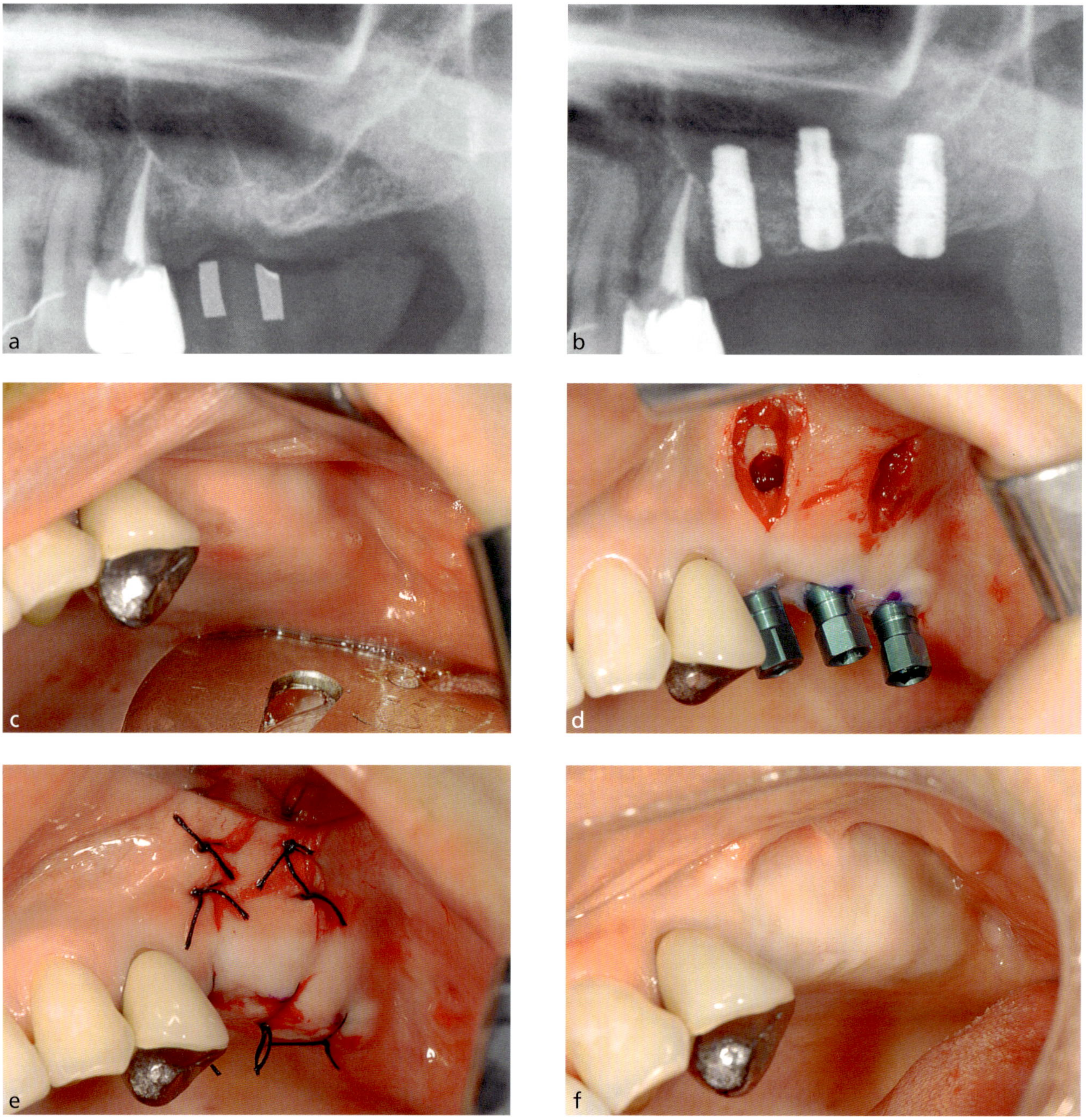

Fig 14-11 Two access bone windows on the lateral wall of the sinus are recommended when patients receive more than two implants within the unilateral maxillary sinus, using a method of sinus membrane elevation to avoid perforation of the antral membrane. (a) Panoramic radiograph of a patient with missing posterior teeth in the maxillary left region. (b) Postoperative radiograph. (c) Intraoral view. (d) View of the implants immediately after placement in the maxillary sinus using two access bone windows on the lateral wall of the sinus. (e) Immediate postoperative intraoral view. (f) Intraoral view after a 4-month healing period.

Height of new bone formation possible using sinus membrane elevation

There are reports of successful bone formation using the sinus floor elevation technique, which involves elevating the maxillary sinus membrane without adjunctive grafting material.[5,6] To our knowledge, there are no reports that have addressed the level of new bone formation made possible by this procedure. Using CT and dental X-ray studies, the present authors evaluated the endosinus bone gain and crestal peri-implant bone loss 4 months after implantation in nine patients whose implants were inserted more than 4 mm

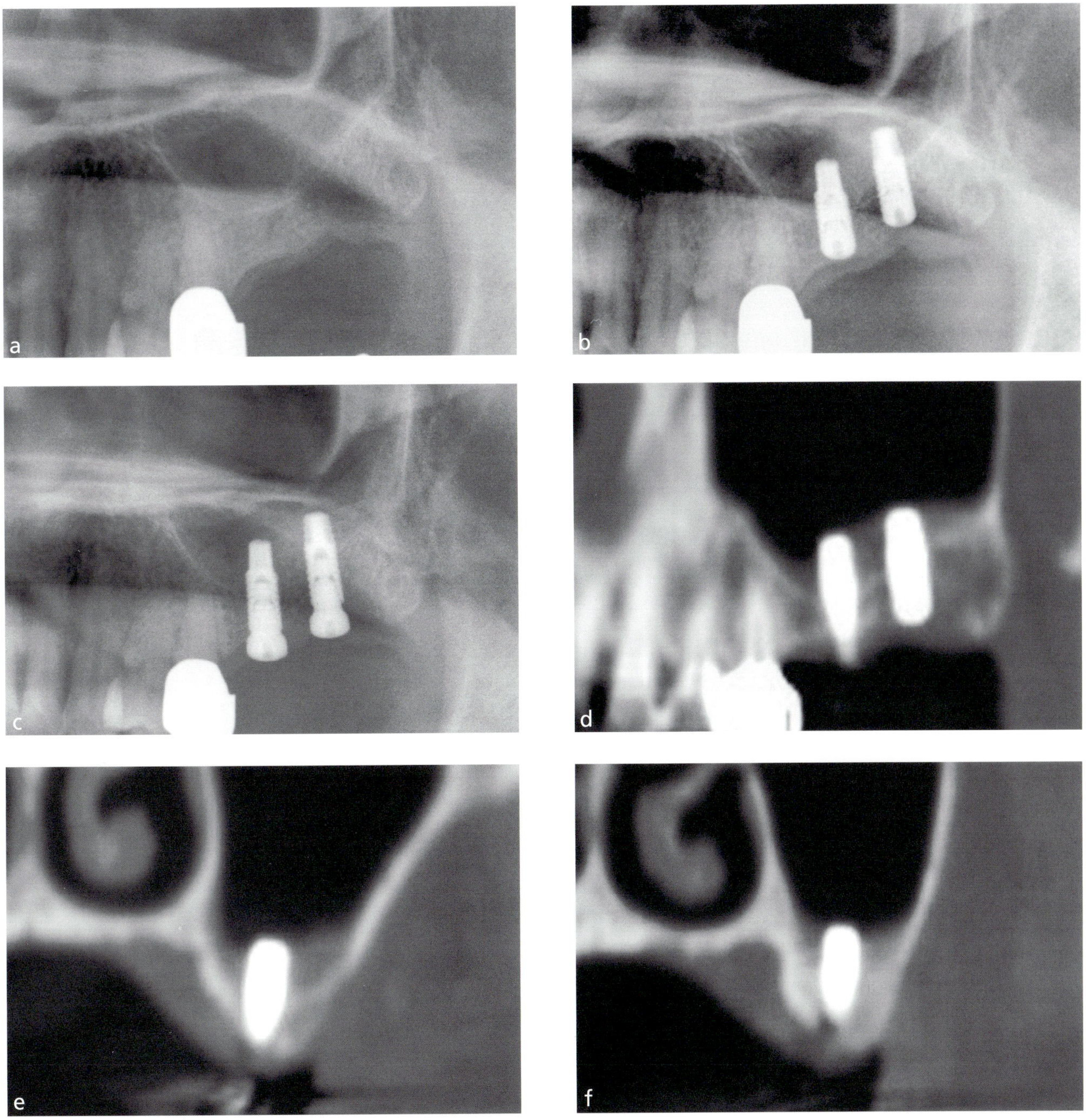

Fig 14-12 A patient with mucosal elevation of the maxillary sinus and simultaneous flapless implant surgery. (a) Radiograph of the patient with the missing maxillary molars. (b) Radiograph taken immediately after surgery. Two implants (4 mm in diameter and 10 mm in length) were placed in the left maxillary sinus in such a way that they protruded 4 or 5 mm into the maxillary sinus after sinus membrane elevation. (c) Panoramic radiograph after 4 months. (d–f) Postoperative CT images after 4 months. They show radiographic evidence of ossification in the elevated sinus area for all implants.

(range 4–6 mm) into the maxillary sinus after sinus membrane elevation.[8] All implants gained endosinus bone. The mean endosinus bone gain was 3.5 ± 0.6 mm (range 2.9–4.8 mm). The extent of crestal peri-implant bone loss was small, with a mean of 0.1 ± 0.1 mm.

The postoperative CT images showed tent-like bone formation around the implants. This suggests that a tent-like figure is drawn by the sinus membrane from the apical surface of the implant, and new bone formation occurs in the space created by this sinus membrane tent (Figs 14-12 to 14-14). Therefore, it is important to find techniques that enable the membrane to remain elevated at its new position in order to achieve more bone formation. Lundgren et al.[2] used a method of suturing the sinus membrane

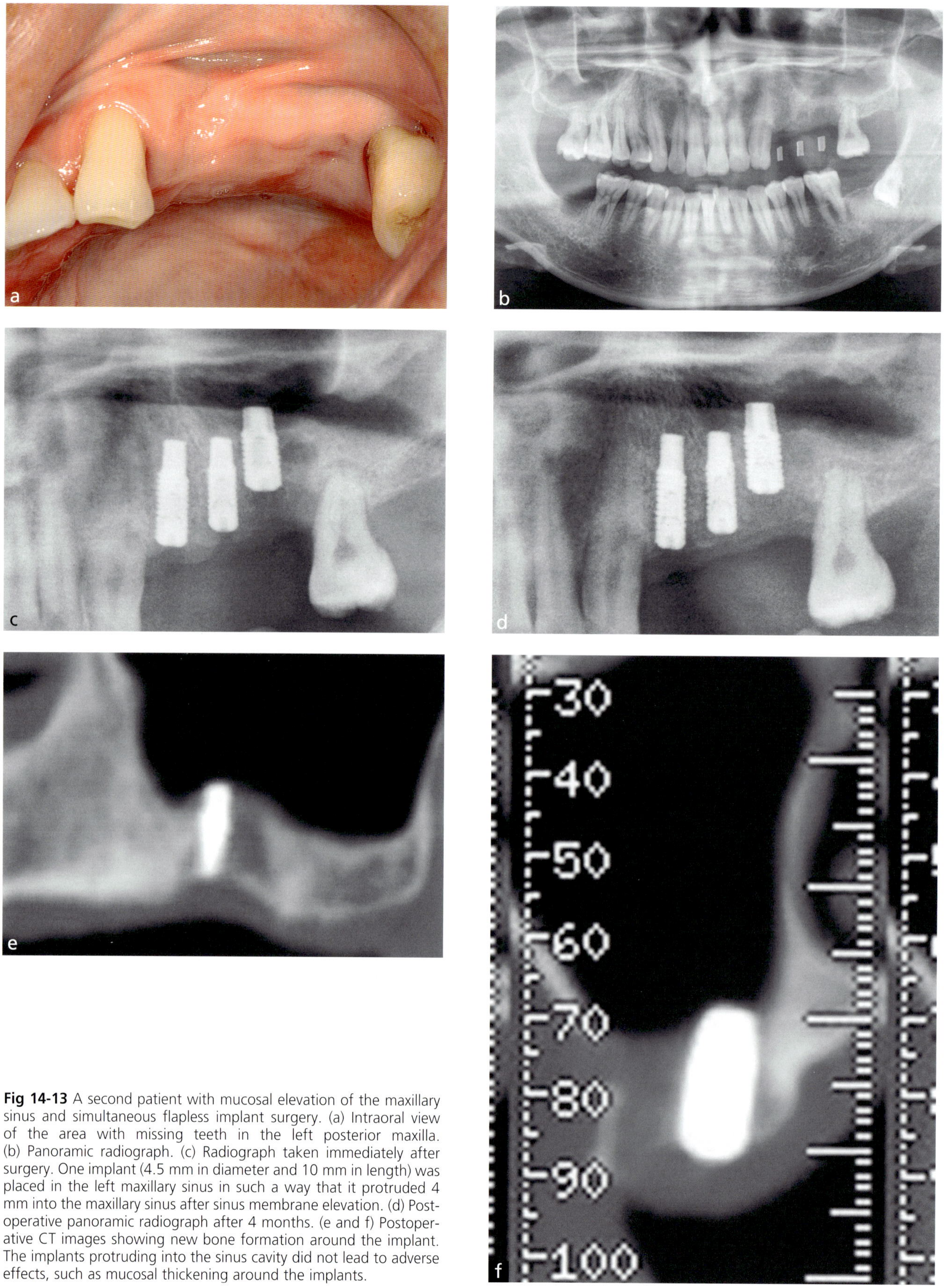

Fig 14-13 A second patient with mucosal elevation of the maxillary sinus and simultaneous flapless implant surgery. (a) Intraoral view of the area with missing teeth in the left posterior maxilla. (b) Panoramic radiograph. (c) Radiograph taken immediately after surgery. One implant (4.5 mm in diameter and 10 mm in length) was placed in the left maxillary sinus in such a way that it protruded 4 mm into the maxillary sinus after sinus membrane elevation. (d) Postoperative panoramic radiograph after 4 months. (e and f) Postoperative CT images showing new bone formation around the implant. The implants protruding into the sinus cavity did not lead to adverse effects, such as mucosal thickening around the implants.

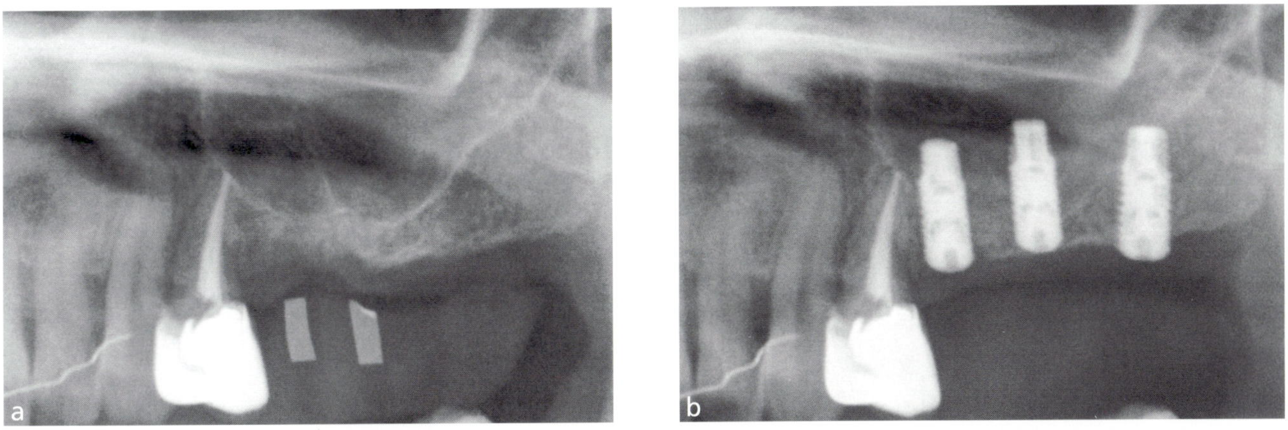

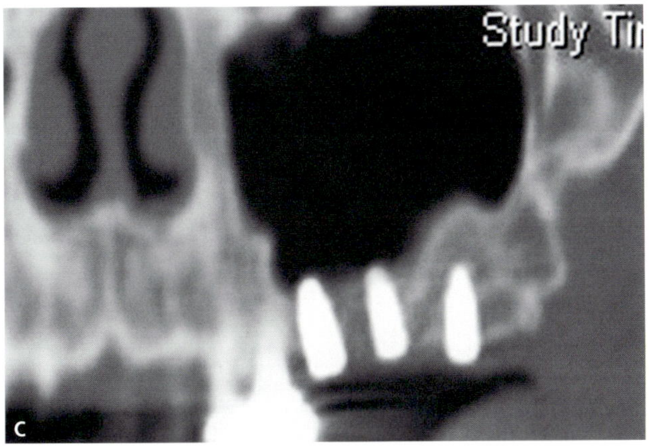

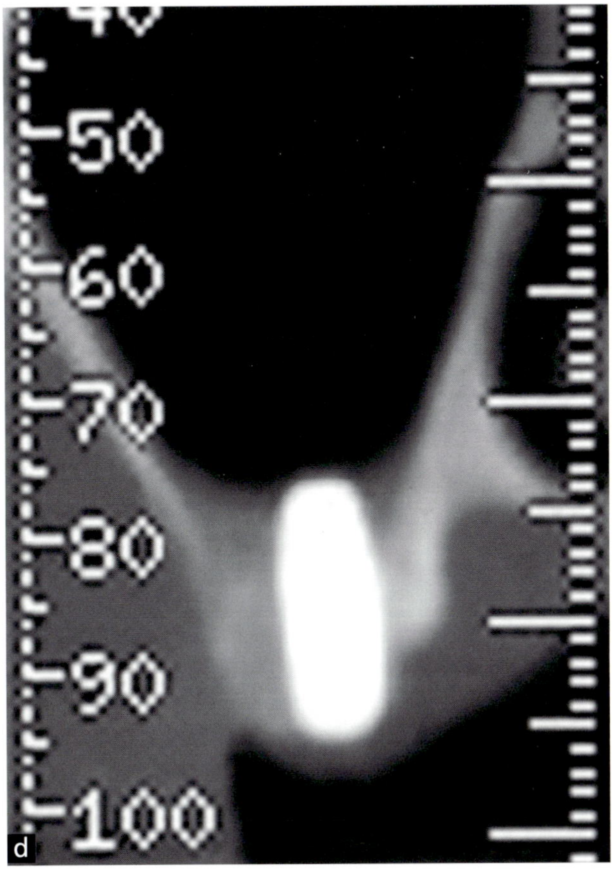

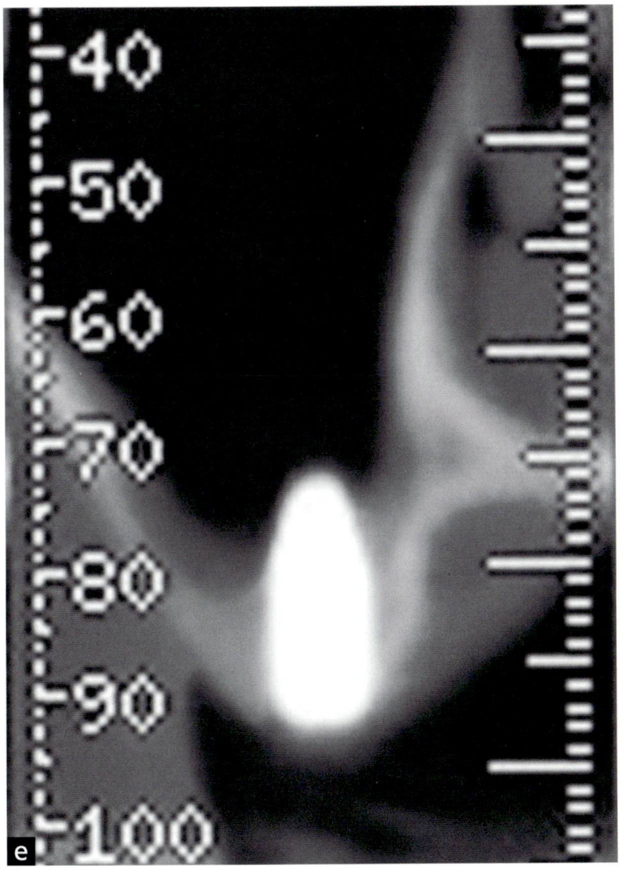

Fig 14-14 A third patient with mucosal elevation of the maxillary sinus and simultaneous flapless implant surgery. (a) Radiograph of the implant site. (b) Radiograph taken immediately after implant placement. Two implants (4.0 mm in diameter and 10 mm in length) were placed in the left maxillary sinus in such a way that they protruded 4 or 6 mm into the maxillary sinus after sinus membrane elevation. (c–e) Radiographs taken after 4 months. Evidence of ossification in the elevated sinus area was observed in all implants. The sides of the implants were covered with bone, but no bone tissue was observed at the apical implant surface.

to the sinus wall after elevating the membrane. However, suturing the membrane with a needle and thread is impossible for the elevated sinus membrane through the small access bone window with limited access.

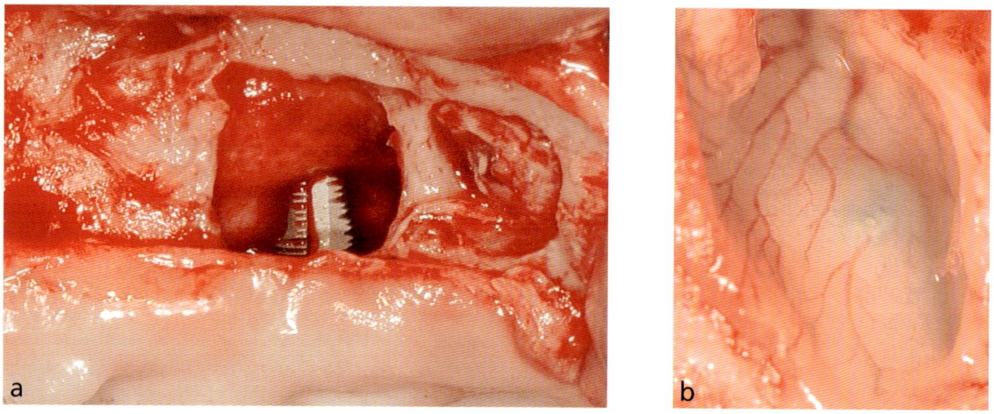

Fig 14-15 (a) An implant was placed in such a manner that it protruded 4 mm into the maxillary sinus after sinus membrane elevation. (b) The maxillary sinus 6 months after implant placement. The part of the implant that had been introduced into the sinus cavity is fully covered with an intact sinus membrane.

Effect of length of implant protrusion into the sinus cavity

An animal experiment was carried out to evaluate the effects of the length of implant protrusion into the sinus cavity after sinus membrane elevation on the height of new bone formation in the sinus.

Implants were placed bilaterally in the maxillary sinus of six adult mongrel dogs in such a manner that they protruded 4 or 8 mm into the maxillary sinus after sinus membrane elevation. The animals were sacrificed 6 months after surgery and the maxillary sinus was examined by optical microscopy.

A gross examination of the sides containing the implant protruding by 4 mm revealed an intact sinus membrane that was flush with the apical implant surface (Fig 14-15). On each of the 8 mm protruding implants, the part of the implant that had been introduced into the sinus cavity was not fully covered with intact sinus membrane (Fig 14-16). The membrane was also very thin and pale. In two sinuses with 8 mm protruding implants, the membrane was perforated at the apical segment of the implants. Debris accumulated on the surface of the apical sections exposed to the sinus cavity (Fig 14-17).

The average heights of newly formed bone in the sinus for the 4 mm protruding implant group were 3.3 mm and 0.7 mm on the buccal and palatal sides of the implants, respectively. The average heights for the 8 mm protruding implant group were 3.2 mm and 0.6 mm, respectively. The difference between the two groups was not statistically significant ($P > .05$). Therefore, the 8 mm protruding implant group did not demonstrate greater bone formation than the 4 mm protruding implant group (Figs 14-18 and 14-19). This suggests that when implants protrude into the sinus floor after sinus membrane elevation without introducing a grafting material, the length of protrusion implants into the sinus cavity is not related to the height of new bone in the sinus.

Interestingly, in two sinuses with an implant protruding by 8 mm, the membrane was perforated at the apical segment of the implant. It appears that the membrane did not have sufficient strength to resist the elastic pull of the high protruding implants.

A tent-like figure was formed by the sinus membrane from the apical surface of the implant, and new bone formation occurred in the space created by the sinus membrane tent. The maxillary sinus membrane drooped more on the palatal side than on the buccal side. For this reason, more bone was generated on the buccal side than on the palatal side. It appears that positive intrasinus air pressure caused by respiration might make the sinus membrane fall down on to the implant.

Overall, the amount of bone heights that can be gained in the maxillary sinus after sinus membrane elevation are approximately 3.3 mm and 0.7 mm on the buccal and palatal sides of the implants, respectively, regardless of the implant length.

Effect of venous blood inserted into the sinus cavity

Use of the patient's own venous blood to treat posterior maxillary atrophy appears attractive based on its theoretical advantages, which include the ease of procurement and application, a lack of adjunctive grafting materials, and the presence of growth factors in the blood platelet.[9-12] For these reasons, Hatano et al.[4] filled the sinus cavity below the lifted sinus membrane with peripheral venous blood.

However, our animal study showed that the space filled with autologous venous blood collapsed and the sinus membrane fell down on to the implant (Fig 4-20). As a result, only a small amount of new bone formation

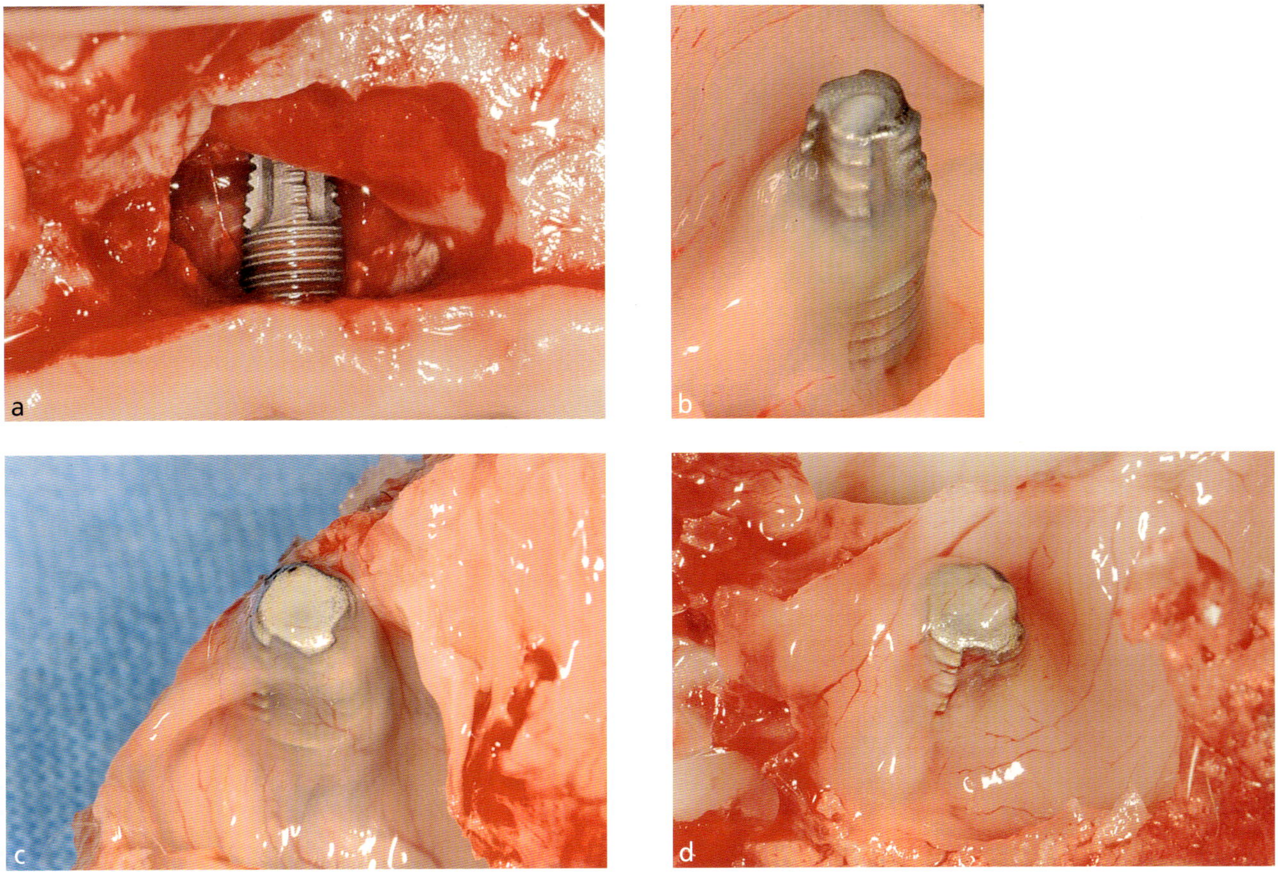

Fig 14-16 (a) An implant was placed in such a manner that it protruded 8 mm into the maxillary sinus after sinus membrane elevation. (b–d) The maxillary sinus 6 months after implant placement. The part of the implant that had been introduced into the sinus cavity is not fully covered with an intact sinus membrane. The membrane is very thin and pale.

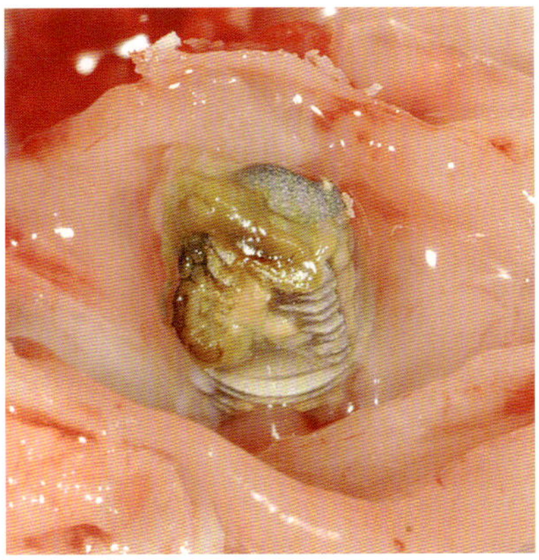

Fig 14-17 On the 8 mm protruding implant, the membrane was perforated at the apical segment of the implants. Debris accumulates on the surface of the apical sections exposed to the sinus cavity.

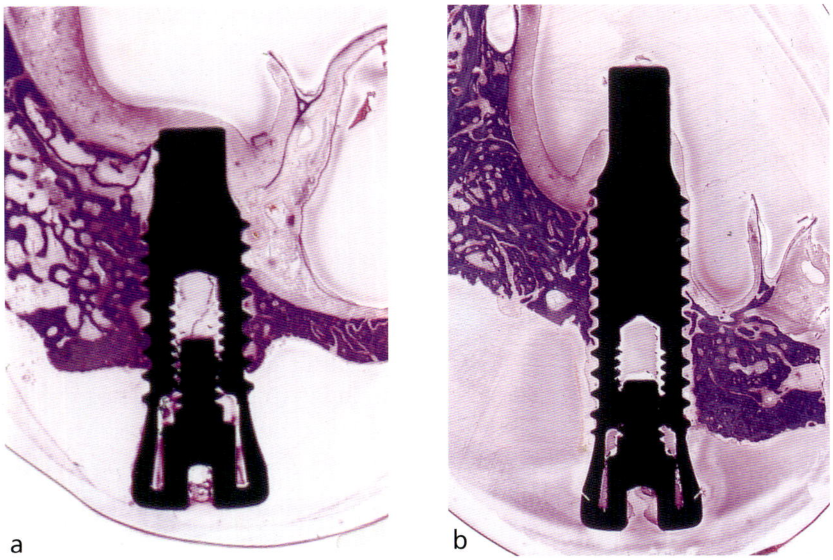

Fig 14-18 Histological views of (a) 4 mm, and (b) 8 mm protruding implant.

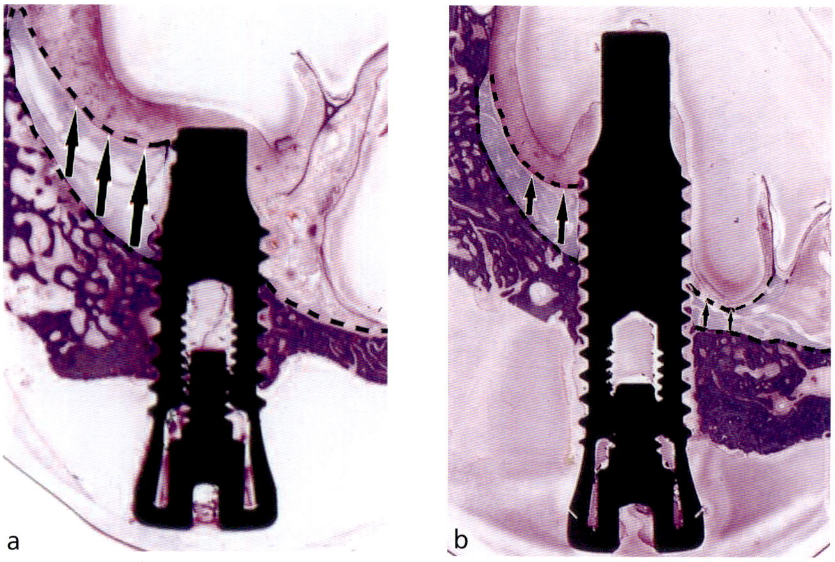

Fig 14-19 Histological views of implants protruding by (a) 4 mm and (b) 8 mm. The length of the protrusion into the sinus cavity is not related to the height of new bone in the sinus.

occurred in the space created by the collapsed membrane. The average height of newly formed bone around the implants in the sinus was 2.7 ± 0.7 mm on the buccal side and 0.6 ± 0.3 mm on the palatal side. One possible explanation for this finding is that the blood clot might degrade too quickly to facilitate the formation of new bone in the maxillary sinus. Another factor may be that sinus air pressure within the maxillary sinus cavity causes the sinus membrane to fall down on to the implant.[4,13] Therefore, to enhance bone formation in the maxillary sinus floor using sinus membrane elevation and venous blood, additional graft materials that enable the membrane to remain in the elevated position are necessary.

Attainable rate of osseointegration after sinus membrane elevation

The bone–implant contact occurs not only in the portion of the implant that is placed on the original alveolar ridge but also in new bone. The rate of osseointegration was higher in the former than in the latter. The average osseointegration rate was only 27.0% at 6 months when 10 mm long implants were inserted in the maxillary sinus using the method of sinus membrane elevation, where 5 mm of vertical bone remained between the residual crest of bone and the floor of the maxillary sinus (Fig 14-21). This suggests a deficiency in the strength required for clinical function because a minimum osseointegration rate of 40% is considered necessary for the clinical functioning of implant fixtures.[14–17] Accordingly, it is recommended that the sinus membrane elevation procedure be used when more than 8 mm of vertical bone is present.

Histology of the elevated mucosa of the maxillary sinus

The normal physiology of the maxillary sinus is strongly dependent on the proper functioning of both the maxillary ostium and the mucosal lining. The maxillary ostium is located in the superior aspect of the medial wall. This structure is the main opening through which the maxillary sinus drains its secretions into the nasal cavity. The maxillary sinus is lined with the Schniederian membrane, which consists of ciliated epithelium. The key to a normal sinus physiological condition is proper functioning of the cilia, which are the main component of the mucociliary transport system.[13,18] Cilia work to move contaminants toward the maxillary ostium and then to the nasopharynx. The mucociliary function of the respiratory epithelium is an important defense against viruses and bacteria, as well as other foreign material in inhaled air. Therefore, the pathogenesis of sinusitis is usually a change in the sinus ostium patency or mucociliary function.

While it has been shown that the sinus mucosa remains healthy after maxillary sinus floor augmentation using grafting material,[19,20] the literature provides few details of the morphology of the sinus membrane after its elevation without the use of adjunctive graft materials. An animal experiment was carried out to evaluate histological changes in the sinus membrane after sinus membrane elevation, and the simultaneous insertion of dental implants without additional grafting material.[21,22]

The insertion of dental implants into the maxillary sinus cavity barely affects the maxillary ostium, which is located far from the surgical field in the upper portion of the medial wall. However, our concern was that implant

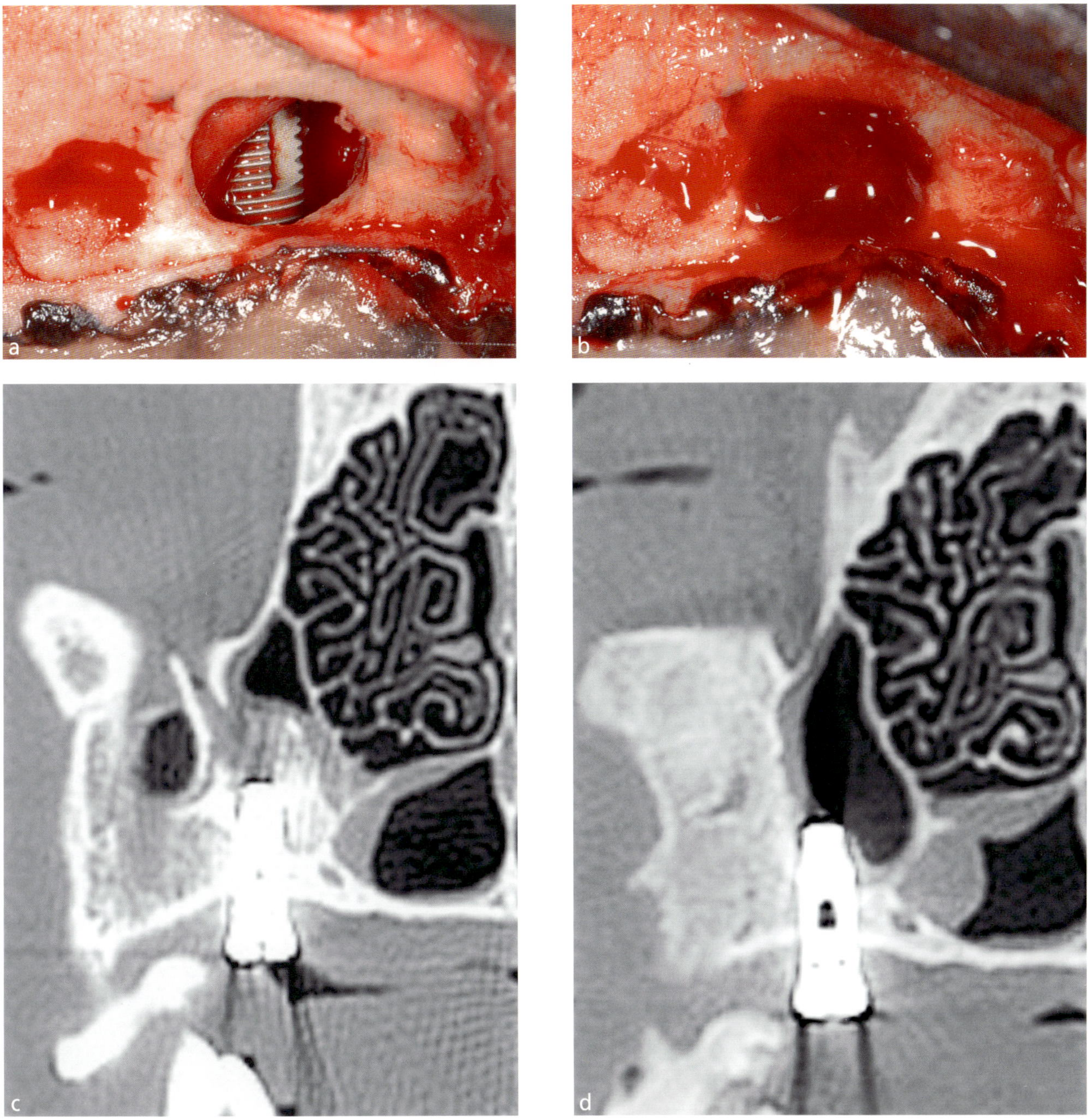

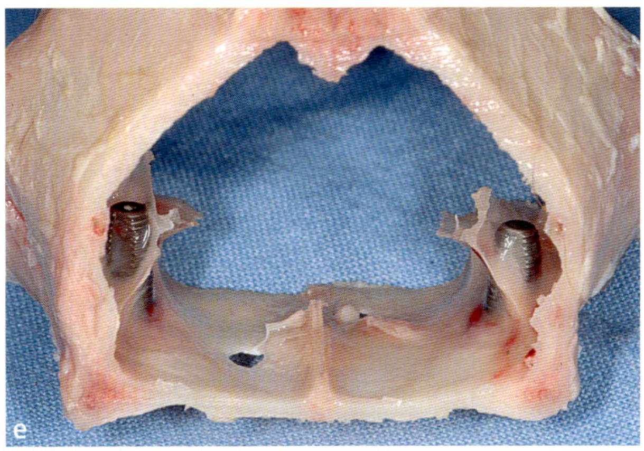

Fig 14-20 (a and b) After elevation of the sinus membrane and protruding an implant into the sinus cavity, the sinus cavity below the lifted sinus membrane was not filled with venous blood on one side of the maxillary sinus, but was filled with venous blood on the other side. (c) CT image taken after 2 days. (d) CT image taken after 6 months. The majority of the space filled with autologous venous blood was collapsed and the sinus membrane had fallen down on to the implant. (e) View of a specimen after 6 months showing only a small amount of new bone formation in the space created by the collapsed membrane.

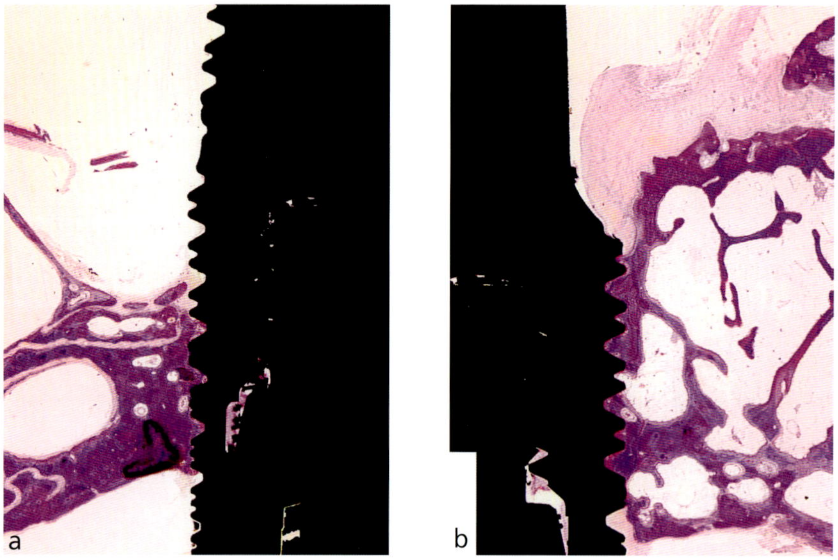

Fig 14-21 (a and b) The average osseointegration rate was only 27.0% at 6 months when 10 mm long implants were inserted in the maxillary sinus using sinus membrane elevation and simultaneous flapless implant surgery with 5 mm of vertical bone remaining between the residual crest of the bone and the floor of the maxillary sinus.

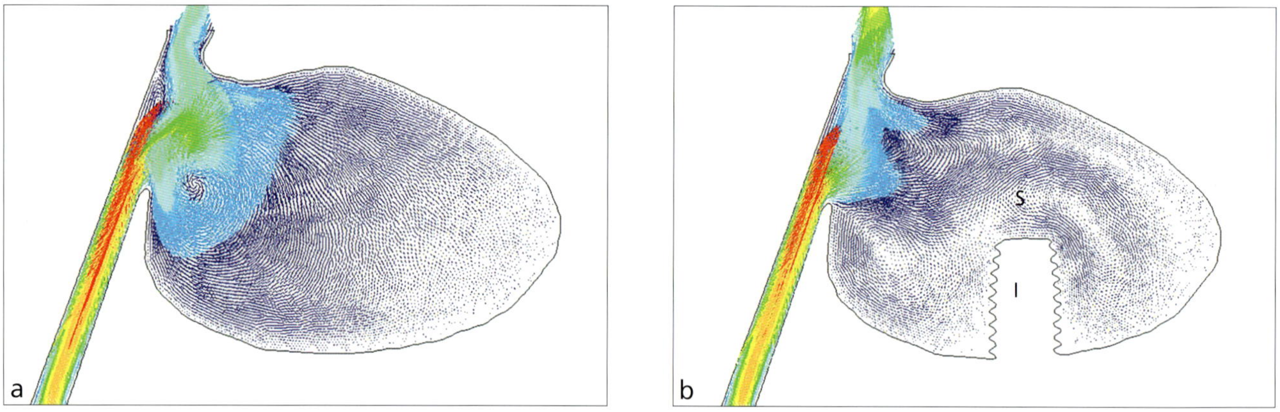

Fig 14-22 (a and b) Implant extension (I) into the maxillary sinus cavity (S) may alter sinus airflow.

extension into the maxillary sinus cavity might disturb the mucociliary function of the antral mucosa, alter the sinus airflow, and be a source of chronic inflammation and sinusitis (Fig 14-22).[23–25] Therefore, the experiment was performed to determine whether implant extension into the maxillary sinus cavity is a source of chronic inflammation and sinusitis.

In six dogs, an implant was placed unilaterally in the maxillary sinus in such a manner that it protruded 5 mm into the maxillary sinus after sinus membrane elevation. On the opposite side, the maxillary sinus was left untreated as a control. The animals were sacrificed 6 months after surgery. The mucosal samples were harvested at the laterocaudal antral wall and examined by optical microscopy as well as scanning and transmission electronic microscopy (Fig 14-23).

Gross examination of the sinuses containing the 5 mm protruding implants showed that the sinus membrane was intact with no signs of infection in any maxillary sinus cavity (Fig 14-24). In addition, all implants were integrated within the surrounding bone. This suggests that the insertion of dental implants into the maxillary sinus cavity does not cause maxillary sinus inflammation or hinder osseointegration of the implants. On microscopic examination of the sinuses containing a 5 mm protruding implant, the sinus membrane appeared to be morphologically intact (Fig 14-25). It did not show any change in the number of glands and goblet cells inside the mucosa. Both transmission and scanning electron microscopy showed that the sinus membrane exhibited a normal epithelial lining with ciliated cells, goblet cells, and basal cells (Figs 14-26 and 14-27).

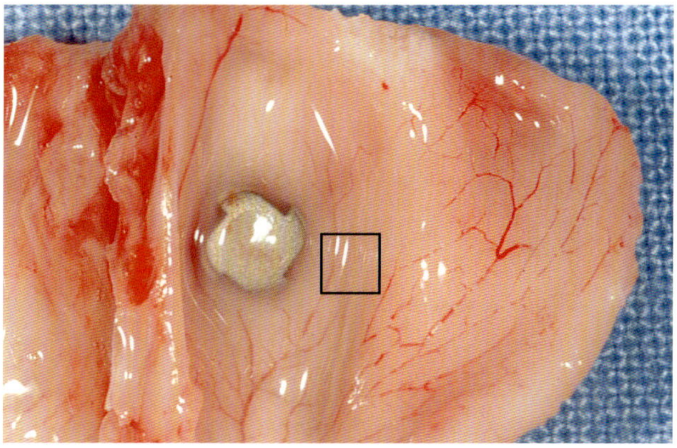

Fig 14-23 Mucosal samples were harvested at the laterocaudal antral wall of the maxillary sinus and examined by optical microscopy and scanning and transmission electronic microscopy.

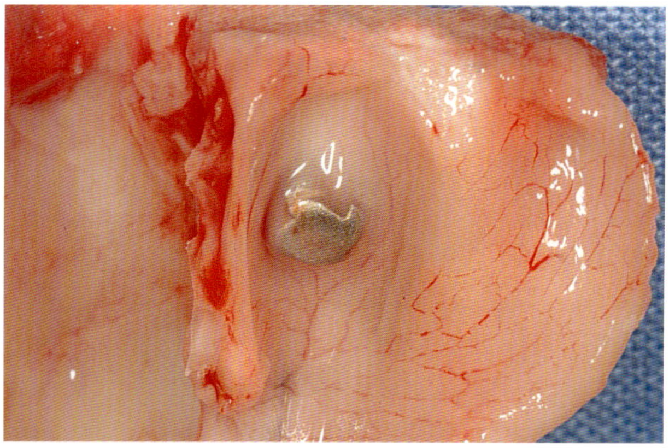

Fig 14-24 Photograph of the maxillary sinus showing the sinus mucosa covering the protruding 5 mm implant 6 months after surgery.

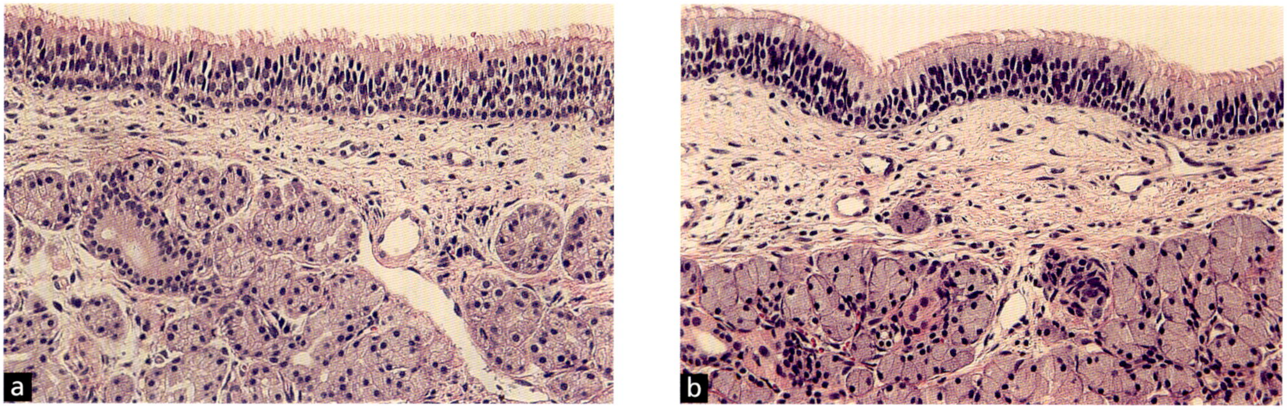

Fig 14-25 Optical micrographs of the maxillary sinus mucosa: (a) untreated sinus, and (b) sinus with the 5 mm protruding implant. The sinus membrane appears to be morphologically intact on both sides. There was no difference in the thickness of either the epithelium or the connective tissue between the untreated and 5 mm protruding implant sides.

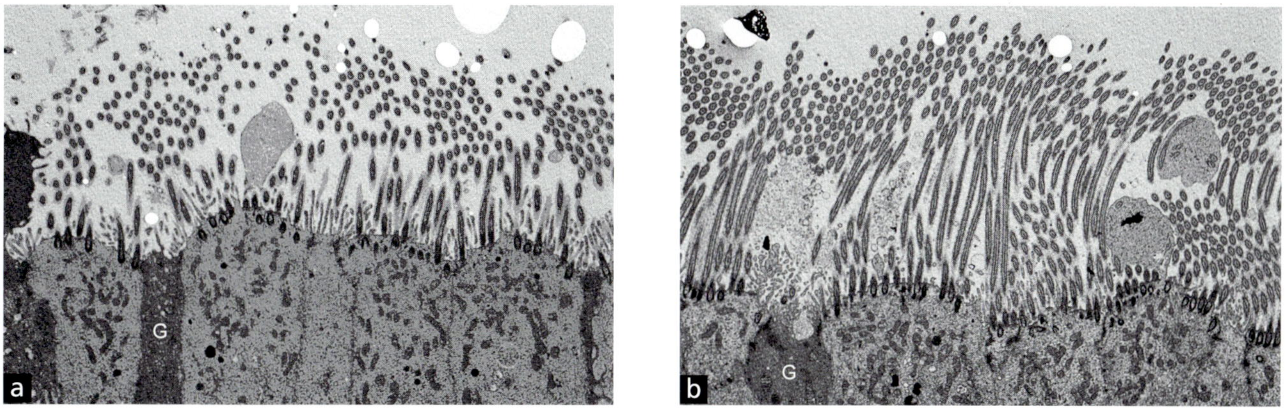

Fig 14-26 Transmission electron micrographs of the maxillary sinus mucosa: (a) untreated sinus, and (b) sinus with the 5 mm protruding implant. Both sinuses show a normal epithelial lining with ciliated cells, goblet cells (G), and basal cells. There is no difference in the number of goblet cells between the untreated and 5 mm protruding implant sides.

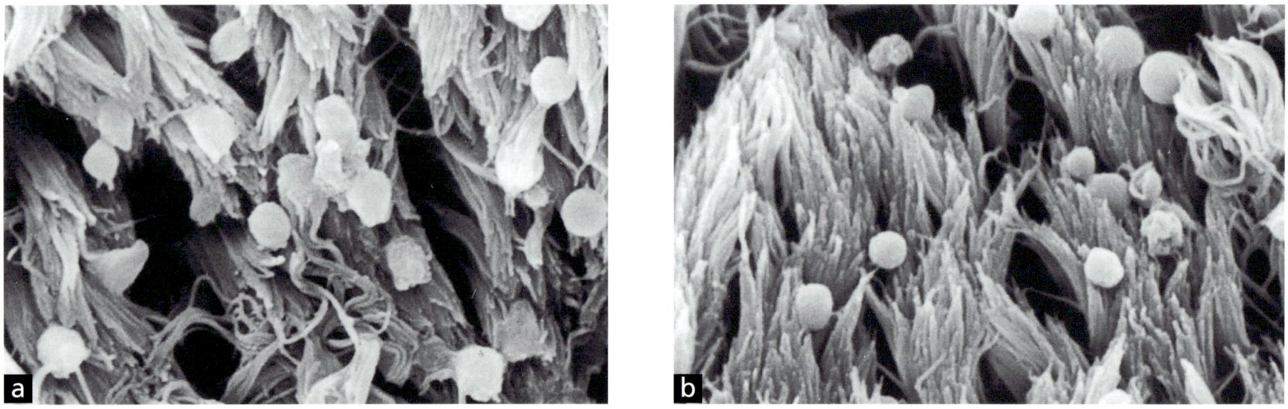

Fig 14-27 Scanning electron micrographs of the maxillary sinus mucosa: (a) untreated sinus, and (b) sinus with the 5 mm protruding implant. The luminal surface of the mucosa shows interspersed goblet cells and the extensive presence of ciliated cells on both sides. The cilia are all arrayed synchronously, leaning in the same direction. There is no ultrastructural difference between the untreated and 5 mm protruding implant sides.

Overall, the surgical procedure by which implants are inserted into the sinus cavity by elevating the sinus membrane without adding any graft material appears to have little effect on the histological characteristics of the sinus membrane. The experimental results appear to confirm that the maxillary sinus mucosa can adapt adequately to the changes induced by implants protruding into the maxillary sinus cavity. However, it should be noted that this finding may be true only if the sinus mucosa is elevated without perforation.

Advantages and disadvantages

Advantages

- Approximately 3 mm of bone height on the buccal side of the implants can be gained in the maxillary sinus after sinus membrane elevation without adding graft material.
- It is possible to elevate the sinus membrane using a small bone window, 5 mm in diameter. The window can be created using a small vertical incision on the buccal cortical plate, approximately 8 mm away from the implant placement sites.
- This minimally invasive technique using small incisions and a small bone window has the advantage of a more conservative surgical entry and less postoperative morbidity, thereby shortening the surgery time and minimizing postoperative pain, edema, and infection.
- Use of a submerged mini-incision implant procedure protects implants during the early postsurgical period.
- Mini-incision implant surgery reduces the amount of bone loss of the crest during the initial healing period, thereby contributing to enhanced implant stability.
- The method of sinus membrane elevation has the advantage of enhancing implant primary stability through bicortical anchorage because implants can be placed deeper by going through the cortical bone on the sinus floor.

Disadvantages

- There are limitations in the bone height achieved with the procedure. The bone heights achieved were approximately 3 mm and 0.7 mm on the buccal and palatal sides of the implants, respectively, regardless of the implant length.
- No bone is generated at the apical surface of the implants.
- The excessively high placement of implants in the maxillary sinus causes severe tension to the sinus mucosa, possibly leading to mucosal perforation.
- The procedure is indicated only when the remaining bone can guarantee primary stability of the implants.
- An attainable osseointegration rate in new bone generated using the procedure is quite low during the 6-month healing period.

Considerations related to surgery

- The implant can be pushed easily into the sinus proper and displaced into the sinus when the remaining bone cannot ensure primary stability of the implant. Therefore, it is prudent to delay implant insertion when primary stability of the implant cannot be guaranteed. Placement of implants should be deferred after sinus bone grafting.
- Sinus bone grafting is indicated in order to obtain more than 4 mm of bone height in the sinus floor. Maxillary

sinus bone grafting is described in more detail in Chapter 15.
- Care should be taken not to damage the sinus membrane when the sinus membrane is elevated through a 5 mm access bone window. In addition, care should be taken not to damage the elevated mucosa by drills while preparing the implant sites.
- The attainable osseointegration rate in new bone generated after sinus membrane elevation is quite low during the 6-month healing period. Therefore, it is prudent to submerge the implants and wait longer to uncover the implant.

Further observations on the procedure

New bone can form in the maxillary sinus when the sinus membrane is elevated and the implant is inserted simultaneously without using adjunctive grafting material.[1–3] However, the results of the authors' experiments show that the maximum amount of bone height that can be gained in the maxillary sinus after sinus membrane elevation is approximately 3 mm on the buccal side of the implants, regardless of the implant length. The length of the implants protruding into the sinus cavity is not related to the height of new bone in the sinus. Therefore, it is prudent to attempt to gain 3 mm of bone height in the maxillary sinus using the sinus membrane elevation procedure without adjunctive grafting material.

However, maxillary sinus bone grafting can contribute more to long-term implant stability than the sinus membrane elevation procedure if more than 4 mm of bone augmentation in the maxillary sinus is necessary to place the implants. According to Friberg et al.,[26] 69 out of 4623 implants failed before mounting the prosthesis; 46 of the failed implants were only 7 mm long (the shortest implant). This suggests that implant failure is related to the bone height. Therefore, in order to place a sufficiently long implant in posterior maxillary sites that receive the greatest load, it is prudent to use the sinus membrane elevation procedure without adjunctive grafting material when more than 8 mm of vertical bone is present.

Summary

It is possible to elevate the sinus membrane using a small bone window, 5 mm in diameter, and protrude implants into the sinus cavity simultaneously with the sinus membrane elevation. Approximately 3 mm of bone height on the buccal side of the implants can be achieved in the maxillary sinus using this procedure.

References

1. Winter AA, Pollack AS, Odrich RB. Sinus/alveolar crest tenting (SACT): a new technique for implant placement in atrophic maxillary ridges without bone grafting or membranes. Int J Periodontic Restorative Dent 2003;23:557–565.
2. Lundgren S, Andersson S, Gualini F, Sennerby L. Bone reformation with sinus membrane elevation: a new surgical technique for maxillary sinus floor augmentation. Clin Implant Dent Relat Res 2004;6:165–173.
3. Leblebicioglu B, Ersanli S, Karabuda C, Tosun T, Gokdeniz H. Radiographic evaluation of dental implants placed using an osteotome technique. J Periodontol 2005;76:385–390.
4. Hatano N, Sennerby L, Lundgren S. Maxillary sinus augmentation using sinus membrane elevation and peripheral venous blood for implant-supported rehabilitation of the atrophic posterior maxilla: case series. Clin Implant Dent Relat Res 2007;9:150–155.
5. Lundgren S, Andersson S, Gualini F, Sennerby L. Bone reformation with sinus membrane elevation: a new surgical technique for maxillary sinus floor augmentation. Clin Implant Dent Relat Res 2004;6:165–173.
6. Palma VC, Magro-Filho O, Oliveira JA, Lundgren S, Salata LA, Sennerby L. Bone reformation and implant integration following maxillary sinus membrane elevation: an experimental study in primates. Clin Implant Dent Relat Res 2006;8:11–24.
7. Gruber R, Kandler B, Fürst G, Fischer MB, Watzek G. Porcine sinus mucosa holds cells that respond to bone morphogenetic protein BMP-6 and BMP-7 with increased osteogenic differentiation in vitro. Clin Oral Implants Res 2004;15:575–580.
8. Jeong SM, Choi BH, Li J, Xuan F. A retrospective study of the effects of sinus membrane elevation on bone formation around implants placed in the maxillary sinus cavity. Oral Surg Oral Med Oral Pathol Oral Radiol Endod 2009;107:364–368.
9. Sanchez AR, Sheridan PJ, Kupp LI. Is platelet-rich plasma the perfect enhancement factor? A current review. Int J Oral Maxillofac Implants 2003;18:93–103.
10. Ganio C, Tenewitz FE, Wilson RC, Maules BG. The treatment of chronic nonhealing wounds using autologous platelet-derived growth factors. J Foot Ankle Surg 1993;32:263–268.
11. Okuda K, Kawase T, Momose M et al. Platelet-rich plasma contains high levels of platelet-derived growth factor and transforming growth factor-β and modulates the proliferation of periodontally related cells in vitro. J Periodontol 2003;74:849–857.
12. Thorn JJ, Sørensen H, Weis-Fogh U, Andersen M. Autologous fibrin glue with growth factors in reconstructive maxillofacial surgery. Int J Oral Maxillofac Surg 2004;33:95–100.
13. Amble FR, Lindberg SO, McCaffrey TV. Mucociliary function and endothelins 1, 2, and 3. Otolarygol Head Neck Surg 1993; 109:634–645.
14. Keller JC, Young FA, Natiella JR. Quantitative bone remodeling resulting from the use of porous dental implants. J Biomed Mater Res 1987;21:305.
15. Buser D, Schenk RK, Skinemann S. Influence of surface characteristics on bone integration of titanium implants: a histomorphometric study in miniature pigs. J Biomed Mater Res 1991;25:889.
16. Gottlander M, Albrektsson T. Histomorphometric studies of hydroxyapatite-coated and uncoated CP titanium threaded implants in bone. Int J Oral Maxillofac Implants 1991;6:399–404.
17. Weinlander M, Kenney EB, Lekovic V. Histomorphometry of bone opposition around three types of endosseous dental implants. Int J Oral Maxillofac Implants 1992;7:491.
18. William E, Bolger M, Clifford A. Paranasal sinus bony anatomic variations and mucosal abnormalities: CT analysis for endoscopic sinus surgery. Laryngoscope 1991;101:56–59.
19. Bravetti P, Membre H, Marchal L, Jankowski R. Histologic changes in the sinus membrane after maxillary sinus augmentation in goats. J Oral Maxillofac Surg 1998;56:1170–1176.

20. Timmenga NM, Raghoebar GM, Liem RSB, van Weissenbruch R, Manson WL, Vissink A. Effects of maxillary sinus floor elevation surgery on the maxillary sinus physiology. Eur J Oral Sci 2003;111:189–197.

21. Sul SH, Choi BH, Li J, Jeong SM, Xuan F. The effects of sinus membrane elevation on bone formation around implants placed in the maxillary sinus cavity: an experimental study. Oral Surg Oral Med Oral Pathol Oral Radiol Endod 2008;105:684–687.

22. Sul SH, Choi BH, Li J, Jeong SM, Xuan F. Histological changes in the maxillary sinus membrane after sinus membrane elevation and the simultaneous insertion of dental implants without the use of grafting materials. Oral Surg Oral Med Oral Pathol Oral Radiol Endod 2008;105:e1–e5.

23. Watelet JB, Bachert C, Gevaert P, Cauwenberge P. Wound healing of the nasal and paranasal mucosa: a review. Am J Rhinol 2002;16:77–84.

24. Westrin KM, Stierna P, Carlsoo B. Mucosal fine structure in experimental sinusitis. Ann Otol Rhinol Laryngol 1993;102:639–645.

25. Raghoebar GM, Weissenbruch R, Vissink A. Rhino-sinusitis related to endosseous implants extending into the nasal cavity: a case report. Int J Oral Maxillofac Surg 2004;33:312–314.

26. Friberg B, Jemt T, Lekholm U. Early failures in 4641 consecutively placed Brånemark dental implants: a study from stage 1 surgery to the connection of completed prostheses. Int J Oral Maxillofac Implants 1991;6:142–146.

CHAPTER

15

Maxillary Sinus Bone Grafting

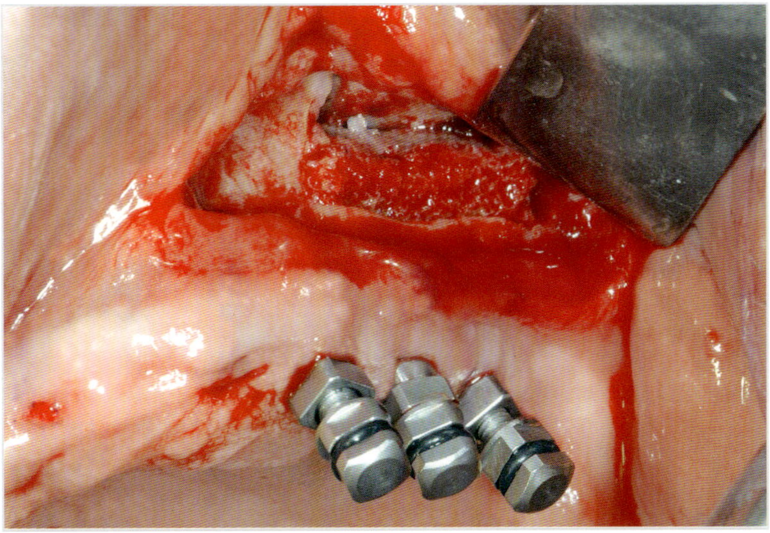

Key point

It is possible to use flapless implant surgery even when a maxillary sinus bone graft is indicated.

Overview

In the posterior maxilla, implant placement may be problematic because the alveolar process tends to resorb with age, and the maxillary sinus becomes larger (Fig 15-1). As there is little bone volume available in this region, sinus floor elevation has become an important procedure in peri-implant grafting.[1] The bone quality is poorest in the posterior maxilla than in any other intraoral region, which compromises the initial implant stability. Because implant success after loading in the posterior maxilla is reduced in implants under 10 mm in length, it is logical to plan longer implants in the region. In general, implants of 4 mm diameter should be at least 12 mm in length when the bone density is poor.[2] This normally provides an adequate bone–implant contact to dissipate the loads applied to the prosthesis. Various maxillary sinus floor augmentation techniques have been proposed to gain adequate bone height for implants with adequate length in this region. This chapter addresses flapless implant surgery performed together with maxillary sinus bone grafting techniques.

Review of the literature

Since its development by Tatum and colleagues,[1,3] sinus bone graft surgery has become a predictable treatment that augments bone to a height of 20 mm. However, success rates between 75% and 97% have been reported for implant placement performed simultaneously with sinus bone grafting,[4–7] highlighting the need for a more effective surgical method. Misch[2] stopped simultaneous implant placement with sinus bone grafting in 1993 owing to the frequent implant failure caused by postoperative complications. In particular, the implants present in the grafting material make the treatment of infections difficult.

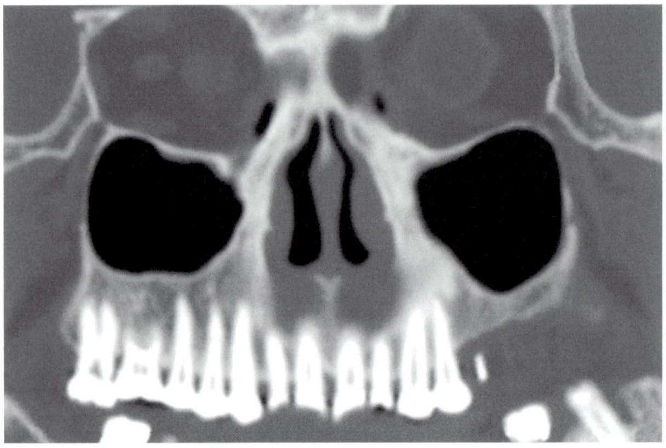

Fig 15-1 In the posterior maxilla, implant placement may be problematic because the alveolar process tends to resorb with age and the maxillary sinus becomes larger.

Classification and features of autogenous bone

The autogenous bone grafts used in sinus floor augmentation are typically harvested from the iliac bone crest.[8–11] The bone can be harvested in either block or particulate form. A block bone can be classified as cortical, cancellous, or corticocancellous.

- *Cortical* block bone has excellent initial mechanical strength but a deficient blood supply, which takes a long time for initial revascularization. This type is suitable for the grafting of a site requiring an initial mechanical load.
- *Cancellous* block bone has the advantage of rapid initial revascularization but poor mechanical strength.
- *Corticocancellous* block bone contains both cortical and cancellous bone, and has the advantages of each type of bone.

Therefore, the present authors prefer to use corticocancellous block bone. Corticocancellous block bone grafts offer significant benefits over particulate bone grafts, such as strength for primary implant stability and rapid bone regeneration, because of the remodeling capacity of cancellous bone.

Comparison of corticocancellous block with particulate bone grafts

There is some controversy regarding bone healing around dental implants when they are installed simultaneously with either a corticocancellous block or particulate bone grafts for maxillary sinus floor augmentation.

Some studies have reported that particle bone offers better results because it enables prompt bone remodeling. Other studies have reported no significant difference in bone grafting between the two types of bone.[12] We have found that, when corticocancellous blocks were used for sinus grafting (Fig 15-2), both the percentage of direct implant–bone contact and the height of newly formed bone on the sinus floor were significantly greater than when corticocancellous particulate bone grafts were used (Figs 15-3 and 15-4). The average osseointegration was significantly higher in the block group (56.7 ± 15.2%) than in the particulate group (32.1 ± 13.1%; $P < .05$) (Fig 15-5). The height of the newly formed bone in the augmented area was greater in the block group (12.3 ± 2.6 mm) than in the particulate group (9.7 ± 2.5 mm; $P < .05$).

These results are in accordance with those reported by Lew et al.,[13] who used the canine ilium as a model site and placed implants through either a corticocancellous block or particulate bone grafts and compared the relative rates and extent of osseointegration of the dental implants. They demonstrated that block bone grafts could increase the rate of bone formation.

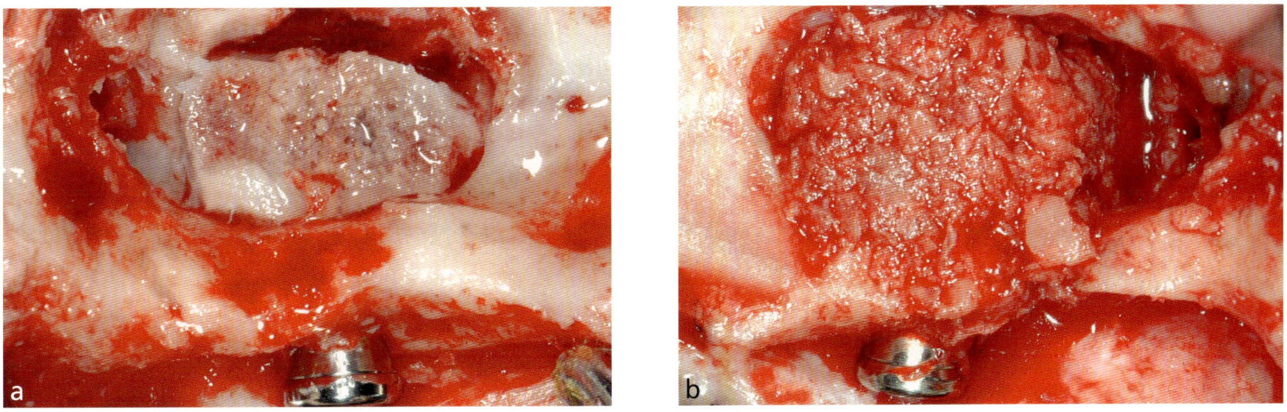

Fig 15-2 (a and b) Comparison of corticocancellous block and particulate bone grafts in maxillary sinus floor augmentation. Six adult mongrel dogs were used in this experiment. After creation of a 1 cm × 2 cm bone window, the mucous membranes were elevated bilaterally. On one side of the maxillary sinus, the resultant space between the membrane and sinus floor was filled with corticocancellous block bone. On the opposite side, a corticocancellous particulate bone was grafted. Two dental implants were placed in the grafting material bilaterally through the maxillary sinus floor. See also Figs 15-3 to 15-5.

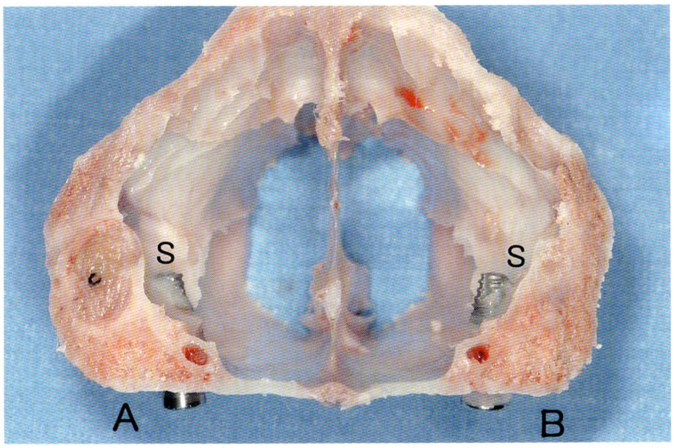

Fig 15-3 The maxillary sinuses (S) 6 months after surgery, showing the augmented area and implant. The height of the newly formed bone in the augmented area was greater in the block bone side (A) than in the particulate bone side (B).

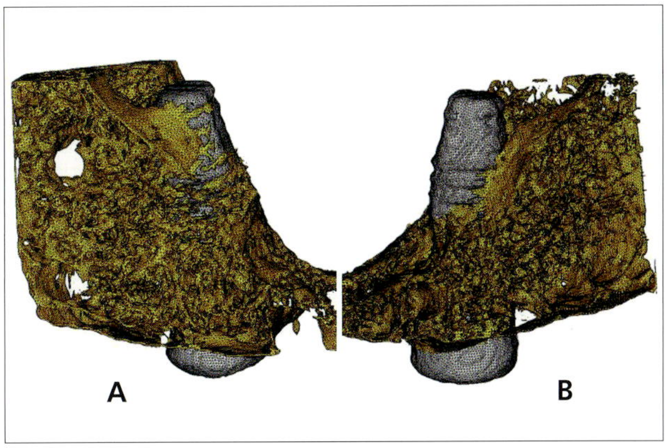

Fig 15-4 Three-dimensional micro-CT images showing the bone (yellow) around the implants (gray), for the block bone side (A) and particulate bone side (B). The mean heights of the newly formed bone in the augmented area were 12.3 mm on the block side and 9.7 mm on the particulate side.

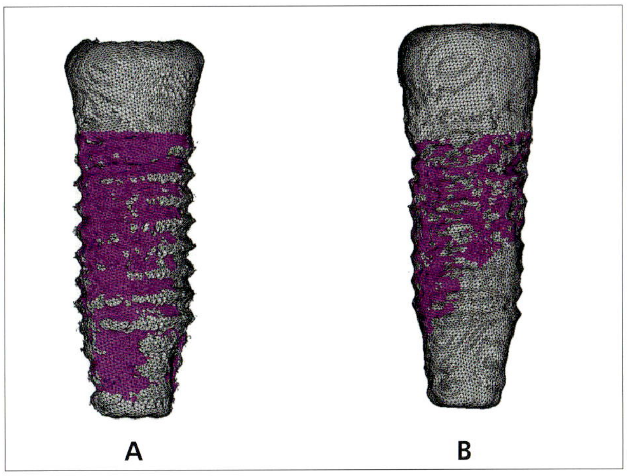

Fig 15-5 Three-dimensional micro-CT overview of the bone–implant contact area (purple) around the implant surface (gray), for the block bone side (A) and particulate bone side (B). The mean bone–implant contact was 56.7% on the block side and 32.1% on the particulate side.

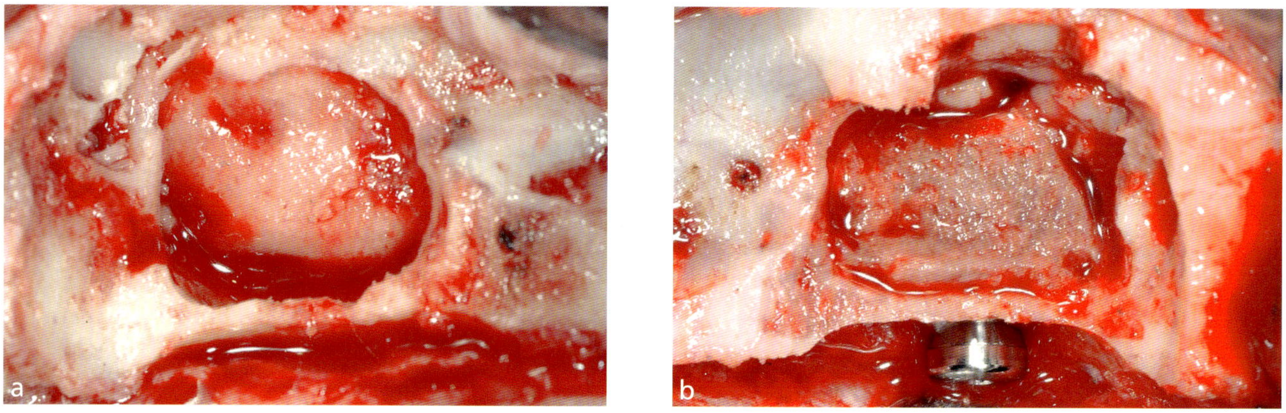

Fig 15-6 (a and b) Primary stability of implants can be achieved with a corticocancellous block iliac bone graft in the maxillary sinus floor, even if the available height is just 1 mm.

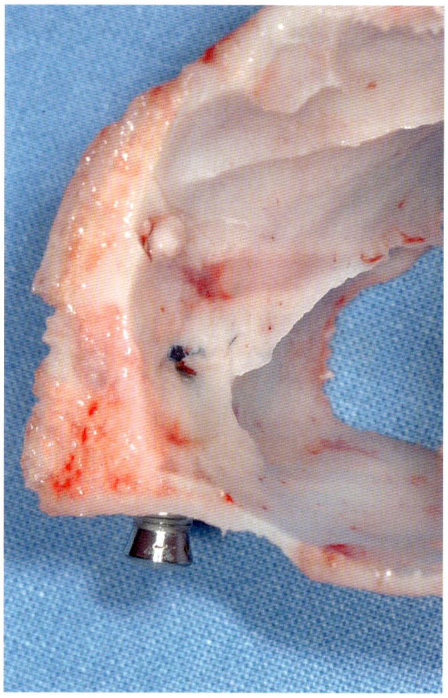

Fig 15-7 Specimen showing block autogenous iliac bone grafting with immediate mini-incision implant placement for 1 mm of maxillary sinus floor bone, 6 months after surgery. The implant is covered with the augmented bone and integrated within the bone.

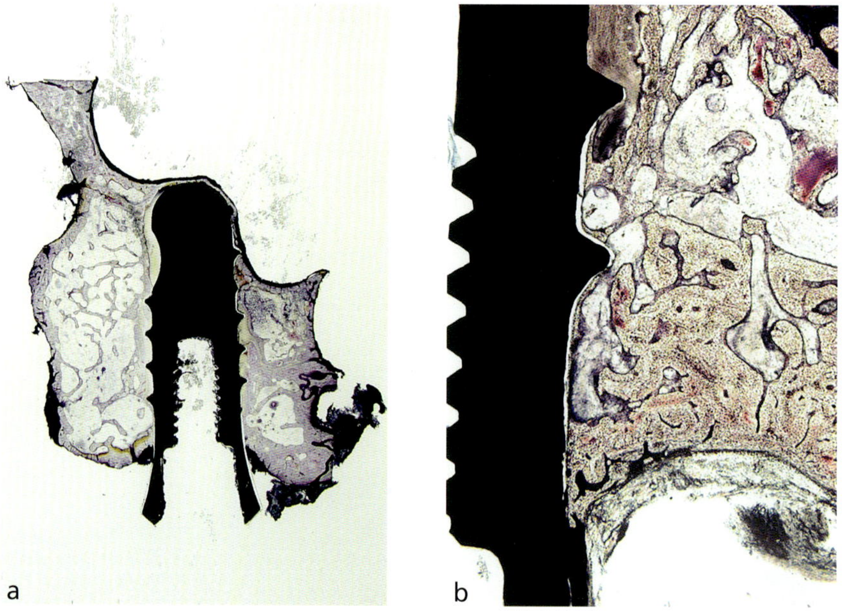

Fig 15-8 (a and b) Block autogenous iliac bone grafting with immediate mini-incision implant placement for 1 mm of maxillary sinus floor bone. Microscopic examination 6 months after surgery revealed bone tissue around the implant with an osseointegration rate of 54%.

Advantages of block-type autogenous iliac bone grafting

Corticocancellous block bone grafts offer significant benefits over particulate bone grafts in that they are strong and can be shaped to match the host site. They provide structural rigidity, which is often required when simultaneously placing implants because rigidity allows for accurate implant placement independent of the thickness of the sinus floor. The primary stability of implants, which is decisive for proper osseointegration, can be achieved even if the available height is 1–2 mm (Figs 15-6 to 15-9).

Traditionally, corticocancellous block bone grafts were believed to maintain more of their bulk than cancellous particulate bone grafts. We have found that corticocancellous block grafts maintain the bulk better than corticocancellous particulate grafts when placed in the sinus. Block-type autogenous iliac bone can provide sufficient bone for placing a long implant with large diameter in the posterior maxillary site (Fig 15-10), which can contribute to long-term implant stability in the posterior maxilla, where the bone quality is poorest.[14]

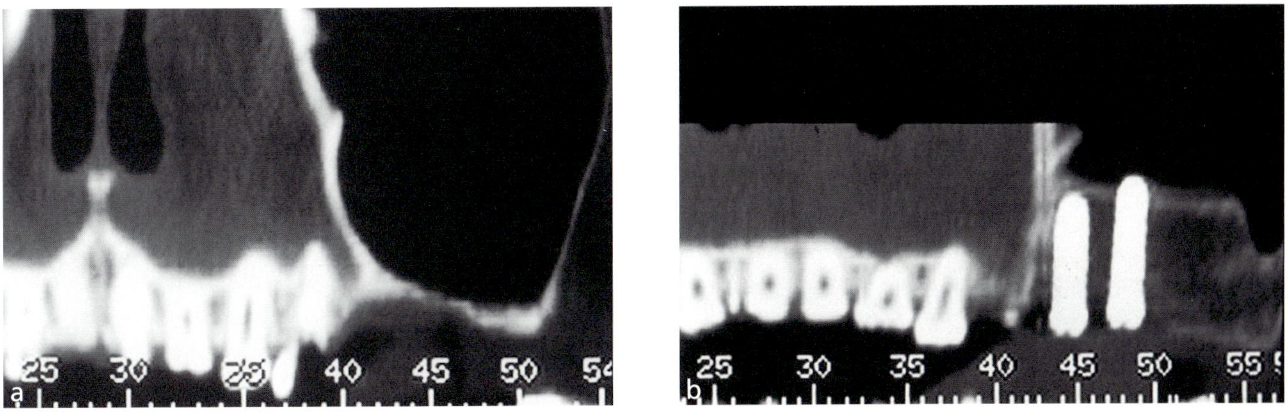

Fig 15-9 (a) Radiograph of a patient before surgery, showing 1 mm of maxillary sinus floor bone and missing maxillary molars. (b) Panoramic radiograph 6 months after surgery. Two implants placed in the left maxillary sinus simultaneously with block autogenous iliac bone grafting show radiographic evidence of ossification.

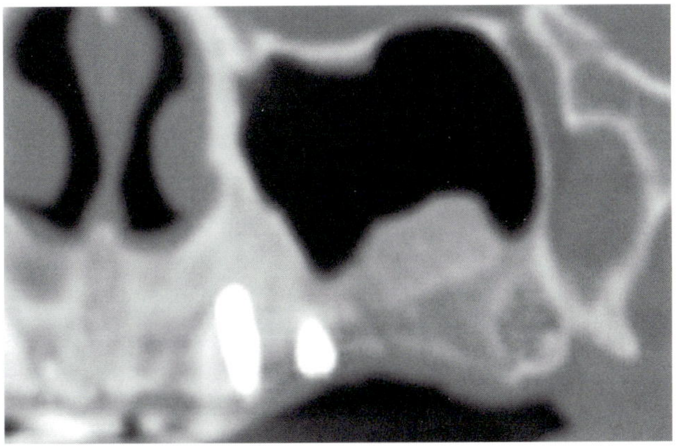

Fig 15-10 Computerized tomography shows that the block-type autogenous iliac bone graft in the maxillary sinus cavity can provide sufficient bone for placing a long implant in the posterior maxillary site.

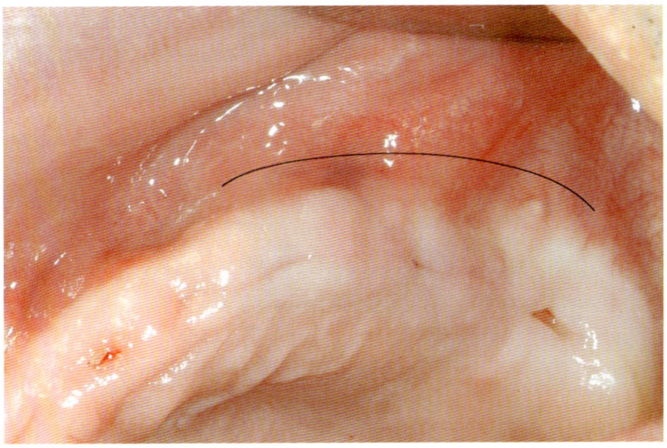

Fig 15-11 Incision for accessing the maxillary sinus wall.

Block autogenous iliac bone grafting with immediate mini-incision implant placement

This procedure is indicated when simultaneous implant placement and sinus bone grafting is performed in cases where there is less than 5 mm of vertical bone available below the maxillary sinus floor.

The incisions

Two separate incisions are made, one to access the maxillary sinus and the other to place the mini-incision implants. To access the maxillary sinus, a horizontal incision is made on the buccal cortical plate of the maxillary sinus horizontally with the alveolar crest approximately 10 mm away from the crest (Fig 15-11). The full-thickness mucoperiosteal flap is reflected to expose the lateral wall of the maxillary sinus.

Access window

Following Tatum's lateral approach, the lateral-access window is delineated using a round bur. The inferior score line of the access window is placed above the level of the horizontal incision line or approximately 2–5 mm above the level of the antral floor. The size of the access window is 15–20 mm in length and 10–15 mm in height (Fig 15-12). The corners of the access window are usually round instead of at right or acute angles. If the corner angles are too sharp, membrane perforation can occur from the use of a surgical curette at the corner or during infracture of the lateral wall.

Where there is thick lateral-wall bone, the outline of the access window is scored first using a no. 6 round carbide bur, which scratches the bone to indicate the overall window dimensions. Once the access window is delineated with the carbide bur, the bur is followed with a no. 4 round diamond bur to scratch the outline until a bluish hue is observed below the bur (Fig 15-13). If the bur

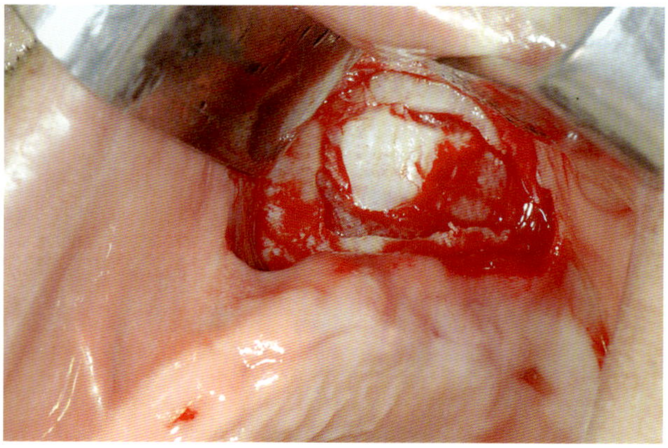

Fig 15-12 Access window in the lateral wall of the maxillary sinus.

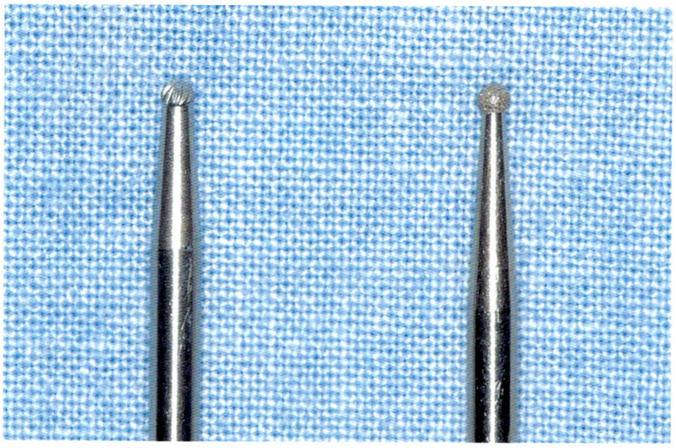

Fig 15-13 A no. 6 round carbide bur (left) and a no. 4 round diamond bur (right). Carbide burs will tear the membrane more readily if they inadvertently come into contact with the sinus membrane, whereas diamond burs minimize damage to the membrane.

inadvertently comes into contact with the sinus membrane, carbide burs tear it more readily, whereas diamond burs minimize damage to the sinus membrane.

A flat-ended metal punch is placed over the access window. A mallet is then used to gently tap the instrument and cause a greenstick fracture of the access window from the surrounding bone. A surgical curette is introduced along the margin of the window. The sinus membrane is then elevated above the maxillary sinus floor. The sinus membrane can be elevated easily from the antral walls because it has few elastic fibers and is not attached to the cortical wall. The periosteal elevator and curettes further reflect the membrane off the anterior vertical wall, floor, and medial vertical wall. Once in the final position, the window bone is positioned as part of the superior wall of the graft site. The sinus membrane is elevated to a height of at least 15 mm from the sinus floor. This allows proper placement of block-type bone in the sinus and the proper height for implant placement.

Block bone harvesting from the iliac crest

The iliac crest is widely accepted as the donor site of choice for obtaining a large bone volume (Fig 15-14). The anterior iliac crest is preferred, because it allows thick tricortical harvesting. In addition, the bone width at the crest of the ilium is often greater in the anterior region compared with the midcrestal anatomy. A 6 cm transverse incision is made alongside the iliac crest. An incision directly over the prominence of the iliac crest is avoided because of the likely irritation from clothing or seat belts. The incision must remain at least 2 cm lateral to the anterior superior iliac spine in order to avoid damage to the lateral femoral cutaneous nerve, which can, rarely, course through this area. Electrocautery is used for hemostasis as well as to dissect through the subcutaneous tissues to the facia overlying the ilium. The inner table of the iliac crest is exposed by a subperiosteal dissection. A corticocancellous block bone is harvested from the ilium using an oscillating saw. The site is closed after placing a suction drain below the facia exiting away from the wound.

Grafting of block bone in the sinus

The block bone is shaped to fit in the maxillary sinus. The bone block is placed in the sinus with the cortical layer on the bottom in order to allow the cortical layer of the bone graft to be perforated with implants during implant placement (Fig 15-15).

Implant placement

After grafting the block bone, the sinus implants are placed using a mini-incision procedure (Fig 15-16). A crestal mini-incision, approximately 5 mm horizontally to the alveolar crest, is made at the center of the implant site and local undermining of the gingiva is then performed. The amount of undermining at the implant site does not exceed 5 mm and falls within the range of a large-diameter implant. When implants are inserted, the block bone is stabilized using bone-holding forceps or a small clamp. The implants are inserted through the alveolar bone into the graft. Once the implant is placed inside the block bone, it is secured together with the bone. The remaining space on the floor of the maxillary sinus between the iliac bone block and alveolar crest is filled with additional cancellous bone harvested from the ilium.

After placement of the implant fixture, a cover screw is connected and the incised gingiva is sutured to submerge the fixture. Finally, the incision for accessing the maxillary sinus is sutured (Figs 15-17 and 15-18).

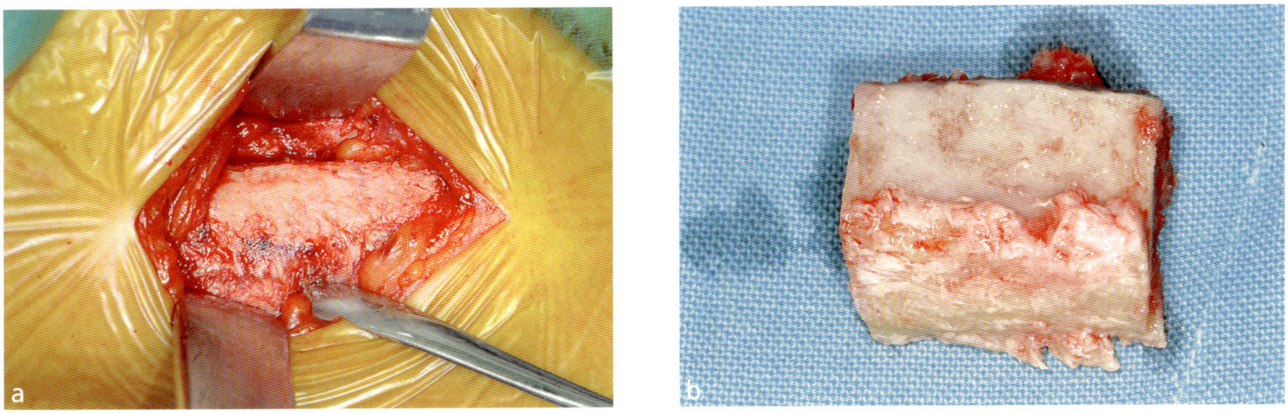

Fig 15-14 (a and b) Corticocancellous block bone is harvested from the ilium.

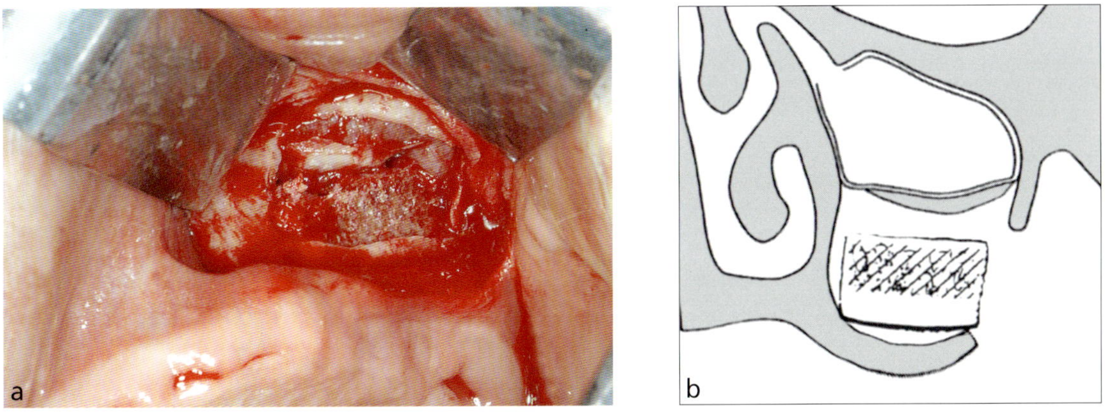

Fig 15-15 (a and b) Corticocancellous block bone is placed in the sinus with the cortical layer on the bottom to allow the cortical layer of the graft to be perforated with implants during implant placement.

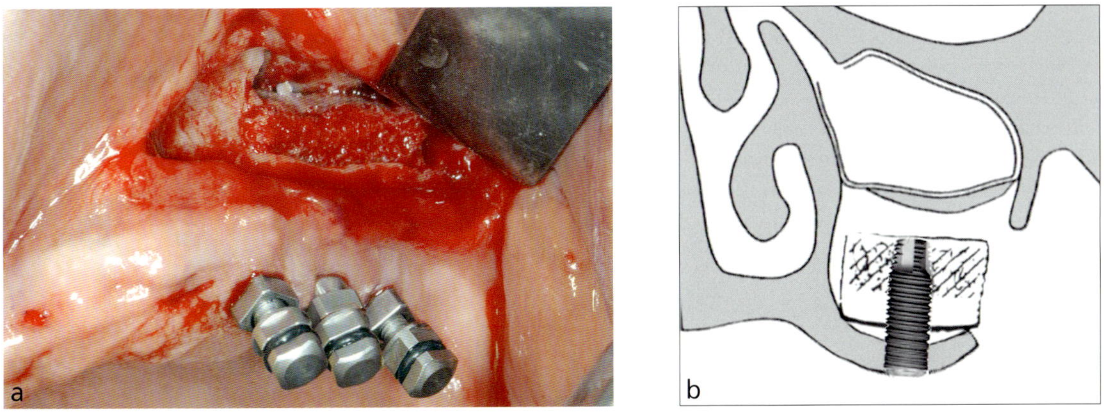

Fig 15-16 (a and b) A crestal mini-incision approximately 5 mm horizontally to the alveolar crest is made at the center of the implant site and local undermining of the gingiva is then performed. The implants are inserted through the alveolar bone into the graft.

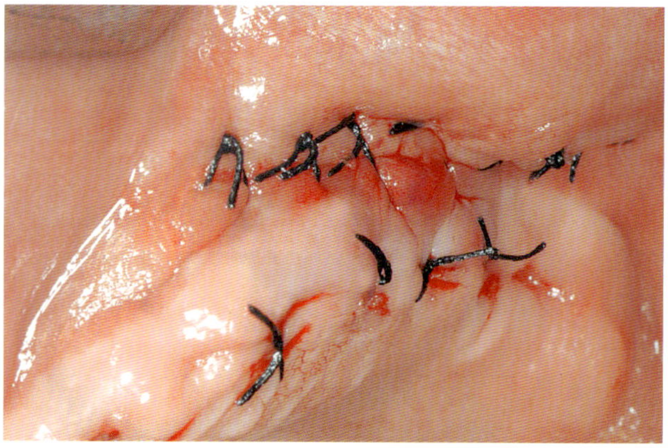

Fig 15-17 After fixture placement, the incised gingiva is sutured in order to submerge the fixture, and the incision for accessing the maxillary sinus is sutured.

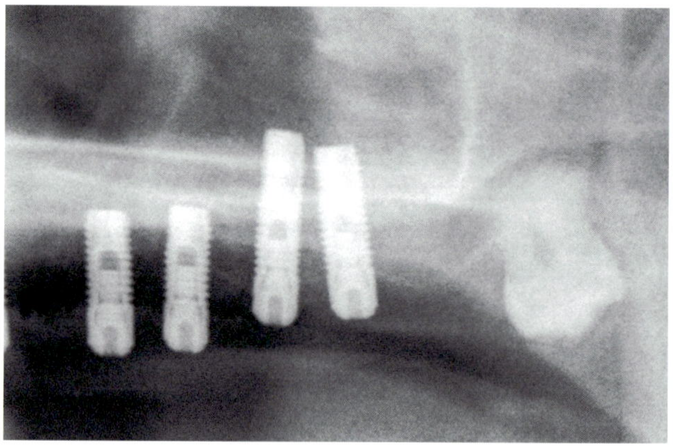

Fig 15-18 Radiograph of the patient in Fig 15-16 taken immediately after surgery.

Procedure to uncover the implants

During the initial healing period, the implant is covered with soft tissue to create a favorable environment for the peri-implant bone as well as to reduce the risk of loading or movement. The implant is uncovered 4–6 months after bone grafting, with immediate implant placement.

Success rate

The authors achieved a 100% success rate based on a 1–3-year follow-up of 28 implants placed in 10 patients (Figs 15-19 and 15-20). This success rate is significantly higher than those reported in the literature (75–97%). Radiographic evidence of ossification in the elevated sinus area was observed in all 10 patients. Computerized tomography showed that all sides of the implants, including the apical implant surface, were covered completely with bone. The extent of crestal peri-implant bone loss was small, with a mean of 0.2 mm. The approach of performing block iliac bone grafting simultaneously with mini-incision implant placement in the maxillary sinus results in improved healing because there were no complications from implant placement. Mini-incision implant surgery is a predictable procedure with a high success rate. For that reason, the authors prefer to perform mini-incision implant surgery simultaneously with block iliac bone grafting in the maxillary sinus when there is less than 5 mm of vertical bone between the residual crest of bone and the floor of the maxillary sinus.

Advantages and disadvantages

Advantages

Inserting the implants using mini-incision procedures at the same time as block iliac bone grafting has the following advantages:

- There is no need for additional surgery, as there is with delayed implant placement.
- The block bone graft can be fixed when the implants are inserted simultaneously inside the bone. The cortical bone in the sinus floor and that of the block bone secure the implants firmly, providing stability for the implants and bone fragment. As a result, it is not necessary to fix the bone fragment with additional screws.
- Immediate stability of the implant can be achieved, if more than 1 mm of pre-existing bone is present below the sinus in the vertical direction.
- The approach allows the placement of implants in the ideal position and at the required angulation.
- The block bone can be shaped to fit in the anatomical structures of the maxillary sinus.
- Compared with a particulate bone graft, a block bone graft increases the graft bone–implant contact area, enhances osseointegration of implants, and increases the height of newly formed bone in the maxillary sinus because of the low rate of bone resorption.
- The blood supply entering the graft bone from the alveolar ridge can be affected when soft tissue flaps are reflected from the alveolar ridge for implant placement. However, the blood supply can be preserved when implants are placed using mini-incision procedures.
- Mini-incision implant surgery reduces the risk of infection.
- Crestal bone loss that occurs during the early period after surgery may have a fatal impact on the stability of implants and block bones in the maxillary sinus when there is very little vertical bone remaining between the residual crest of the bone and the floor of the maxillary sinus. Mini-incision implant surgery reduces the bone loss of the crest.
- The use of the submerged mini-incision procedure protects the implants and block bone during initial healing after implant placement and improves the environment for bone growth.

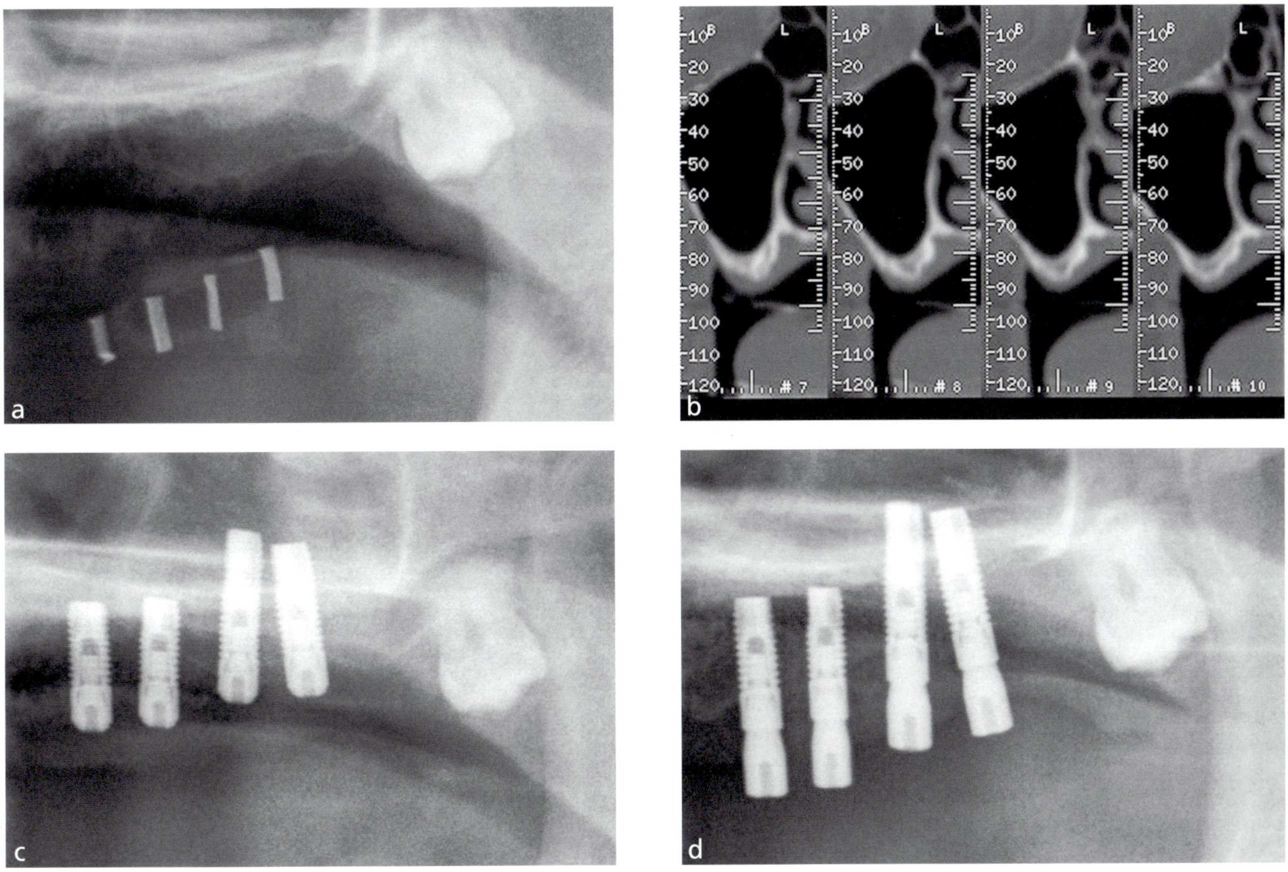

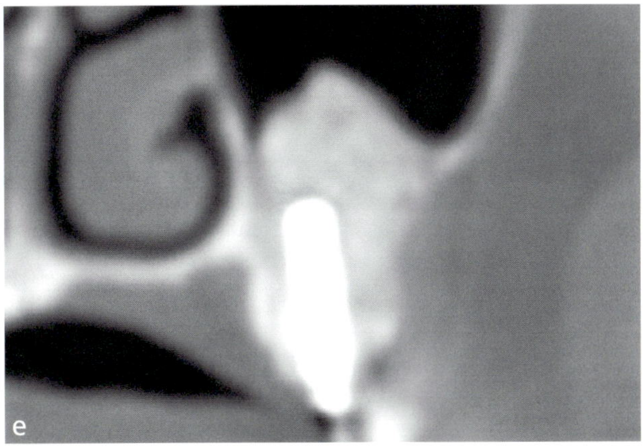

Fig 15-19 A patient with block autogenous iliac bone graft and simultaneous mini-incision implant placement. (a) Radiograph of the patient with the missing maxillary molars. (b) CT image of the patient. (c) Radiograph taken immediately after surgery. Two implants (4 mm in diameter and 13 mm and 15 mm in length) were placed simultaneously with block autogenous iliac bone grafting in the left maxillary sinus. (d and e) Radiographs after 6 months. Evidence of ossification in the augmented sinus area is present; all sides of the implants are covered with bone, even at the apical implant surface.

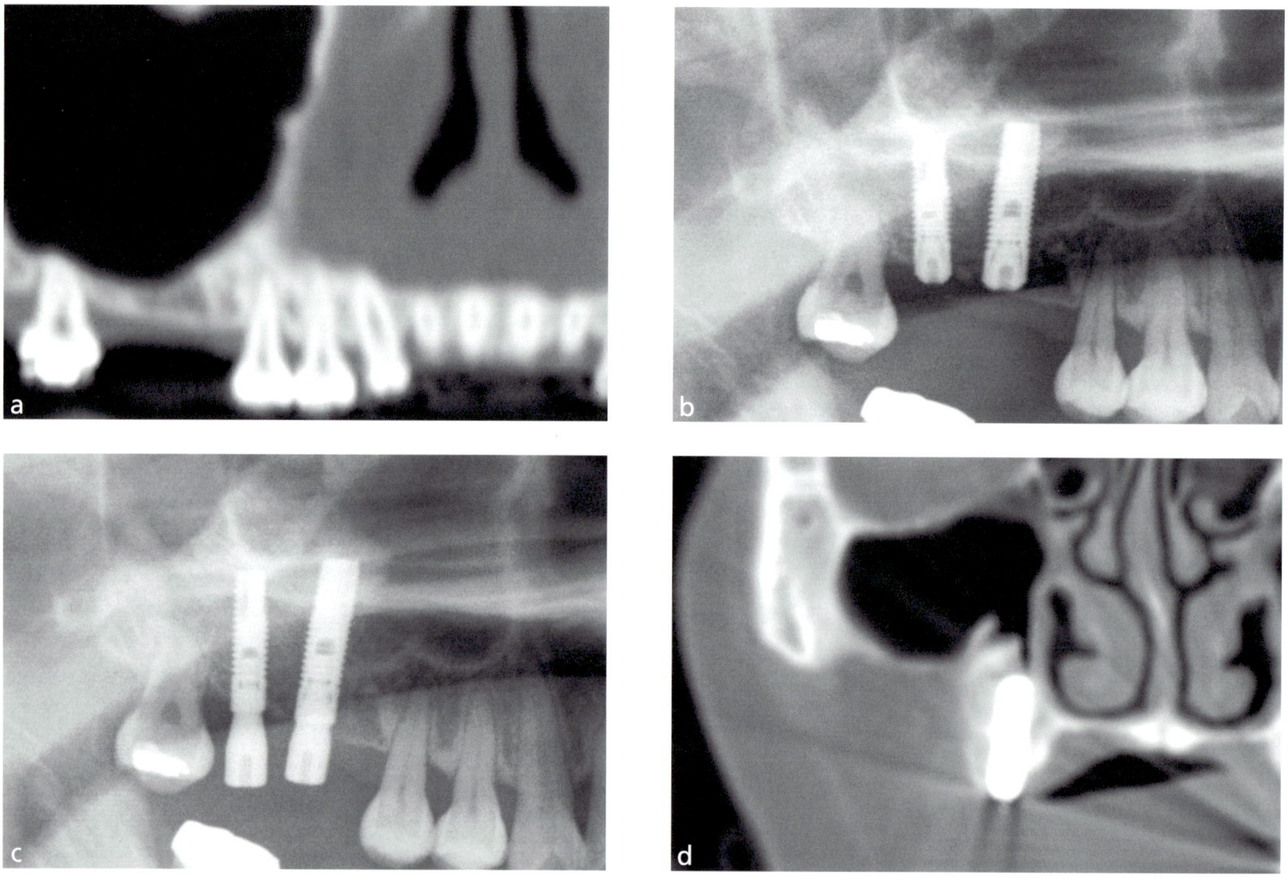

Fig 15-20 A second patient with block autogenous iliac bone grafting and simultaneous mini-incision implant placement. (a) Radiograph of the patient with the missing right maxillary molars. (b) Radiograph taken immediately after surgery. Two implants (3.4 mm and 4.0 mm in diameter and 13 mm and 15 mm in length, respectively) were placed simultaneously with block autogenous iliac bone grafting in the right maxillary sinus. (c and d) Radiographs after 6 months. The implants are totally covered with bone.

Disadvantages

The insertion of implants using mini-incision procedures at the same time as the block iliac bone graft has the following disadvantages:

- Additional surgery is required to harvest the autogenous bone grafts.
- General anesthesia and hospitalization are necessary.
- Morbidity and postoperative pain can occur at the donor site.

Bio-Oss® particle sinus graft with immediate or delayed flapless implant placement

The use of autogenous block iliac bone grafts as fillers for maxillary sinus augmentation procedures is considered the gold standard, with the main disadvantage being its limited availability. Bone grafts have the disadvantage of patient morbidity associated with graft procurement. Many investigators have proposed a range of allografts and xenografts as substitutes for autogenous bone grafts. Among the suggested grafts, anorganic bovine bone (Bio-Oss®) is one of the most popular biomaterials used for sinus elevation surgery.[12,15–17] Bio-Oss® particle grafting and immediate or delayed implant placement in sinus augmentation procedures have been reported to yield favorable results.[15,18–23]

Indications

Bio-Oss® particle sinus graft with immediate or delayed flapless implant placement is indicated when 5–10 mm of vertical bone is present (Fig 15-21). Flapless implant placement is performed at the same time as the sinus graft procedure when the remaining bone can ensure the primary stability of implants. However, when it does not allow primary implant

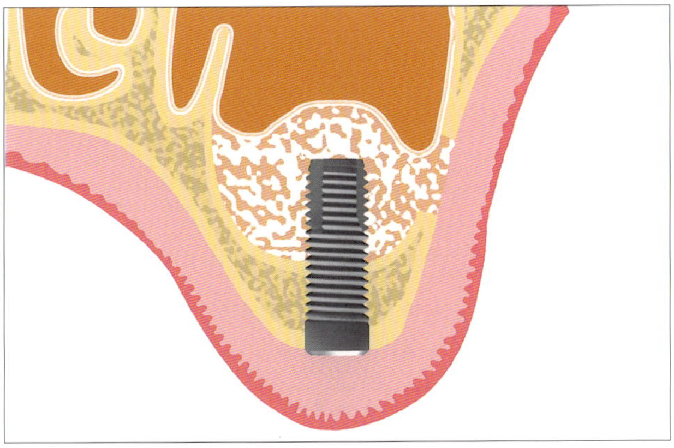

Fig 15-21 Illustration of Bio-Oss® particle sinus graft with flapless implant placement.

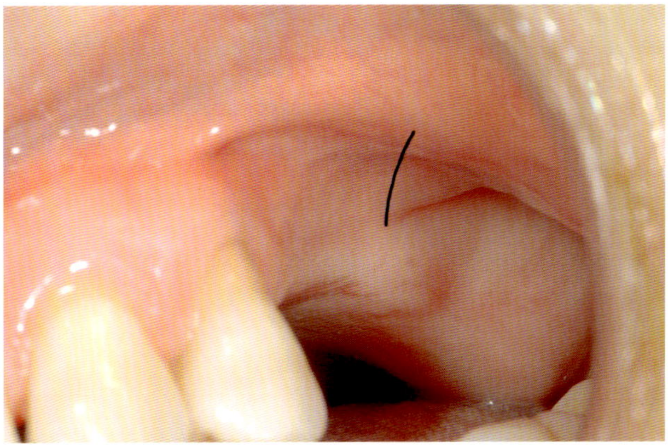

Fig 15-22 To access the maxillary sinus, a vertical incision approximately 8 mm in length is made on the buccal cortical plate approximately 8 mm away from the alveolar crest. See also Figs 15-23 to 15-28.

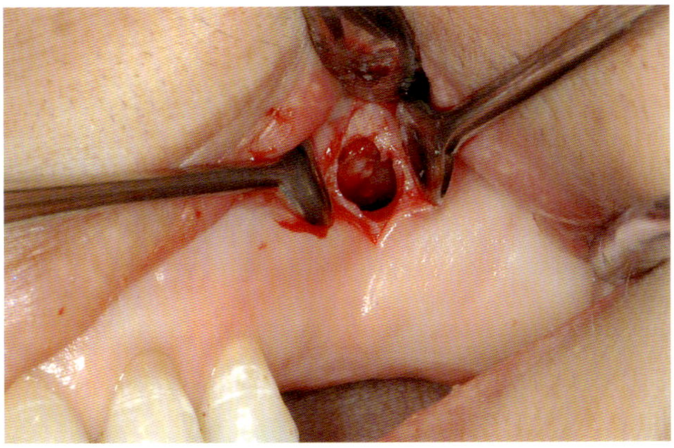

Fig 15-23 A 5 mm diameter hole made in the lateral sinus wall with a round bur.

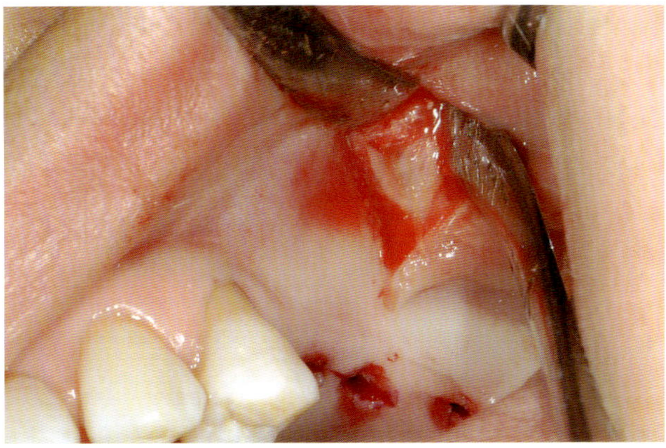

Fig 15-24 The Bio-Oss® particle and autologous fibrin composite grafting is performed through the small bone window.

stability, flapless implant placement should be delayed until 6–10 months after the Bio-Oss® particle sinus graft. A minimum residual bone height of 5 mm is considered necessary for the primary stability of implant fixtures.[24,25]

The incisions

Two separate incisions are made, one for accessing the maxillary sinus and the other for placing the mini-incision implants. To access the maxillary sinus, a vertical incision, approximately 8 mm in length, is made on the buccal cortical plate approximately 8 mm away from the alveolar crest (Fig 15-22). A mucoperiosteal flap is reflected to expose the lateral wall of the maxillary sinus.

Access window

A 5 mm diameter hole is made in the lateral sinus wall with a round bur, taking care to avoid perforating the sinus membrane (Fig 15-23). The hole is made approximately 2–5 mm above the level of the antral floor. The sinus membrane is then elevated above the maxillary sinus floor using small curettes.

Grafting of Bio-Oss® particle in the sinus

Bio-Oss® particle grafting in the sinus is performed through the small bone window (Fig 15-24). In order to prevent the Bio-Oss® particles from dispersing, the particles are mixed with autologous fibrin gel made from autologous blood. The addition of autologous fibrin gel can enhance the hardening of the granular grafting material and help to reduce the amount of Bio-Oss® particles used. The mixture is introduced to the peri-implant defects through the bone window. An amalgam carrier is used to place the mixture on the sinus floor effectively. The mixture is then molded into the desired contour.

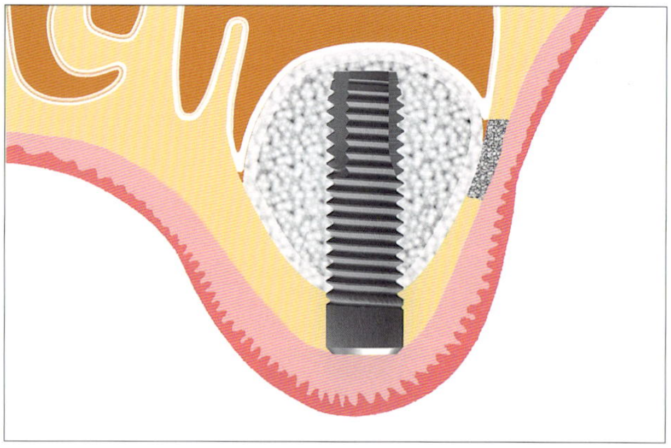

Fig 15-25 After implant placement, a piece of Bio-Oss® block is impacted into the window to close it. This prevents the graft material from escaping from the sinus cavity and the fibrous tissue from invading into the graft.

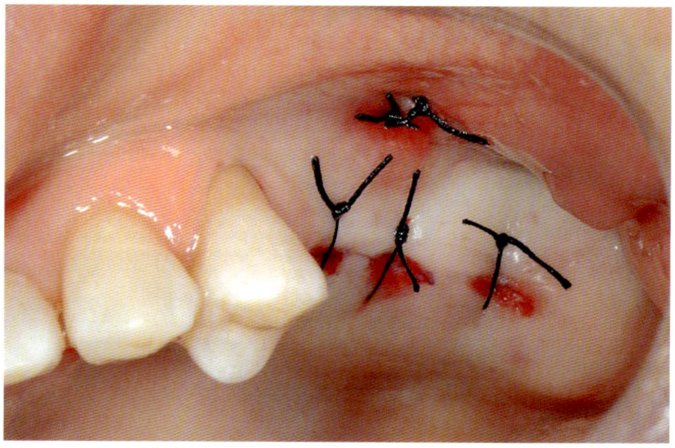

Fig 15-26 Intraoral view of the patient immediately after surgery.

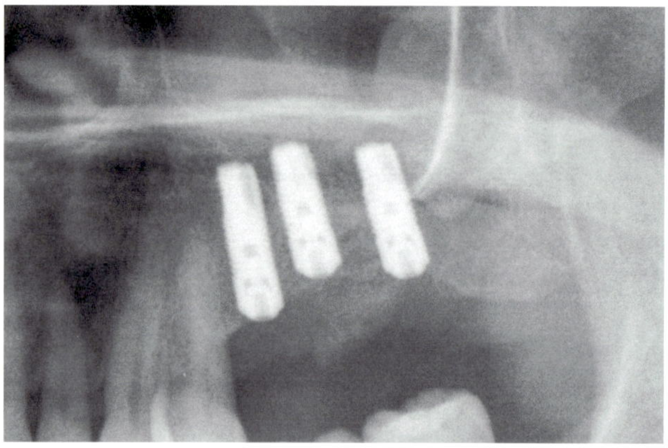

Fig 15-27 Radiograph taken immediately after surgery.

Implant placement

After elevation of the sinus membrane, the implants are placed using a mini-incision procedure. A crestal mini-incision, approximately 5 mm horizontally with the alveolar crest, is made at the center of the implant site and local undermining of the gingiva is then performed. Implant osteotomy is prepared to the appropriate final diameter, beyond the antral floor. In patients with poor bone quality, a 2 mm pilot drill is used to prepare the initial osteotomy, and an osteotome is then used to prepare the osteotomy.

After preparation of the implant site, the implant is threaded into the osteotomy and extends into the graft site. After implant placement, a piece of Bio-Oss® block is impacted into the window to close it (Fig 15-25). This prevents both the graft material from escaping from the sinus cavity and the fibrous tissue from invading into the graft. The mucoperiosteal flap is replaced and sutured.

After a cover screw is connected, the crestal mini-incision is sutured to submerge the fixture (Fig 15-26). A post-insertion radiograph is made to identify the implant depth (Fig 15-27).

Attainable osseointegration rate from Bio-Oss® particle grafting

Postoperative CT images show dome-like bone formation around the implants (Fig 15-28). However, there is some concern that the attainable osseointegration rate from Bio-Oss® particle grafting might be insufficient to achieve the strength required for the clinical function of the implants.

Based on the authors' animal experiment results, when implants were inserted at the same time as the Bio-Oss® particle grafting in the maxillary sinus, all implants had been integrated clinically and radiographically within the augmented bone at 6 months (Fig 15-29 and 15-30). Histological examination revealed that the grafted particles were surrounded by a layer of newly formed bone (Fig 15-31). However, the new bone was generally not in direct contact with the implants (Fig 15-32). As a result, the average osseointegration rate was only 29.3%. This suggests a deficiency in the strength needed for the clinical function because a minimum osseointegration rate of 40% is considered necessary for the clinical functioning of implant fixtures.[26–29]

After 6 months or longer, the area grafted with Bio-Oss® particles had more new bone around the particles and adjacent implants, showing enhanced osseointegration with time (Fig 15-33).[12,30] Accordingly, it is optimal to have a 1-year healing period to improve the ability to withstand the loading forces transmitted by the implants. However, the healing period is still too long before the required osseointegration and bone density is obtained for clinical functioning of implants. In the future, technical development will be necessary to produce rapid bone formation around the implants and to enhance osseointegration in the early stage.

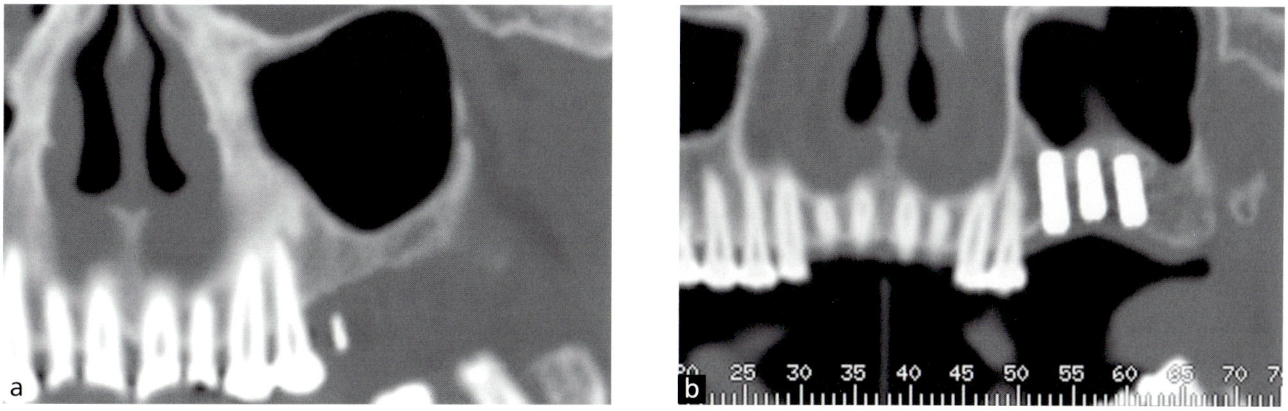

Fig 15-28 CT images of the patient in Fig 15-27: (a) before surgery and (b) after surgery. There is dome-like bone formation around the implants.

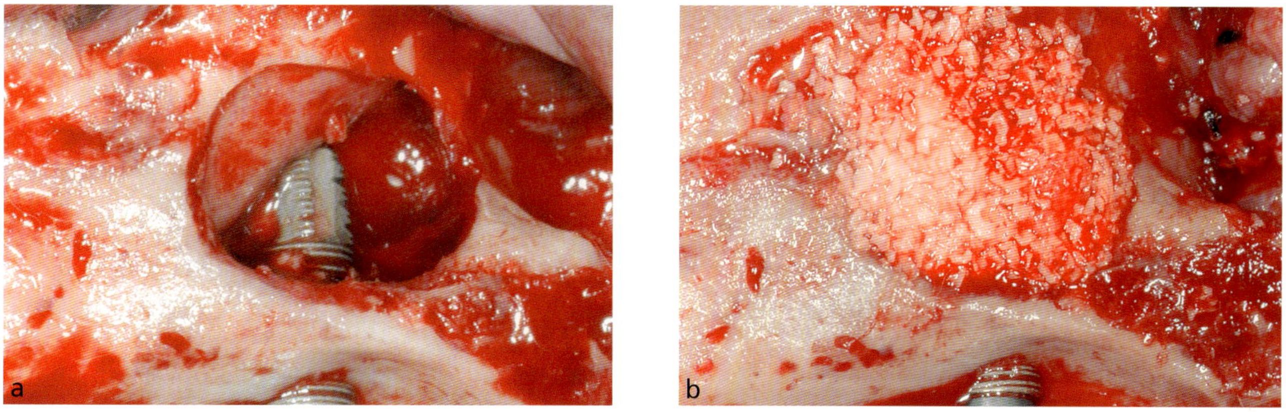

Fig 15-29 In an animal experiment using six adult mongrel dogs, implants were inserted into the sinus cavity on one side of the maxillary sinus after sinus membrane elevation. On the opposite side, implants were inserted at the same time as the Bio-Oss® particle and autologous fibrin composite grafting in the maxillary sinus. See also Figs 15-30 to 15-33.

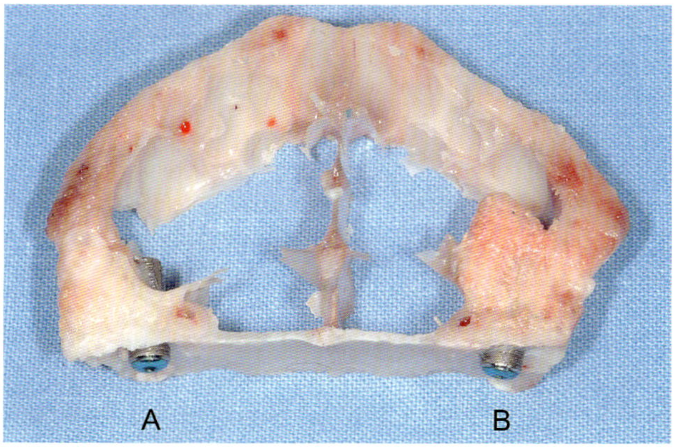

Fig 15-30 A specimen 6 months after surgery, showing the sinus membrane elevation side (A) and the Bio-Oss® particle and autologous fibrin composite grafting side (B).

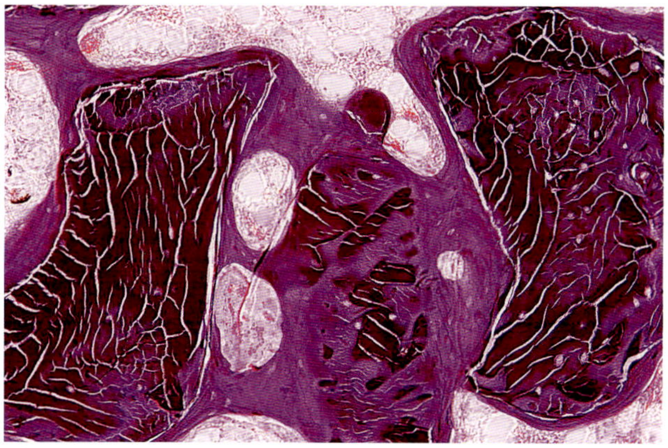

Fig 15-31 The grafted Bio-Oss® particles were surrounded by a layer of newly formed bone. Note that particles were in the process of resorption and newly formed bone was in contact with the trabeculae of residual particles.

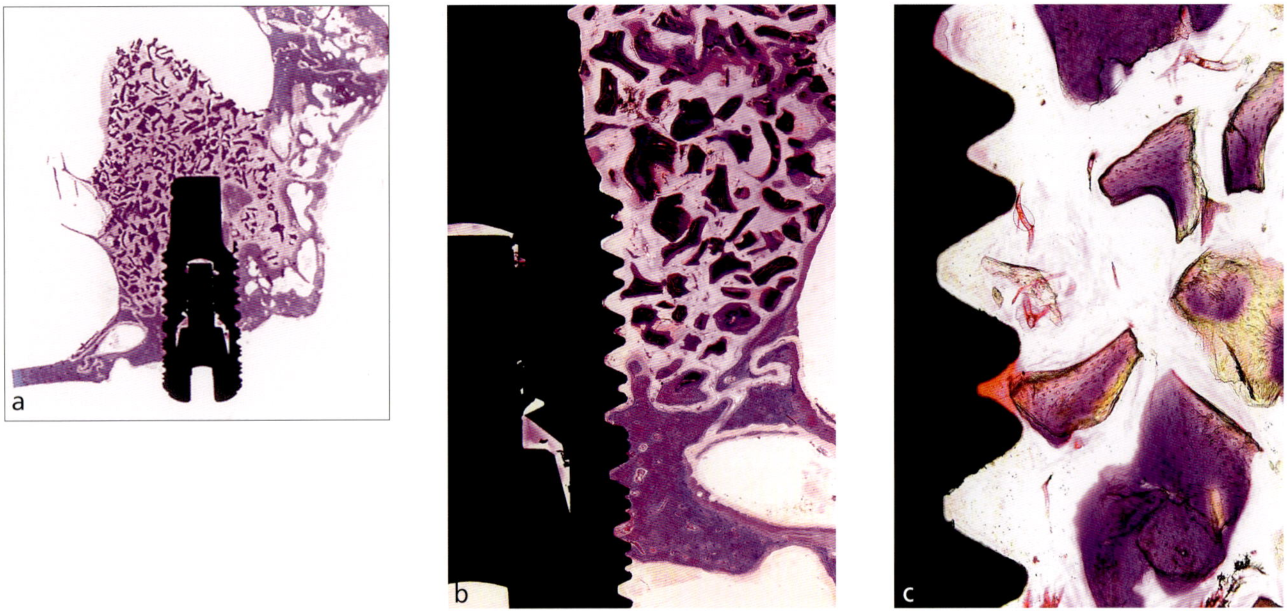

Fig 15-32 New bone surrounding the grafted Bio-Oss® particles is generally not in direct contact with the implants.

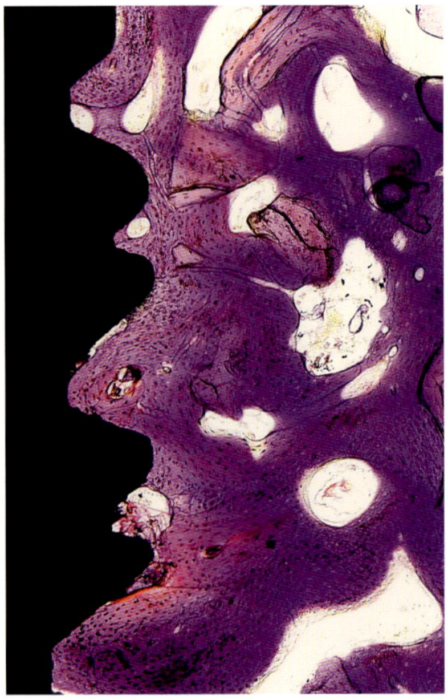

Fig 15-33 After 1 year, the area grafted with Bio-Oss® particles has more new bone around the particles and adjacent implants, showing enhanced osseointegration with time.

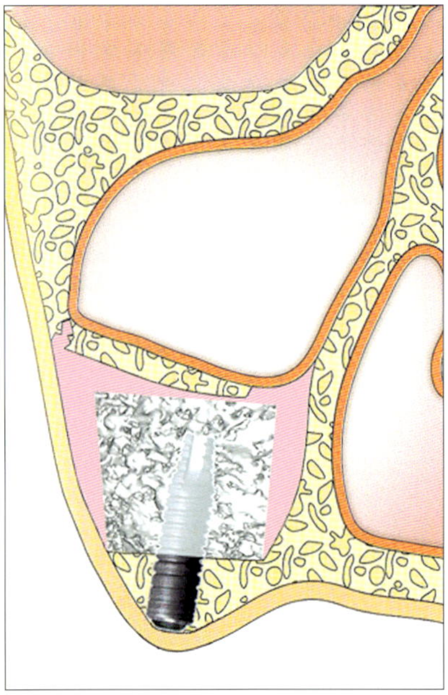

Fig 15-34 Illustration of a Bio-Oss® block sinus graft with immediate flapless implant placement.

Bio-Oss® block sinus graft with immediate or delayed flapless implant placement

Bio-Oss® block sinus graft with immediate or delayed flapless implant placement is indicated when there is less than 5 mm remaining between the residual crest of bone and the floor of the maxillary sinus. One of the main advantages of a block-type graft material is that the block bone can be shaped to fit in the anatomical structure of the recipient site. However, a Bio-Oss® block bone is so brittle and weak that it cannot provide sufficient mechanical force for primary stability of implants. Accordingly, immediate flapless implant placement in the maxillary sinus may be performed at the same time as the sinus graft procedure when the remaining bone can ensure primary stability (Fig 15-34). When it does not allow primary implant stability, flapless implant placement should be delayed by 6–10 months after the Bio-Oss® block sinus graft. The Bio-Oss® block sinus graft procedure is similar to the block autogenous iliac bone graft procedure, except for the graft material.

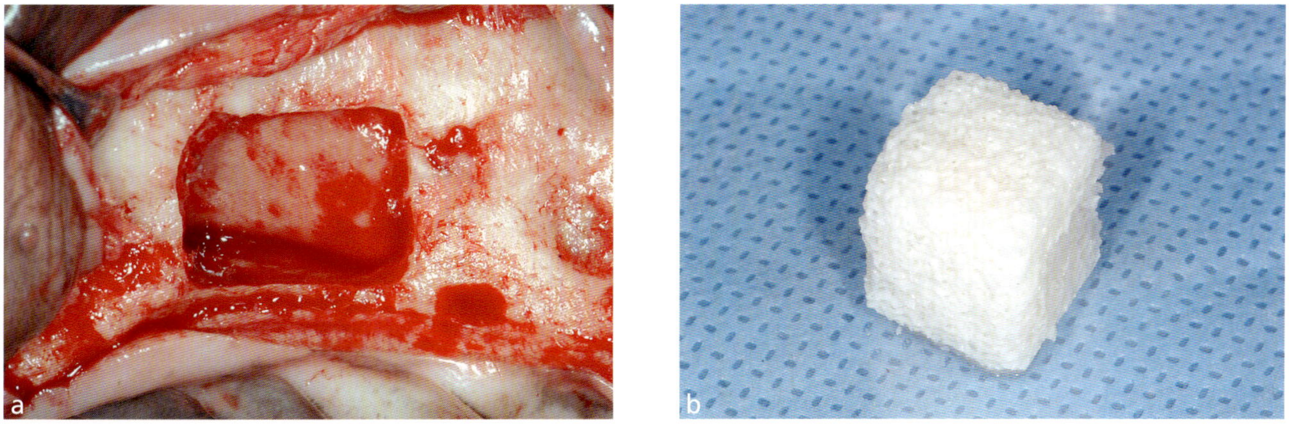

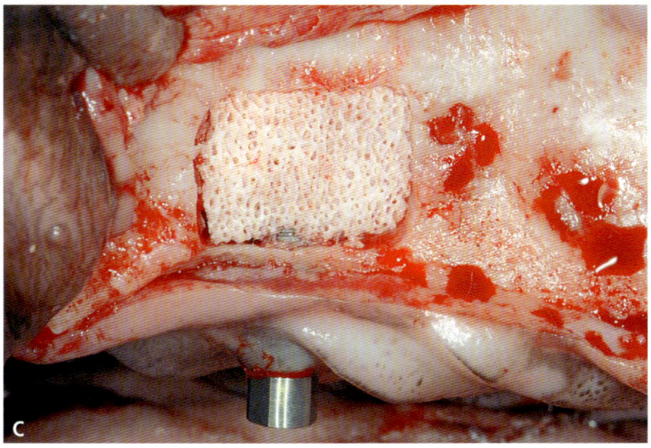

Fig 15-35 An animal experiment was performed to evaluate Bio-Oss® block grafting in the maxillary sinus. (a) Maxillary sinus membrane elevation. (b) A Bio-Oss® block. (c) Implant inserted simultaneously.

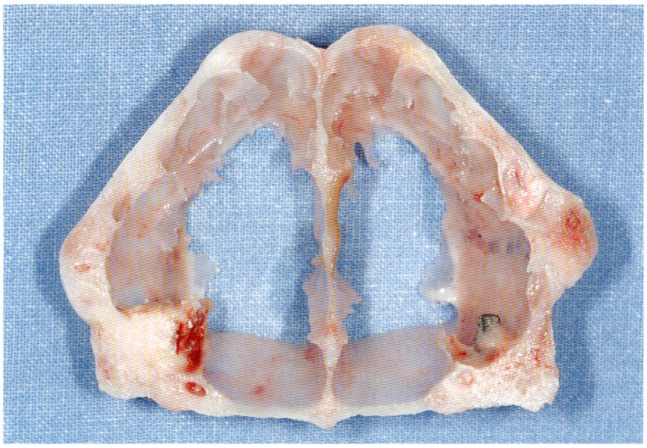

Fig 15-36 Specimen of the maxillary sinus of a dog 6 months after surgery. Newly formed bone was more abundant with the sinus augmentation procedure with Bio-Oss® block grafting (left) than without (right).

Based on the authors' animal experiment, when implants were inserted in the maxillary sinus at the same time as Bio-Oss® block grafting (Fig 15-35), all implants were integrated clinically and radiographically within the augmented bone at 6 months (Fig 15-36). Histological examination showed that new bone formation was evident surrounding the mineral particles in direct connection with the newly formed bone and implants (Fig 15-37). The average osseointegration rate was 45.7% at 6 months. The area grafted with a Bio-Oss® block had more new bone around the implants than those with the Bio-Oss® particles.

Healing of the sinus graft

Many local variables affect sinus graft maturation, including the healing time, graft materials, and graft volume, all of which are related to the speed and amount of new bone formation. The healing time is perhaps the most significant value. The amount of new bone increases continuously with time. More new bone is formed as more time has elapsed from a sinus graft.[31] The materials in the sinus graft affect the rate of bone formation. Bone formation is fastest and most complete with autogenous bone, occuring within the first 4–6 months, followed by Bio-Oss® (6–10 months) and alloplasts (24 months).

Our animal experiments have shown that more new bone formed in 6 months with Bio-Oss® particles, when bone marrow stem cells and bone morphogenic protein 2 (BMP-2) were mixed with the Bio-Oss® particles (Fig 15-38). The time required to form new bone is closely related to the graft volume. A large volume of the graft material placed into the sinus requires a longer time before implant insertion. Therefore, the sinus graft volume should be appropriate. Autogenous fibrin gel helps to prevent the Bio-Oss® particles from dispersing, meaning that less sinus graft material is needed to obtain sufficient vertical height of the material to place the implant (Fig 15-39). In terms of structural rigidity, Bio-Oss® block grafts have benefits over Bio-Oss® particulate grafts, because they are strong and can be shaped to match the host site.

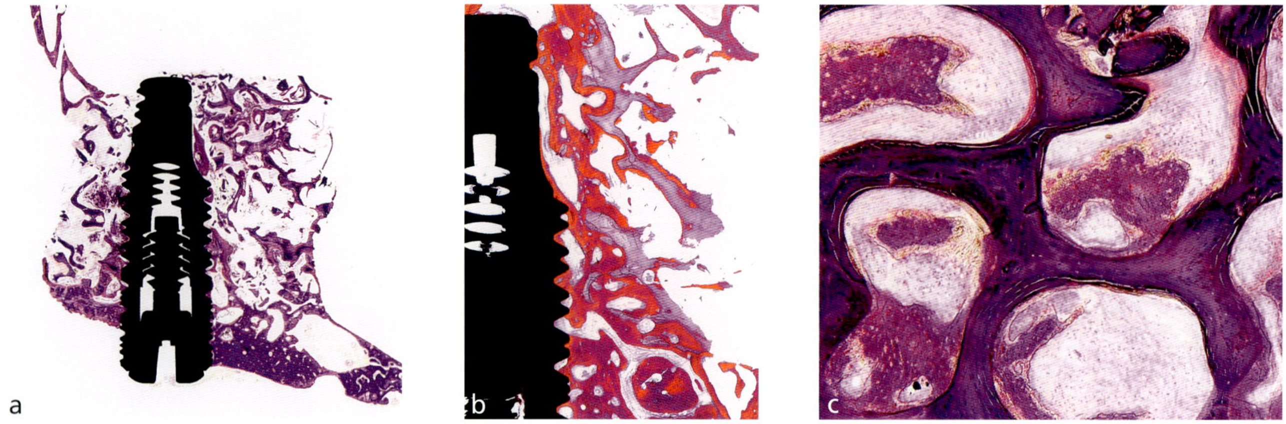

Fig 15-37 (a–c) Histological examination shows new bone formation surrounding the mineral particles in direct connection with the newly formed bone and implants. The average osseointegration rate was 44.5% at 6 months.

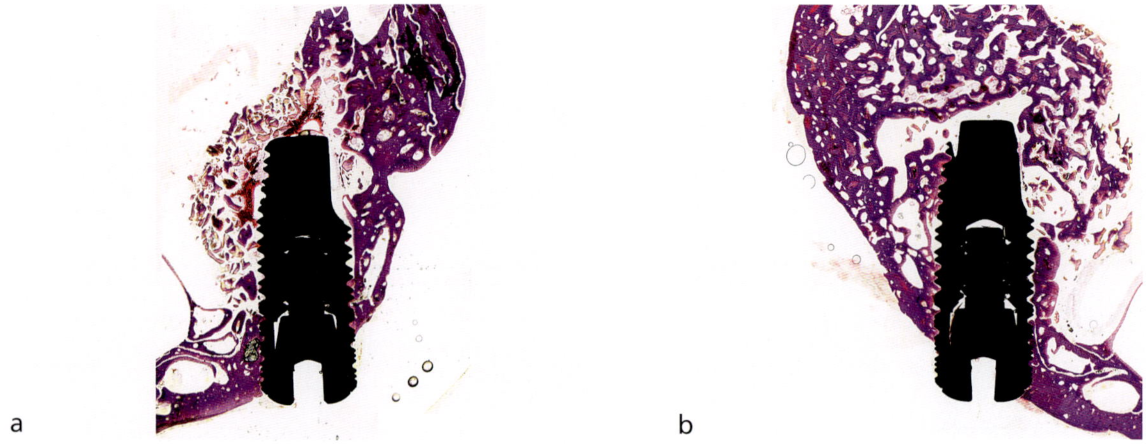

Fig 15-38 (a) Grafting with Bio-Oss® particle and autologous fibrin composite. (b) Grafting with Bio-Oss® particle, bone marrow stem cells, bone morphogenic protein 2 (BMP-2), and autologous fibrin composite. More new bone formed in 6 months when bone marrow stem cells and BMP-2 were added.

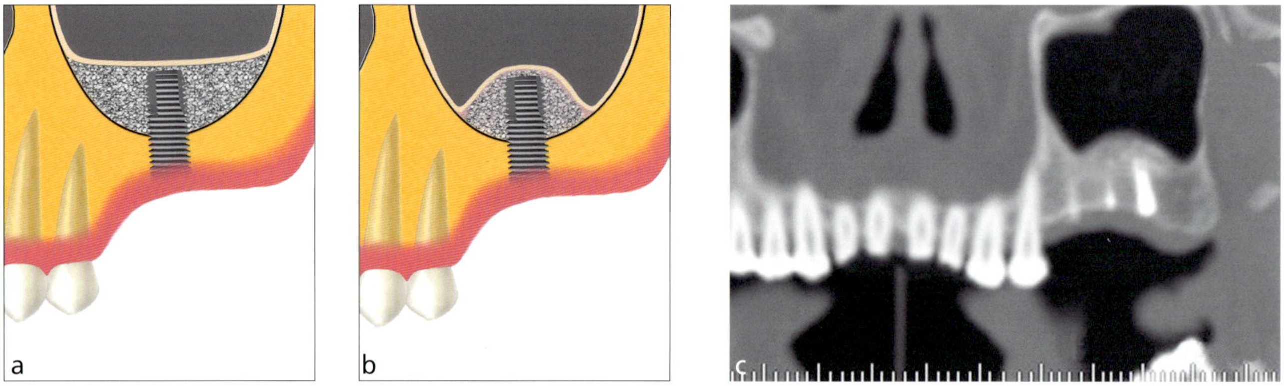

Fig 15-39 Illustrations of a sinus graft using (a) Bio-Oss® particles alone and (b) mixed with autologous fibrin gel. (c) Postoperative CT images showing dome-like bone formation around the implants. The addition of autologous fibrin gel can help to reduce the amount of Bio-Oss® particles required.

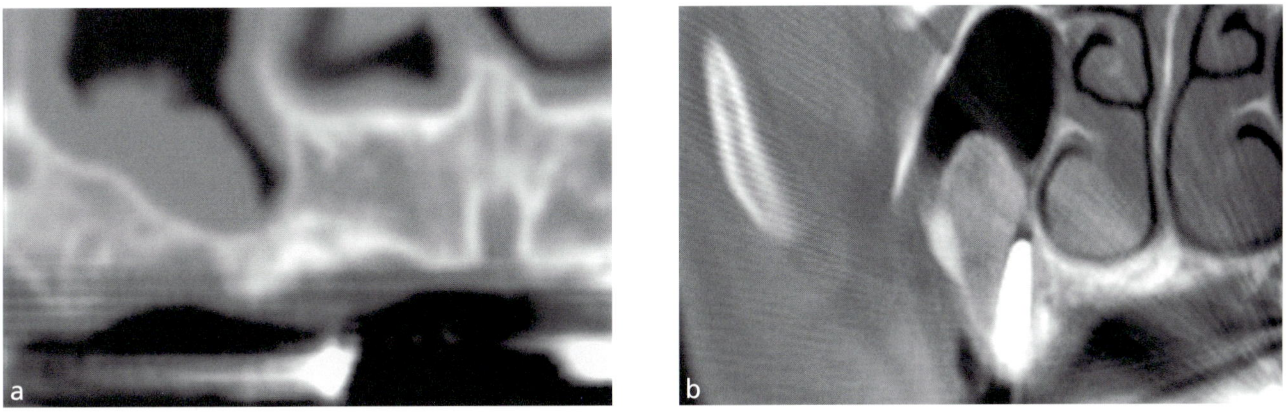

Fig 15-40 (a) A patient with preexisting antral mucosa thickening in the right maxillary sinus with clinical signs of sinusitis at the time of surgery. (b) The symptoms vanished and CT showed complete recovery of the antral mucosa 6 months after the maxillary sinus floor elevation surgery with block autogenous iliac bone grafting.

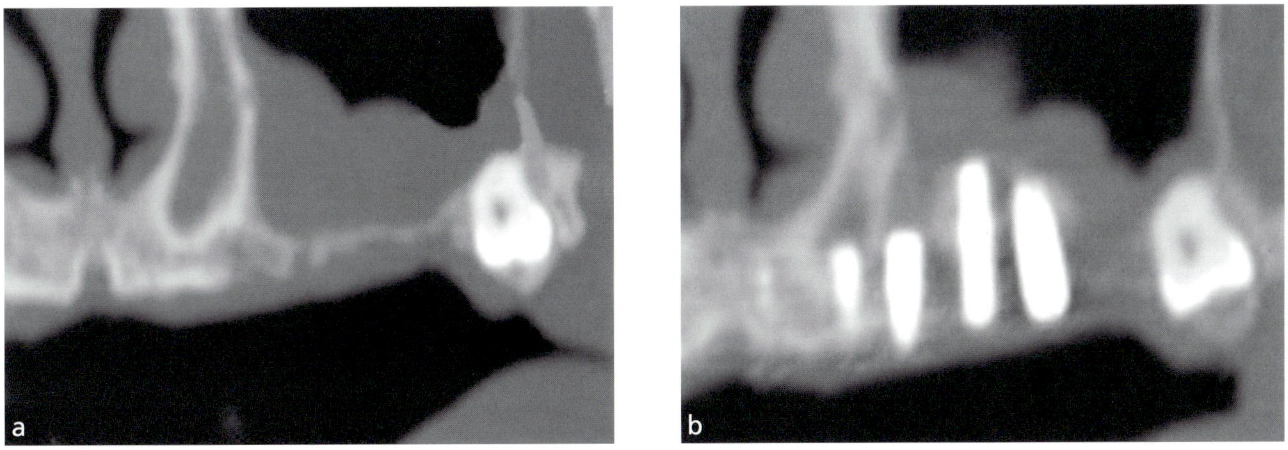

Fig 15-41 (a) A patient with preexisting antral mucosa thickening at the time of surgery. (b) Postoperative CT showed the presence of a thickened sinus mucosa 6 months after maxillary sinus floor elevation surgery with block autogenous iliac bone grafting.

Effects of sinus augmentation procedures on maxillary sinus function

The maxillary sinus is lined with mucosa, which consists of the pseudostratified, ciliated columnar epithelium containing ciliated columnar epithelial cells, nonciliated columnar cells, basal cells, goblet cells, and seromucinous cells. The thickness of the normal sinus mucosa varies, but it is generally between 0.3 and 0.8 mm. Pseudostratified columnar cells have 50–200 cilia per cell, which beat toward the ostium to help to clear the mucus produced from the mucous and serous glands. Most of the glands are located close to the ostium.

Maxillary sinus floor elevation surgery with bone grafts has little influence on functioning of the maxillary sinus. The maxillary sinus mucosa seems to adapt adequately to the changes induced by the elevation procedure. In some patients with preexisting antral mucosa thickening and clinical signs of sinusitis at the time of surgery, the symptoms vanished and CT showed complete recovery of the antral mucosa after 6 months (Figs 15-40), whereas other patients showed the presence of preexisting antral mucosa thickening after surgery (Fig 15-41). This might result from the lifted sinus floor propelling mucoid fluid to drain through the ostium of the maxillary sinus. However, when a thickened sinus mucosa is present, care should be taken not to block the maxillary ostium with the lifted sinus mucosa and not to overfill the sinus, which would result in a blockage of the ostium. The normal physiology of the maxillary sinus is strongly dependent on the proper functioning of both the maxillary ostium and the mucosal lining.[32,33] Accordingly, placement of graft material into the maxillary sinus cavity should not affect the maxillary ostium, which is located in the upper portion of the medial wall.

Complications

Membrane perforations

The most common complication during sinus graft surgery is tearing or creation of an opening in the sinus membrane (Fig 15-42). A sinus perforation can increase the risk of short-term complications. There is greater risk of bacterial penetration into the graft material through a torn membrane. Mucus can invade the graft and affect the amount of bone formation. Graft material may leak through the tear into the sinus proper, which can become a source of infection or may migrate and close off the ostium to the nose and create a favorable environment for infection. In terms of preventing graft material from leaking through the torn membrane into the sinus proper, block bone grafts offer significant benefits over particulate bone grafts, in that the former provide structural rigidity and are not dispersed.

A number of approaches have been assessed to seal a perforation (Figs 15-43 to 15-45) and prevent contamina-

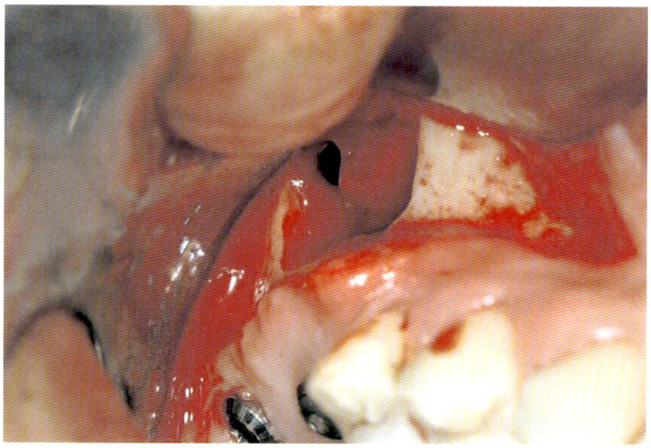

Fig 15-42 A sinus membrane perforation.

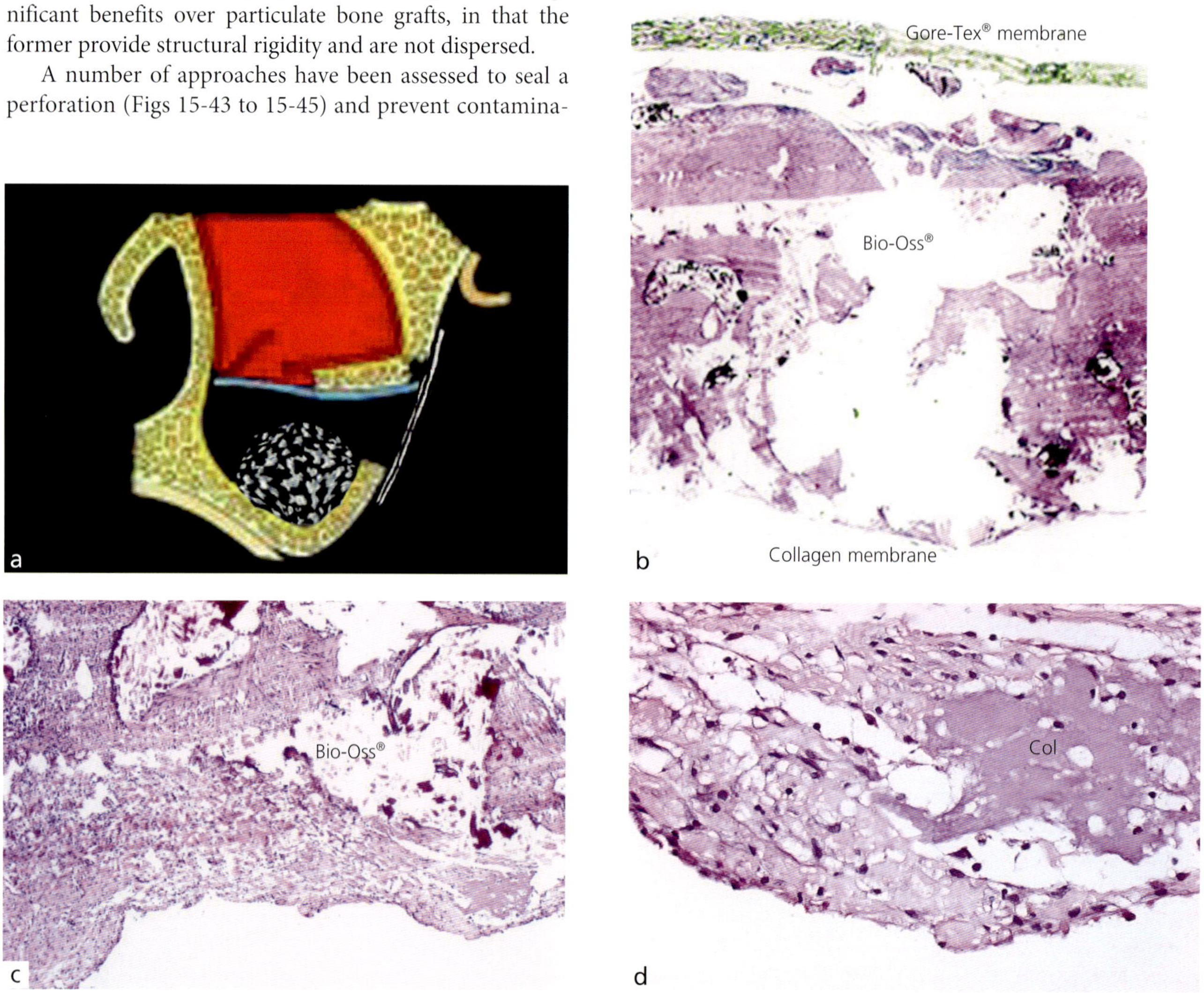

Fig 15-43 An animal experiment using dogs was performed to assess the efficacy of collagen membranes in the management of large perforations of the maxillary sinus membrane occurring during sinus lifts. After elevation of the sinus membrane in the maxillary sinuses, a laceration (about 2 cm in length) was made in the membrane. (a and b) The laceration was covered with a bioabsorbable collagen membrane (CollaTape®) to form a new ceiling. Subsequently, space obtained by elevating the sinus membrane on both sides was filled with Bio-Oss® particles. The fenestration of the buccal plate was subsequently closed by placing an expanded polytetrafluoroethylene (e-PTFE) membrane (Gore-Tex®). Wounded areas were biopsied 2 weeks after surgery for a microscopic evaluation of the antral membrane. (c and d) Histological examination showed extensive fibrosis and complete loss of the surface epithelium in the previous perforation site. Col – collagen membrane

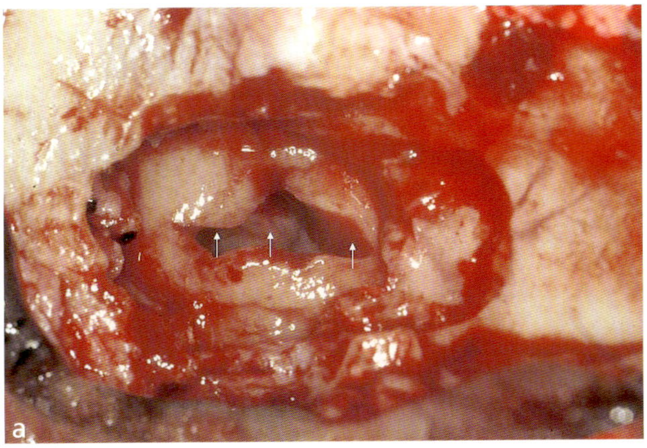

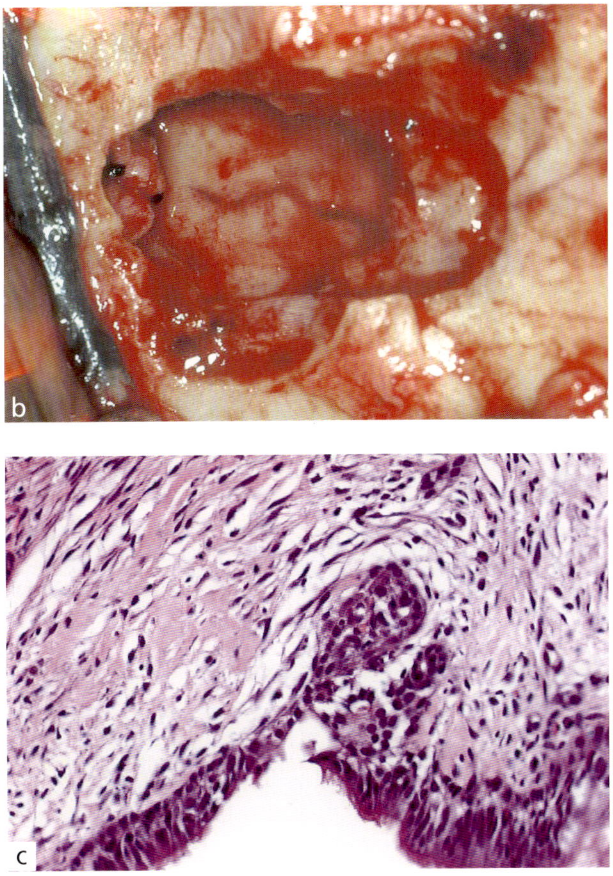

Fig 15-44 An animal experiment using dogs was performed to assess the efficacy of autologous fibrin glue in the management of large perforations of the maxillary sinus membrane occurring during sinus lifts. (a and b) After elevation of the sinus membrane in maxillary sinuses, a laceration (about 2.0 cm in length) was made in the membrane. The laceration was repaired with autologous fibrin glue. Wounded areas were biopsied 2 weeks after the operation for microscopic evaluation of the antral membrane. (c) Histological examination showed newly formed continuous epithelium across the previous perforation site on the autologous fibrin glue side.

tion of the grafts from the mucus and extrusion of graft material into the sinus proper. Suggested techniques, include the use of collagen membranes (e.g., CollaTape®)[34–37] and fibrin glues.[38] Collagen membranes are used to cover perforations and autologous fibrin glue is used to close sinus membrane perforations hermetically with adhesive strength.

Based on the authors' animal experiment results,[39] although the collagen membranes act as a barrier between the sinus antrum and the site of graft placement, extensive fibrous connective tissue formation can occur in wounds treated in this manner (Fig 15-43). However, normal sinus membrane healing was observed with epithelialization when sinus membrane perforations were closed with fibrin glue (Fig 15-44). As a result, the authors prefer the use of fibrin glue to repair sinus membrane perforations. Commercially available fibrin glues include Tisseel (Immuno, Vienna, Austria; Fig 15-45) and Beriplast® (Behring, Germany). Autogenous fibrin glue can be made from the patient's own blood by a process that requires approximately 60–90 minutes for preparation using an ethanol precipitation technique (Figs 15-46 and 15-47). Therefore, if the use of autologous fibrin glue is necessary, it will be helpful to withdraw a small sample of autologous blood (20 mL) before surgery.

Incision line opening

Incision line opening occurs commonly when implants are inserted at the same time as bone grafting in the maxillary sinus after making an incision into the gingiva of the alveolar crest. Incision line opening can increase the risk of infection, which can lead to failure of the implants and bone grafts. For this reason, Misch[40] recommends performing delayed implant placement after sinus graft healing.

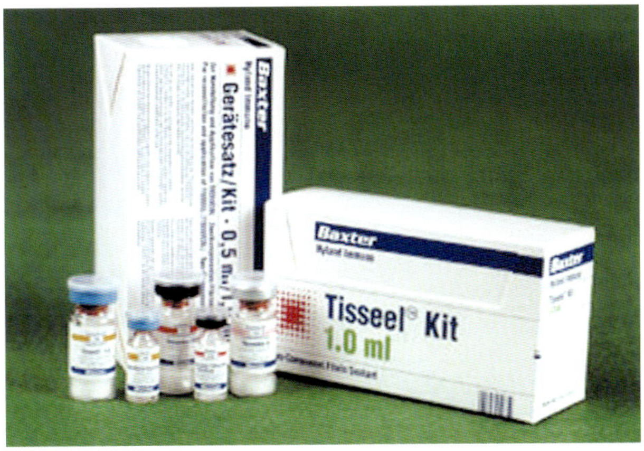

Fig 15-45 Tisseel kit.

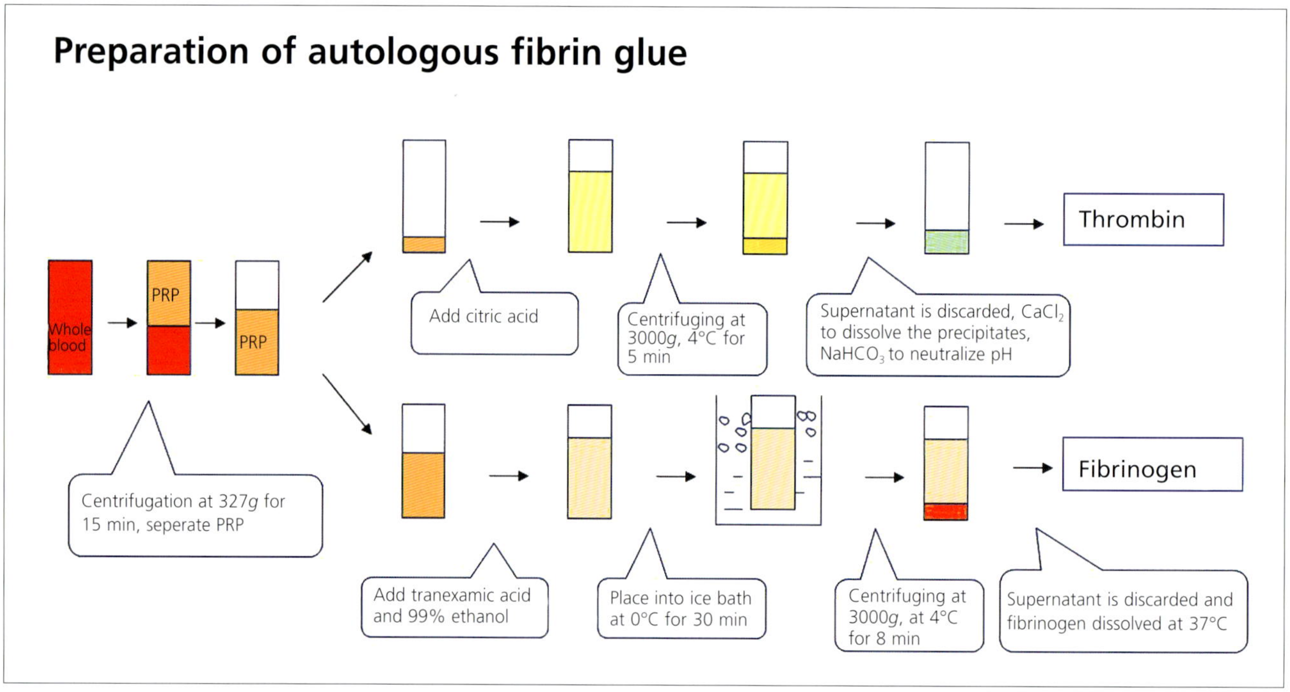

Fig 15-46 In order to prepare autologous fibrin glue, 20 mL of autologous blood is withdrawn before surgery. The blood is centrifuged for 15 minutes at 327*g* to separate the platelet-rich plasma (PRP). To 7.5 mL of PRP, 240 µL of transexamic acid and 900 µL of ethanol are added, and incubated in an ice-water bath for 20–30 minutes. The precipitated fibrinogen is separated by centrifugation at 3000*g* for 8 minutes at 0–4°C. After discarding the supernatant, the fibrinogen precipitate is re-dissolved at 37°C and then diluted to 50% with 0.9% NaCl. A thrombin solution is then prepared using the remaining PRP. To 2.5 mL of the remaining PRP, 22.5 mL of citric acid is added, and the mixture is then centrifuged at 3000*g* for 5 minutes at 4°C. After discarding the supernatant, the precipitate is dissolved in 150 µL of $CaCl_2$ (0.1 M) and the pH adjusted to 7 by adding 100 µL of $NaHCO_3$. After clot formation, the thrombin solution is collected and diluted to 10% with 0.05 M $CaCl_2$. The fibrin glue is formed by mixing the fibrinogen and thrombin solutions at a 3:1 (vol/vol) ratio.

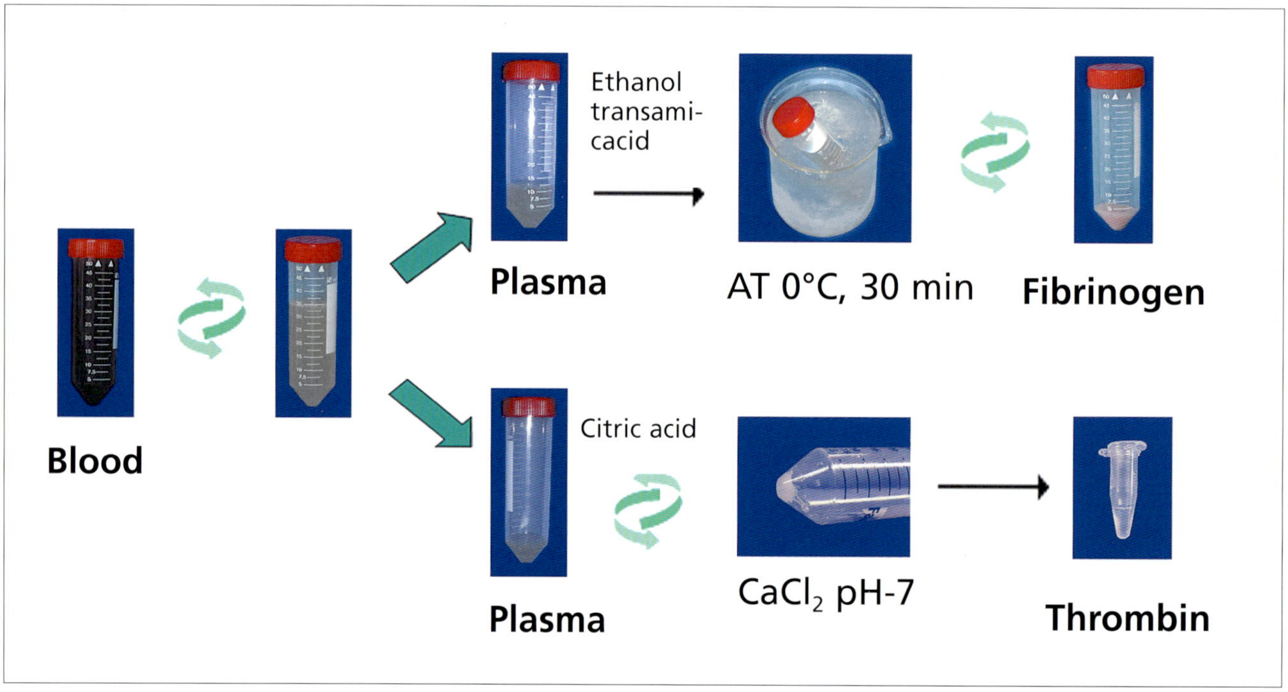

Fig 15-47 The method for preparing the autologous fibrin glue.

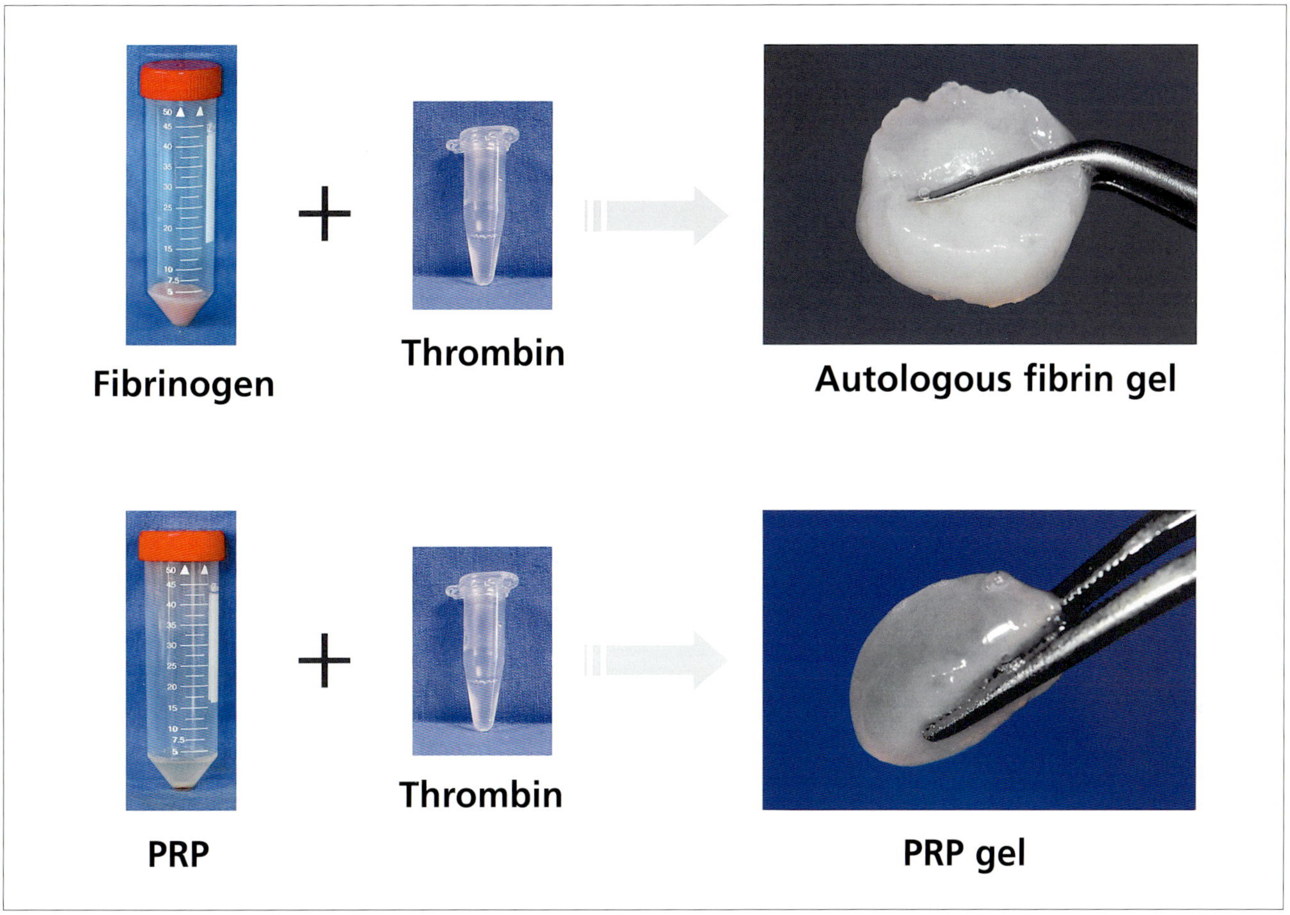

Fig 15-48 Comparison of the gels formed from the platelet-rich plasma (PRP) or the autologous fibrin glue. The autologous fibrin gel is harder and more bulky than the PRP gel.

In the authors' experience, postoperative complications can be avoided when two separate incisions are made – one to access the maxillary sinus and the other to place the mini-incision implants. This is because mini-incision implant placement in the maxillary sinus results in good healing around the implants and does not cause complications related to incision line opening.

Summary

When there is insufficient vertical bone available below the maxillary sinus floor, a treatment approach to the posterior maxilla is based on the available bone height between the floor of the antrum and the crest of the residual ridge in the region of the ideal implant locations. The following treatment options are available for the edentulous posterior maxilla. A particle bone sinus graft with immediate or delayed flapless implant placement is indicated when there is 5–10 mm of vertical bone present. A block bone sinus graft with immediate or delayed flapless implant placement is indicated when <5 mm remains between the residual crest of the bone and the floor of the maxillary sinus. To access the maxillary sinus, an incision for the approach is made on the buccal cortical plate of the maxillary sinus away from the alveolar crest. These procedures ensure favorable conditions for flapless implant surgery in the alveolar crest.

References

1. Tatum OH. Maxillary and sinus implant reconstruction. Dent Clin North Am 1986;30:207–229.
2. Misch CE. Contemporary Implant Dentistry, ed 2. St Louis, MO: Mosby, 1999:397–407.
3. Tatum OH, Lebowitz MS, Tatum CA, Borgner RA. Sinus augmentation: rationale, development, long-term results. NY St Dent J 1993;43–48.
4. Boyne PJ, James RA. Grafting of the maxillary sinus floor with autogenous marrow and bone. J Oral Surg 1980;38:613–616.
5. Wood RM, Moore DL. Grafting of the maxillary sinus with intraorally harvested autogenous bone prior to implant placement. Int J Oral Maxillofac Implants 1988;3:209–214.

6. Jensen J, Simonsen EK, Sindet-Petersen S. Reconstruction of the severely resorbed maxilla with bone grafting and osseointegrated implants: a preliminary report. J Oral Maxillofac Surg 1990;48:27–32.
7. Raghoebar GM, Brouwer TJ, Reintsema H. Augmentation of the maxillary sinus floor with autogenous bone for the placement of endosseous implants: a preliminary report. J Oral Maxillofac Surg 1993;51:1198–1203.
8. Pejrone G, Lorenzett M, Mottati M, Valente G, Schierano GM. Sinus floor augmentation with autogenous iliac bone block grafts: a histological and histomorphometrical report on the two-step surgical technique. Int J Oral Maxillofac Surg 2002;31:383–388.
9. Peleg M, Garg AK, Misch CM, Mazor Z. Maxillary sinus and ridge augmentations using a surface-derived autogenous bone graft. J Oral Maxillofac Surg 2004;62:1535–1544.
10. Keller EE, Triplett WW. Iliac bone grafting: review of 160 consecutive cases. J Oral Maxillofac Surg 1987;45:11–14.
11. Block MS, Kent JN. Sinus augmentation for dental implants: the use of autogenous bone. J Oral Maxillofac Surg 1997;55:1281–1286.
12. Haas R, Donath K, Födinger M, Watzek G. Bone hydroxyapatite for maxillary sinus grafting: comparative histomorphometric findings in sheep. Clin Oral Implants Res 1998;9:107–116.
13. Lew D, Marino AA, Startzell JM, Keller JC. A comparative study of osseointegration of titanium implants in corticocancellous block and corticocancellous chip grafts in canine ilium. J Oral Maxillofac Surg 1994;52:952–958.
14. Friberg B, Jemt T, Lekholm U. Early failures in 4641 consecutively placed Brånemark dental implants: a study from stage 1 surgery to the connection of completed prostheses. Int J Oral Maxillofac Implants 1991;6:142–146.
15. Wentzel AC, Stich H, Caffesse RG. Bone apposition onto oral implants in the sinus area filled with different grafting materials. Clin Oral Implants Res 1995;6:155–163.
16. Hürzeler MB, Kirsch A, Ackermann KL, Quinones CR. Reconstruction of the severely resorbed maxilla with dental implants in the augmented maxillary sinus: a 5-year clinical investigation. Int J Oral Maxillofac Implants 1996;11:466–475.
17. Valentini P, Abensur D, Densari D, Graziani JN, Hämmerle CHF. Histological evaluation of Bio-Oss® in a 2-stage sinus floor elevation and implantation. Clin Oral Implants Res 1998;9:59–64.
18. Boyne PJ. Host response to intraosseous implants placed in HA grafted mandibles. Mater Res Soc Symp Proc 1989;110:219–227.
19. Klinge B, Alberius P, Isaksson S, Jönsson J. Osseous response to implanted natural bone mineral and synthetic hydroxyapatite ceramic in the repair of experimental skull bone defects. J Oral Maxillofac Surg 1992;50:241–249.
20. Boyne PJ. Analysis of performance of root-form endosseous implants placed in the maxillary sinus. J Long Term Effects Med Implants 1993;3:143–159.
21. Jensen SS, Aaboe M, Pinholt EM, Hjorting-Hansen E, Melsen F, Ruyter IE. Tissue reaction and material characteristics of four bone substitutes. Int J Oral Maxillofac Implants 1996;11:55–66.
22. Smiler DG, Johnson PW, Lozada JL et al. Sinus lift grafts and endosseous implants: treatment of the atrophic posterior maxilla. Dent Clin North Am 1992;36:151–186.
23. Nentwig GH, Nick I, Helmke U. Implantation in a narrow alveolar process: diagnosis, classification and operative procedure. Zeit Zahn Implants 1993;9:156–159.
24. Jensen OT, Greer RO. Immediate placement of osseointegrating implants into the maxillary sinus augmented with mineralized cancellous allograft and Gore-Tex: second-stage surgical and histological findings. In: Laney WR, Tolman DE (eds). Tissue Integration in Oral, Orthopedic, and Maxillofacial Reconstruction. Chicago, IL: Quintessence, 1992:321–333.
25. Jensen OT. Guided bone graft augmentation. In: Buser D, Dahlin C, Schenk RK (eds). Guided Bone Regeneration in Implant Dentistry. Chicago, IL: Quintessence, 1992:235–264.
26. Keller JC, Young FA, Natiella JR. Quantitative bone remodelling resulting from the use of porous dental implants. J Biomed Mater Res 1987;21:305
27. Buser D, Schenk RK, Skinemann S. Influence of surface characteristics on bone integration of titanium implants: a histomorphometric study in miniature pigs. J Biomed Mater Res 1991;25:889
28. Gottlander M, Albrektsson. Histomorphometric studies of hydroxyapatite-coated and uncoated CP titanium threaded implants in bone. Int J Oral Maxillofac Implants 1991;6:399.
29. Weinlander M, Kenney EB, Lekovic V. Histomorphometry of bone opposition around three types of endosseous dental implants. Int J Oral Maxillofac Implants 1992;7:491.
30. Haas R, Haidvogl D, Donath K, Watzek G. Freeze-dried homogenous and heterogenous bone for sinus augmentation in sheep. I: Histological findings. Clin Oral Implants Res 2002;13:396–404.
31. Froum SJ, Wallace SS, Elian N. Comparison of mineralized cancellous bone allograft (Puros) and anorganic bovine bone matrix (Bio-Oss®) for sinus augmentation: histomorphometry at 26 to 32 weeks after grafting. Int J Periodont Restor Dent 2006;26:543–551.
32. Amble FR, Lindberg SO, McCaffrey TV. Mucociliary function and endothelins 1, 2, and 3. Otolarygol Head Neck Surg 1993;109:634–645.
33. William E, Bolger M, Clifford A. Paranasal sinus bony anatomic variations and mucosal abnormalities: CT analysis for endoscopic sinus surgery. Laryngoscope 1991;101:56–61.
34. Proussaefs P, Lozada J, Kim J. Effects of sealing the perforated sinus membrane with a resorbable collagen membrane: a pilot study in humans. J Oral Implantol 2003;29:235–241.
35. Aimetti M, Romagnoli R, Ricci G, Massei G. Maxillary sinus elevation: the effect of macrolacerations and microlacerations of the sinus membrane as determined by endoscopy. Int J Periodont Restor Dent 2001;21:581–589.
36. Pikos MA. Maxillary sinus membrane repair: report of a technique for large perforations. Implant Dent 1999;8:29–34.
37. Proussaefs P, Lozada J, Kim J, Rohrer MD. Repair of the perforated sinus membrane with a resorbable collagen membrane: a human study. Int J Oral Maxillofac Implants 2004;19:413–420.
38. Sullivan SM, Bulard RA, Meaders R, Patterson MK. The use of fibrin adhesive in sinus lift procedures. Oral Surg Oral Med Oral Pathol Oral Radiol Endod 1997;84:616–619.
39. Choi BH, Zhu SJ, Jung JH, Lee SH, Huh JY. The use of autologous fibrin glue for closing sinus membrane perforations during sinus lifts. Oral Surg Oral Med Oral Pathol Oral Radiol Endod 2006; 101:150–154.
40. Misch CE. Contemporary Implant Dentistry, ed 3. St Louis, MO: Mosby, 2008:68–91.

CHAPTER

16

Clinical Cases

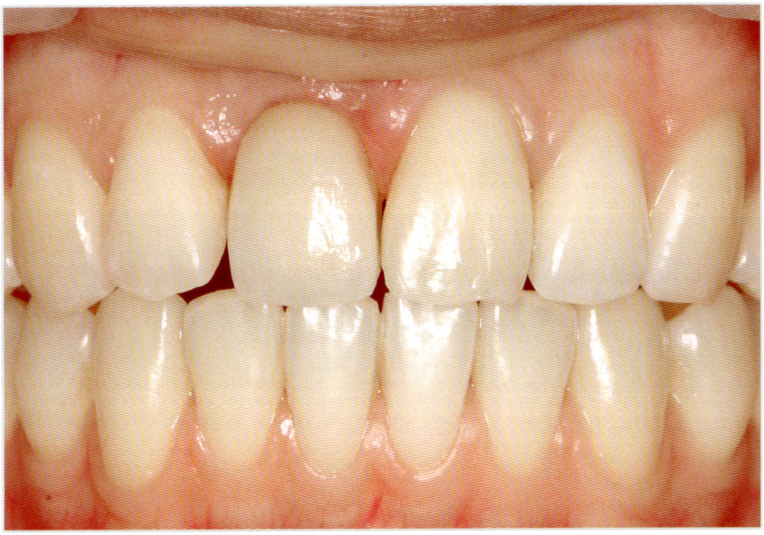

Key point

There are few cases in which flapless implant surgery cannot be applied.

Case 1: Flapless implant placement in the mandibular molar region

Case 2: Flapless implant placement in the maxillary anterior and maxillary first molar regions

Case 3: Flapless implant placement in the maxillary central incisor region after orthodontic treatment

Case 4: Socket lift and simultaneous flapless implant placement in the maxillary molar region

Case 5: Flapless implant placement and application of progressive loading in the mandibular molar region

Case 6: Flapless implant placement for a heavy smoker and drinker

Case 7: Flapless implant placement for a 76-year-old patient

Case 1: Flapless implant placement in the mandibular molar region

A 29-year-old woman visited the clinic for implant placement in the mandibular left second molar region. The height between the maxillary antagonist tooth and the alveolar crest mucosa in the missing tooth area was approximately 5 mm. The height from the inferior alveolar nerve to the alveolar crest was approximately 15 mm. The width of the alveolar crest bone was sufficient for implant placement. Implant placement was accomplished with the flapless method using a soft tissue punch technique. An Osstem Implant fixture (GSII; Seoul, Korea; 4.5 mm × 13 mm) was inserted after preparing the implant site, and then a permucosal healing abutment with a height of 4.5 mm × 3 mm was connected to the fixture. During the implant placement, bone quality was at the D2 level, and the insertion torque was 38 Ncm. The perio-test value of the implant measured immediately after implant placement was –1. After the surgery, the patient performed meticulous plaque control. Three months after placement, implant prosthetic treatment was initiated. The superstructure was fabricated with a gold crown as in the adjacent tooth. The probing depth around the implant that was evaluated 6 months after the prosthetic treatment was 1.0–2.0 mm. No gingival bleeding was observed during the probing. The peri-implant mucosa remained healthy following prosthetic treatment.

Comment

During flapless implant surgery, the mucosa was punched with a soft tissue punch with a diameter 1.5 mm narrower than the implant fixture. As a result, the peri-implant mucosa was in tight contact with the implant after placement, and the peri-implant mucosa healed quickly. Immediately after implant placement, the patient could clean the implant surfaces using meticulous plaque control methods. The meticulous plaque control played a crucial role in promoting health in the peri-implant mucosa and preventing peri-implant bone loss. The good condition of the peri-implant mucosa might be the basis for successful implant treatment.

Table 16-1-1 Peri-implant bone loss at intervals.

	3 months	4 months	6 months	12 months
37	0.1 mm	0.2 mm	0.2 mm	0.2 mm

Table 16-1-2 Insertion torques and perio-test values at intervals.

	Insertion torque (Nm)	0 months	3 months	12 months
37	38	–1	–3	–4

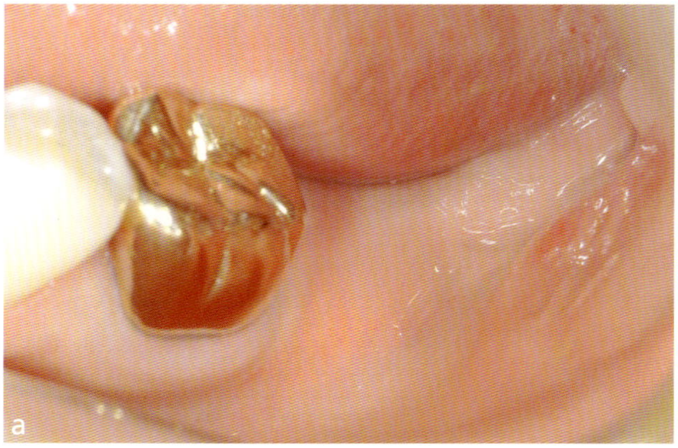

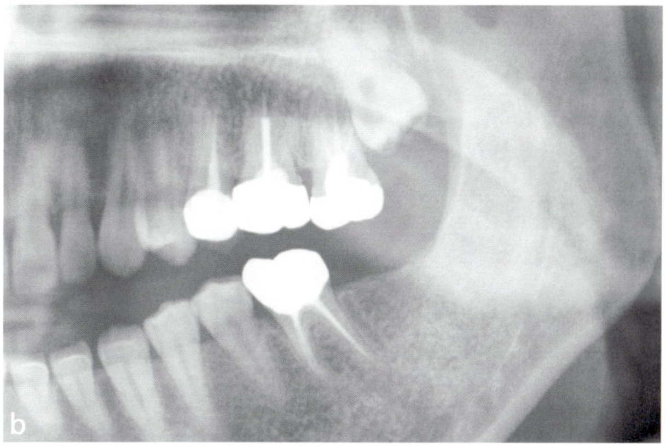

Fig 16-1-1 (a and b) The condition of the patient at the first visit.

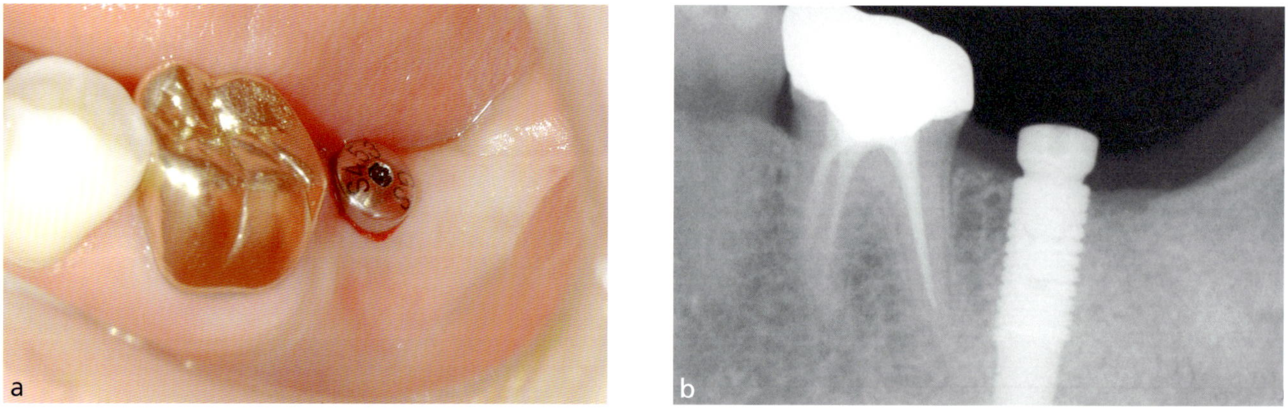

Fig 16-1-2 (a and b) Intraoral view and radiograph immediately after implant placement.

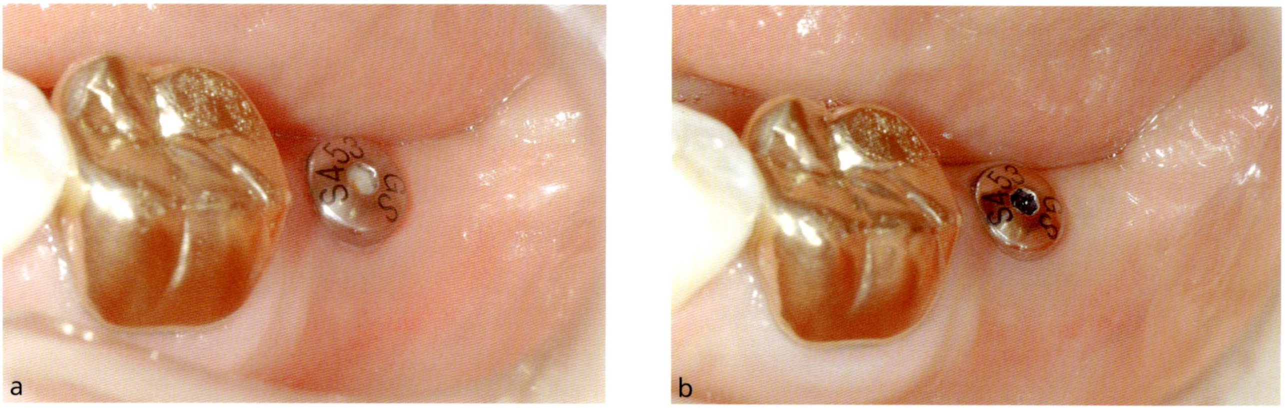

Fig 16-1-3 (a and b) Intraoral views 2 and 4 weeks after implant placement.

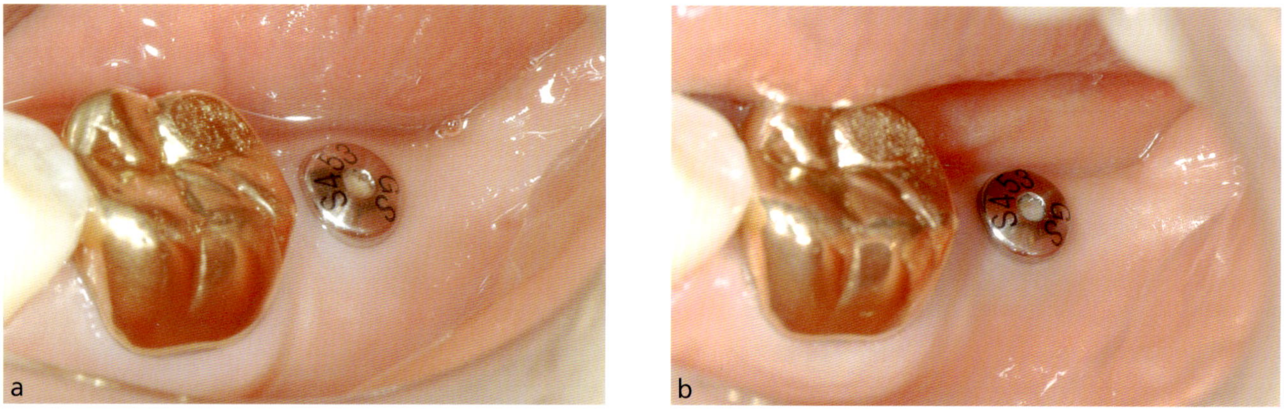

Fig 16-1-4 (a and b) Intraoral views 2 and 3 months after implant placement.

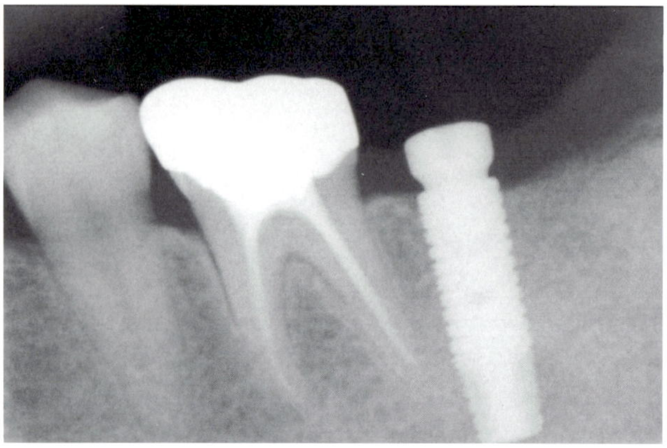

Fig 16-1-5 Radiograph 3 months after implant placement.

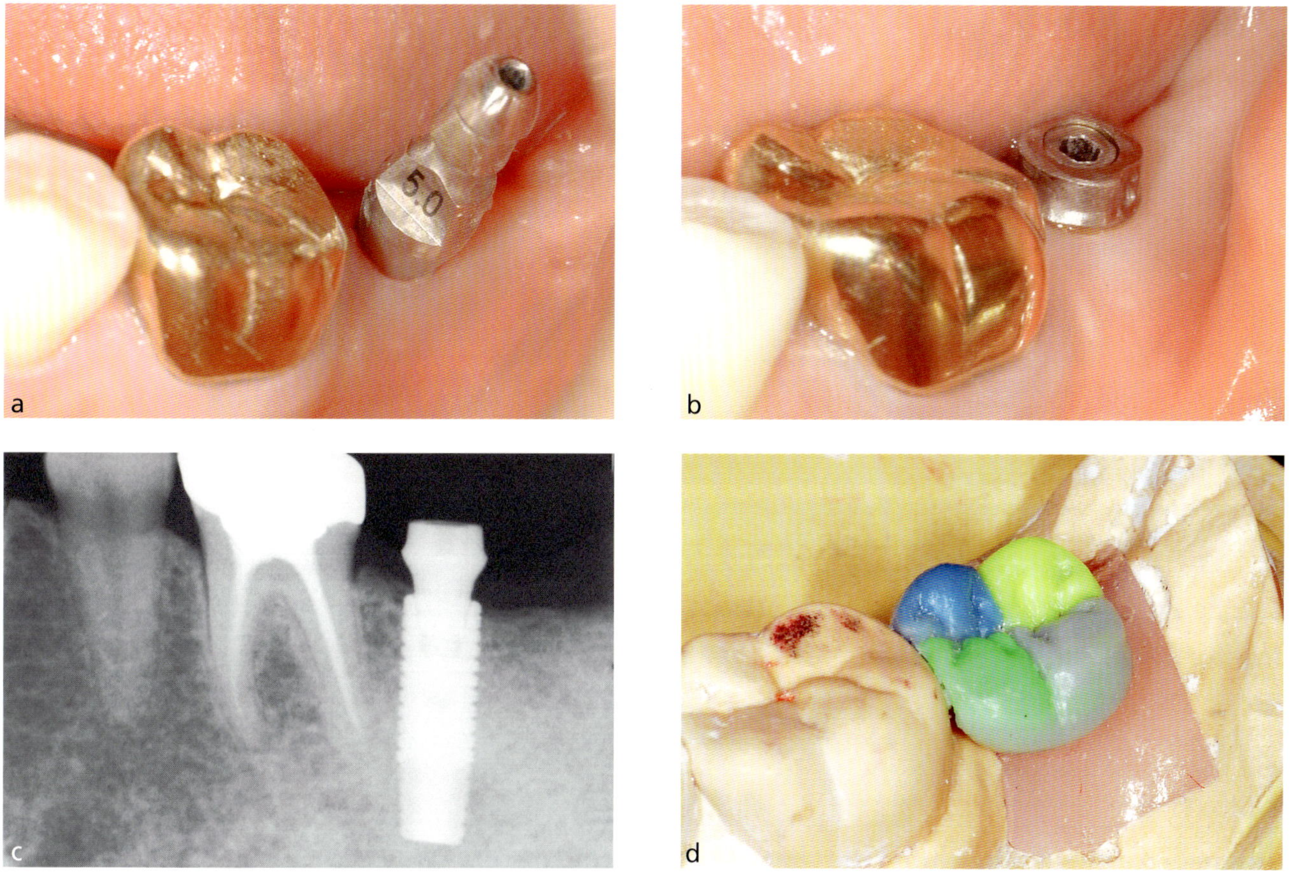

Fig 16-1-6 (a–d) Prosthesis fabrication 3 months after implant placement.

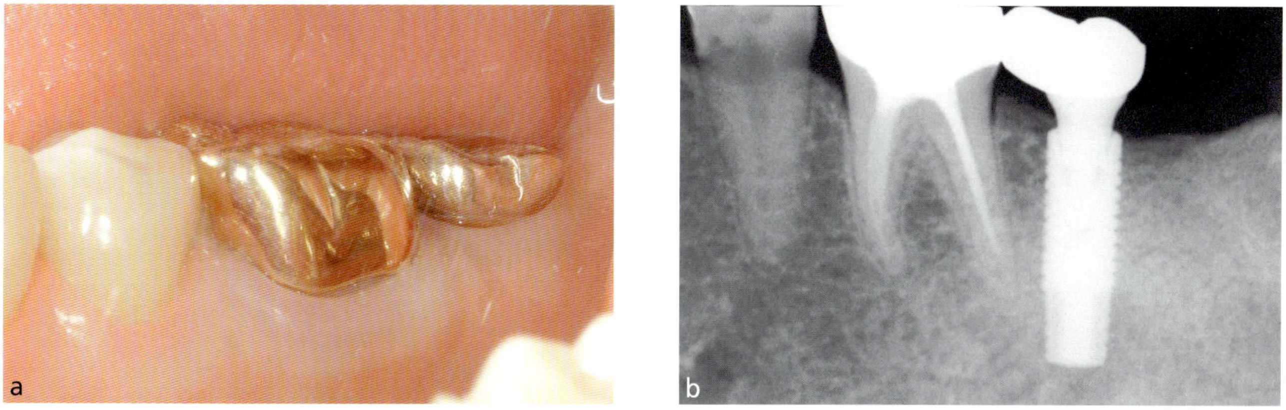

Fig 16-1-7 (a and b) Intraoral view and radiograph 6 months after implant placement

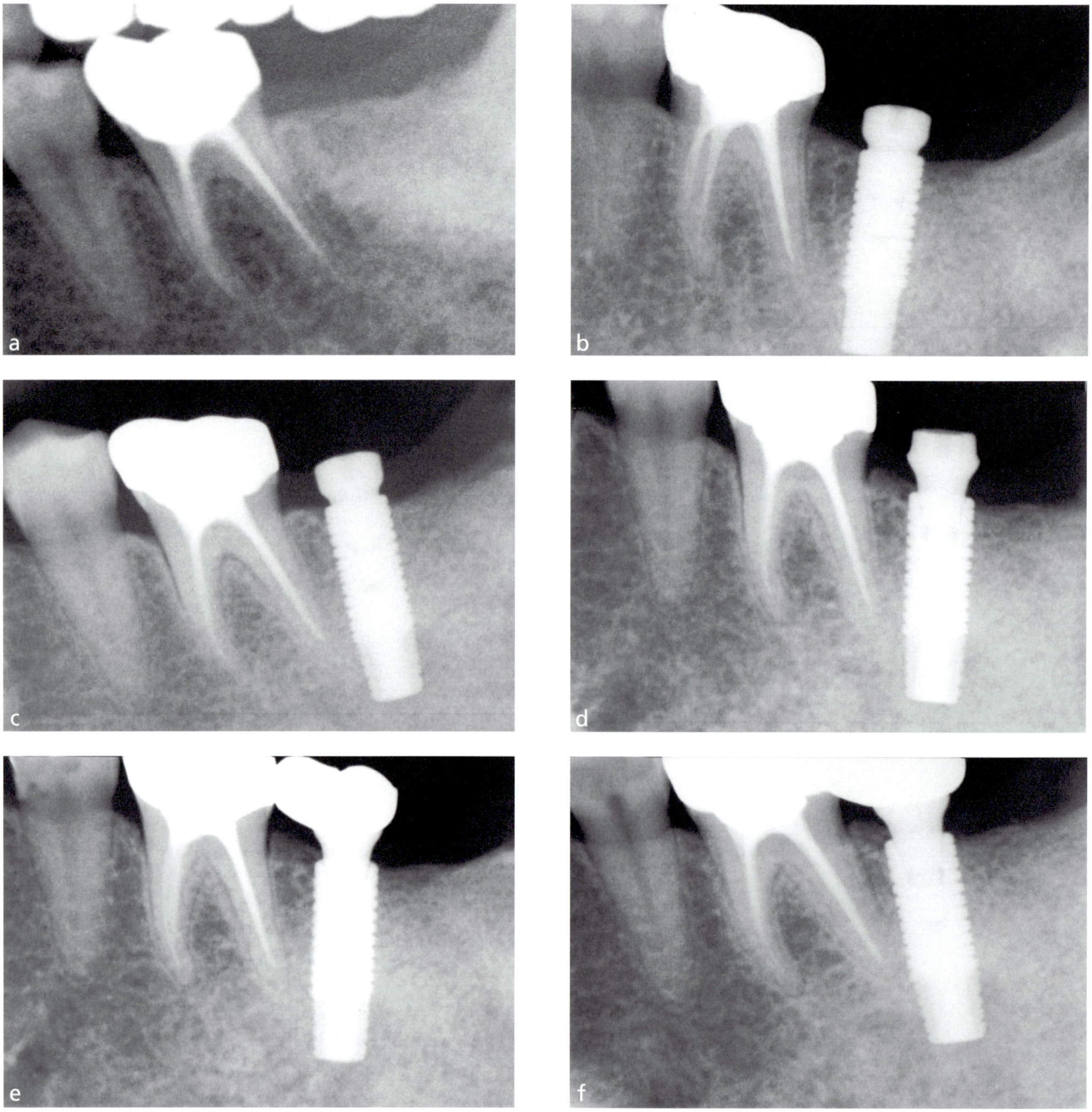

Fig 16-1-8 (a–f) Radiographs of peri-implant bone at intervals.

Case 2: Flapless implant placement in the maxillary anterior and maxillary first molar regions

A 41-year-old man visited the clinic for implant placement in the maxillary left lateral incisor and first molar regions. The mesiodistal distance of the sites with missing teeth was 6 mm at the maxillary left incisor site and 7 mm at the maxillary left first molar site. The bone height from the alveolar crest to the antral floor measured at the maxillary left first molar site was approximately 14 mm. A sufficient width of alveolar crest bone was present at both sites. Two Osstem Implant fixtures (GSII 4.0 mm × 13 mm and 4.5 mm × 13 mm) were placed at the lateral incisor and the first molar sites using flapless implant surgery. Flapless implant placement was performed using a mini-incision technique. At the time of implant placement, both sites clinically showed D3-level bone quality. The insertion torques were 37 Ncm for the lateral incisor implant and 22 Ncm for the first molar implant. The perio-test value of the implant measured immediately after implant placement was 0 for the lateral incisor implant and −2 for the first molar implant. The patient had hypertension, but no postoperative bleeding occurred. Aside from a little dull pain in the surgery site for a day, the patient did not experience any other discomfort. One week after surgery, the suture was removed. The implant covered with soft tissue at the first-stage surgery was not exposed prior to stage II uncovering. The uncovering was performed 4 months after the implant placement using a mini-incision technique. The perio-test values of the implants measured immediately after the stage II uncovering were −2 for the lateral incisor implant and −3 for the first molar implant. A temporary prosthesis was mounted on the healing abutment. Three months later, the final prosthesis was completed. At a follow-up evaluation performed 12 months after implant placement, peri-implant bone loss was 0.2 mm, the probing depth around the implants was 1.0–1.5 mm, and no inflammation was found in the peri-implant mucosa. The interdental papilla was also well maintained.

Comment

After flapless implant surgery, the original height of the bone and the mucosa around the implants was well maintained. Thus, an esthetically successful result was obtained. The flapless procedure was extremely advantageous in terms of esthetics. The implant stability improved over time.

Table 16-2-1 Peri-implant bone loss at intervals.

	3 months	5 months	12 months
22	0.1 mm	0.2 mm	0.2 mm
26	0.0 mm	0.1 mm	0.1 mm

Table 16-2-2 Insertion torques and perio-test values at intervals.

	Insertion torque (Nm)	0 months	4 months	12 months
22	37	−0	−2	−3
26	22	−2	−3	−3

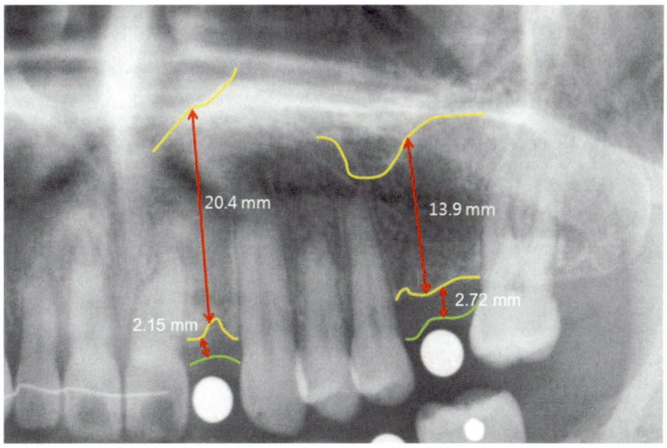

Fig 16-2-1 The condition of the patient at the first visit.

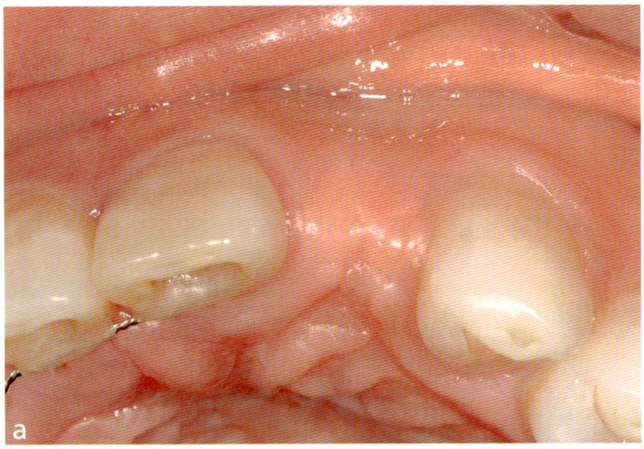
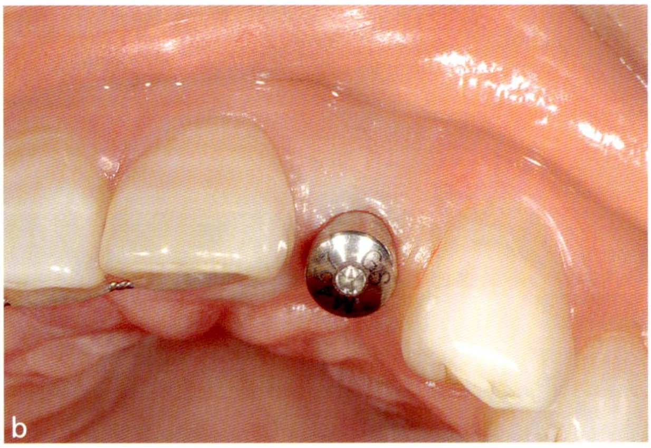
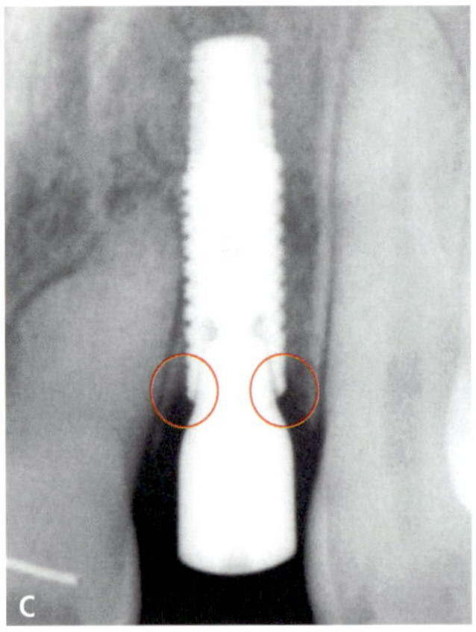

Fig 16-2-2 (a) Intraoral view 2 weeks after implant placement in the maxillary left lateral incisor region using a mini-incision technique. (b) Intraoral view after the stage II uncovering using a mini-incision technique. (c) Radiograph taken immediately after the uncovering procedure. Note that the original height of the peri-implant bone is well maintained.

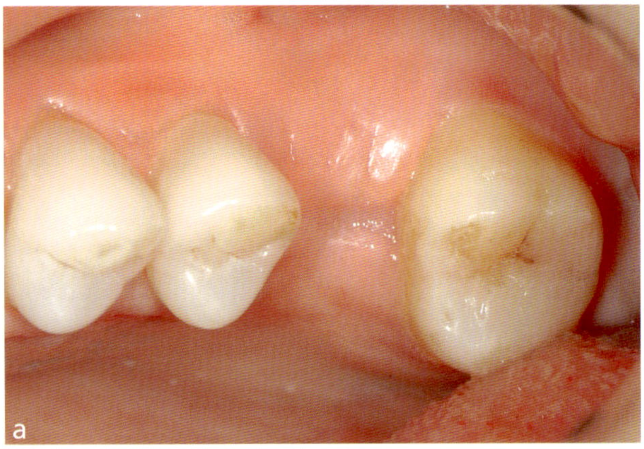
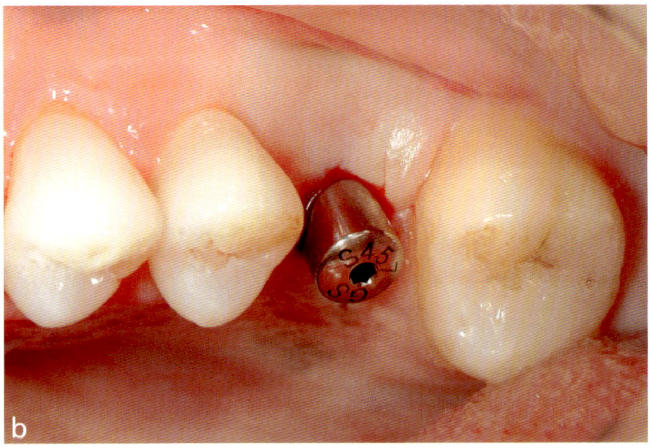
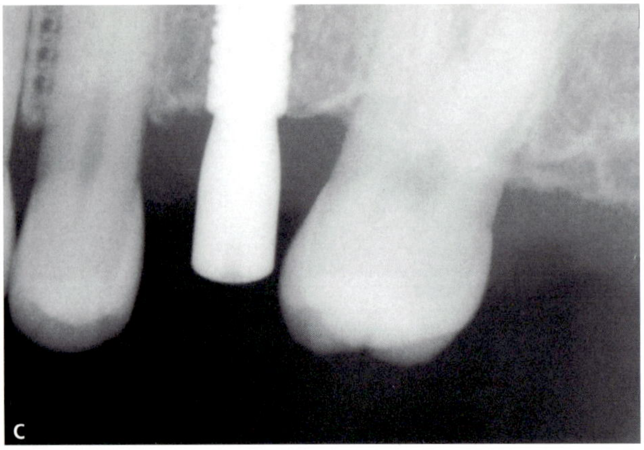

Fig 16-2-3 (a) Intraoral view 2 weeks after implant placement in the maxillary first molar region using a mini-incision technique. (b) Intraoral view after the stage II uncovering using a mini-incision technique. (c) Radiograph taken immediately after the uncovering procedure. Note that the original height of the peri-implant bone is well maintained.

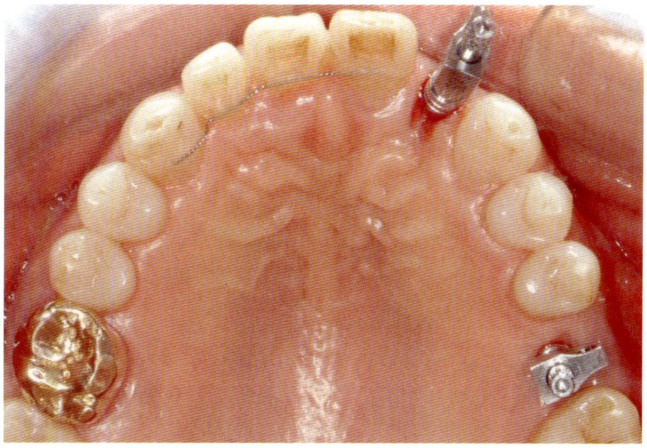

Fig 16-2-4 One month after the stage II uncovering, impressions are taken for temporary prosthetic treatment.

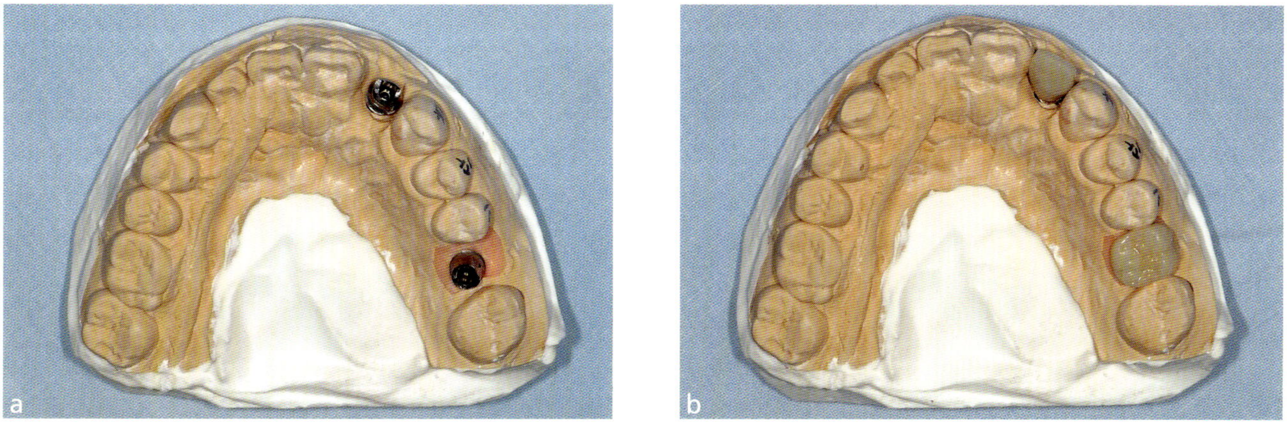

Fig 16-2-5 (a and b) A temporary prosthesis is made.

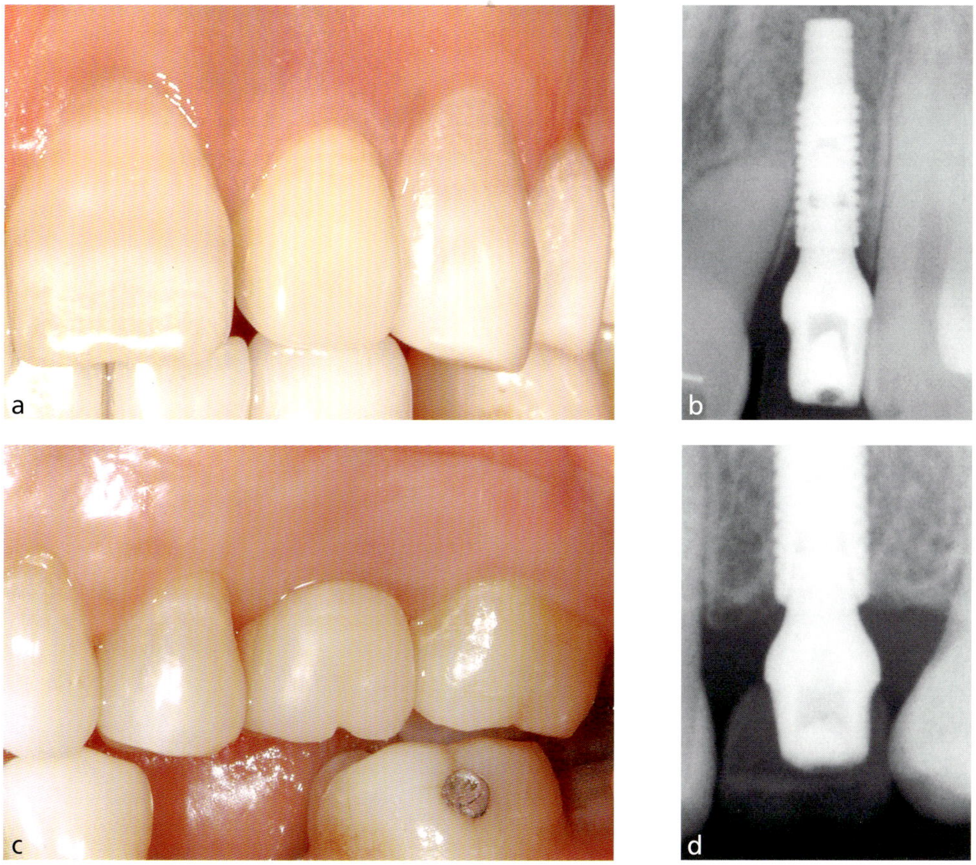

Fig 16-2-6 (a–d) Intraoral views and radiographs after the temporary prosthesis are mounted. Note that the original form of the interdental papillae is well maintained.

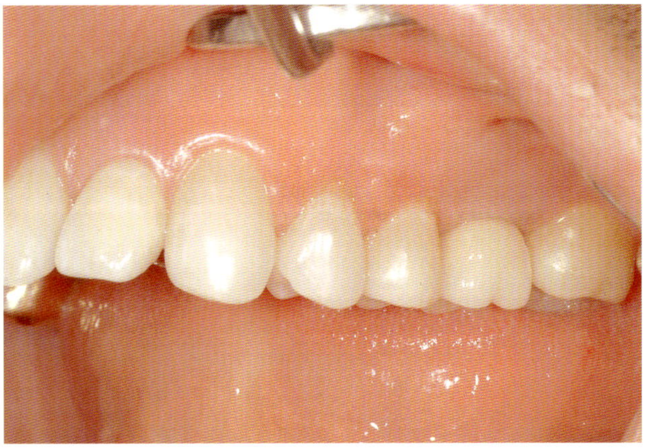

Fig 16-2-7 Intraoral view 1 year after the final prosthetic treatment.

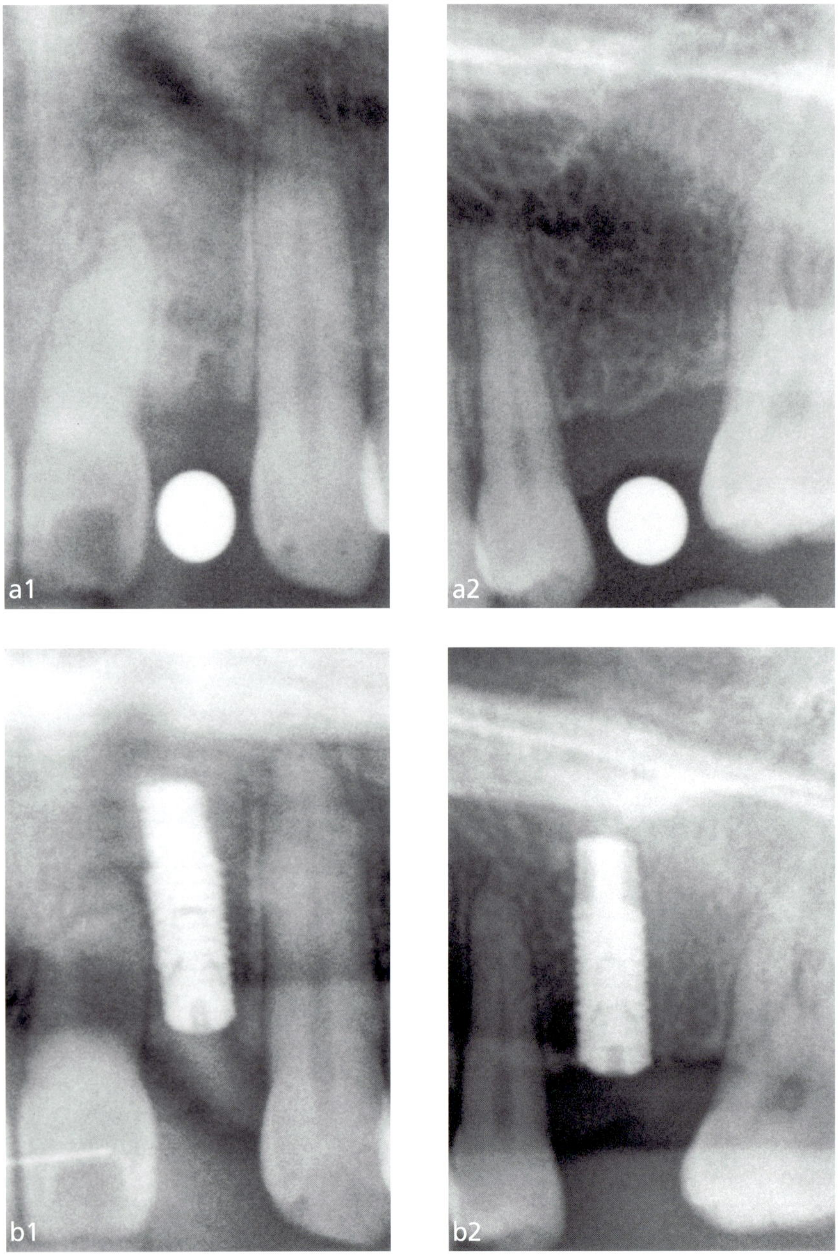

Fig 16-2-8 (a1/2–e1/2) Radiographs of the peri-implant bone at intervals.

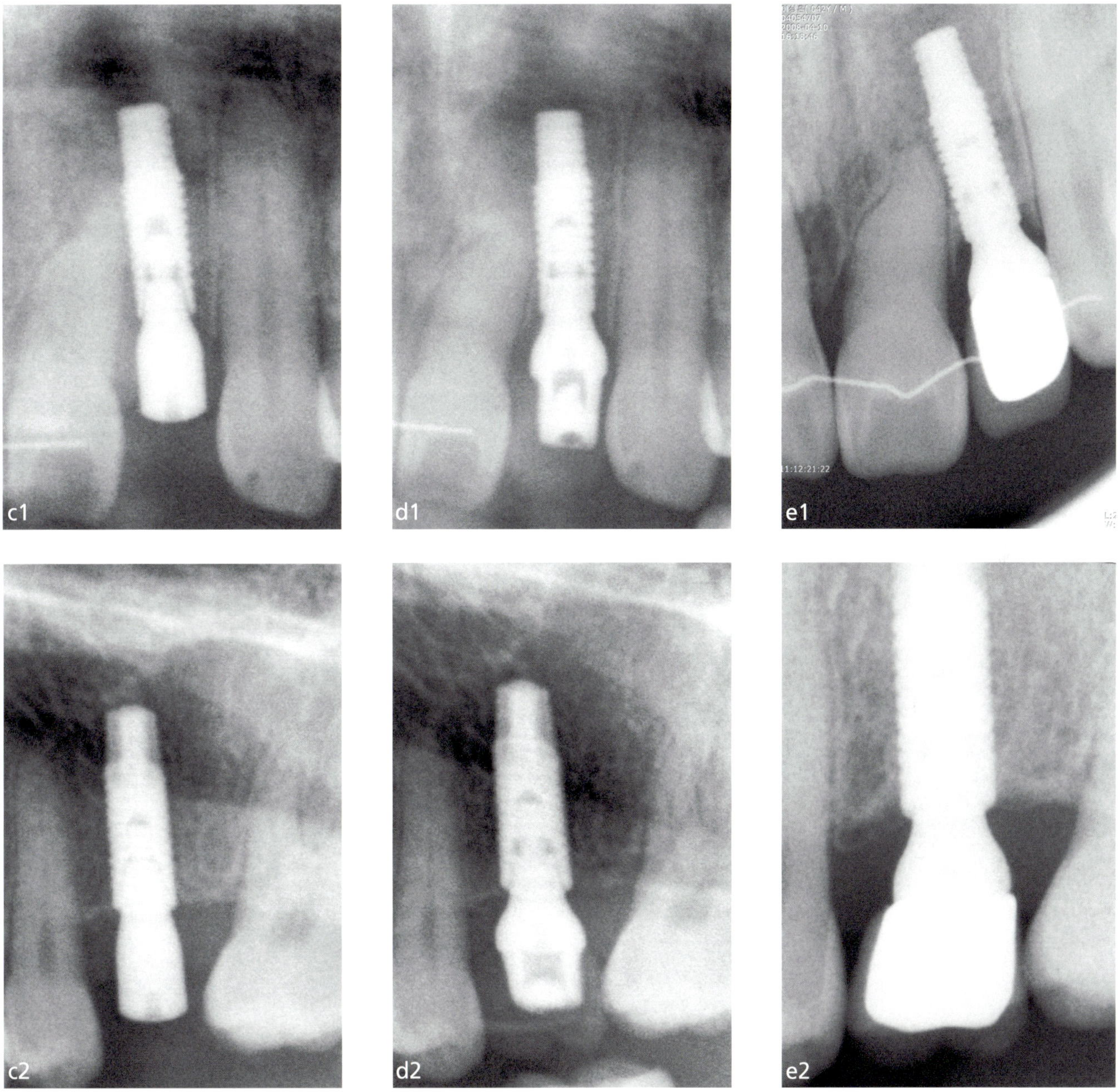

Fig 16-2-8 *(cont.)*

Case 3: Flapless implant placement in the maxillary central incisor region after orthodontic treatment

A 16-year-old female visited the clinic because of a fractured maxillary right central incisor. Six months earlier, she had injured the tooth during exercise. The maxillary right central incisor was invaginated deeply into the alveolar bone owing to the injury. As a result, the vertical dimension of the alveolar process on the region was lowered. In addition, tooth discoloration and root resorption were observed. The space of the maxillary right central incisor had also narrowed. Orthodontic treatment preceded implant placement. After the orthodontic treatment, the fractured central incisor was extracted. One month later, an Astra implant (3.5 mm × 11 mm) was placed on the central incisor site using flapless implant surgery. The flapless implant surgery was performed using a mini-incision technique. At the time of implant placement, the mucosal thickness of the placement site was approximately 5 mm, and the soft tissue along the edentulous crest was at the level of the interdental papillae. An implant was inserted with an insertion torque of 40 Ncm. A long healing abutment was connected, and the implant was nonsubmerged. The perio-test value of the implant measured immediately after implant placement was –1. Four months after implant placement, gingivoplasty was performed to sculpt the crest of the ridge and form a scalloped emergence profile around the abutment. The contour of the midfacial position of the gingival margin was 1 mm more incisal than the contour of the adjacent teeth. A temporary prosthesis was then mounted. One month after prosthesis placement, the gingival contour was corrected by the gingival shrinkage. At the time of the routine checkup 16 months after final prosthesis placement, the gingival margin was maintained at the same level as the adjacent tooth. The dental papillae were also kept in good condition without exhibiting black interproximal spaces. Bone loss was minimal (0.4 mm), and the peri-implant sulcus depth was 1.0–2.0 mm. No bleeding occurred during probing into the peri-implant sulcus.

Comment

In the case of the intruded fractured anterior tooth, positional restoration of the vertical height of both the crestal bone and the gingival margin was carried out through the orthodontic treatment, and then the fractured tooth was extracted. The shape of the gingival margin was enhanced using both flapless implant surgery and gingivoplasty. To make up for the imperfect gingivoplasty, gingival formation was completed through gingival pressure using a temporary prosthesis. Even though the implant was placed in the site with a mucosal thickness of 5 mm, the peri-implant crest bone height was well maintained, and the adjacent soft tissue also remained healthy.

Table 16-3-1 Peri-implant bone loss at intervals.

	4 months	6 months	12 months	20 months
11	0.2 mm	0.2 mm	0.3 mm	0.3 mm

Table 16-3-2 Insertion torques and perio-test values at intervals.

	Insertion torque (Nm)	0 months	4 months	20 months
11	40	–1	–2	–2

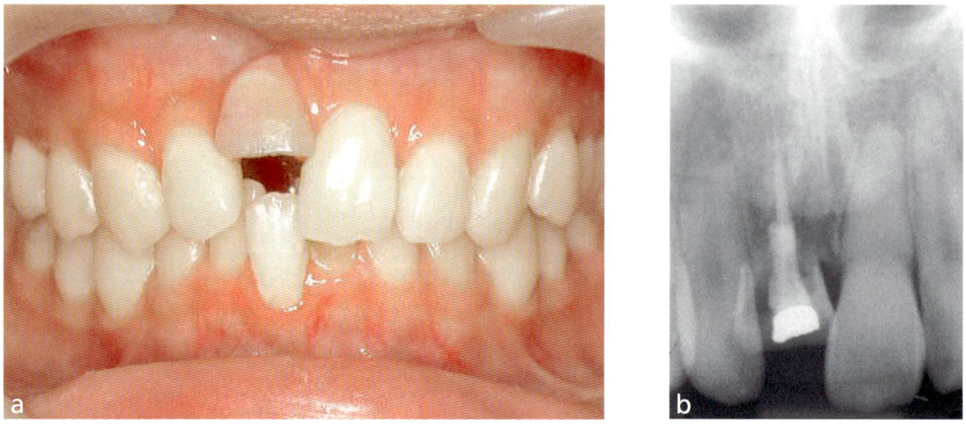

Fig 16-3-1 (a and b) The condition of the patient at the first visit.

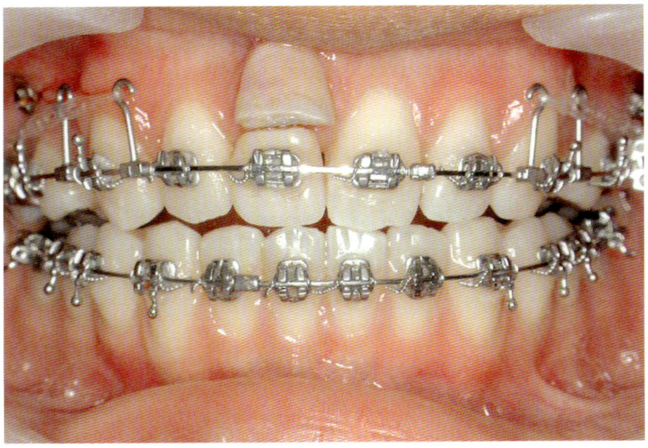

Fig 16-3-2 Orthodontic treatment is carried out to restore the vertical height of both the crestal bone and the gingival margin.

Fig 16-3-3 After the orthodontic treatment, an Astra implant (3.5 mm × 11 mm) is placed using a mini-incision technique. A long healing abutment is then connected so the implant is nonsubmerged.

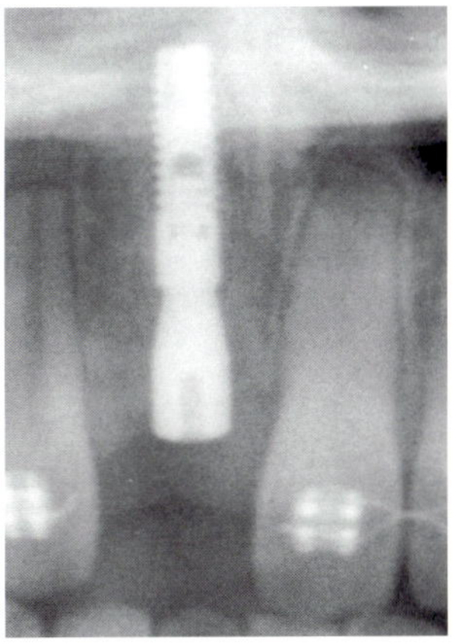

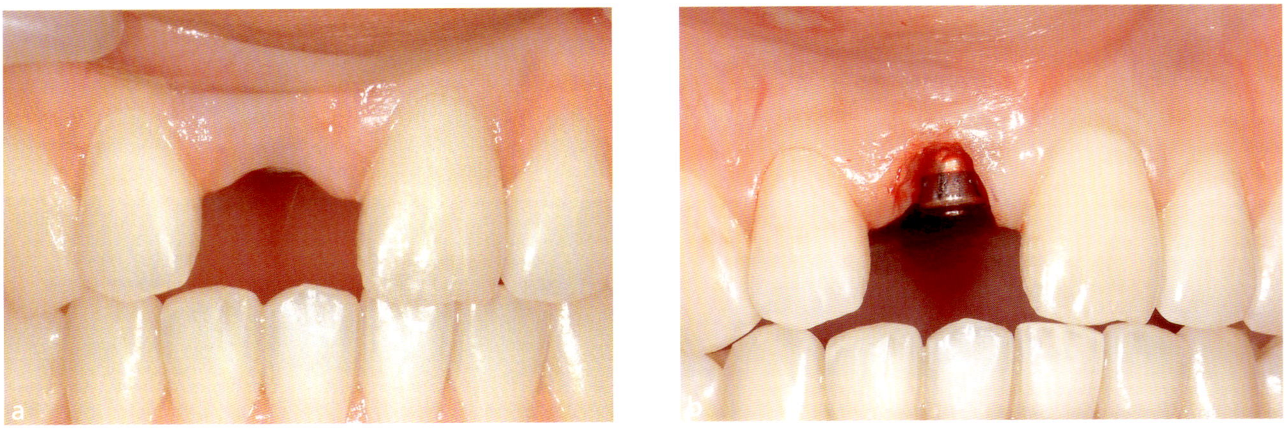

Fig 16-3-4 (a and b) Four months after implant placement, gingivoplasty is performed.

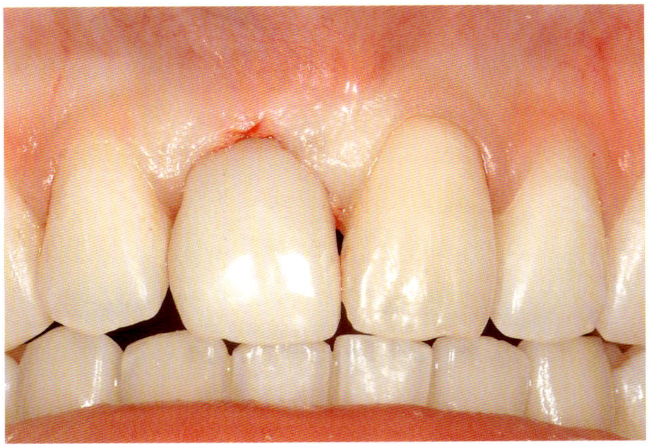

Fig 16-3-5 Intraoral view after temporary prosthesis placement. Note that the contour of the midfacial position of the gingival margin is 1 mm more incisal than the contour of the adjacent teeth.

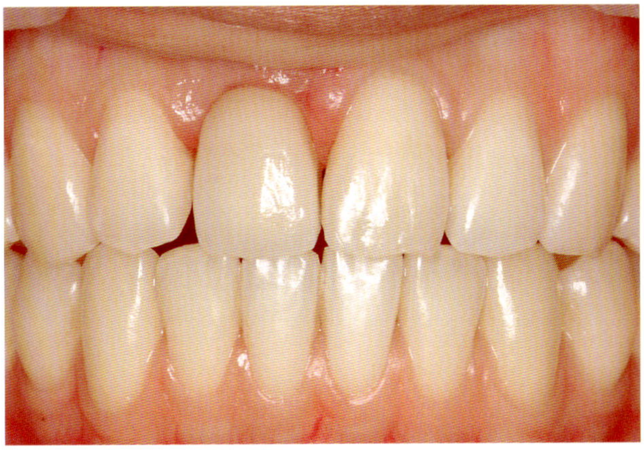

Fig 16-3-6 One month after prosthesis placement, the gingival contour is corrected by the gingival shrinkage.

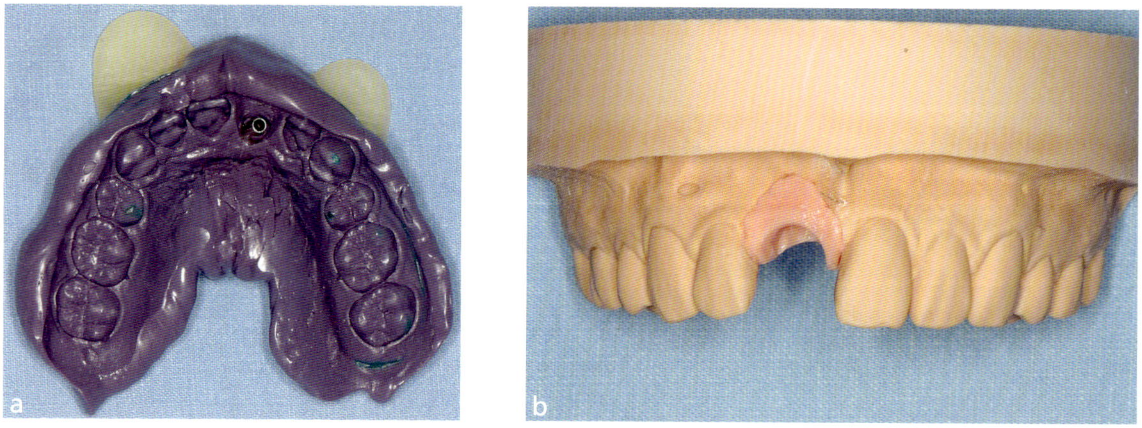

Fig 16-3-7 (a and b) Taking impressions for the final prosthesis.

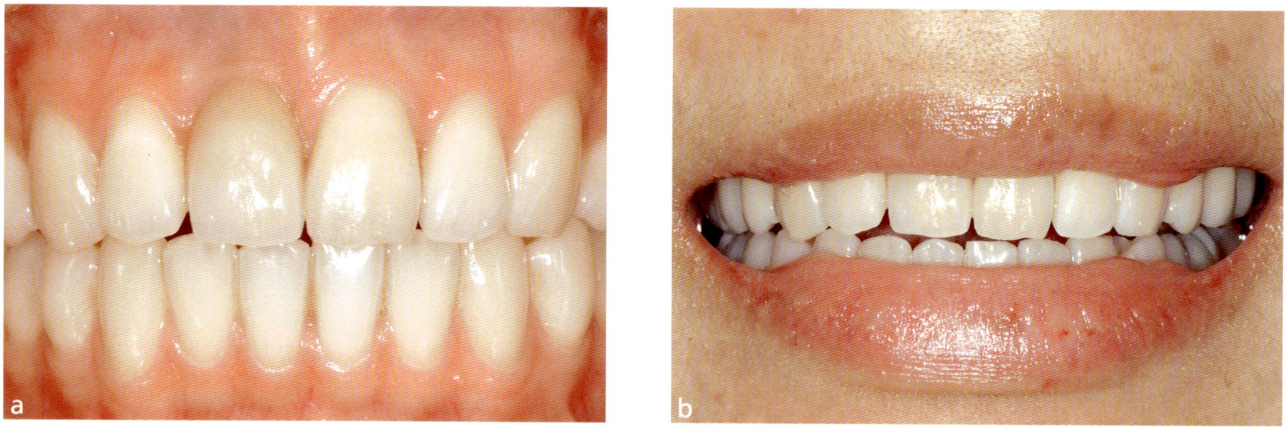

Fig 16-3-8 (a and b) Sixteen months after the final prosthesis, the gingival margin is maintained at the same level as the adjacent tooth. The dental papillae are kept in good condition without showing the black triangle.

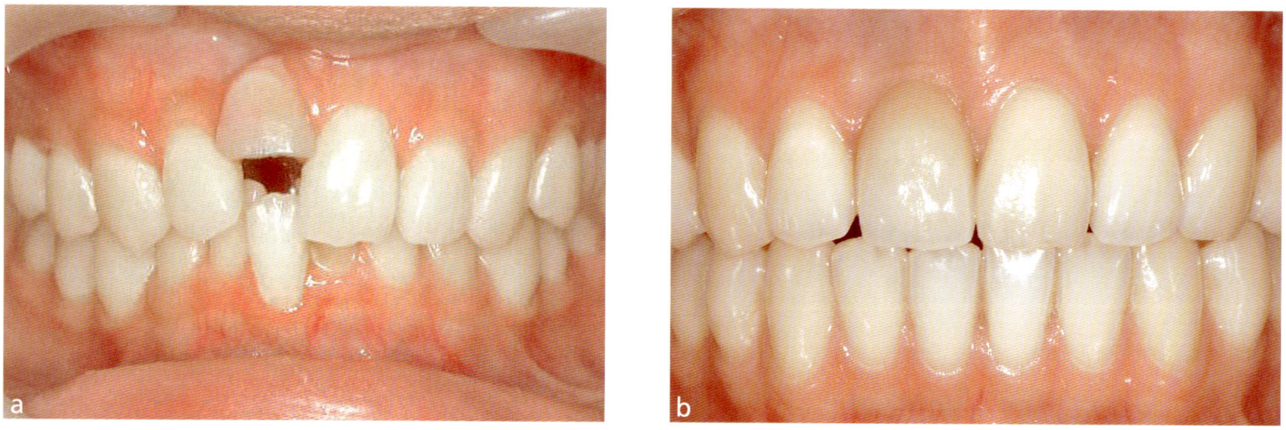

Fig 16-3-9 (a and b) Comparison before and after treatment.

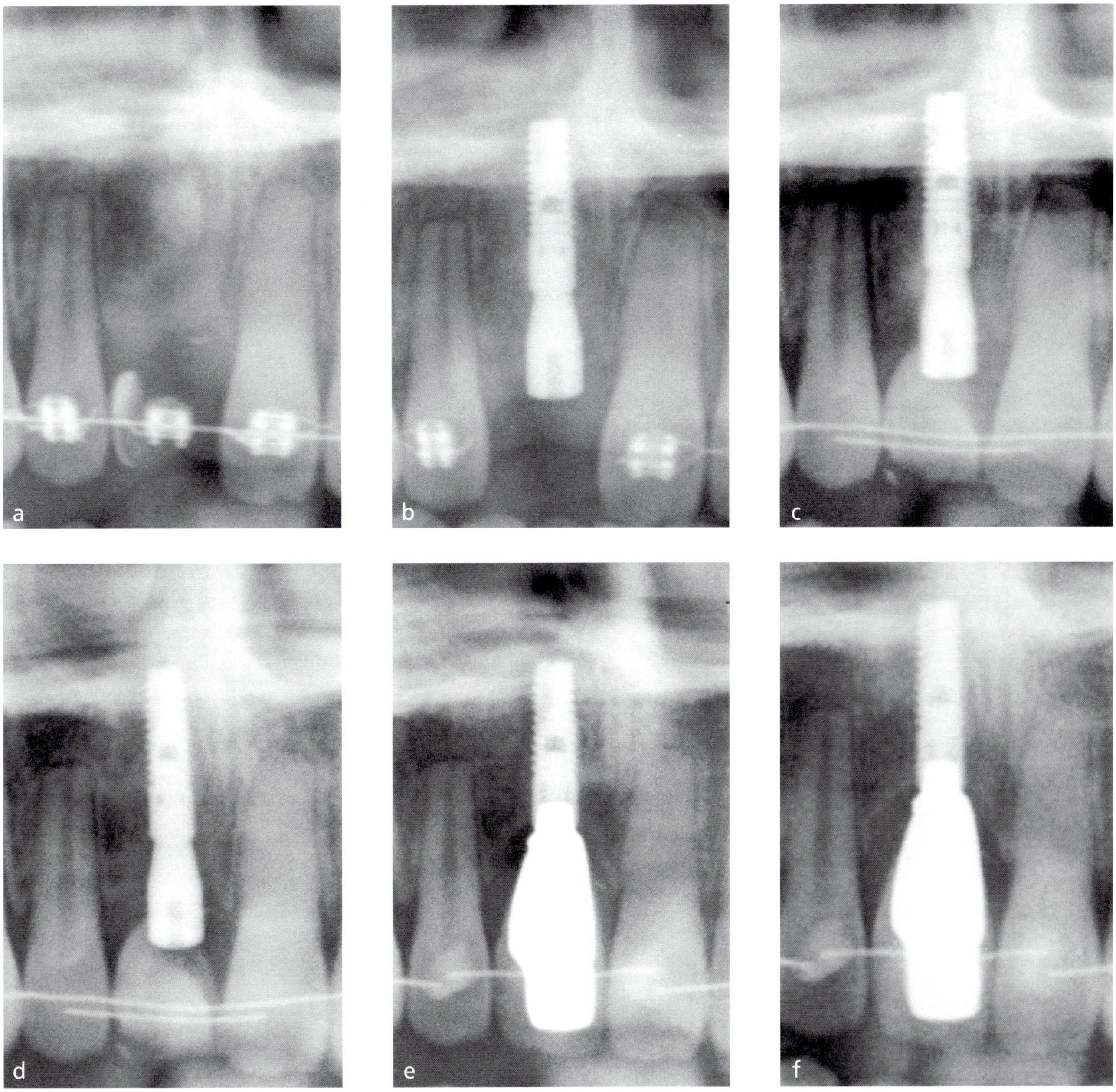

Fig 16-2-10 (a–f) Radiographs of peri-implant bone at intervals.

Case 4: Socket lift and simultaneous flapless implant placement in the maxillary molar region

A 39-year-old woman visited the clinic for implant placement in the maxillary right first molar region. The mesiodistal distance of the site without a tooth was sufficient for implant placement. The bone height from the alveolar crest to the antral floor in the region was approximately 9 mm, and a sufficient width of alveolar crest bone was present. The socket lift within the implant osteotomy and simultaneous flapless implant placement procedures were performed using a mini-incision technique. The socket lift procedure was performed for 2 mm of bone augmentation in the maxillary sinus to place an 11 mm long implant (Osstem implant, GS II 4.5 mm × 11 mm). Immediately after the socket lift, the implant site was evaluated for perforation of the sinus membrane by the Valsalva maneuver (nose-blowing test). At the time of implant placement, the implant site showed D3-level bone quality. The insertion torque was 40 Ncm. The perio-test value of the implant measured immediately after implant placement was –1. A CT scan taken 4 months after implant placement showed augmented bone and a healthy maxillary sinus. The stage II uncovering was performed 4 months after the implant placement using a mini-incision technique. Three weeks after the secondary surgery, a temporary acrylic restoration was mounted for the application of progressive loading. The progressive loading was applied for 4 months, and then the final prosthesis was mounted. At the time of the routine checkup 18 months after the final prosthesis, the sulcus depth was less than 2.0 mm, and the bone loss was less than 0.2 mm. The implant was considered successful.

Comment

In the case of the maxillary posterior site with D3 bone quality and an alveolar ridge height of 9 mm, a socket lift within the implant osteotomy and flapless implant placement procedures were performed simultaneously. After the flapless stage II surgery, a temporary acrylic restoration was used to apply a progressive load to the implant. With these procedures, peri-implant bone loss was minimized in the D3 bone-supporting implant.

Table 16-4-1 Peri-implant bone loss at intervals.

	4 months	6 months	8 months	18 months
16	0.2 mm	0.2 mm	0.2 mm	0.2 mm

Table 16-4-2 Insertion torques and perio-test values at intervals.

	Insertion torque (Nm)	0 months	4 months	18 months
16	40	–1	–3	–3

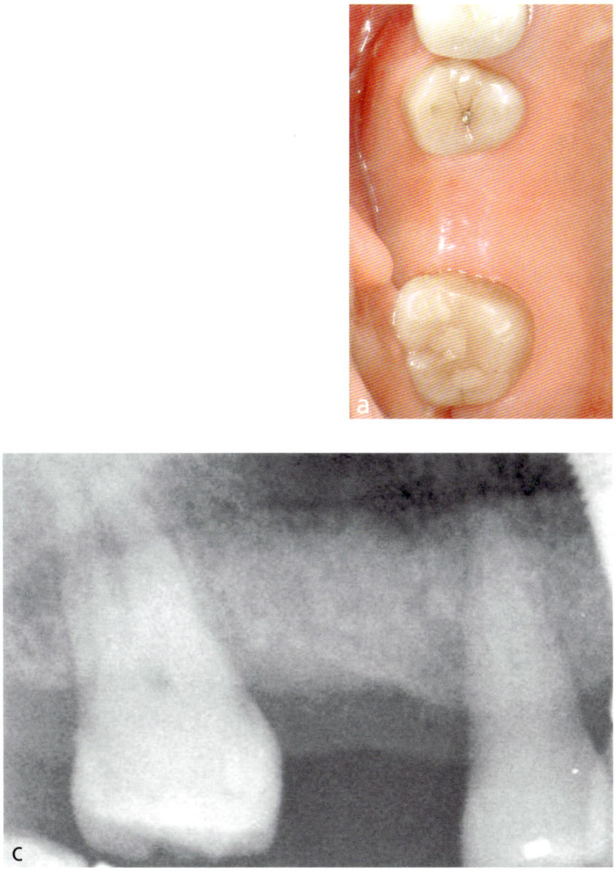

Fig 16-4-1 (a–c) The condition of the patient at the first visit.

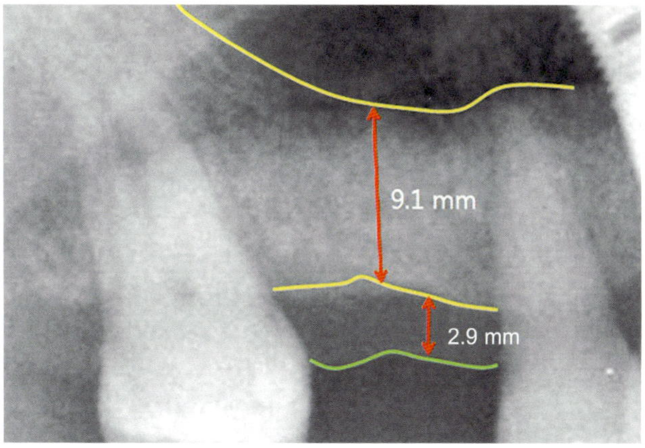

Fig 16-4-2 Radiograph showing the bone height from the alveolar crest to the antral floor and the thickness of the mucosa.

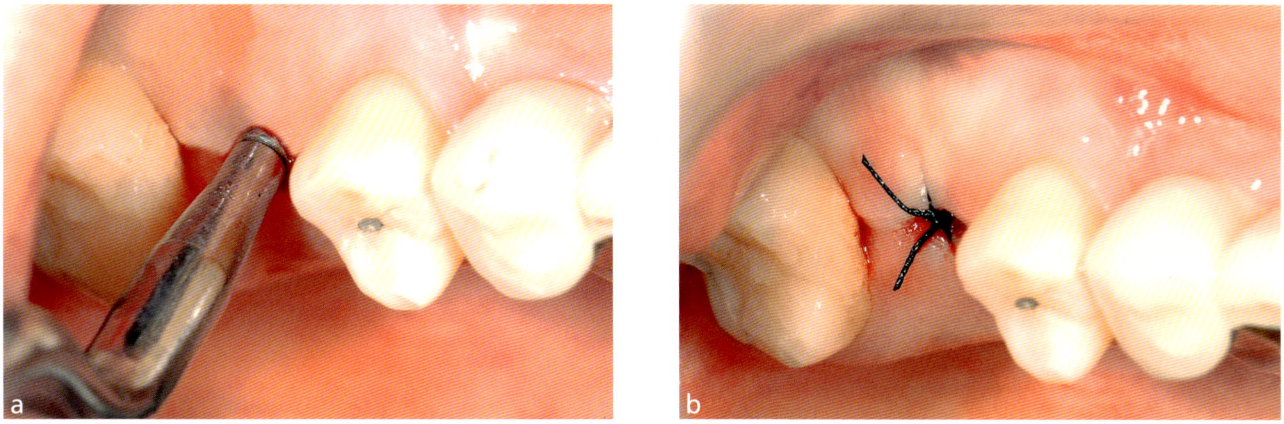

Fig 16-4-3 (a and b) Intraoral view showing the socket lift and the simultaneous flapless implant placement.

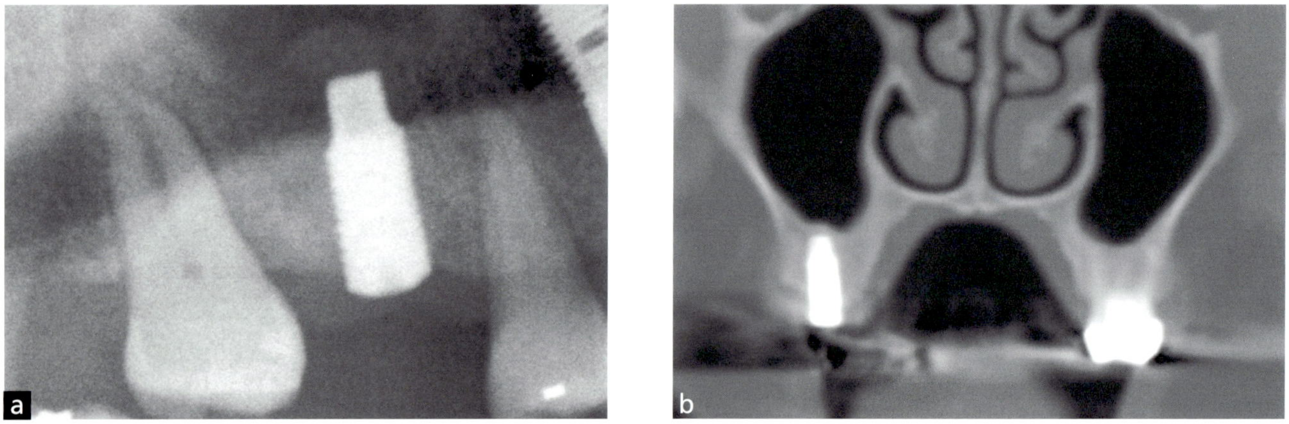

Fig 16-4-4 (a and b) Postoperative radiographs taken after 4 months indicate that bone formed over the apex of the implant, and the maxillary sinus is healthy.

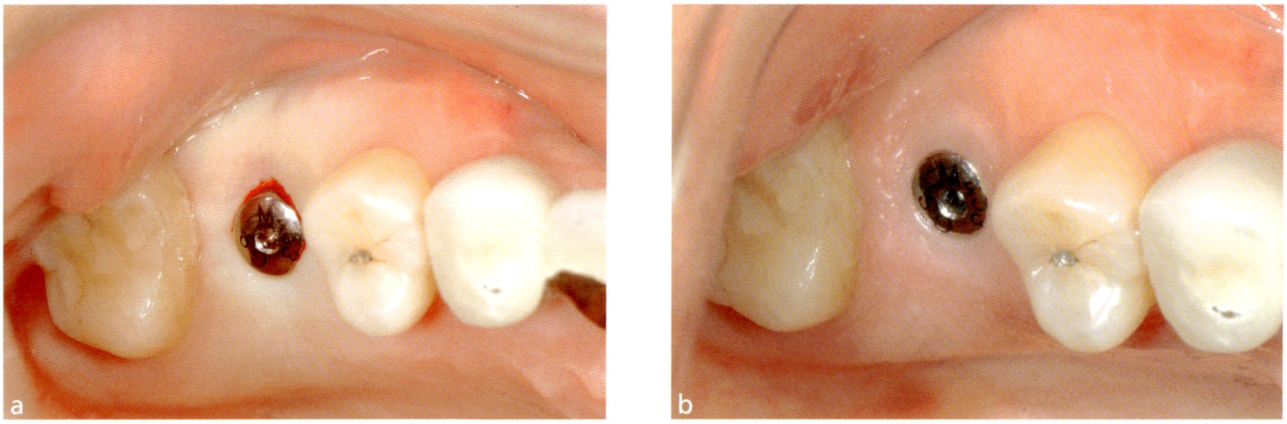

Fig 16-4-5 (a and b) Intraoral views immediately following and 1 month after the stage II uncovering procedure.

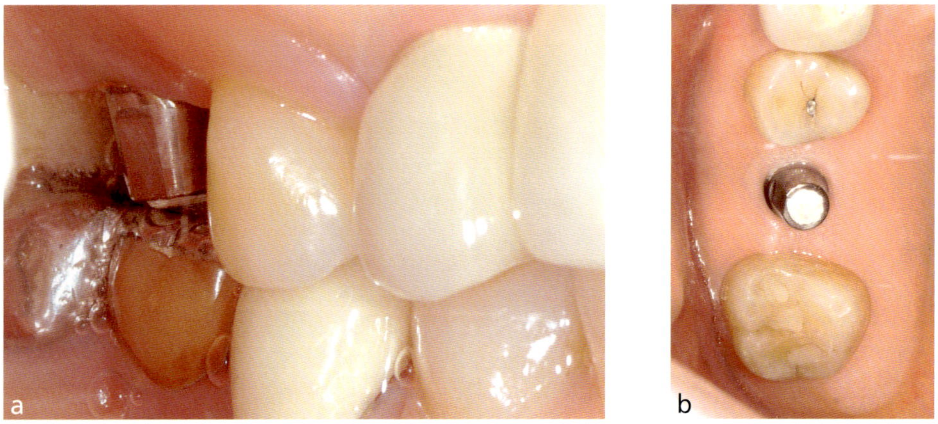

Fig 16-4-6 (a and b) Intraoral views showing a prosthetic abutment connected to the implant fixture.

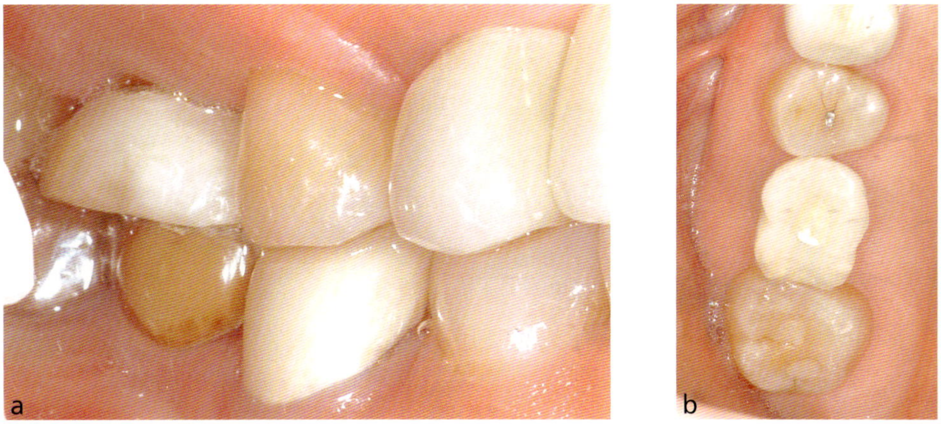

Fig 16-4-7 (a and b) A temporary prosthesis made of resin is mounted, and a progressive load is applied to the implant.

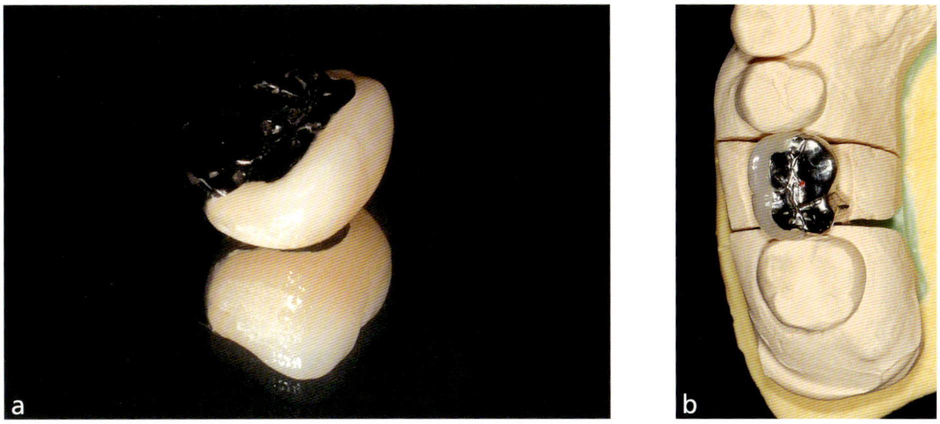

Fig 16-4-8 (a and b) The final prosthesis.

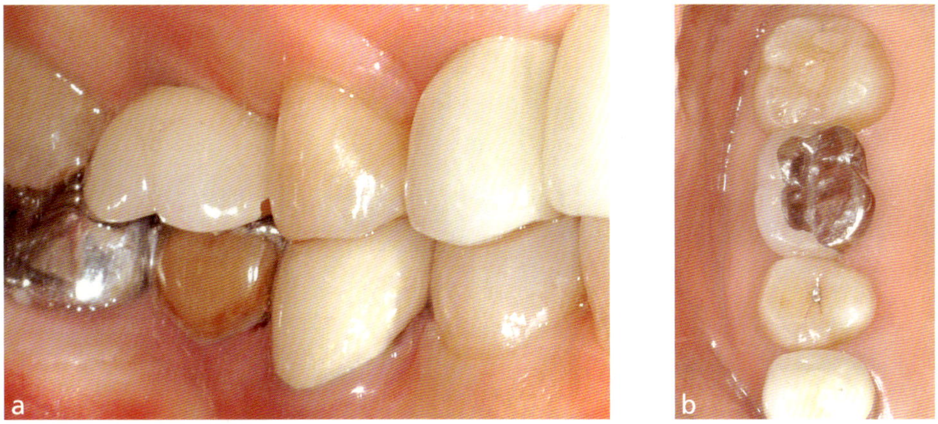

Fig 16-4-9 (a and b) Intraoral views showing the mounted final prosthesis.

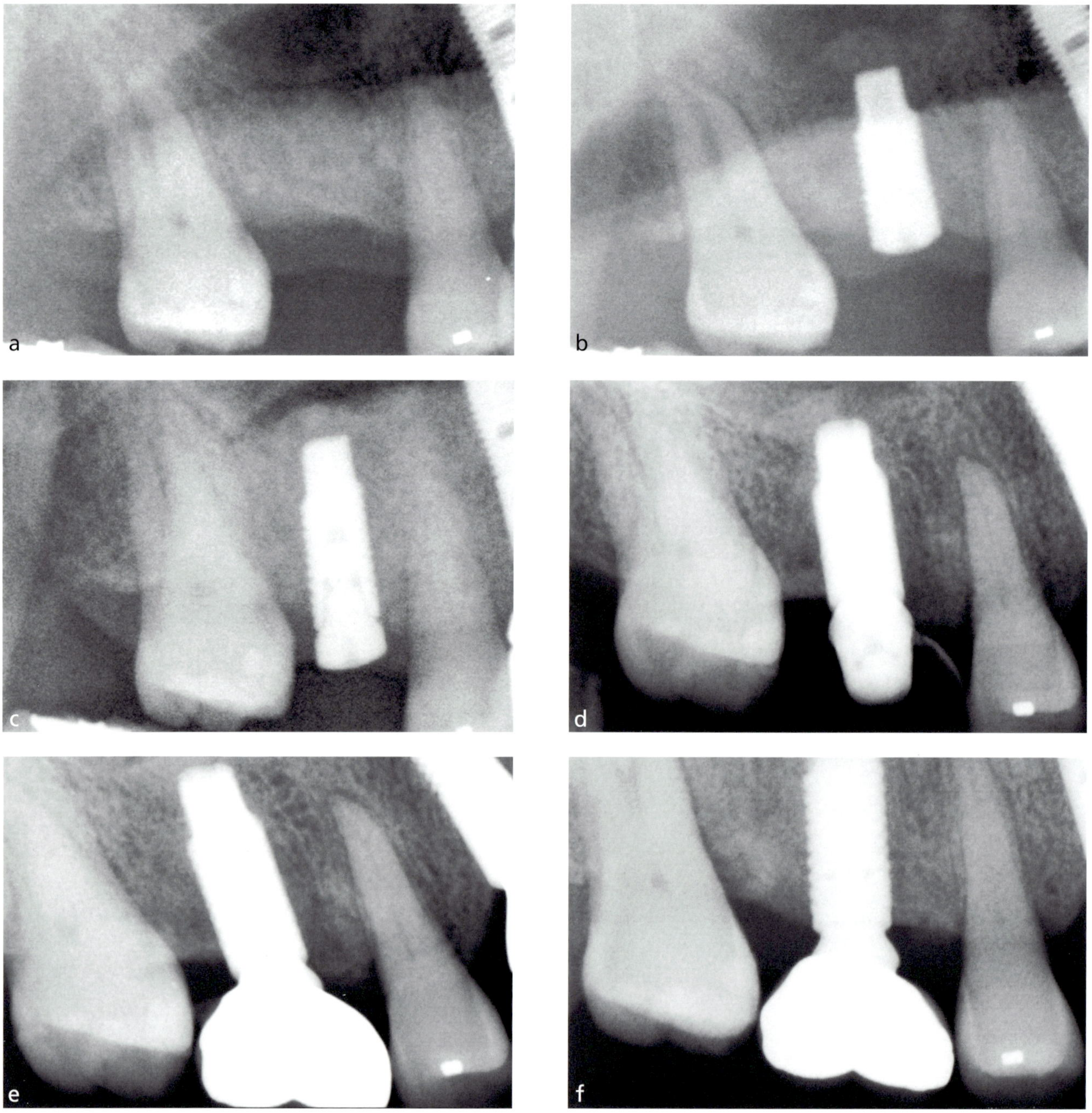

Fig 16-4-10 (a–f) Radiographs of peri-implant bone at intervals.

Case 5: Flapless implant placement and application of progressive loading in the mandibular molar region

A 49-year-old woman visited the clinic complaining of gingival swelling in the mandibular right posterior area. The diagnosis was progressive periodontitis. Since periodontal treatment did not result in any improvement, tooth extraction was carried out for the right mandibular first and second molars. Three months after the extraction, implant placement was planned. A panoramic radiograph taken 3 months following the extraction showed that the heights from the inferior alveolar nerve to the alveolar crest were approximately 13 mm at the first molar site and 10 mm at the second molar site. A short implant (Osstem, GSII 4.5 mm × 8 mm) was placed at the second molar site, and an 11 mm implant was placed at the first molar site. Three months after the placement, a temporary acrylic restoration was mounted for the application of progressive loading. The progressive loading was applied for 2 months, and then the final prosthesis was mounted. At the time of the routine checkup 20 months after final prosthesis, bone loss in the alveolar crest was approximately 0.1–0.2 mm, and sulcus depth was 1.0–1.5 mm. The implant was considered successful.

Comment

If excessive occlusal force is applied to implants, the load is converged on to the alveolar crest, resulting in marginal bone loss around the crestal portion of an implant. Marginal bone loss often occurs during the first year of occlusal loading. To minimize such bone loss, a pretreatment prosthesis was used to gradually load the bone for progressive loading before the fabrication of the final restoration, thus improving the quality of bone. In the case of short implant placement in the mandibular molar regions, flapless implant surgery as well as a progressive load concept contributed to the implant success.

Table 16-5-1 Peri-implant bone loss at intervals.

	3 months	6 months	12 months	20 months
46	0.0 mm	0.0 mm	0.1 mm	0.1 mm
47	0.0 mm	0.1 mm	0.2 mm	0.2 mm

Table 16-5-2 Insertion torques and perio-test values at intervals.

	Insertion torque (Nm)	0 months	3 months	20 months
46	40	−2	−3	−5
47	36	−1	−2	−3

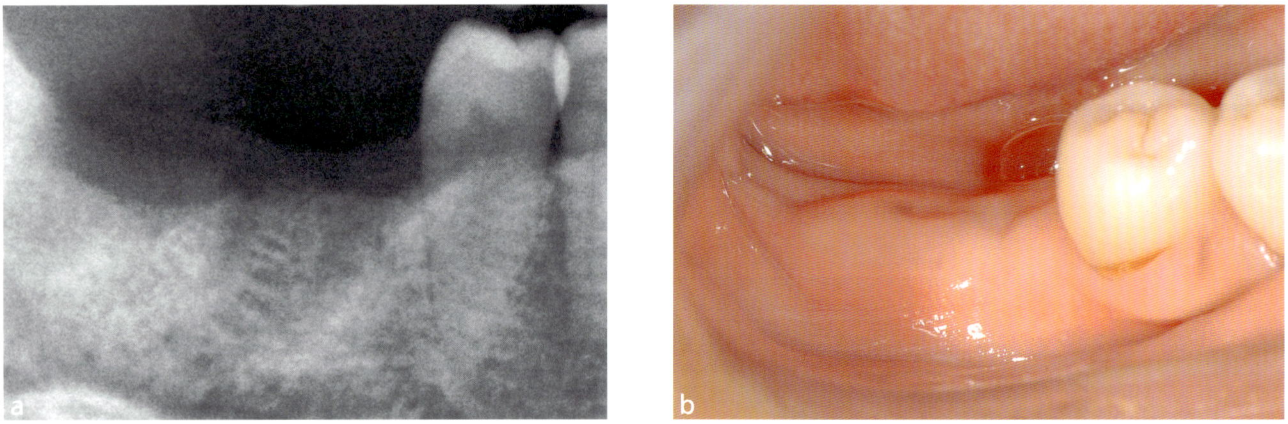

Fig 16-5-1 (a and b) The condition of the patient at the first visit.

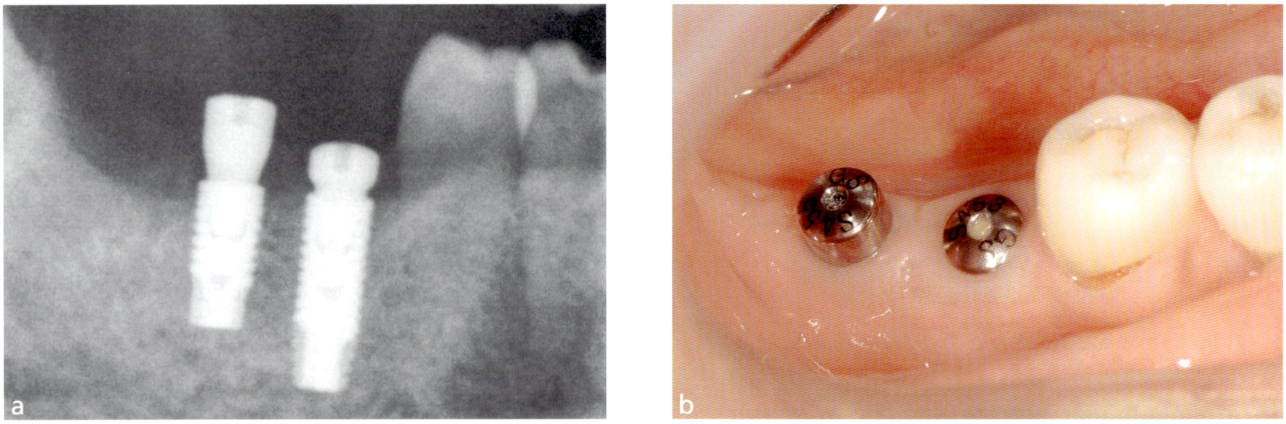

Fig 16-5-2 (a and b) Radiograph and intraoral view immediately after implant placement.

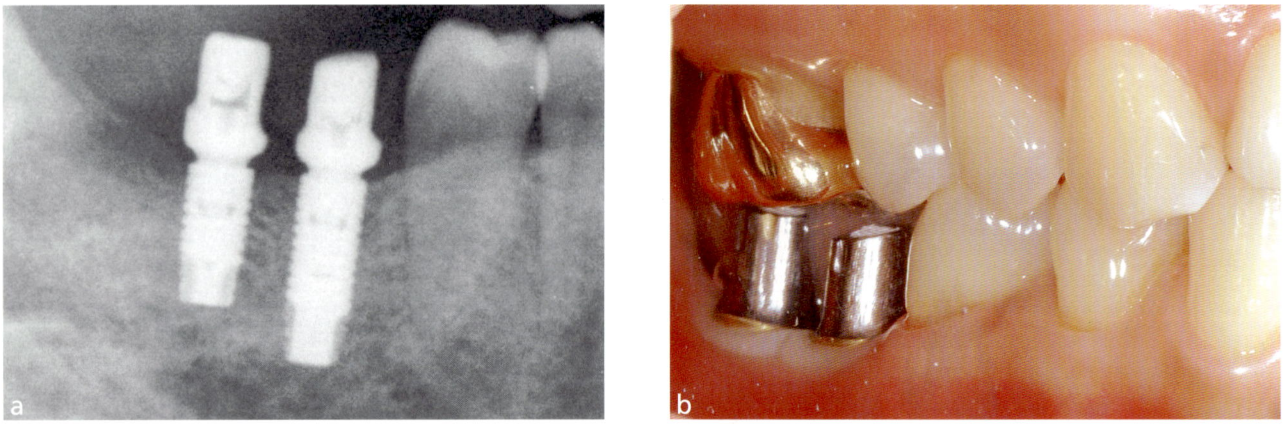

Fig 16-5-3 (a and b) Three months after the placement, a radiograph and an intraoral view showing a prosthetic abutment connected to the implant fixture.

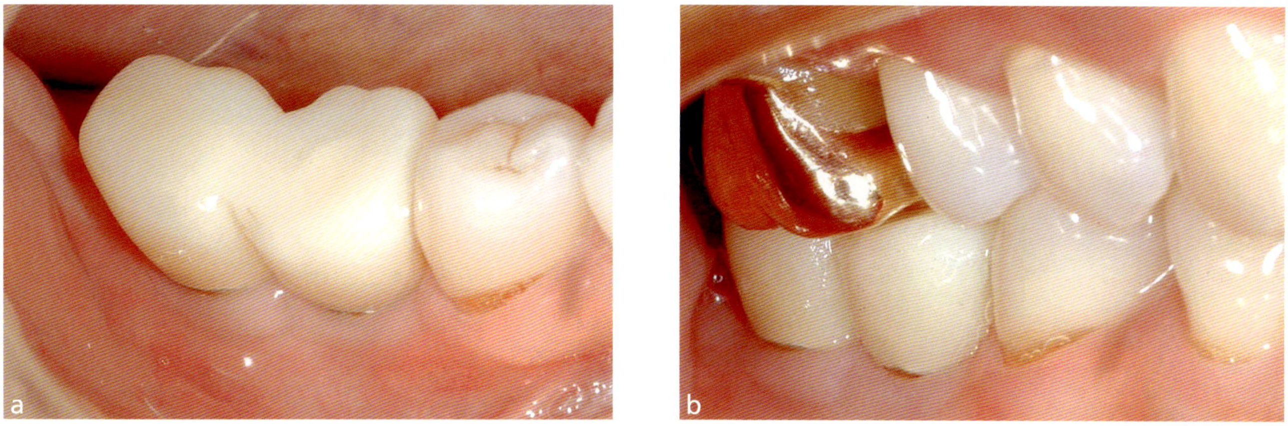

Fig 16-5-4 (a and b) Intraoral views showing the temporary acrylic restoration.

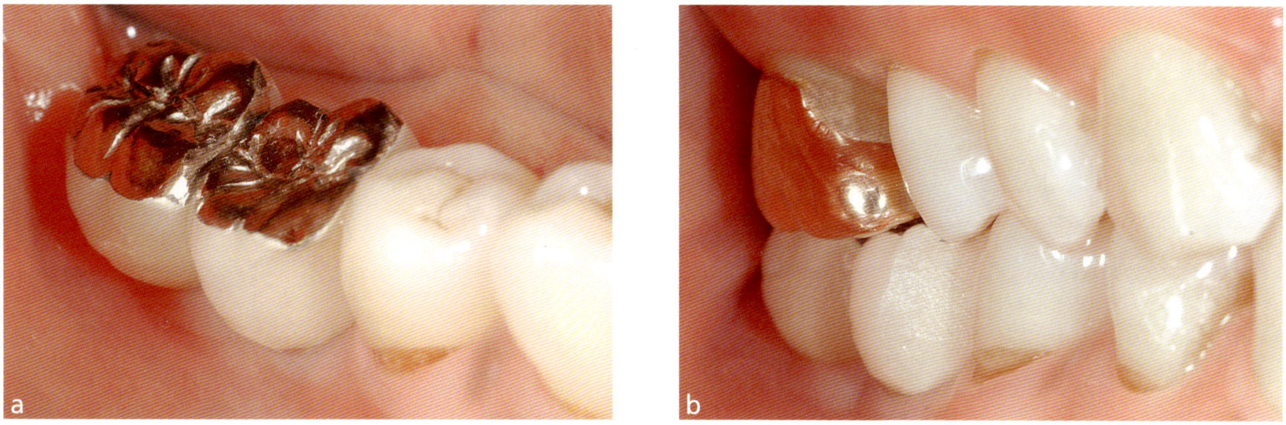

Fig 16-5-5 (a and b) Intraoral views showing the final prosthesis.

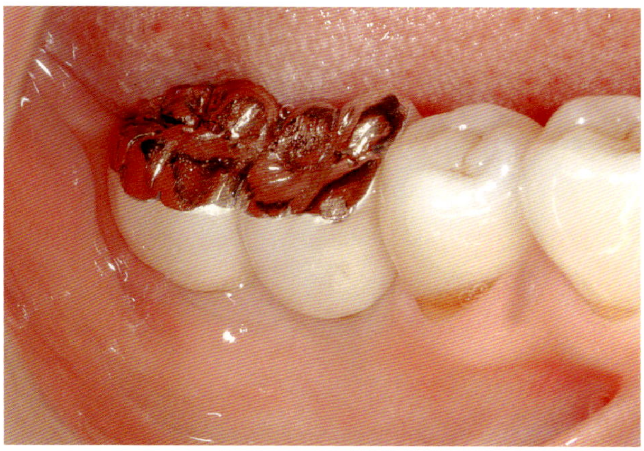

Fig 16-5-6 Intraoral view 20 months after implant placement.

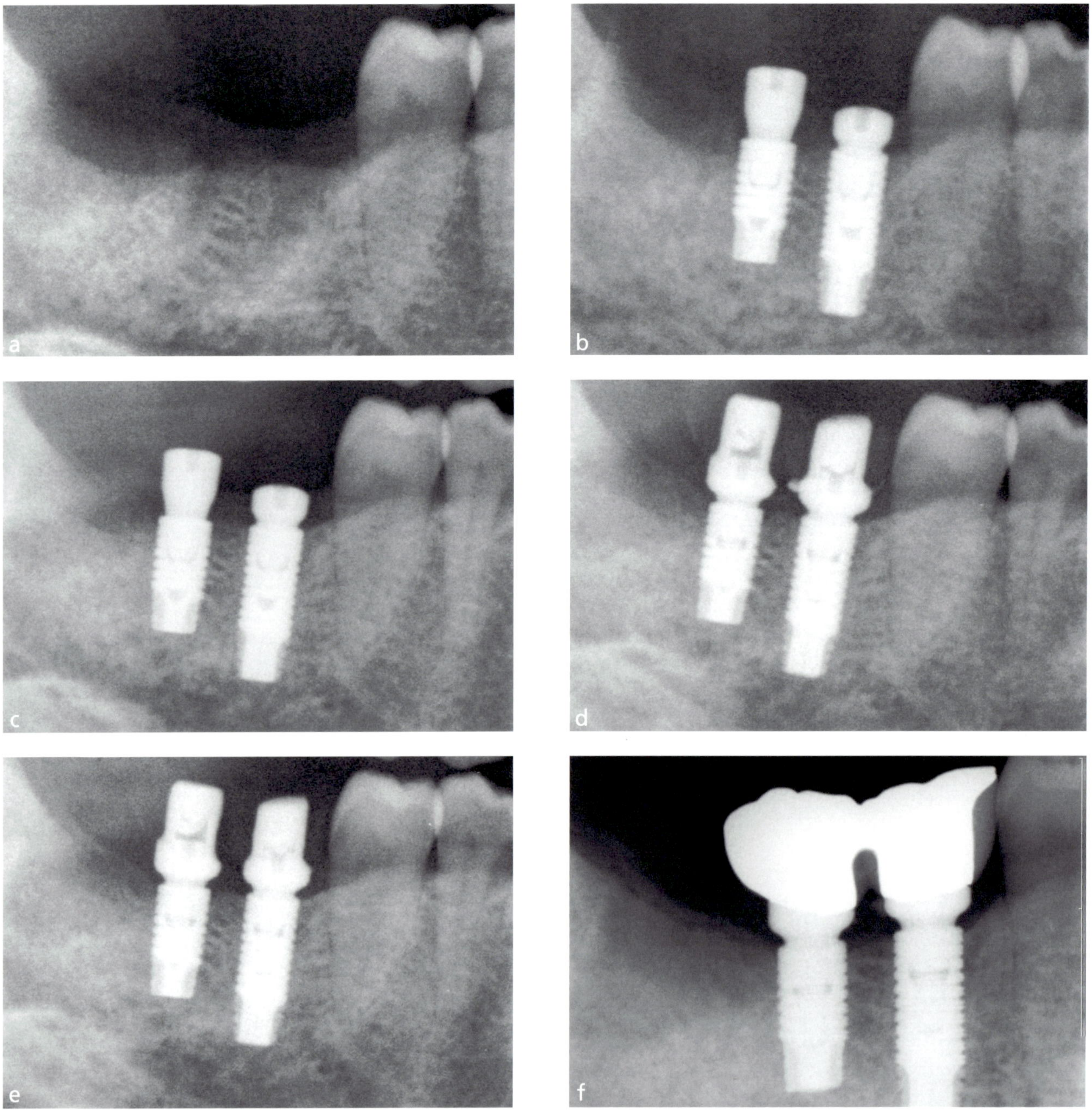

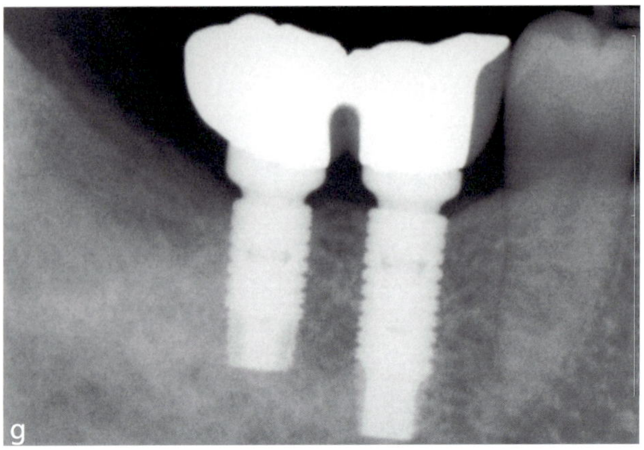

Fig 16-5-7 (a–g) Radiographs of the peri-implant bone at intervals.

Case 6: Flapless implant placement for a heavy smoker and drinker

A 58-year-old man visited the clinic for implant placement in regions that were missing teeth. He had lost multiple teeth through dental caries and periodontitis. Oral hygiene control was very poor. The patient was a heavy smoker and drinker. Implant placement was planned because of his strong demand for implants. The bone height from the alveolar crest to the antral floor was 5 mm at the upper right first molar site. Under general anesthesia, Astra implants were placed in the upper right first molar, upper left first premolar, upper left second premolar, lower left second premolar, lower right first molar, and lower right second molar sites. A simultaneous socket lift procedure was performed at the upper right first molar site. All implants were submerged using a mini-incision technique. At the time of implant placement, the insertion torques were all within the 26–40 Ncm range. The perio-test values of the implants measured immediately after implant placement ranged from −1 to −3. The patient was discharged from the hospital that same day. He did not experience any discomfort caused by postoperative edema or bleeding. One week after the surgery, the suture was removed. The implant covered with soft tissue at the first-stage surgery was not exposed prior to stage II uncovering. The stage II uncovering was performed 4 months after the implant placement using a mini-incision technique. Radiographs taken prior to the secondary surgery showed new bone formation around the implants in the maxillary sinus and also the healthy condition of the sinus. The patient was recalled after prosthetic fabrication every 4–6 months to evaluate his oral hygiene and to educate him about his responsibility to decrease plaque effectively. At a follow-up evaluation performed 24 months after the implant placement, peri-implant bone loss was 0.2 mm, and no inflammation was found in the peri-implant mucosa. The implant was considered successful.

Comment

For a heavy smoker and drinker with poor oral hygiene, the flapless implant surgery was performed using the mini-incision technique, and the implants were submerged. The procedure was successful. The margins of the crowns were placed above the gingival level to make plaque control easy. The patient continued smoking and drinking after the implant placement, but his oral hygiene improved considerably. In the case of a heavy smoker and drinker, flapless implant surgery performed via the mini-incision technique contributed to the implant success.

Table 16-6-1 Peri-implant bone loss at intervals.

	4 months	12 months	18 months	24 months
16	0.1 mm	0.2 mm	0.2 mm	0.3 mm
24	0.1 mm	0.1 mm	0.2 mm	0.2 mm
25	0.2 mm	0.2 mm	0.2 mm	0.2 mm
35	0.2 mm	0.3 mm	0.3 mm	0.3 mm
46	0.0 mm	0.0 mm	0.3 mm	0.3 mm
47	0.1 mm	0.1 mm	0.2 mm	0.2 mm

Table 16-6-2 Insertion torques and perio-test values at intervals.

	Insertion torque (Nm)	0 months	4 months	24 months
16	37	−1	−1	−1
24	26	−2	−3	−2
25	26	−1	−3	−2
35	35	−1	−3	−3
46	40	−3	−6	−6
47	34	−2	−4	−5

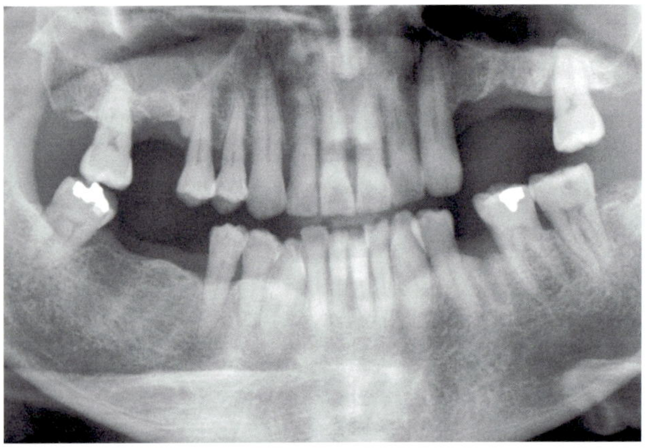

Fig 16-6-1 The condition of the patient at the first visit.

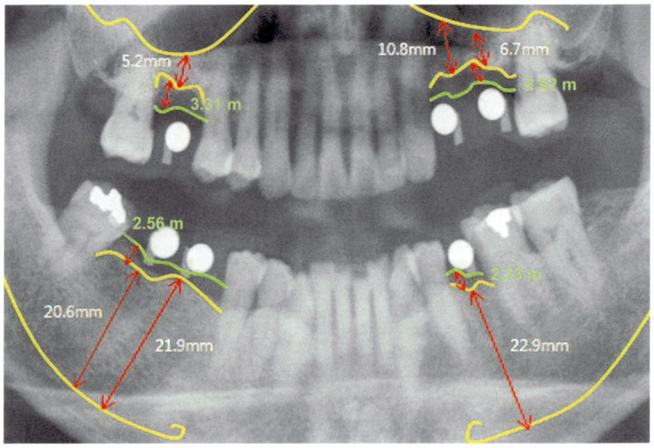

Fig 16-6-2 Radiograph showing the available bone height for implant placement and the thickness of the mucosa.

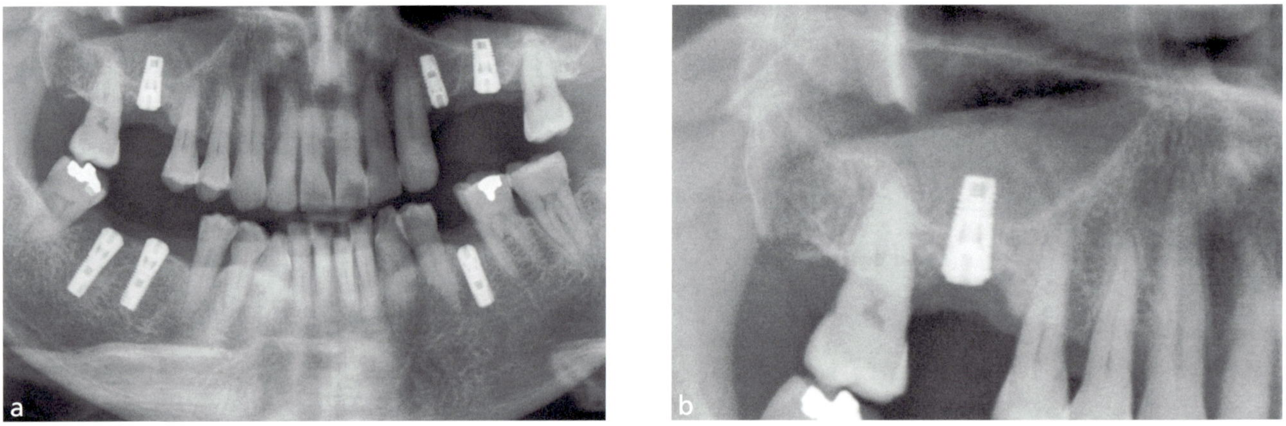

Fig 16-6-3 (a and b) Radiographs taken immediately after implant placement. The socket lift and the flapless implant placement are performed simultaneously at the upper right first molar site.

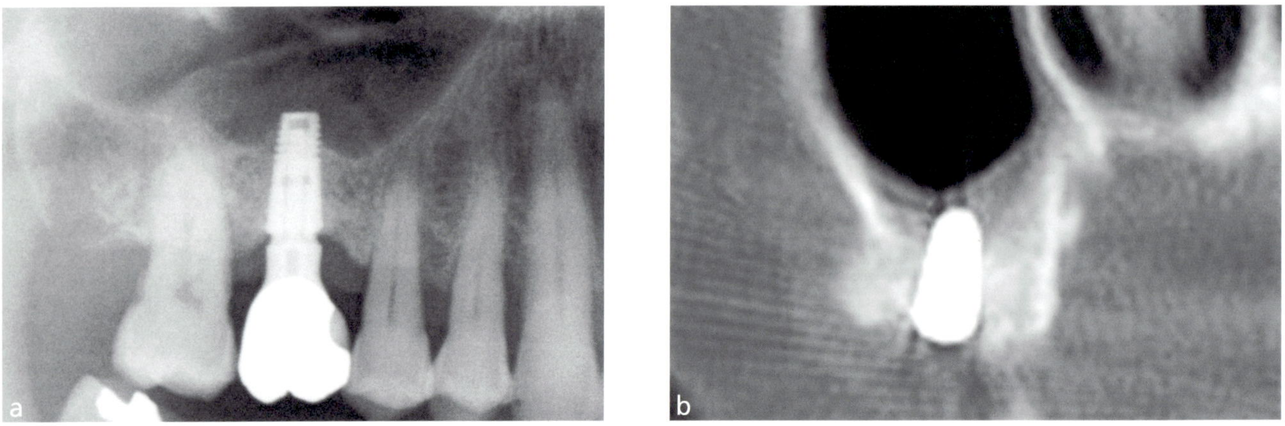

Fig 16-6-4 (a and b) Postoperative radiographs taken after 4 months indicate that bone has formed over the apex of the implant at the upper right first molar site, and the maxillary sinus is healthy.

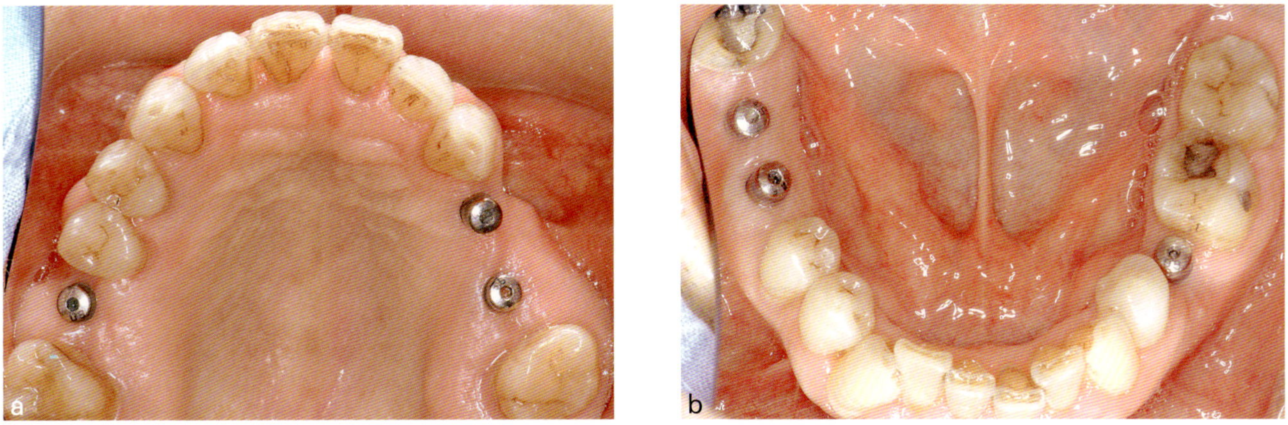

Fig 16-6-5 (a and b) Intraoral views immediately after the stage II uncovering procedure.

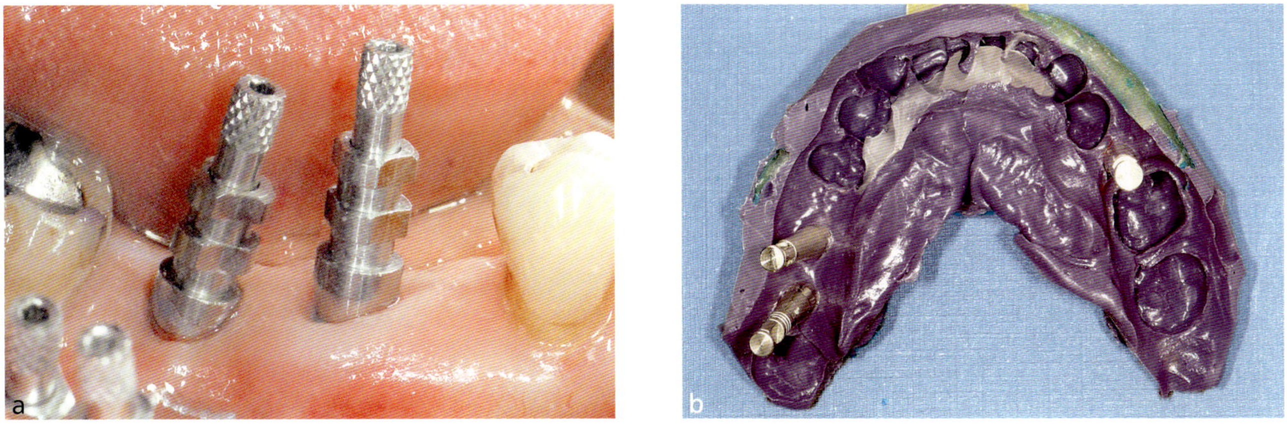

Fig 16-6-6 (a and b) One month after the uncovering procedure, impressions are taken for implant prosthetic treatment.

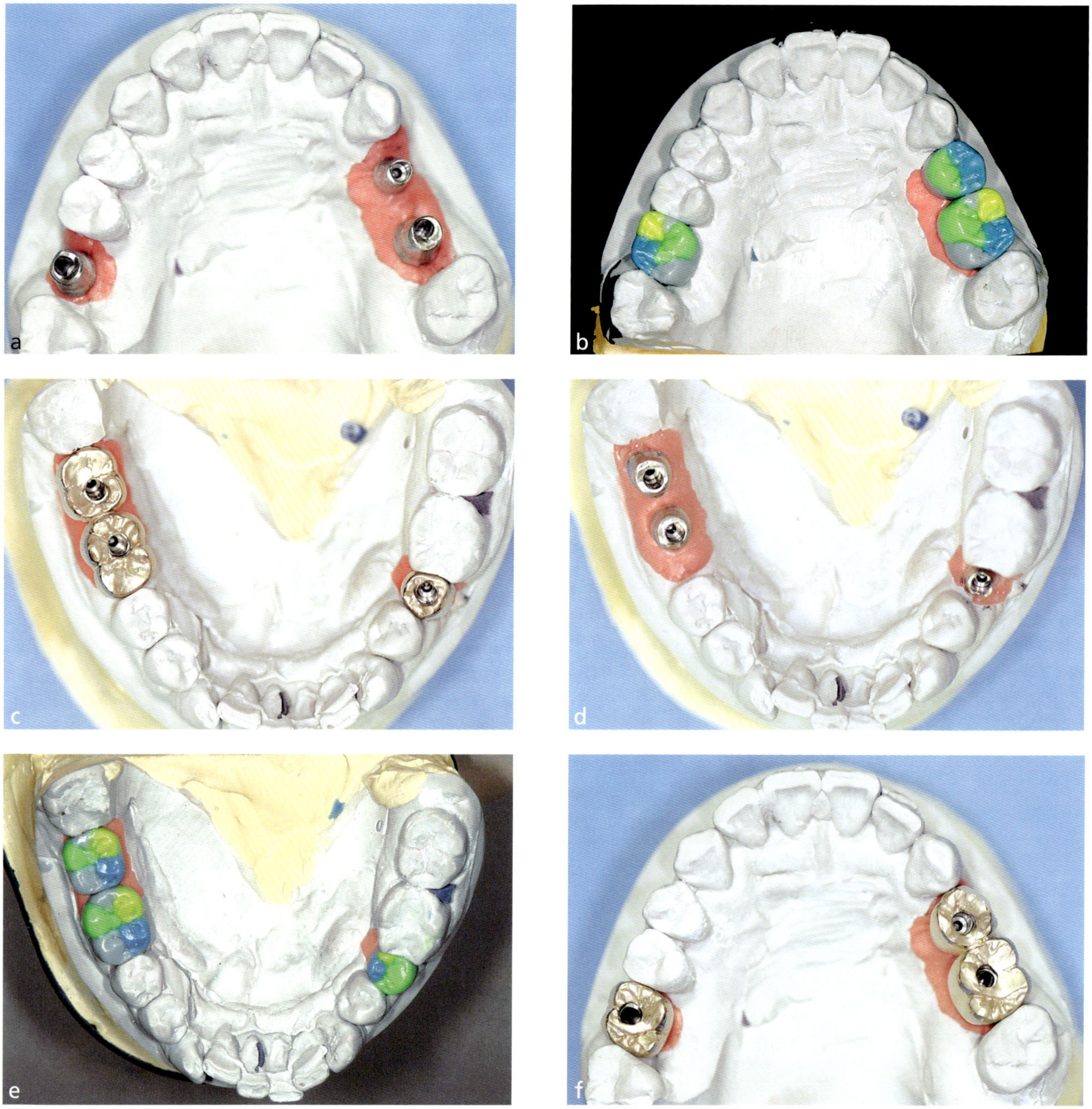

Fig 16-6-7 (a–f) Prostheses are made.

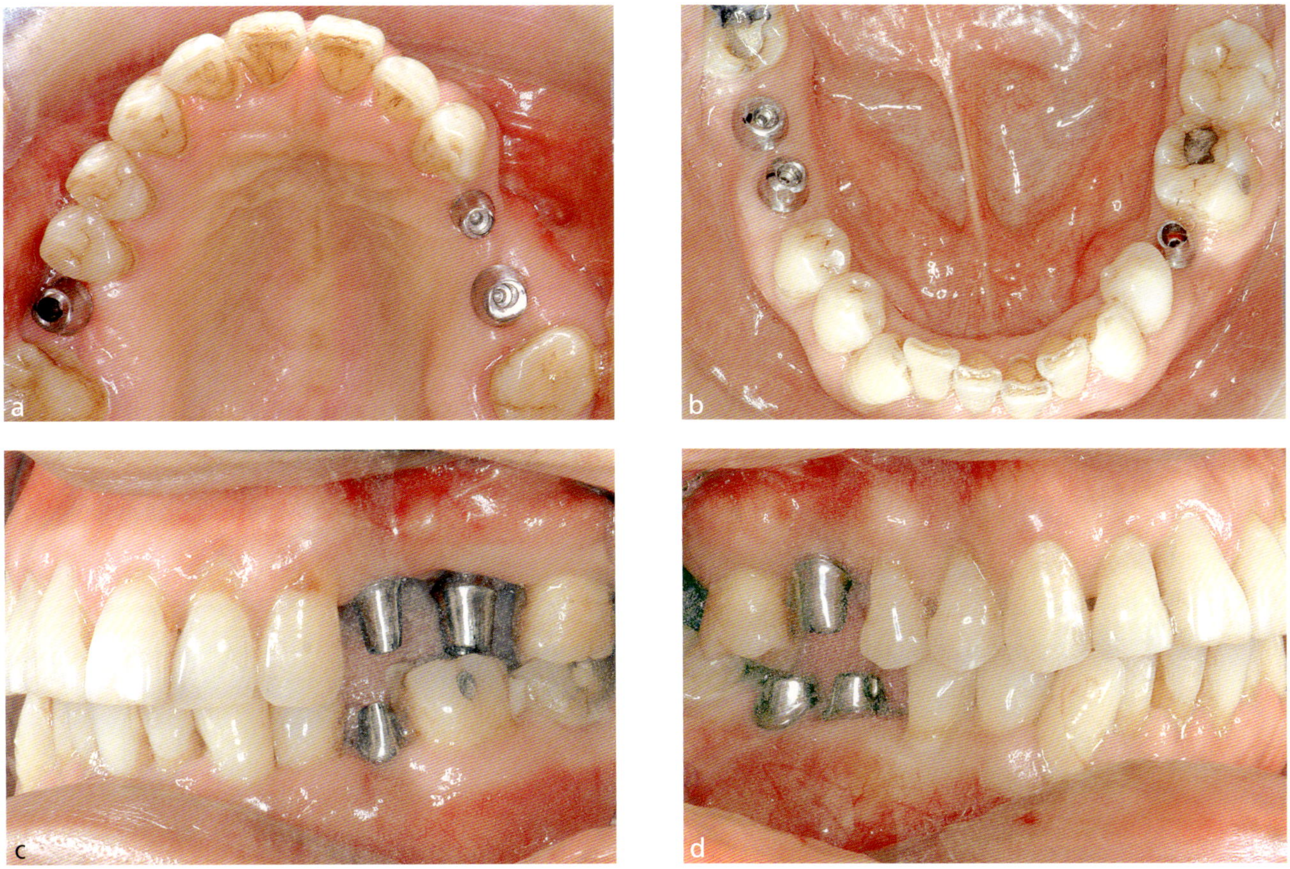

Fig 16-6-8 (a–d) Intraoral views showing a prosthetic abutment connected to the implant fixture.

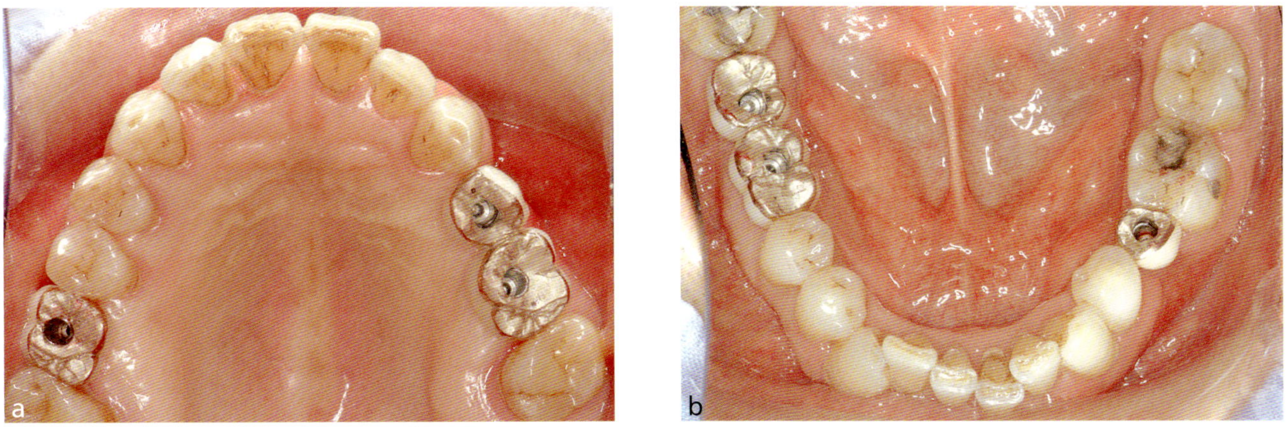

Fig 16-6-9 (a and b) Intraoral view showing the final prosthesis.

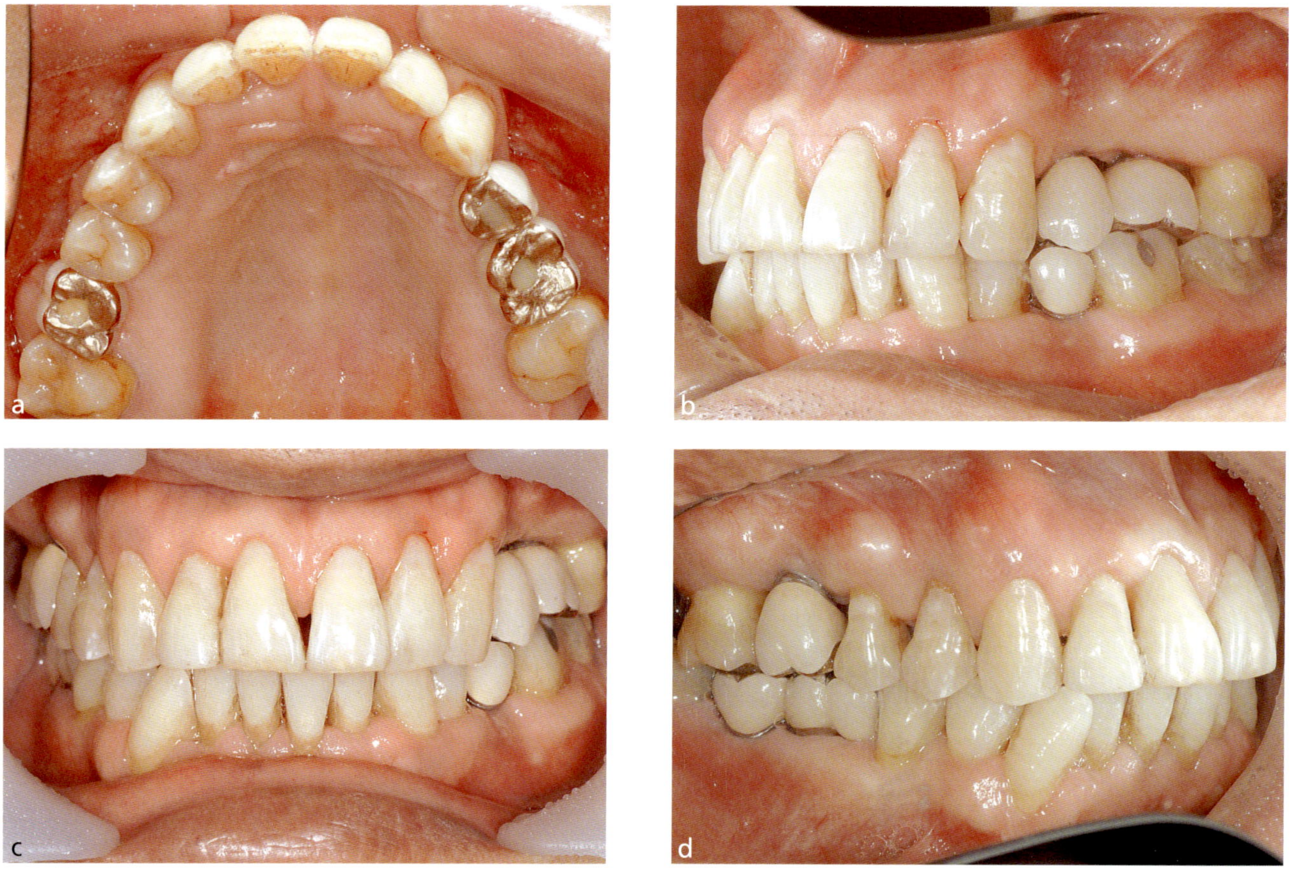

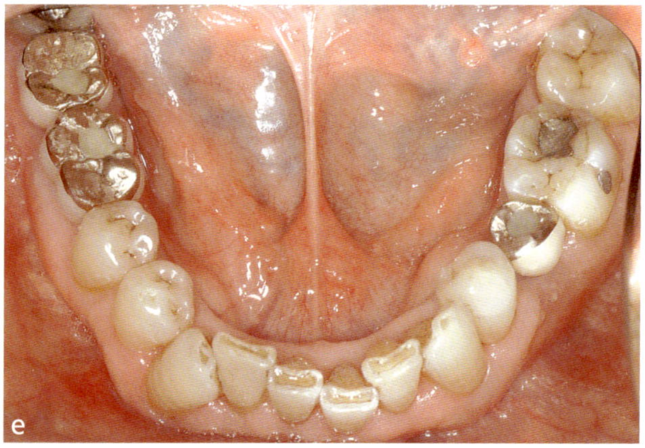

Fig 16-6-10 (a–e) Intraoral views at a follow-up evaluation performed 24 months after the implant placement.

Fig 16-6-11 (a–h) Radiographs of peri-implant bone at intervals.

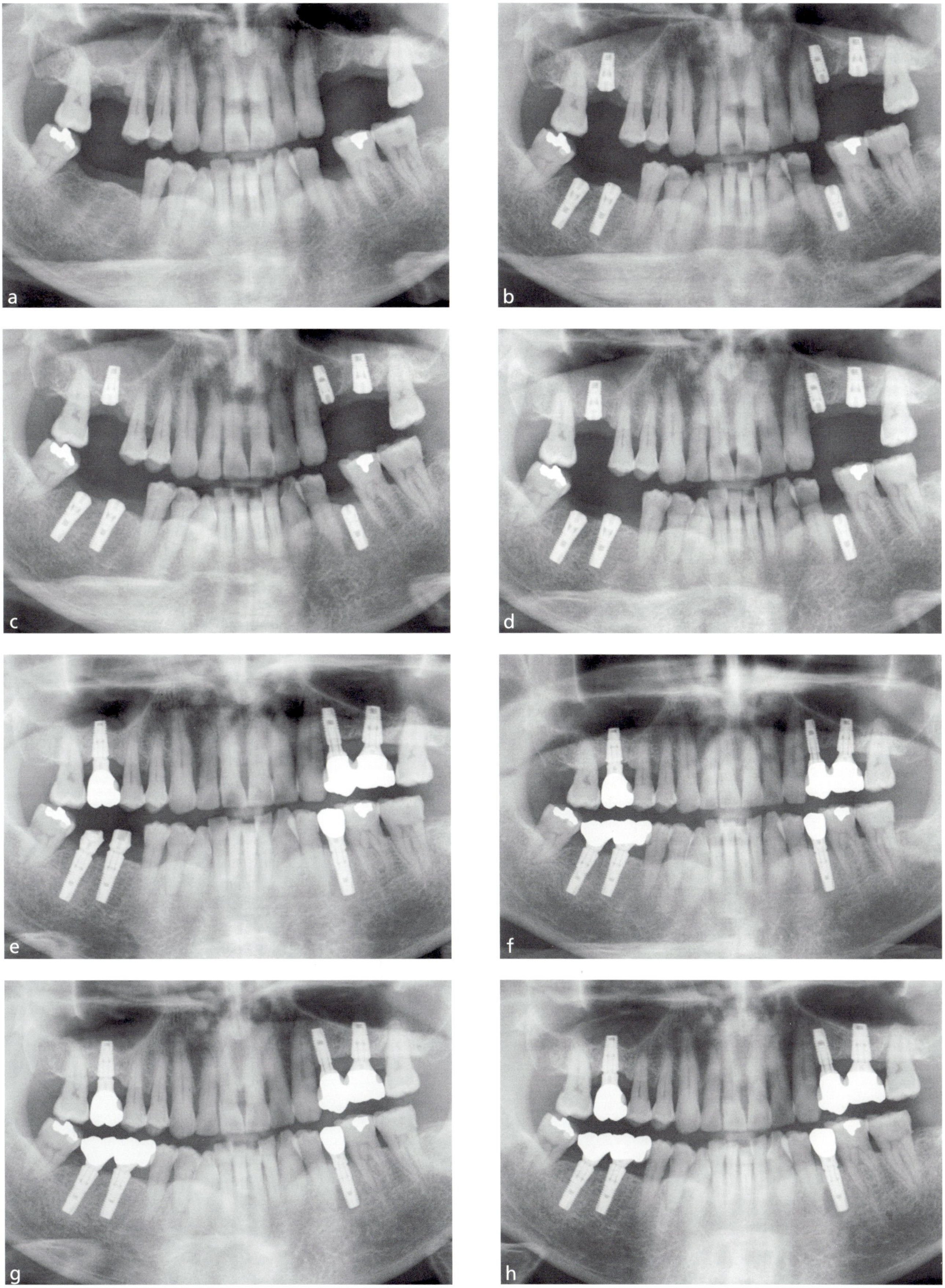
a
b
c
d
e
f
g
h

Case 7:
Flapless implant placement for a 76-year-old patient

A 76-year-old man visited the clinic for implant placement in the lower right posterior region. He was wearing a partial denture in the mandible but was strongly averse to using the denture. His first and second molars and first and second premolars were missing. The height from the inferior alveolar nerve to the alveolar crest in the region was higher than 15 mm. The width of the alveolar crest bone was sufficient for implant placement. Three Osstem implants (GSII 4.0 mm × 13 mm, 4.0 mm × 13 mm, and 4.0 mm × 11 mm) were placed in the region using the soft tissue punch technique, and then a permucosal healing abutment with a height of 4.5 mm × 3 mm was connected to the fixture. At the time of implant placement, bone quality was at the D2 level, and the insertion torques were 30 Ncm for the second premolar implant, 20 Ncm for the first molar implant, and 52 Ncm for the second molar implant. The perio-test values of the implants measured immediately after implant placement ranged from –2 to –3. Three months after placement, these values increased to the –3 to –5 range. A pretreatment prosthesis was used for 2 months to improve the bone quality before the fabrication of the final restoration.

Comment

Despite the patient's advanced age, the flapless implant surgery was successful. The implant stability improved over time. The patient did not experience postoperative discomfort or side-effects. The one-stage surgery saved the elderly patient discomfort and a second surgical procedure. At a follow-up evaluation performed 20 months after the implant placement, the average peri-implant bone loss was 0.2 mm, and no inflammation was found in the peri-implant mucosa. The implant was considered successful.

Table 16-7-1 Peri-implant bone loss at intervals.

	3 months	6 months	12 months	20 months
45	0.1 mm	0.2 mm	0.2 mm	0.2 mm
46	0.1 mm	0.1 mm	0.1 mm	0.2 mm
47	0.1 mm	0.2 mm	0.2 mm	0.2 mm

Table 16-6-2 Insertion torques and perio-test values at intervals.

	Insertion torque (Nm)	0 months	3 months	12 months
45	30	–2	–3	–5
46	20	–1	–3	–4
47	52	–4	–5	–5

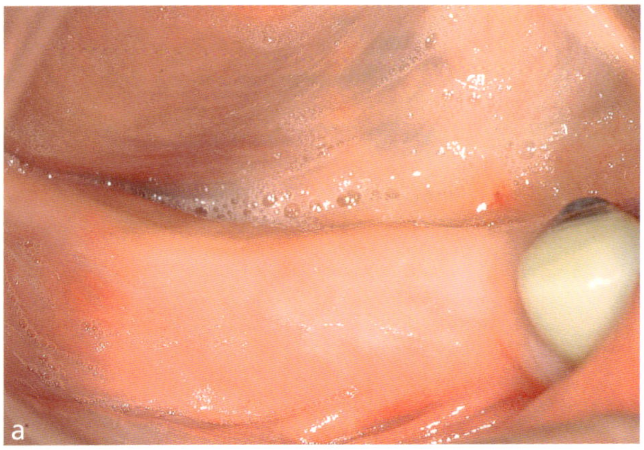

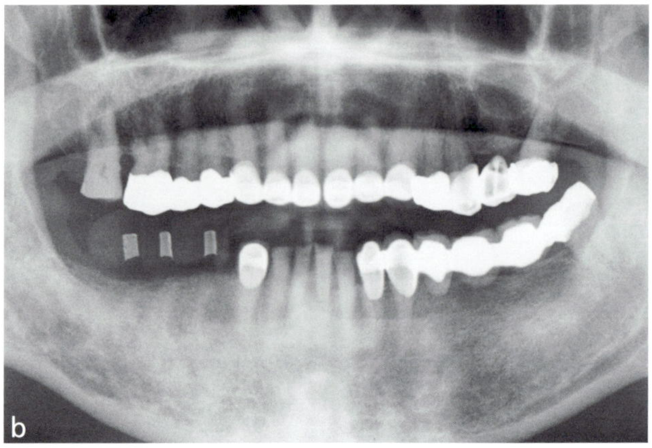

Fig 16-7-1 (a and b) The condition of the patient at the first visit.

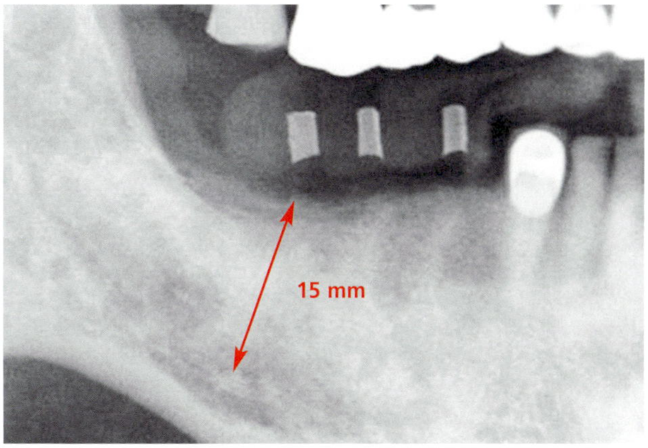

Fig 16-7-2 Radiograph showing the available bone height for implant placement.

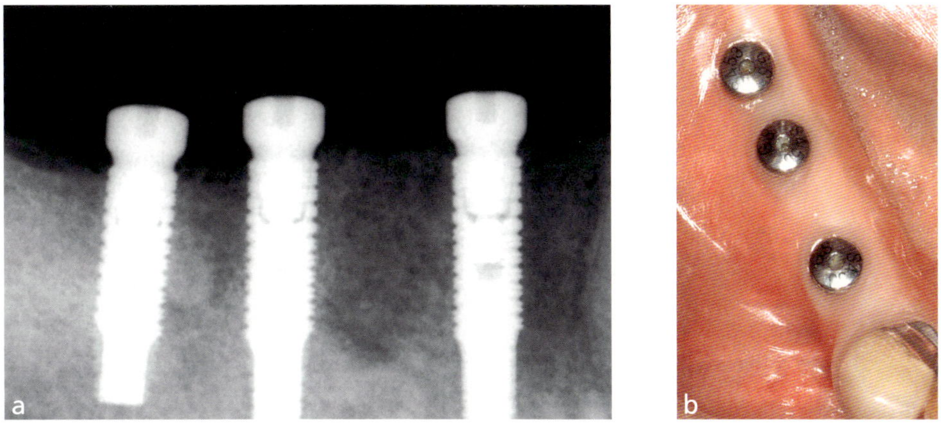

Fig 16-7-3 (a and b) Radiograph and intraoral view taken immediately after implant placement.

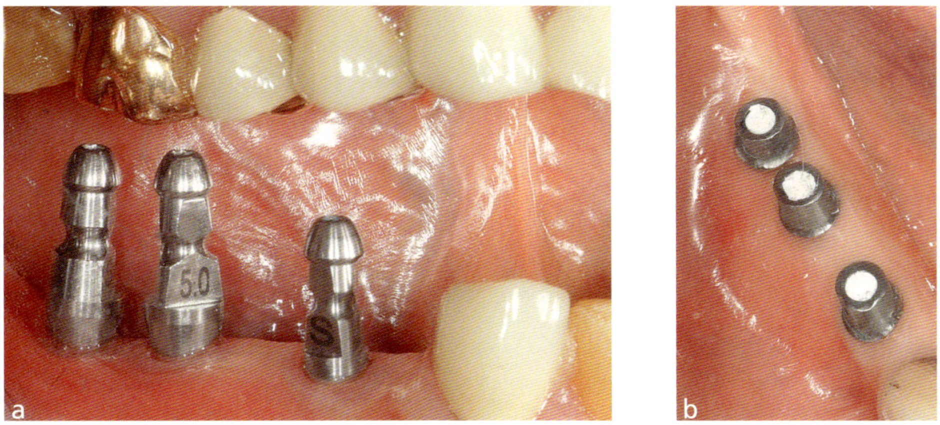

Fig 16-7-4 (a and b) Three months after implant placement, an intraoral view showing transfer abutments.

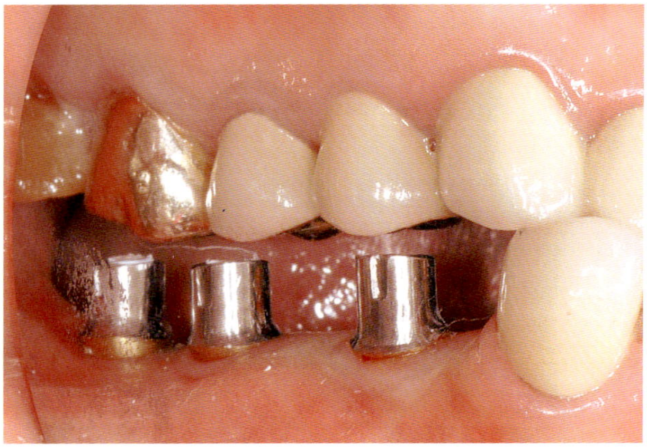

Fig 16-7-5 Intraoral view showing prosthetic abutments connected to the implant fixtures.

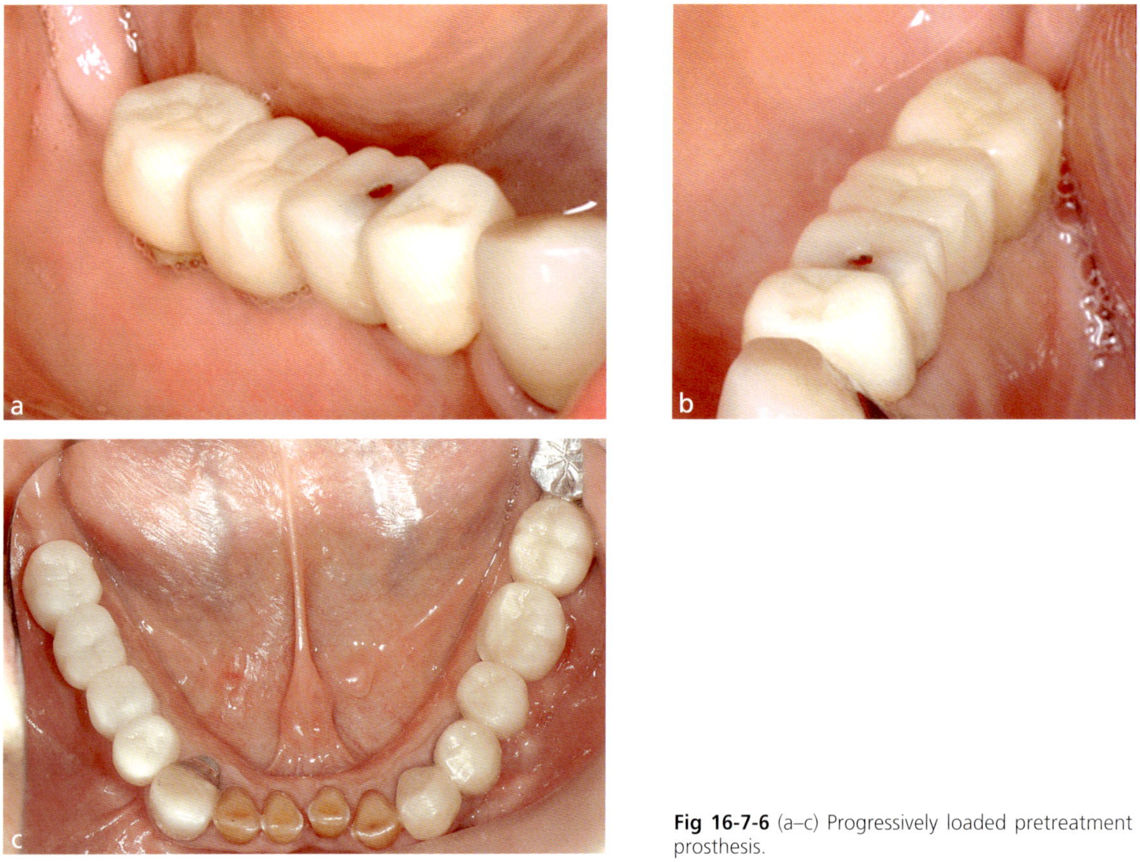

Fig 16-7-6 (a–c) Progressively loaded pretreatment prosthesis.

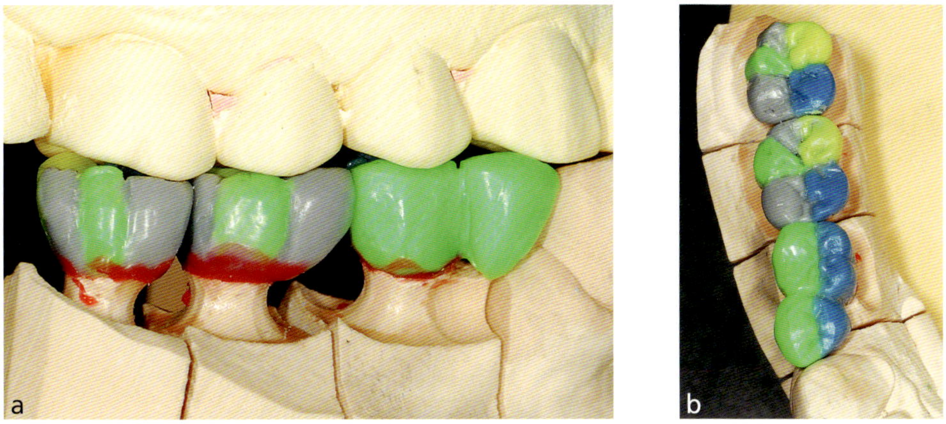

Fig 16-7-7 (a and b) Fabrication of the final prosthesis.

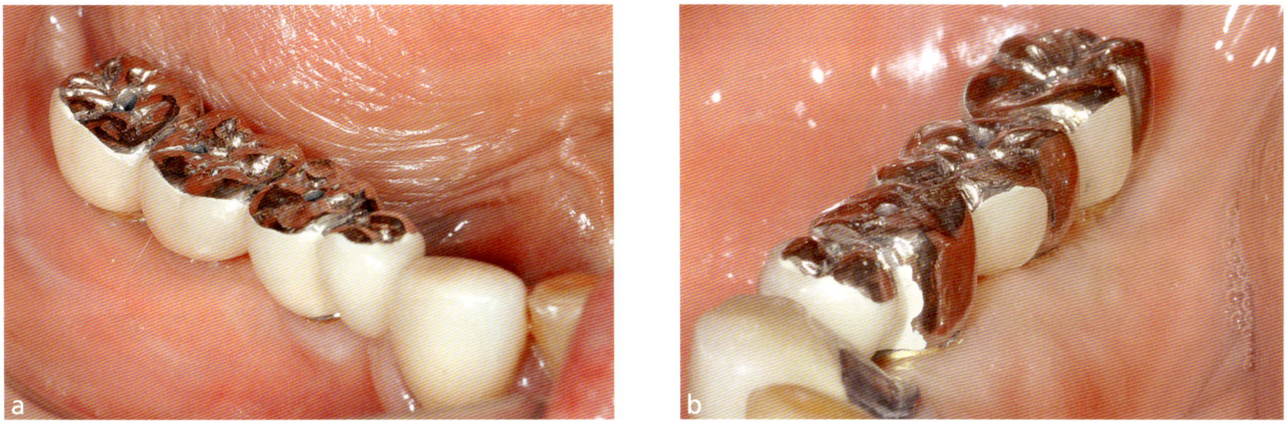

Fig 16-7-8 (a and b) Intraoral views showing the final prosthesis.

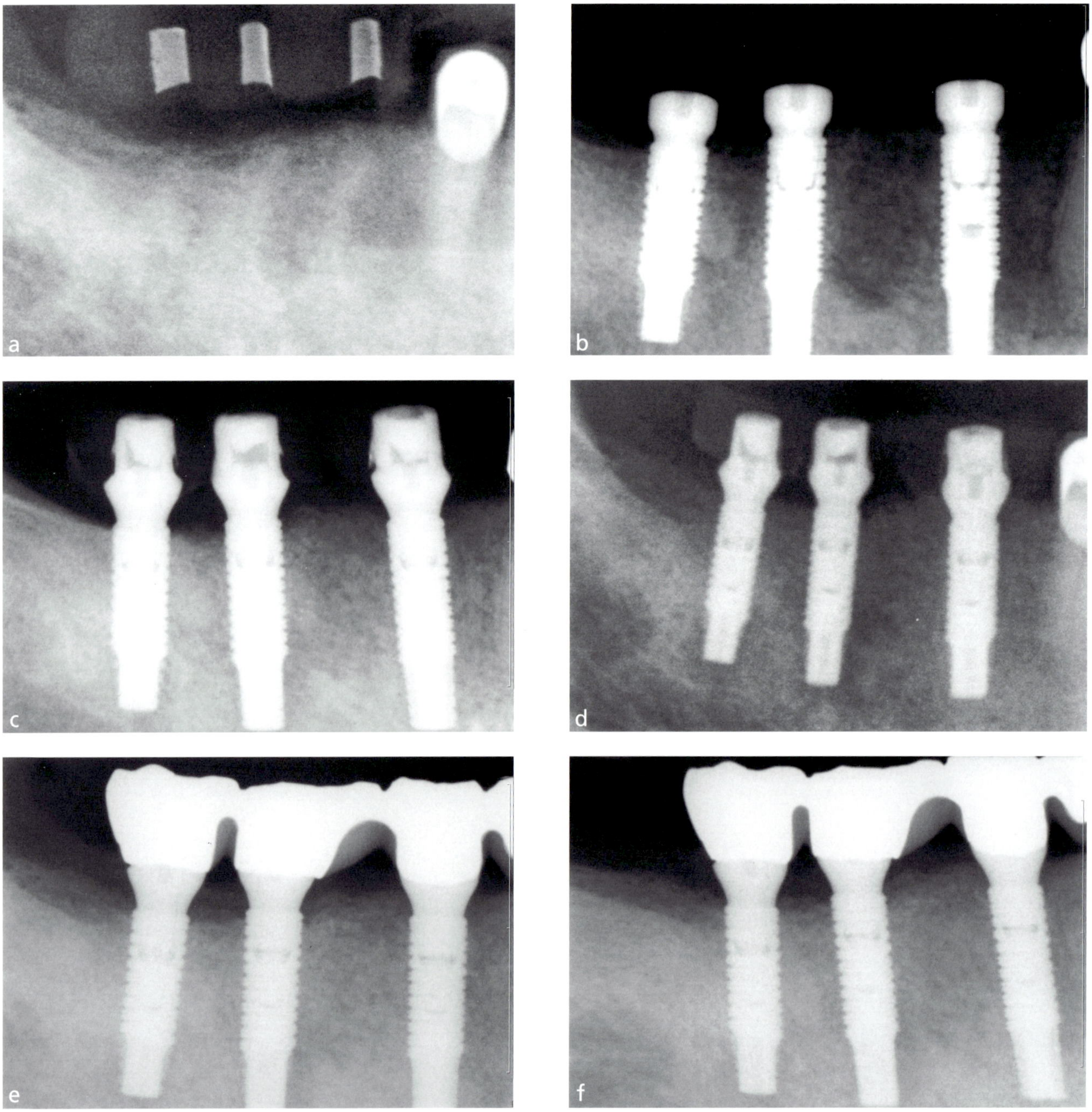

Fig 16-7-9 (a–f) Radiographs of peri-implant bone at intervals.

CHAPTER

17

Flapless Implant Surgery for Specific Implant Systems

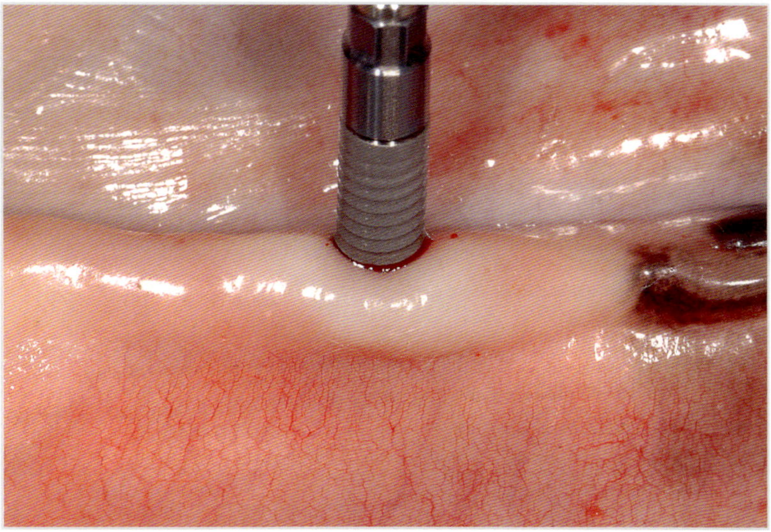

Key point

Flapless implant surgery can be performed even with different implant designs.

Overview

There are many implant body designs available in implant dentistry, which can be categorized as either bone level or soft tissue level types (Fig 17-1). The bone level type has the top surface of the fixture at the bone level so that the fixtures can be either submerged or not submerged at the time of flapless implant placement. The soft tissue level type has its top surface at the soft tissue level so that the coronal portion of the implant is likely to be exposed to the oral cavity at the time of implant placement. Submerging a soft tissue level implant below the soft tissue is difficult using a flapless implant procedure. This chapter addresses a flapless implant procedure using specific implant designs.

Implant body design

The implant body is designed to be placed into the bone to anchor prosthetic components. The implant body has a crest module, body, and apex (Fig 17-2).

The crest module is the portion designed to retain the abutment. There are three types of fixture–abutment relationship (Fig 17-3): a conical connection under the marginal bone, a conical connection above the marginal bone, and a flat-to-flat connection. The conical connection under the marginal bone level transfers the load deeper into the bone, reduces the peak stress, and preserves the marginal bone.[1] It also minimizes the micro-movements and micro-leakage.[2]

The implant crest module has a smooth collar that is often called a "cervical collar." Its dimension varies greatly from one system to another (0–5 mm). The bone level implant type has a short cervical collar, whereas the soft tissue level type has a long cervical collar that facilitates a one-stage surgical approach.

Effect of crest module on marginal bone loss

Hermann et al.[3] placed one-piece implants with a 1.5 mm smooth cervical collar below the bone in dogs. They reported that marginal bone loss occurred in the smooth collar 1.5 mm below the crestal region. Hanggi et al.[4] reported a longer, smooth metal collar with more crestal bone loss. These findings are in accordance with those of an animal study by the present authors. In canine mandibles, Osstem (Seoul, Korea) implants with a short collar, Astra Tech (Mölndal, Sweden) implants with a short collar, and CAMLOG® (Basel, Switzerland) implants with a long collar were placed below the crestal bone and submerged. These three implant designs were observed for 3 months. Marginal bone loss occurred at the smooth collar of the CAMLOG® implant below the crestal bone, which was related directly to the length of the smooth collar submerged (Fig 17-4). Therefore, the smooth cervical collar of the implant should not have an extended smooth area placed below the bone.

Implant designs suitable for flapless implant surgery

Implant systems designed for a one-stage surgical approach may be selected for a soft tissue punch method of flapless implant surgery. For a mini-incision method of flapless implant surgery, implant systems designed for a

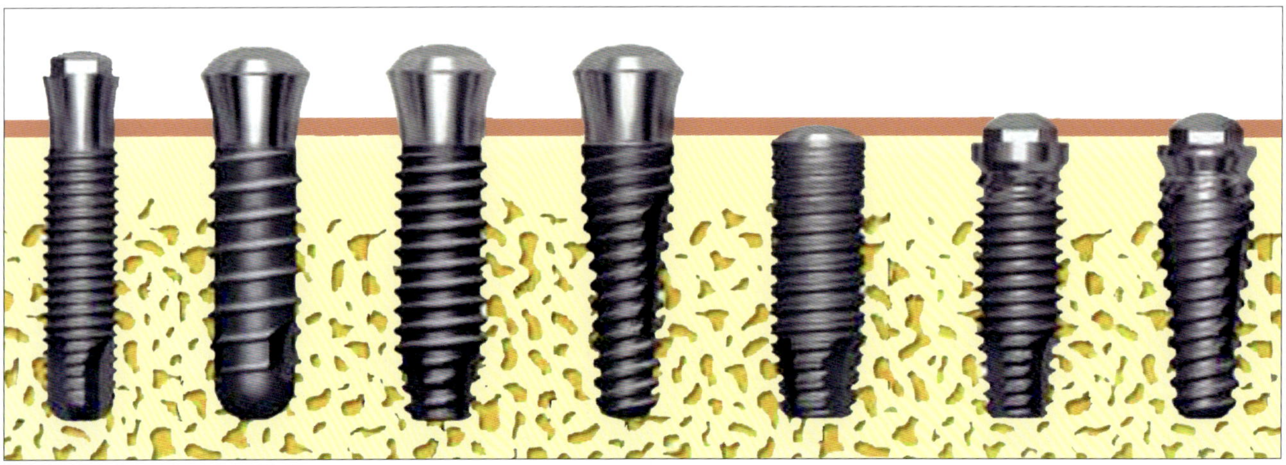

Fig 17-1 Various available implant body designs. They can be categorized as bone level or soft tissue level types.

two-stage surgical approach can be selected, but the implant system should have a low-profile cover screw as well as a shorter cervical collar (Fig 17-5). It is difficult to approximate the tissues required for primary closure of an implant when it has a high-profile cover screw or a longer metal collar. In addition, the risk of implant exposure is greater when the implant is extended further above the bone crest. Therefore, it is prudent to select an implant system for a mini-incision technique, in which the top of implants can be placed at the same level as the alveolar crest (Fig 17-6).

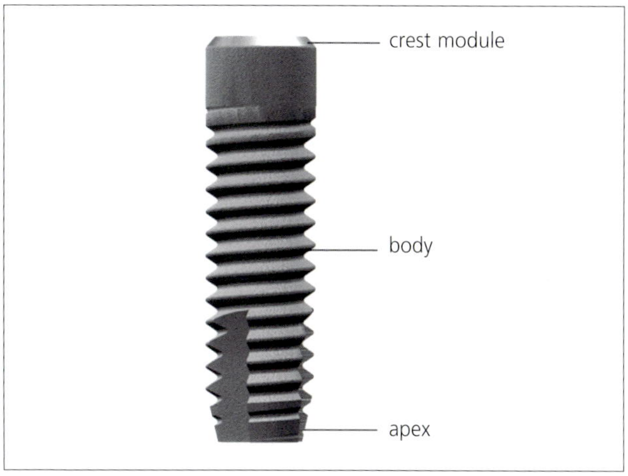

Fig 17-2 The implant body has a crest module, body, and apex.

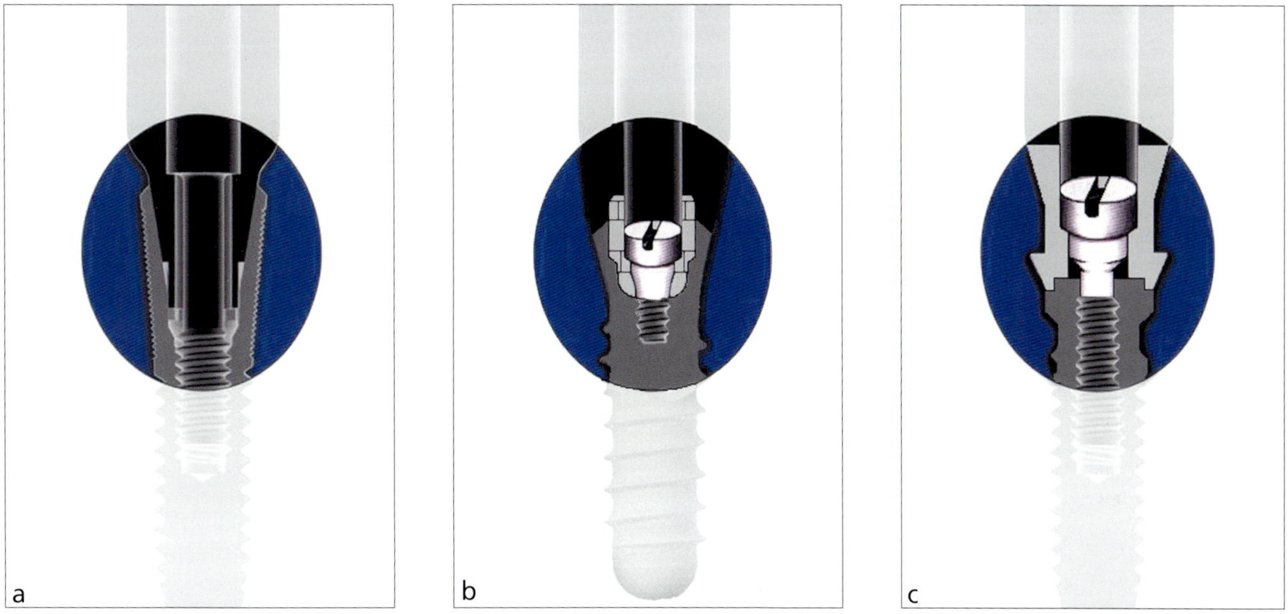

Fig 17-3 Three types of fixture–abutment relationship: (a) conical connection under the marginal bone; (b) conical connection above the marginal bone; (c) flat-to-flat connection above the marginal bone.

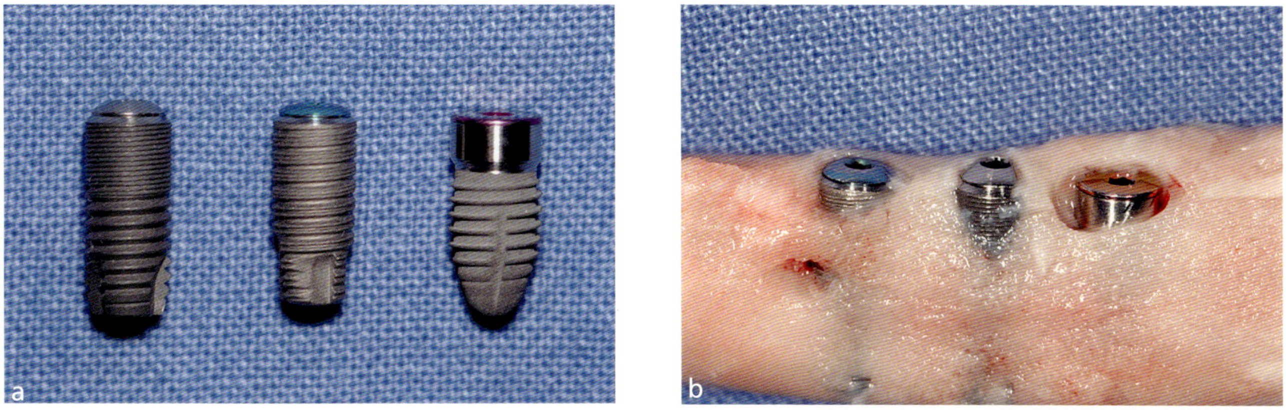

Fig 17-4 (a and b) In canine mandibles, an Osstem implant with a short collar, an Astra Tech implant with a short collar, and a CAMLOG® implant with a long collar (a: left to right) were placed below the crestal bone and submerged. These implant designs were observed for 3 months. Marginal bone loss occurred along the smooth collar of the CAMLOG® implant below the crestal bone, which was related directly to the length of the smooth collar.

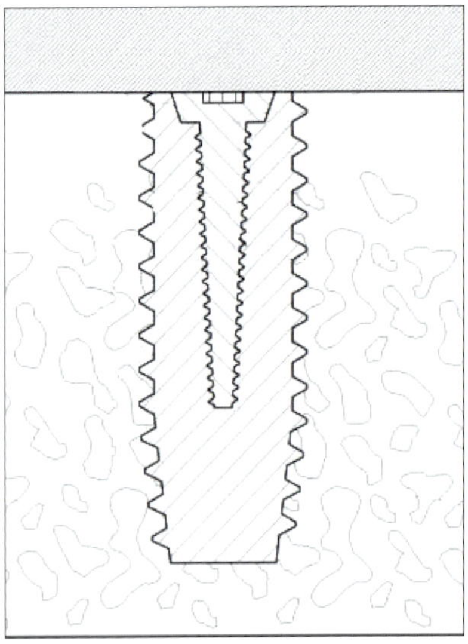

Fig 17-5 This implant design is more specific for the mini-incision submersion procedure because it has no cervical collar.

Most commercially available implant drilling systems are designed for flap implant surgery and may be unsuitable for flapless surgery. The drills for flapless surgery require the protection of the mucosa while drilling, as well as sufficient length to allow for the cutting of bone through the soft tissue. The drills need to have stops or depth lines inscribed on their shanks to control the depth of drilling above the mucosa (Figs 17-7 and 17-8). These depth lines should include a line that is longer than the sum of the fixture length and mucosal thickness. Short-step drills do not allow deep drilling in bone through the soft tissue (Fig 17-9).

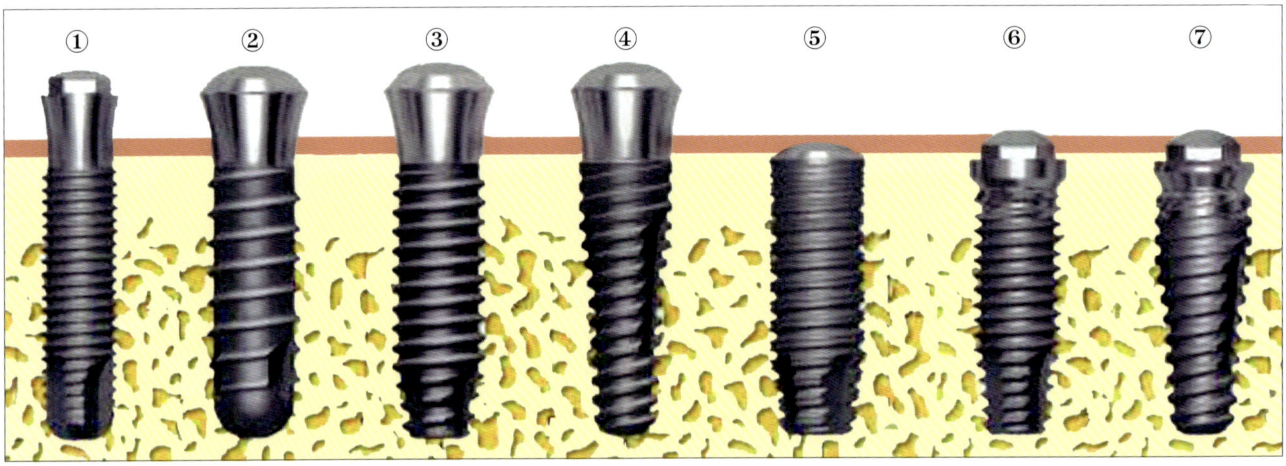

Fig 17-6 For the mini-incision submersion procedure, the implant system should have a low-profile cover screw and a low-profile cervical collar. Among the various types of implant available, the most suitable is no. 5.

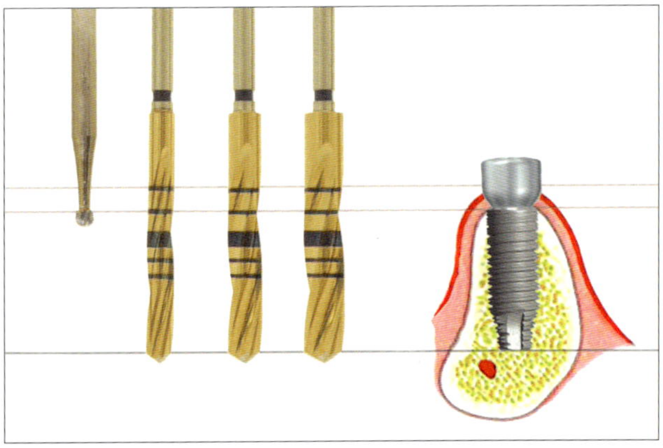

Fig 17-7 Drills for flapless surgery in the mandible. The drills require depth lines inscribed on their shanks to control the drilling depth above the mucosa.

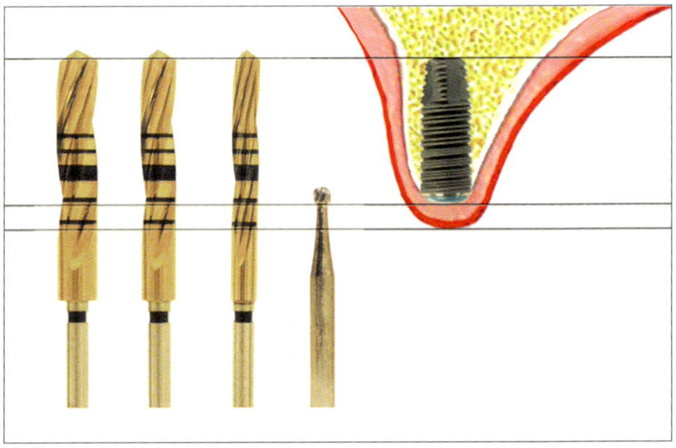

Fig 17-8 Drills for flapless surgery in the maxilla. To control the depth of drilling above the mucosa, the drills require depth lines inscribed on their shanks.

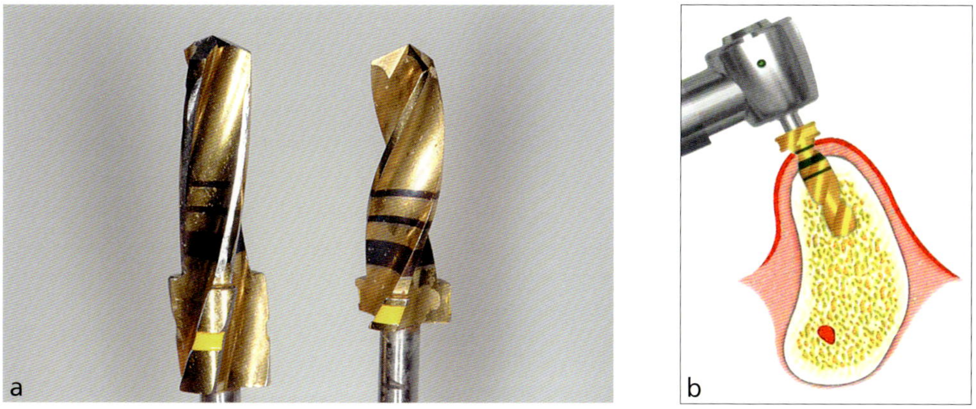

Fig 17-9 (a and b) Short-step drills do not allow deep drilling through the soft tissue.

Flapless implant surgery for Straumann Implants

Straumann (Basel, Switzerland) soft tissue level implants (Fig 17-10) have a smooth neck section, 2.8 mm in length, and are especially suitable for a soft tissue punch method of flapless implant surgery, where the implants are placed at the soft tissue level and not covered with soft tissue during the healing phase. The implants have an internal octagonal connection (Straumann synOcta) with its corresponding prosthetic components above the marginal bone (Fig 17-11). The implants have either sandblasted, large-grit, acid-etched (SLA) surfaces or a chemically enhanced SLActive surface. The SLActive surface, which is hydrophilic, is known to increase earlier blood vessel formation, cellular activity, and bone apposition around the implants better than the standard SLA surface, resulting in significantly earlier implant stability (Fig 17-12).[5–7] Moreover, the SLActive implants stabilize more quickly without flap elevation than with flap elevation. Flapless implant surgery plays a crucial role in enhancing implant stability.

The Straumann soft tissue level implants with long metal collars make it difficult to submerge the implant using a mini-incision flapless procedure. The problem with this design is that it will encourage marginal bone loss if the smooth crest module is placed below the crest of the bone.[8] As a result, this type of implant should be used for a one-stage surgical approach and not to place the smooth cervical collar below the bone when the implants are placed using a flapless procedure.

Recently, a new bone level implant was added to the Straumann® Dental Implant System and is available with diameters of 3.3, 4.1, and 4.8 mm and lengths of 8, 10, 12, and 14 mm (Fig 17-13). The implant has a conical connection with its abutment under the marginal bone (Fig 17-14). The rough surface of the implant extends to the top and its closure screw has a low profile (0 or 0.5 mm height). Therefore, the top of the implant can be placed at

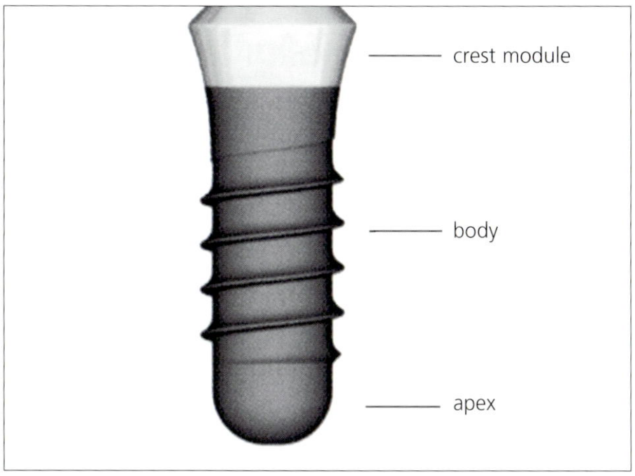

Fig 17-10 Straumann soft tissue level implants.

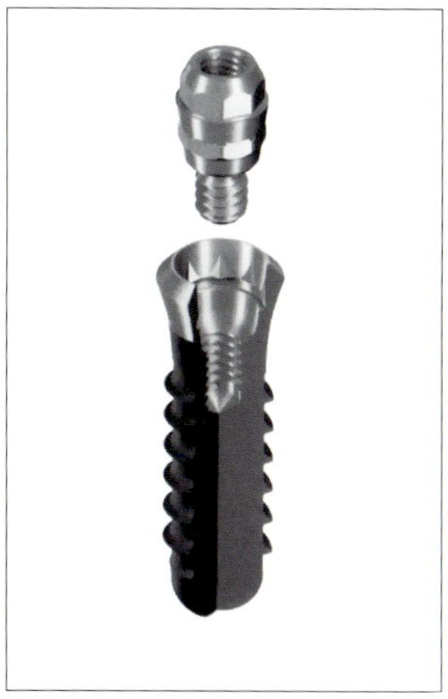

Fig 17-11 The Straumann soft tissue level implant has an internal octagonal connection with its corresponding prosthetic components above the marginal bone.

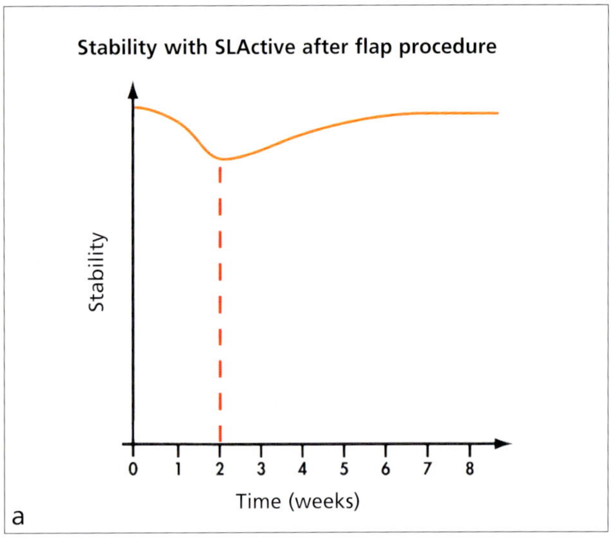

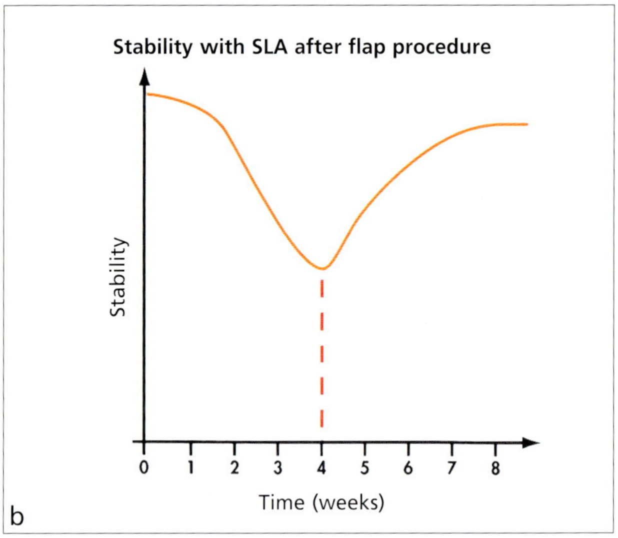

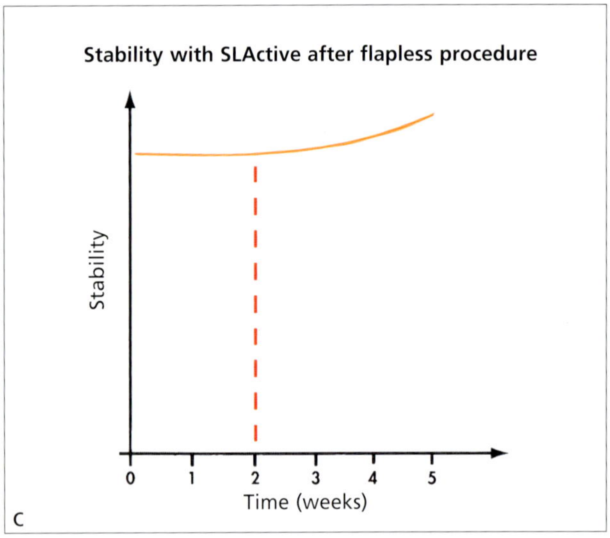

Fig 17-12 (a–c) The SLActive surface increases implant stability earlier than the standard SLA surface. The SLActive implants stabilize more quickly without flap elevation than with flap elevation.

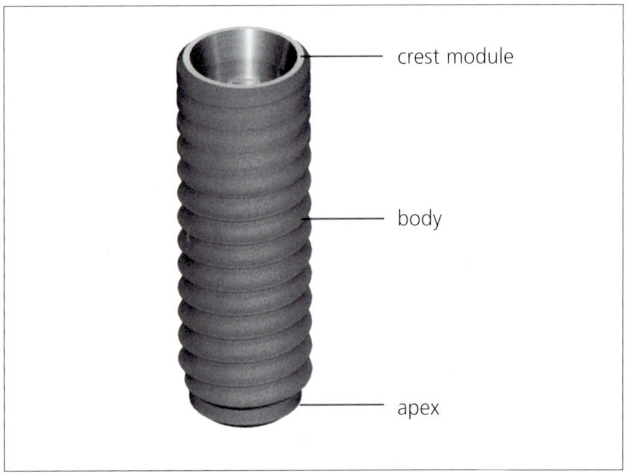

Fig 17-13 Straumann bone level implant.

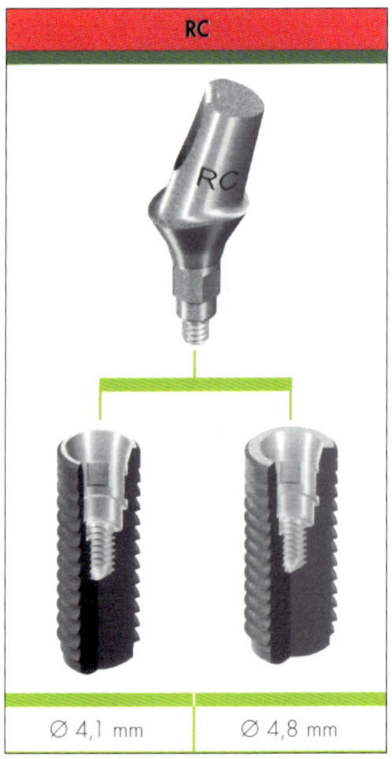

Fig 17-14 The Straumann bone level Implant has a conical connection with its abutment under the marginal bone.

the same level as the alveolar crest. This means that Straumann bone level implants can be submerged easily using a mini-incision flapless procedure. These implants provide intraoperative flexibility in determining whether to use submerged or nonsubmerged flapless procedures. The following surgical method involves the use of bone level implants.

The incision

An incision is made based on the selection of surgical method: mini-incision or soft tissue punch.

- *Incision for the mini-incision technique.* A crestal mini-incision, approximately 5 mm horizontally with the alveolar crest, is made at the center of the implant site (Fig 17-15). Local undermining of the gingiva is then performed (Fig 17-16). During the undermining procedure, the soft tissue on both sides of the incision line is pushed aside to accommodate the drills and implants.
- *Incision for the soft tissue punch technique.* A circumferential incision is made in the gingiva at the center of the implant site using a soft tissue punch (Fig 17-17) and the incised attached gingiva is then removed with a curette (Fig 17-18) or mosquito hemostat (Fig 17-19). The soft tissue punch should be 1.0–1.5 mm narrower than the implant diameter (Fig 17-20). Multiple punches are recommended when more than two implants are placed (Fig 17-21).

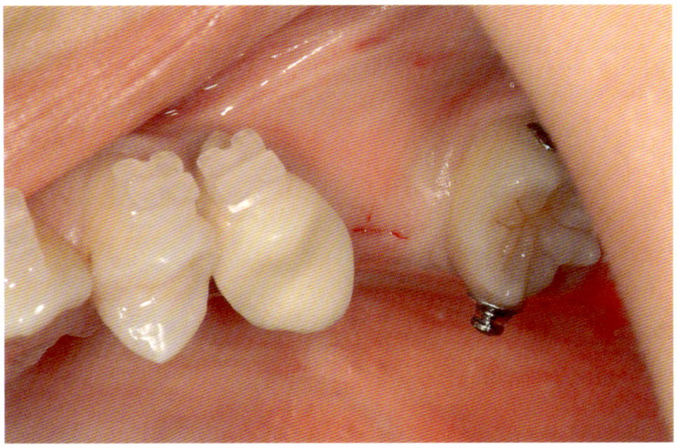

Fig 17-15 For the mini-incision implant placement, a crestal mini-incision, approximately 5 mm in length, is made at the center of the implant site, parallel to the alveolar crest.

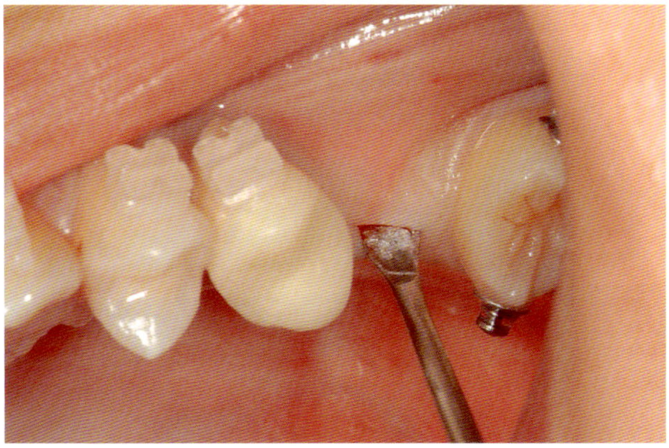

Fig 17-16 Local undermining of the gingiva is performed to allow the entrance of the drill and implants.

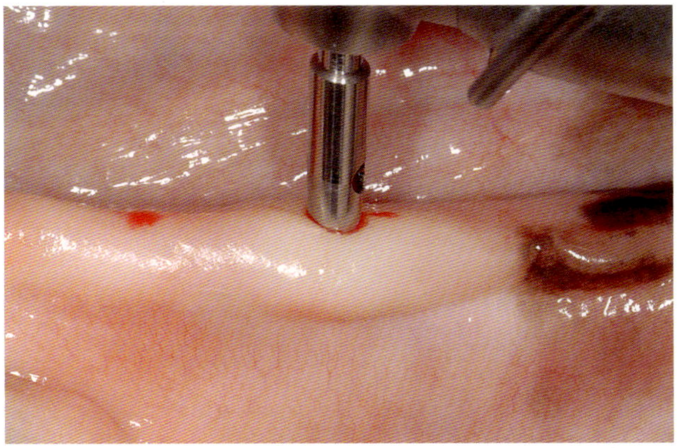

Fig 17-17 For soft tissue punch implant placement, a circumferential incision is made in the gingiva at the center of the implant site using a soft tissue punch. The punch should be 1.0–1.5 mm narrower than the implant diameter.

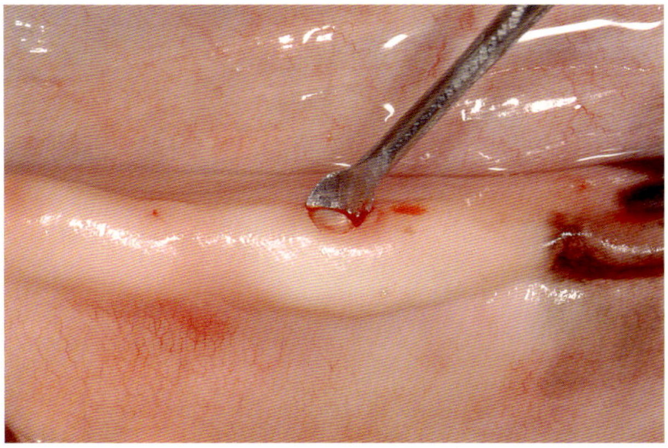

Fig 17-18 Local undermining of the incised attached gingiva is performed using a curette.

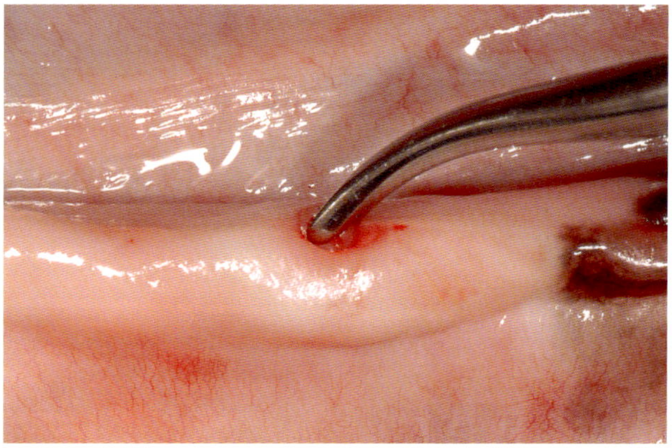

Fig 17-19 The incised attached gingiva is removed with a mosquito hemostat.

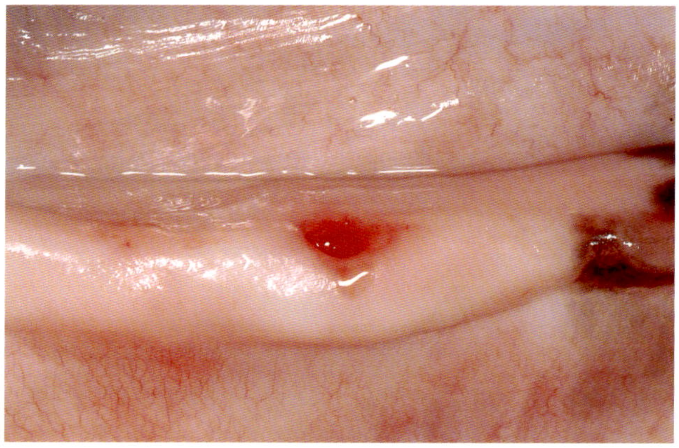

Fig 17-20 The implant site after removing a core of soft tissue over the crestal bone.

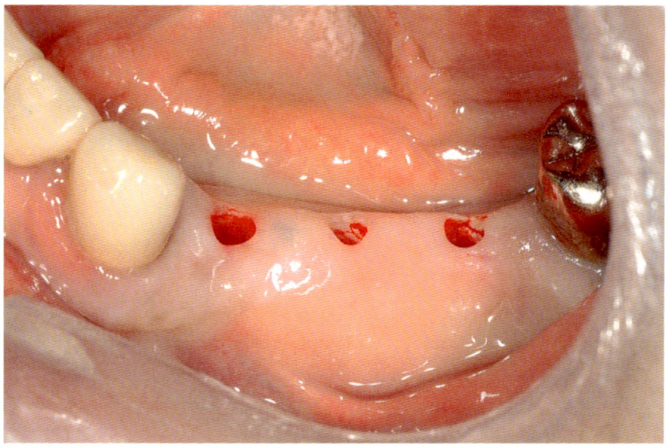

Fig 17-21 Multiple punches are recommended when more than two implants are placed.

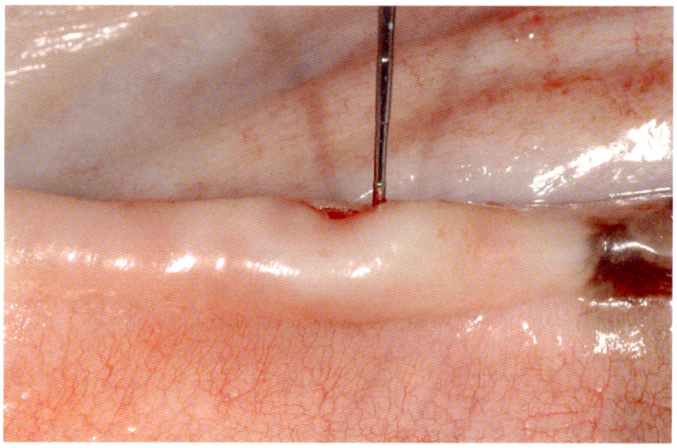

Fig 17-22 The mucosal thickness is measured using a periodontal probe before drilling.

Measurement of the thickness of soft tissue

Before drilling, the mucosal thickness is measured using a periodontal probe or a depth gauge to confirm the height of the mucosa at the implant site (Fig 17-22).

Drilling

The center implant site is marked with a round bur and prepared with a pilot drill for the initial depth of bone preparation of the implant length. The osteotomy preparation proceeds according to the drill sequence (Figs 17-23 to 17-26). Straumann Standard Plus, Tapered Effect, and Bone Level implants require additional profile drilling to prepare the coronal section of the osteotomy (Fig 17-27). The correct use of the profile drill is important for inserting the implant to the planned depth because it has a slightly conical core in the coronal region. The drilling depth above the mucosa is controlled by marks on the drills that correspond to the sum of the length of the implant and the thickness of the mucosa. To protect the adjacent mucosa while drilling, it is advisable to use flapless implant drills with cutting surfaces on their tips and rounded surfaces on the other parts (Figs 17-28 and 17-29).

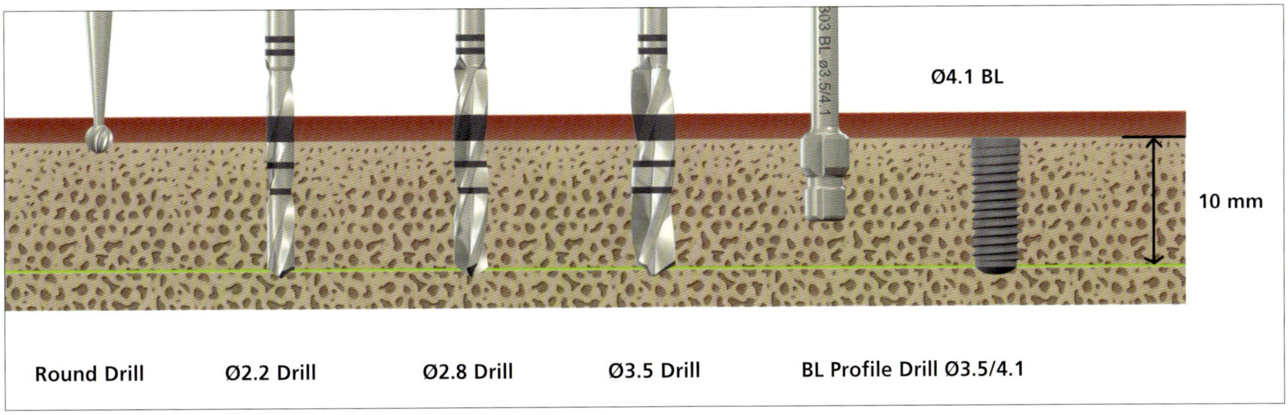

Fig 17-23 Implant site preparation for the Straumann 4.1 mm diameter Bone Level implant.

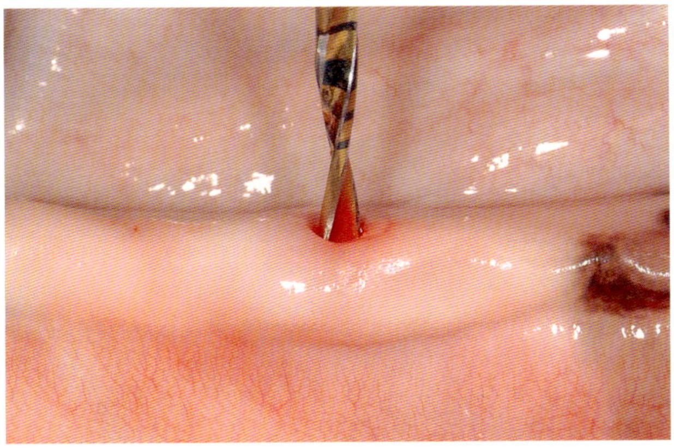

Fig 17-24 A 2.2 mm diameter end-cutting starter drill is used under copious sterile saline.

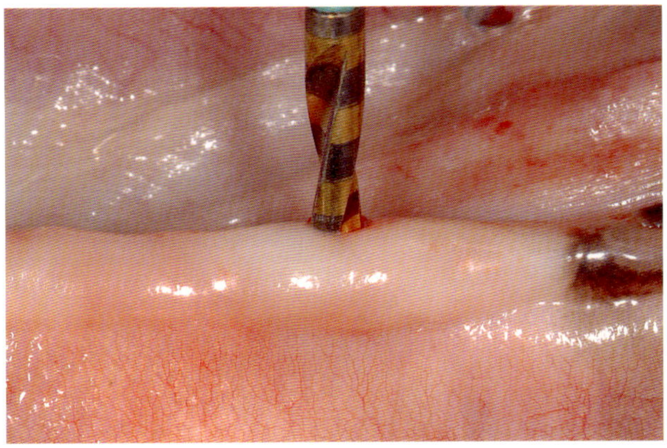

Fig 17-25 A 2.8 mm diameter drill is inserted into the initial osteotomy and prepares the bone.

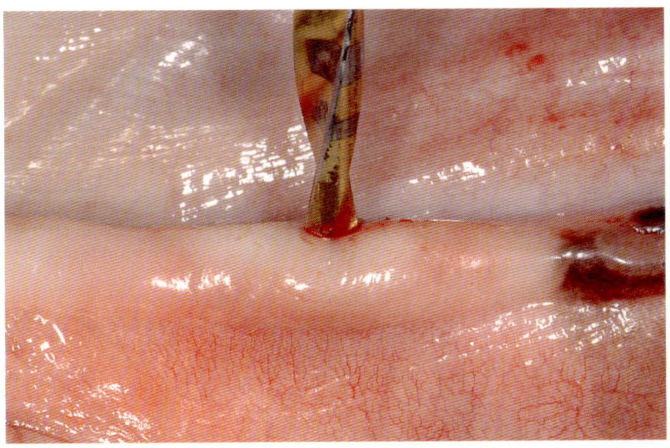

Fig 17-26 A 3.5 mm diameter drill is used to prepare the final diameter for a 4.1 mm bone level implant body.

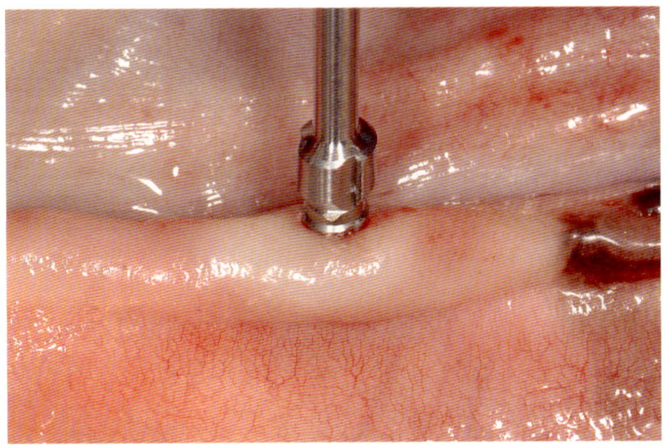

Fig 17-27 A profile drill prepares the coronal section of the osteotomy, as the coronal region of the implant is larger than the implant body.

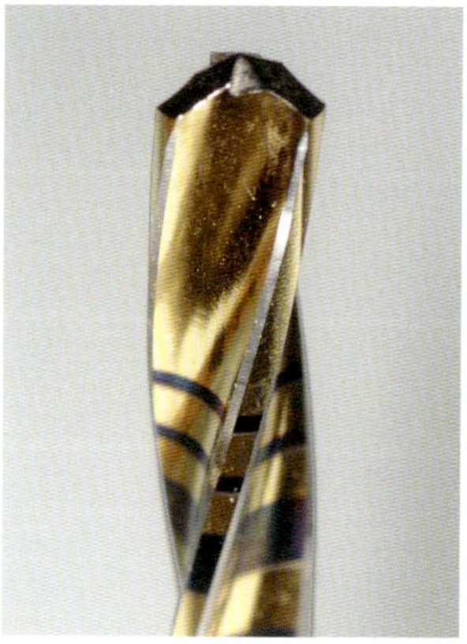

Fig 17-28 A drill for flapless implant surgery has a cutting surface on the tip and rounded surfaces on the other sides.

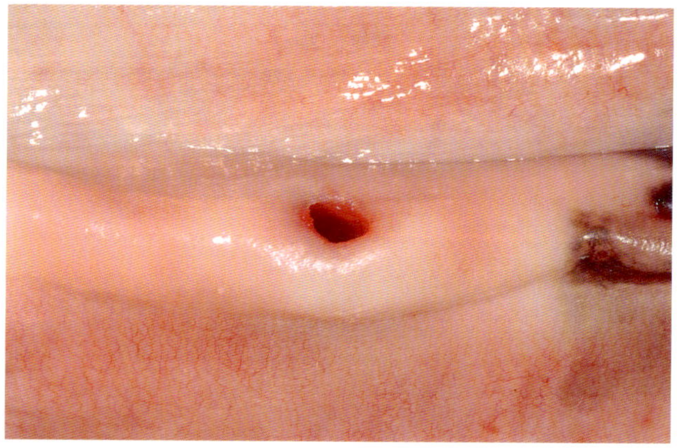

Fig 17-29 The implant site after drilling. Note the adjacent mucosa is well protected while drilling.

Implant placement

A low-speed handpiece (Fig 17-30) or a hand wrench is used to place the implants, which allows more precise implant rotation, and a constant pressure ensures that the implant will progress into the site without a risk of stripping the bone within the threads (Fig 17-31). The insertion torque should not exceed 35 Ncm because excessive pressure at the implant–bone interface at the time of insertion can cause bone loss.[9] The transfer part height is used to control the depth of the implant fixture above the mucosa (Figs 17-32 and 17-33). Immediately after placing bone level implants (Fig 17-34), peri-implant probing around the implant should be performed to confirm that the implant shoulder is located at the level of the bone crest (Fig 17-35).

- *Soft tissue punch technique.* After placement of the implant, a permucosal healing abutment is inserted for the one-stage surgical approach (Fig 17-36). The permucosal healing abutment should extend 1–2 mm above the adjacent mucosa to help to prevent tissue overgrowth during the healing period (Fig 17-37). The permucosal healing abutment should be 1.0–1.5 mm wider than the soft tissue punch in order to ensure close contact between the peri-implant mucosa and the healing abutment.
- *Mini-incision technique.* After placement of the implant, either a low-profile closure screw is inserted into the implant body for the two-stage approach or a permucosal healing abutment is inserted for the one-stage approach (Fig 17-38). For the two-stage approach, the tissues are then approximated over the implant for primary closure. One interrupted suture is sufficient to allow primary closure of the soft tissue (Fig 17-39).

A post-insertion periapical radiograph should be made once the implant is in its final position in order to identify the implant depth, opposing landmarks, adjacent roots, and position of the crest module and crest of the bone (Fig 17-40).

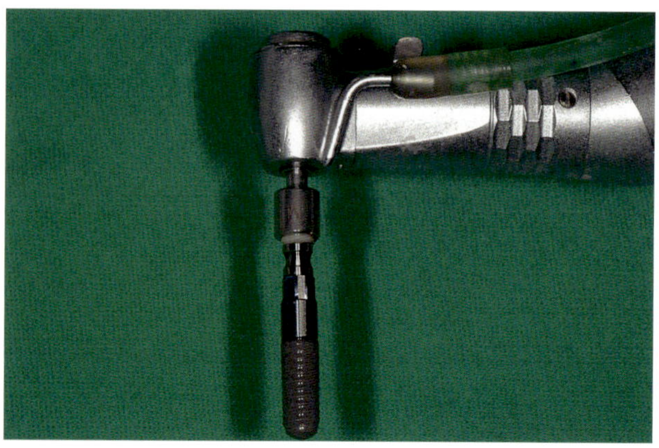

Fig 17-30 A low-speed handpiece is used to place the implant.

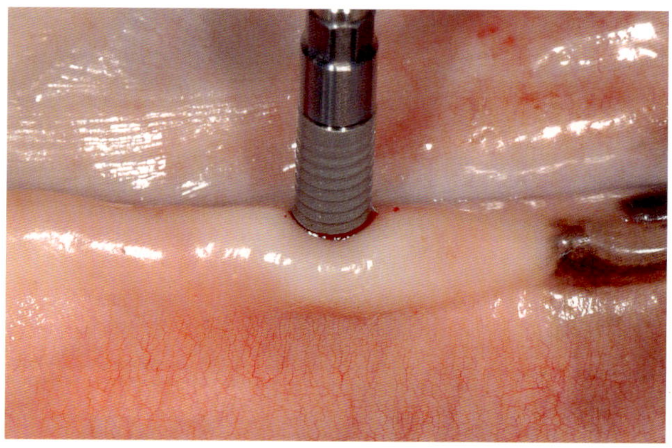

Fig 17-31 The implant is inserted into the osteotomy with a handpiece at reduced speed.

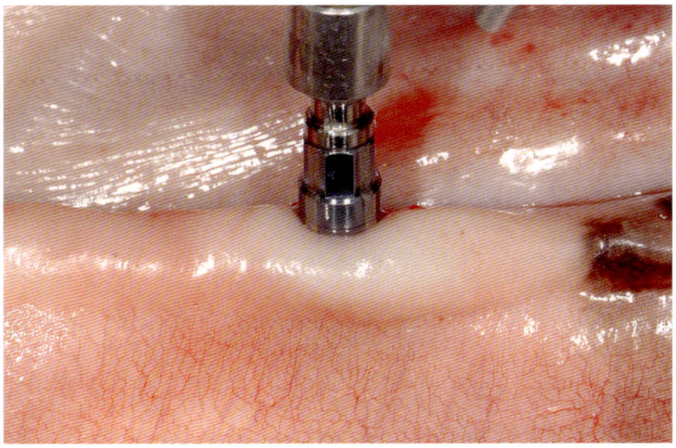

Fig 17-32 The transfer part height is used to control the depth of the implant fixture above the mucosa.

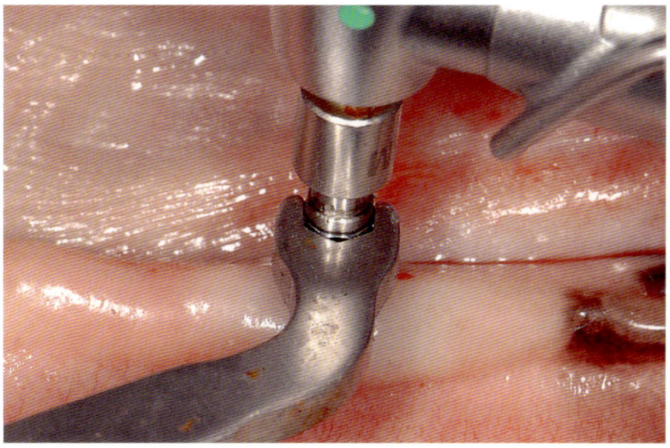

Fig 17-33 The transfer part is removed once the implant is in final position.

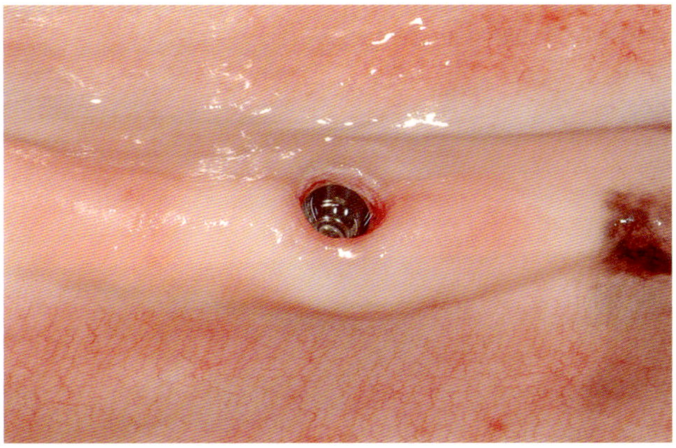

Fig 17-34 The implant shoulder is located apical to the gingival margin.

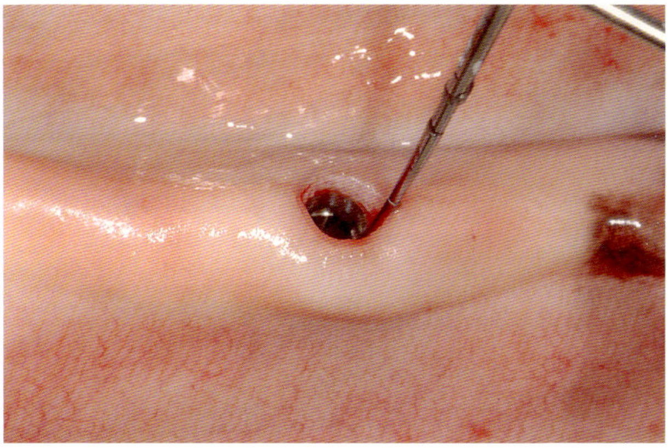

Fig 17-35 Peri-implant probing around the implant is carried out to confirm that the implant shoulder is located at the level of the bone crest.

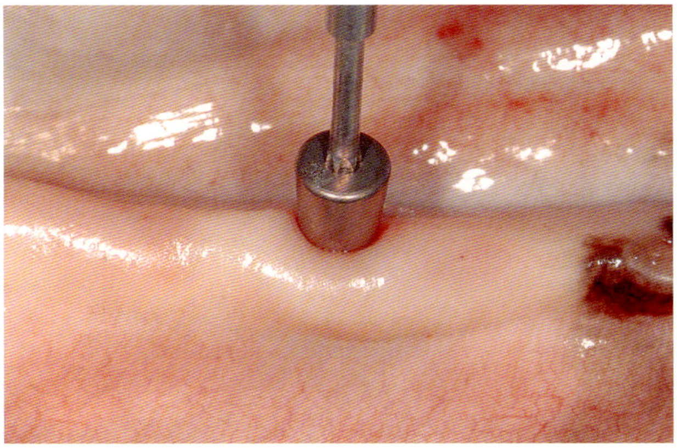

Fig 17-36 After tissue punch implant placement, a permucosal healing abutment is inserted for the one-stage surgical approach.

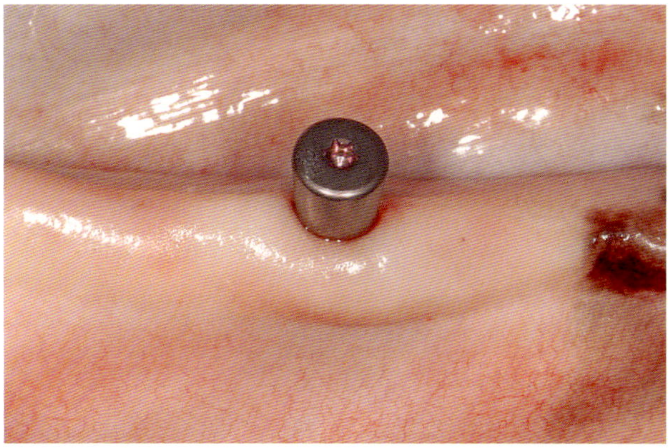

Fig 17-37 The permucosal healing abutment should extend 1–2 mm above the adjacent mucosa to help prevent tissue overgrowth during the healing period.

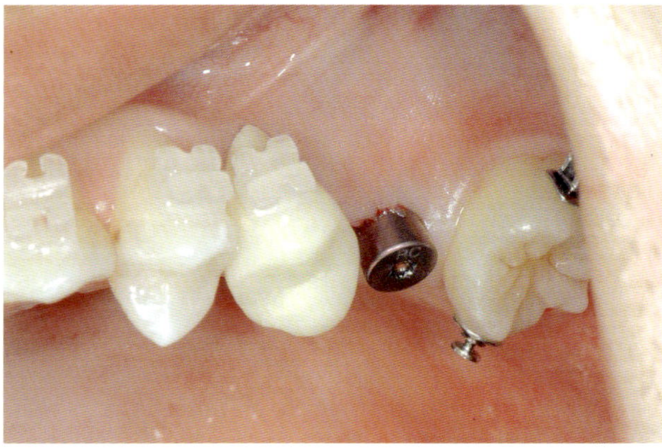

Fig 17-38 After mini-incision implant placement, a permucosal healing abutment is inserted for the one-stage surgical approach.

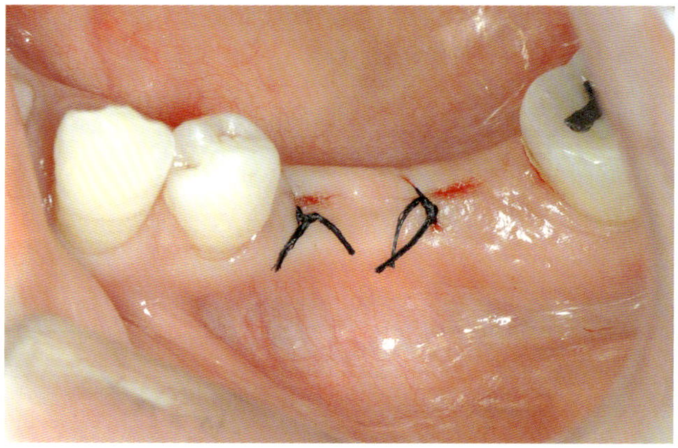

Fig 17-39 After mini-incision implant placement, the tissues are approximated over the implant for the two-stage surgical approach. One interrupted suture is sufficient to allow primary closure of the soft tissue.

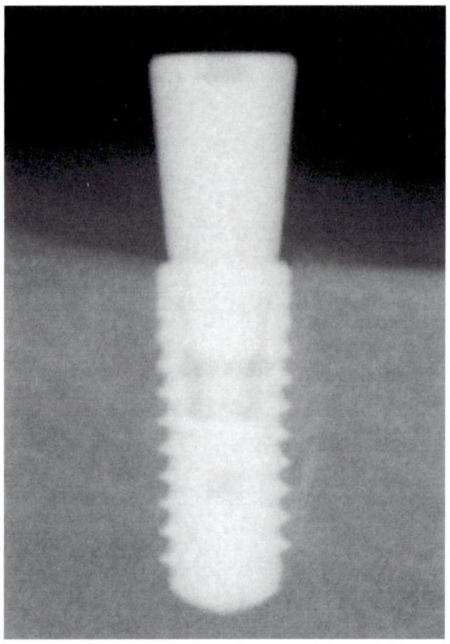

Fig 17-40 Periapical radiograph taken immediately after implant placement.

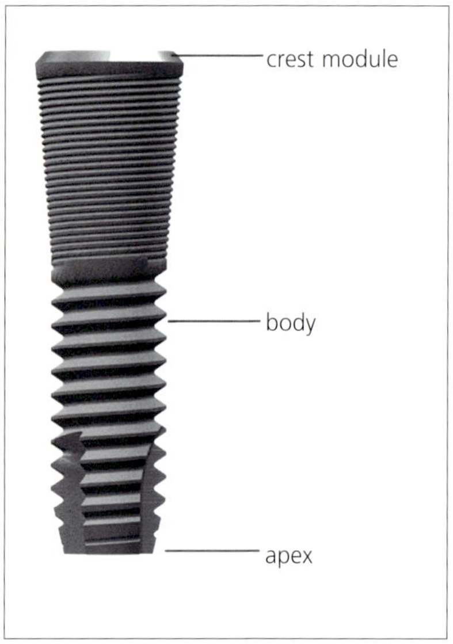

Fig 17-41 The Astra Tech implant.

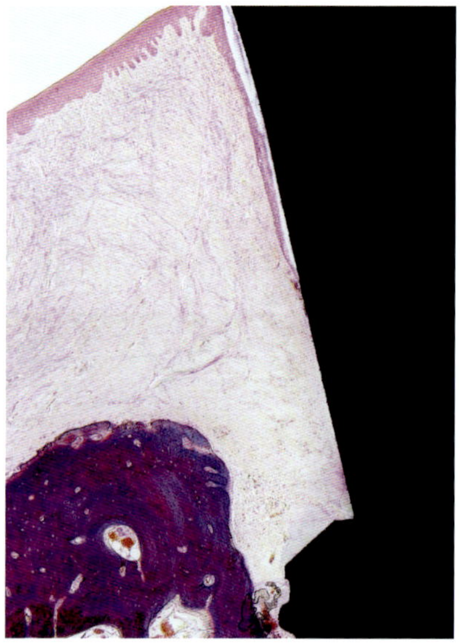

Fig 17-42 The apical extension of the junctional epithelium is above the fixture–abutment border at the Astra implant site.

Suture removal

The suture is removed 1 week after placing the mini-incision implant.

Flapless implant surgery for Astra Tech implants

The Astra Tech implant is a bone level implant type with a short cervical collar, 0.5 mm in height (Fig 17-41). The neck of the implant is designed with micro-threads that offer optimal load distribution and lower stress values considering that the critical point of the implant–bone interface is located at the marginal cortical bone where the peak pressures occur.[10] The implants have a well-defined rough TiOblast™ surface and a conical connection with its abutment under the marginal bone (see Fig 17-3a). The cone-screw abutment has been shown to reduce micro-movement and provide a seal against invasion by microorganisms.[11] Animal experiments have shown that the apical termination of the junctional epithelium is located coronal to the abutment/fixture border using the Astra implant system (Fig 17-42).

Astra Tech implants can be placed using either soft tissue punch or mini-incision flapless methods. There is

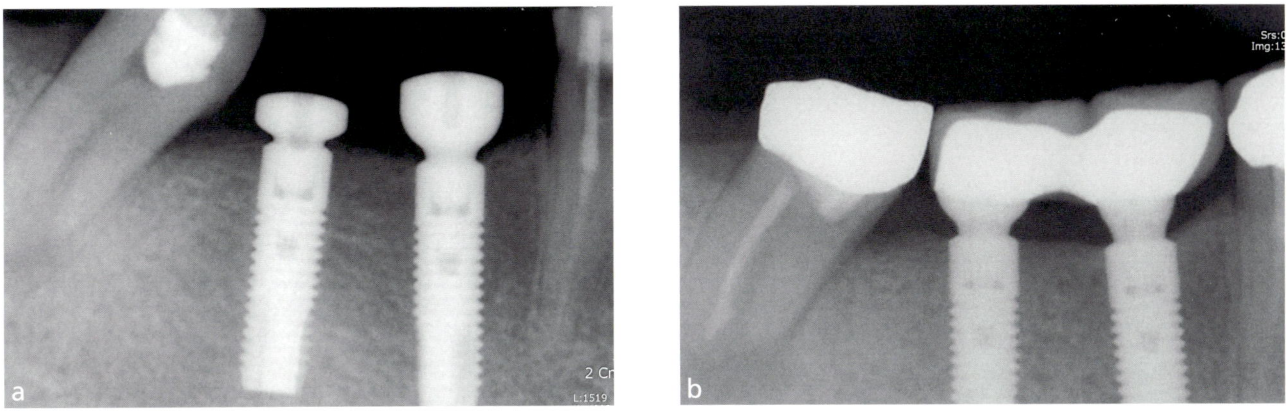

Fig 17-43 Radiographs of the peri-implant bone (a) immediately after and (b) 1 year after flapless implant placement.

intraoperative flexibility to determine whether to use submerged or nonsubmerged flapless procedures. A clinical study, which was carried out to evaluate the failure rates and overall degree of peri-implant bone loss 1 year after flapless implant surgery, showed that osseointegration occurred in all 38 patients with 78 implants with no failures. The bone loss was 0.24 ± 0.21 mm (Fig 17-43).

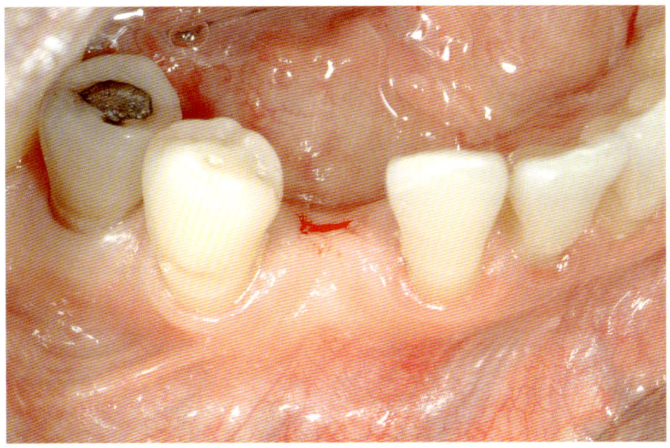

Fig 17-44 A mini-incision.

Flapless implant procedure

An incision is made based on the surgical method: mini-incision (Fig 17-44) or soft tissue punch (Fig 17-45). The osteotomy preparation proceeds according to the drill sequence (Fig 17-46). Conical drills are required for implants with a conical shape in the coronal region, regardless of the bone quality, owing to the conical design of these implants (Fig 17-47). However, conical drills can

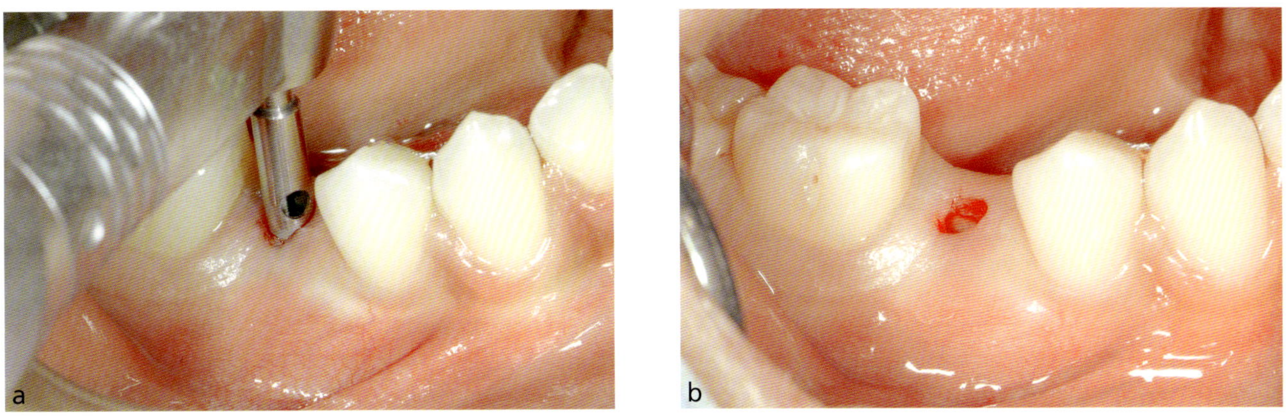

Fig 17-45 Soft tissue punch technique. (a) A circumferential incision is made in the gingiva at the center of the implant site using a soft tissue punch. (b) The incised attached gingiva is then removed.

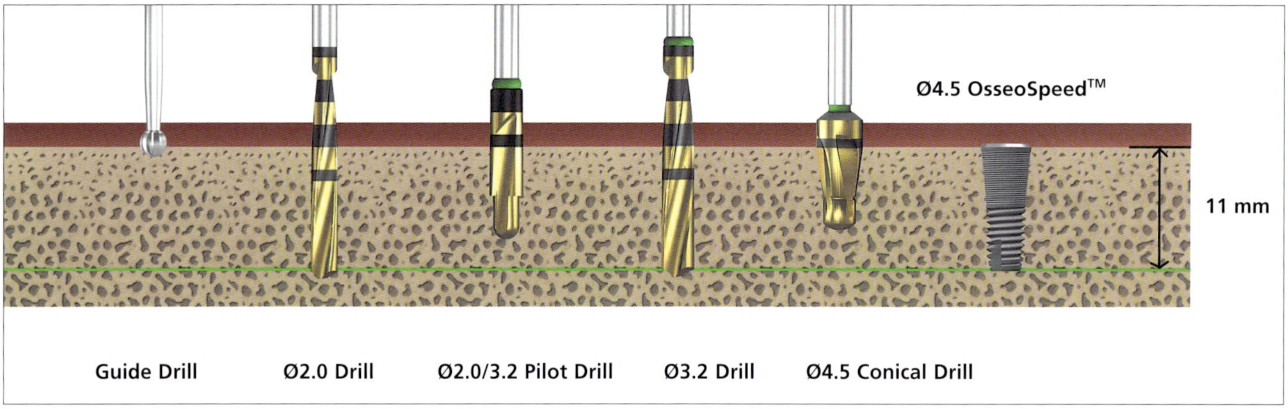

Fig 17-46 Implant site preparation for the Astra Tech 4.5 mm diameter OsseoSpeed™ implants.

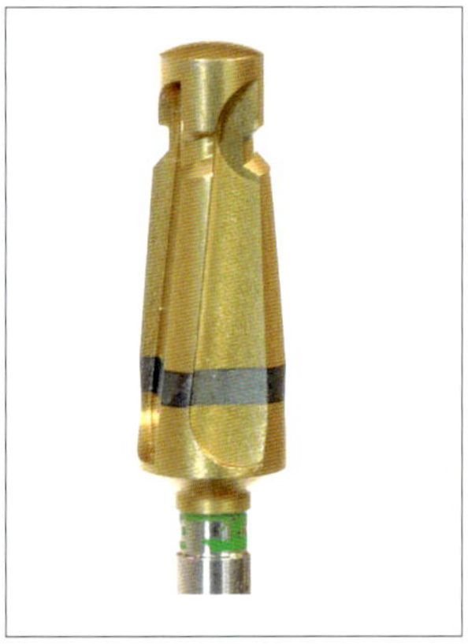

Fig 17-47 A conical drill is required for implants with conical shape in the coronal region. It can cause damage to the soft tissue in deeper preparations because of its wide diameter on the top.

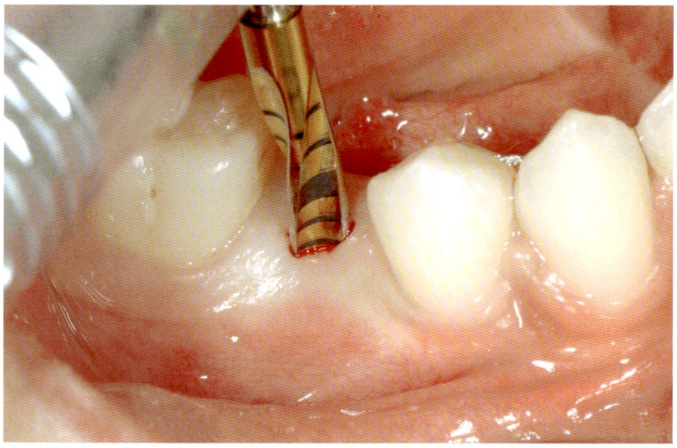

Fig 17-48 The implant site is prepared using a flapless drill.

cause damage to the soft tissue in deeper preparations because of the wide diameter on the top. To protect the adjacent mucosa during drilling, it is advisable to use flapless implant drills with cutting surfaces on their tips and rounded surfaces on their other parts (Fig 17-48). The drilling depth can be controlled above the mucosa by marks on the drills corresponding to the sum of the length of the implant and mucosa thickness.

A low-speed handpiece or a hand wrench is used to place the implants (Fig 17-49). Immediately after implant placement, peri-implant probing around the implant should be carried out to confirm that the implant crest module is located at the level of the bone crest (Figs 17-50 and 17-51).

After implant placement, either a low-profile cover screw is inserted into the implant body for the two-stage approach, or a permucosal healing abutment is inserted for the one-stage approach. For the two-stage approach, the tissues are approximated over the implant for primary closure (Fig 17-52). One interrupted suture is sufficient to allow primary closure of the soft tissue (Fig 17-53). For the one-stage approach, the permucosal healing abutment should extend 1–2 mm above the adjacent mucosa to help to prevent tissue overgrowth during the healing period (Fig 17-54). The permucosal healing abutment should be 1–5 mm wider than the soft tissue punch to ensure close contact between the peri-implant mucosa and healing abutment. The suture is removed 1 week after placing the mini-incision implant.

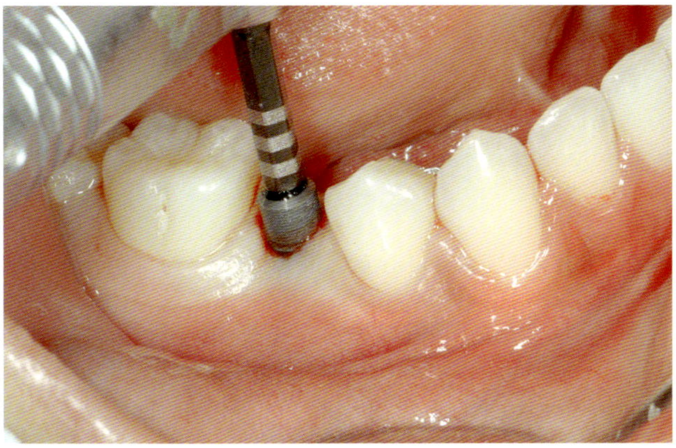

Fig 17-49 A low-speed handpiece is used to place the implant.

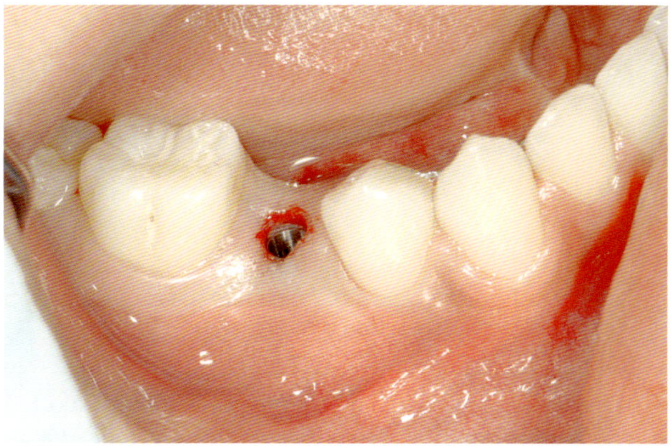

Fig 17-50 The OsseoSpeed™ implant (4.5 mm diameter) is finally positioned.

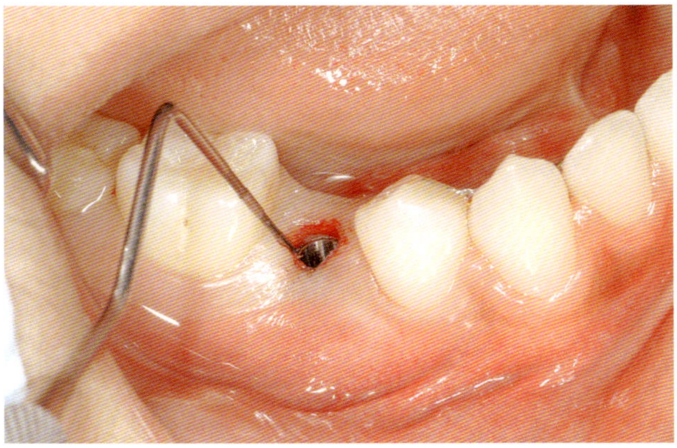

Fig 17-51 Peri-implant probing around the implant is carried out to confirm that the implant shoulder is located at the level of the bone crest.

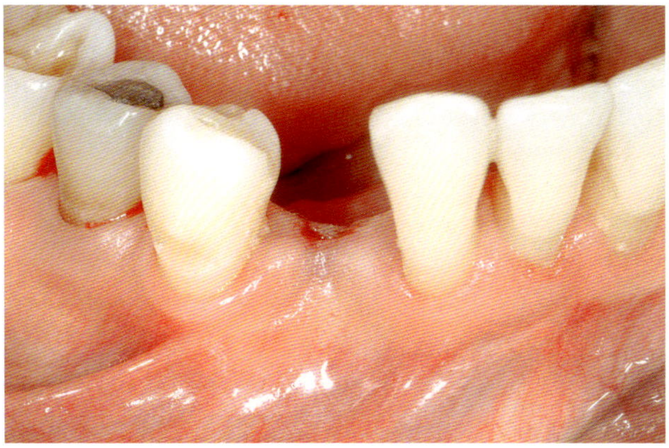

Fig 17-52 The soft tissues are approximated over the implant for primary closure after mini-incision implant placement.

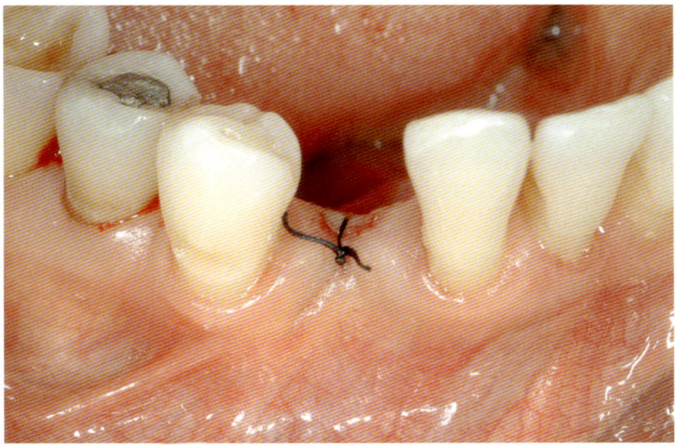

Fig 17-53 One interrupted suture is sufficient to allow primary closure of the soft tissue.

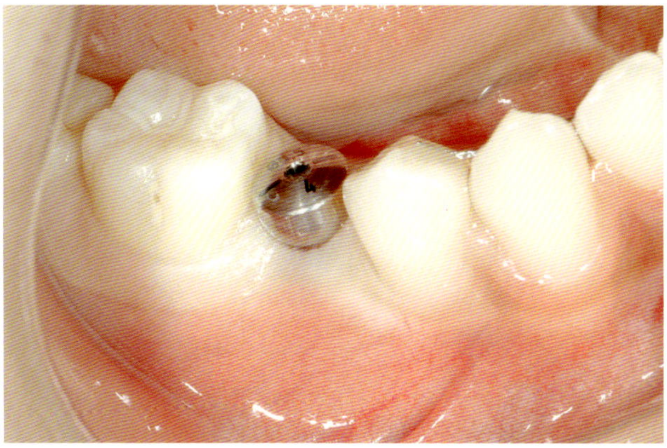

Fig 17-54 Placement of the permucosal healing abutment after tissue punch implant placement.

Flapless implant surgery for Dentsply Friadent implants

The Dentsply Friadent (Mannheim, Germany) implant is available in both bone and soft tissue level types. XiVE S Plus is a bone level type with a short cervical collar, 0.4 mm in height (Fig 17-55). XiVE TG Plus is a soft tissue level type with a 2.5 mm smooth cervical collar and a 2 mm square on the collar (Fig 17-56). XiVE S Plus has an internal hexagonal connection with an abutment under the marginal bone (Fig 17-57), whereas XiVE TG Plus has a square external connection with the corresponding prosthetic component above the marginal bone (Fig 17-58). The implants have two different types of surface: an acid-etched surface in the cervical region for improved adhesion of the subepithelial connective tissue as well as a grit-blasted and high-temperature etched surface in the endosseous region for the attachment of osteoblasts (Fig 17-59). XiVE S Plus can be placed using either a soft tissue punch or mini-incision flapless method. XiVE TG Plus can be nonsubmerged using a soft tissue punch flapless procedure.

Flapless implant procedure

An incision is made based on the surgical method: mini-incision (Fig 17-60) or soft tissue punch. The osteotomy preparation proceeds according to the drill sequence (Fig 17-61). As the implants have a conical shape, they require crestal drilling to prepare the coronal section of the osteotomy. The crestal preparation depth is 2 mm where there is low bone density. In high bone density, the site is prepared to a maximum depth of 6 mm. To protect the adjacent mucosa during drilling, it is advisable to use flapless implant drills with cutting surfaces on their tips and rounded surfaces on their other parts. The drilling depth is controlled above the mucosa by marks on the drills corresponding to the sum of the length of the implant and mucosa thickness (Figs 17-62 and 17-63).

A low-speed handpiece or a hand wrench is used to place the implants (Fig 17-64). Immediately after implant placement, peri-implant probing around the implant should be carried out to confirm that the implant crest module is located at the level of the bone crest (Fig 17-65). After implant placement, either a low-profile cover

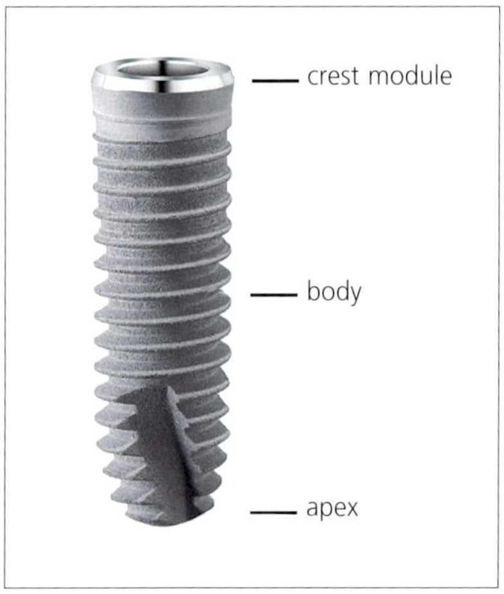

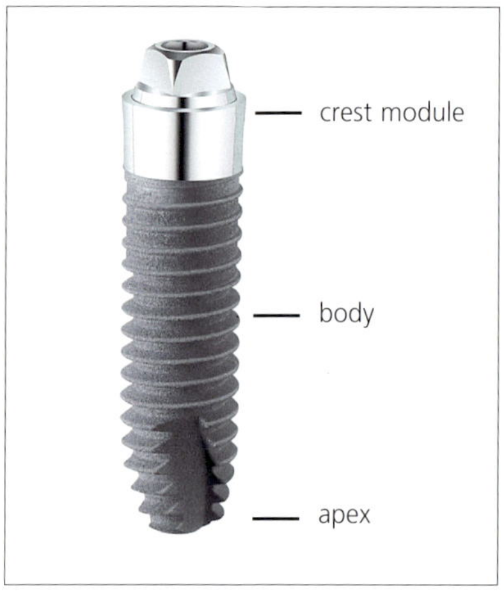

Fig 17-55 *(left)* XiVE S Plus implant.

Fig 17-56 XiVE TG Plus implant.

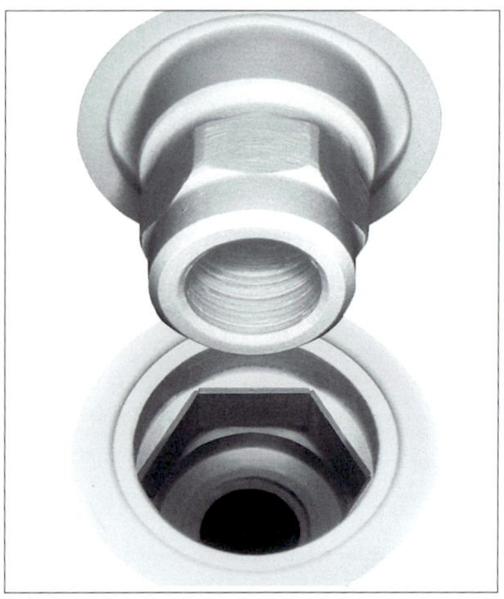

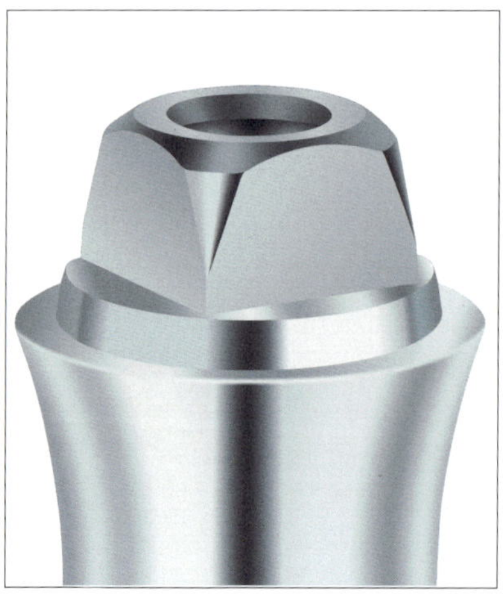

Fig 17-57 *(left)* The implant–abutment connection of XiVE S Plus implants.

Fig 17-58 The implant–abutment connection of XiVE TG Plus implants.

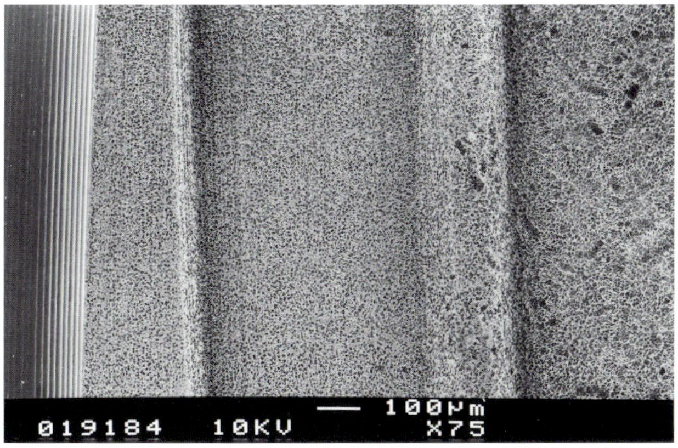

Fig 17-59 The implant surface of XiVE Plus implants.

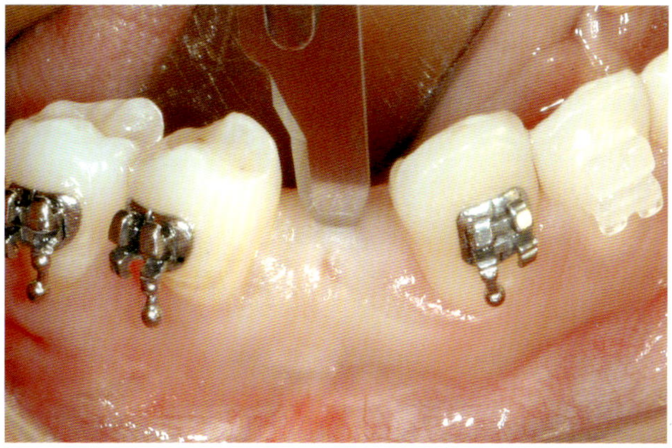

Fig 17-60 A mini-incision.

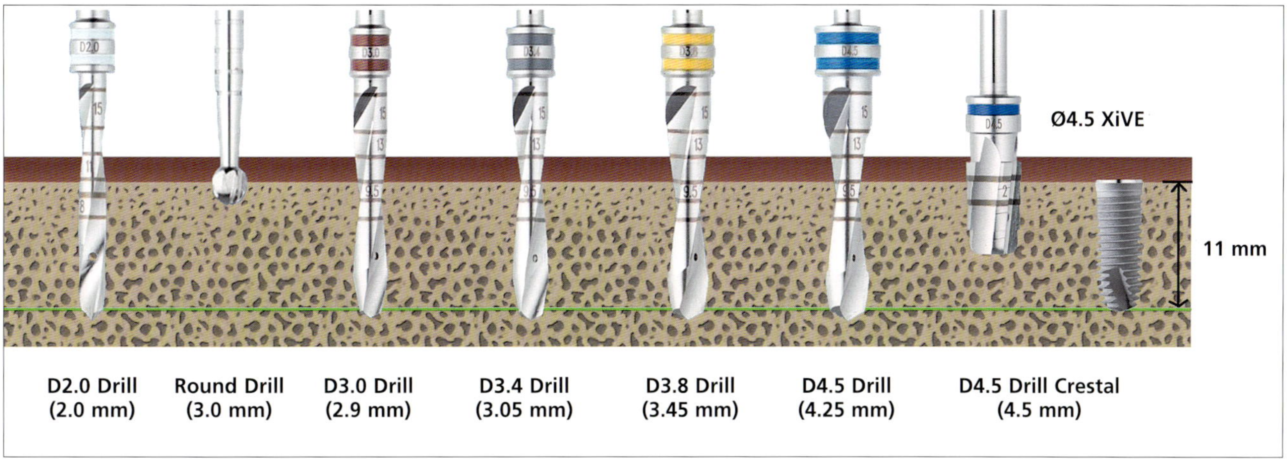

Fig 17-61 Implant site preparation for Dentsply 4.5 mm diameter XiVE S Plus implants.

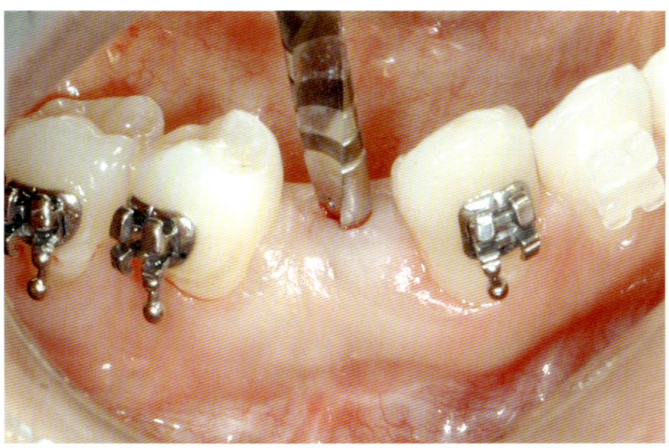

Fig 17-62 The implant site is prepared with XiVE twist drills with increasing diameters.

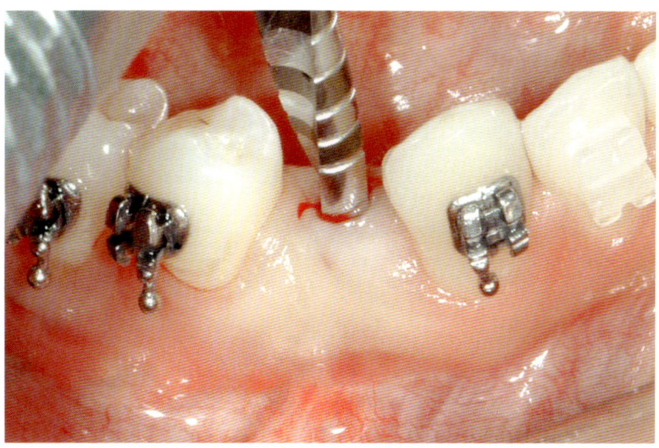

Fig 17-63 The osteotomy is prepared until a diameter of 4.5 mm is reached. The drilling depth is controlled above the mucosa by marks on the drills corresponding to the sum of the length of the implant and mucosa thickness.

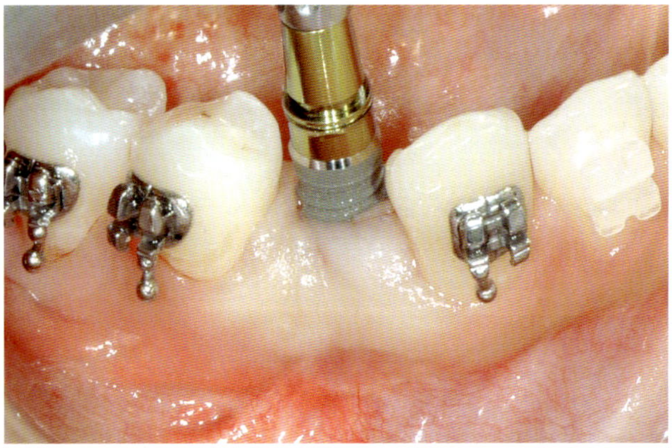

Fig 17-64 The XiVE S Plus implant (4.5 mm diameter) is placed with a low-speed handpiece.

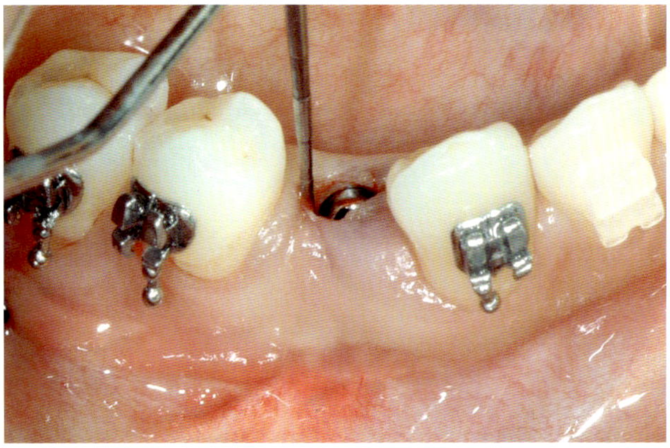

Fig 17-65 Peri-implant probing around the implant is carried out to confirm that the implant shoulder is located at the level of the bone crest.

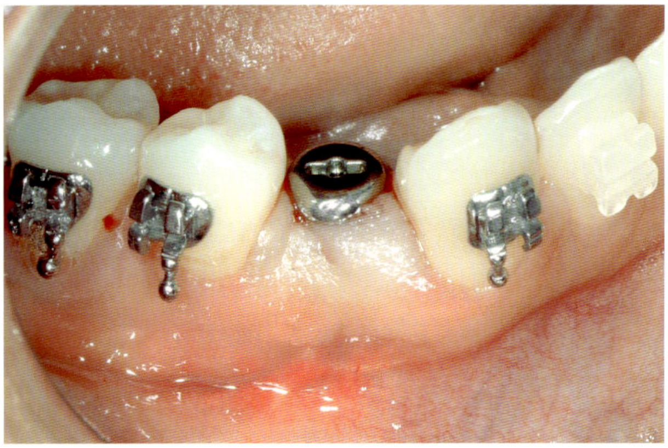

Fig 17-66 Placement of the permucosal healing abutment.

screw is inserted into the implant body for the two-stage approach, or a permucosal healing abutment is inserted for the one-stage approach (Fig 17-66).

Summary

Flapless implant surgery can be performed using various implant systems. Those with a short cervical collar can be selected for either a soft tissue punch or mini-incision technique. However, it is difficult to approximate the tissues required for primary closure of the implant using systems with a long cervical collar. Therefore, it is prudent to select them only for the soft tissue punch technique.

References

1. Palmer RM, Smith BJ, Palmer PH, Floyd PD. A prospective study of Astra single tooth implants. Clin Oral Implant Res 1997;8:173–179.
2. Norton MR. In-vitro evaluation of the strength of the conical implant-to-abutment joint in two commercially available implant systems. J Prosthet Dent 2000;83:567–571.
3. Hermann JS, Cochran DL, Nummikoski PV, Buser D. Crestal bone changes around titanium implants: a radiographic evaluation of unloaded non-submerged and submerged implants in the canine mandible. J. Periodontol 1997;68:1117–1130.
4. Hanggi MP, Hanggi DC, Schoolfield JD. Crestal bone changes around titanium implants. I: A retrospective radiographic evaluation in humans comparing two non-submerged implant designs with different machined collar lengths. J Periodontol 2005;76:791–802.
5. Schwarz F, Herten M, Sager M, Wieland M, Dard M, Becker J. Histological and immunohistochemical analysis of initial and early osseous integration at chemically modified and conventional SLA titanium implants: preliminary results of a pilot study in dogs. Clin Oral Implants Res 2007;18:481–488.
6. Schwarz F, Herten M, Sager M, Wieland M, Dard M, Becker J. Histological and immunohistochemical analysis of initial and early subepithelial connective tissue attachment at chemically modified and conventional SLA titanium implants: a pilot study in dogs. Clin Oral Invest 2007;11:245–255.
7. Oates TW, Valderrama P, Bischof M et al. Enhanced implant stability with a chemically modified SLA surface: a randomized pilot study. Int J Oral Maxillofac Implants 2007;22:755–760.
8. Hammerle CH, Bragger U, Burgin W. The effect of subcrestal placement of the polished surface of ITI implants on marginal soft and hard tissues. Clin Oral Implants Res 1996;7:111–119.
9. Bashutski JD, D'Silva NJ, Wang HL. Implant compression necrosis: current understanding and case report. J Periodontol 2009;80: 700–704.
10. Lee DW, Choi YS, Park KH, Kim CS, Moon IS. Effect of microthread on the maintenance of marginal bone level: a 3-year prospective study. Clin Oral Implants Res 2007;18:465–470.
11. Cooper LF, Scurria MS, Lang LA, Guckes AD, Moriarty JD, Felton DA. Treatment of edentulism using Astra Tech implants and ball abutments to retain mandibular overdentures. Int J Oral Maxillofac Implants 1999;14:646–653.

Index

A

B

I

J

K

L

M

N

O

P